Management of Common Musculoskeletal Disorders

Management of Common Musculoskeletal Disorders

Physical Therapy Principles and Methods
Second Edition

Darlene Hertling, B.S., R.P.T.

Lecturer, Division of Physical Therapy
Department of Rehabilitation Medicine
University of Washington School of Medicine
Seattle, Washington

Randolph M. Kessler, M.D.

With 3 additional contributors

Illustrations by Elizabeth Kessler

A Lippincott
Physical Therapy Title

J. B. Lippincott   *Philadelphia*
Grand Rapids   New York   St. Louis
San Francisco   London   Sydney   Tokyo

Acquisitions Editor: Patricia L. Cleary
Copy Editors: Jeanne Carper and Eileen Cunniffe
Project Editor: Kathy Crown
Indexer: Julia Schwager
Art Director: Susan Hess Blaker
Design Coordinator: Doug Smock
Production Manager: Carol A. Florence
Production Coordinator: Barney Fernandes
Compositor: Progressive Typositors, Inc.
Printer/Binder: The Murray Printing Company

Second Edition

1   3   5   6   4   2

Library of Congress Cataloging-in-Publication Data
Hertling, Darlene.
    Management of common musculoskeletal disorders: physical therapy principles and methods/Darlene Hertling, Randolph M. Kessler; with three contributors; illustrations by Elizabeth Kessler. — 2nd ed.
        p.   cm.
    Kessler's name appears first on previous ed.
    Includes bibliographies and index.
    ISBN 0-397-54805-2 (soft)
    1. Physical therapy.   2. Musculoskeletal system — Diseases — Patients — Rehabilitation.   I. Kessler, Randolph M.   II. Title. [DNLM: 1. Bone Diseases — therapy.   2. Muscular Diseases — therapy.   3. Physical Therapy.   WE 140 H574m]
RM700.H48   1990
616.7'062 — dc19
DNLM/DLC   89-2309
for Library of Congress   CIP

To Max, Tess, Tera
Gunter, Sonja, and Dieter

Contributors

MITCHELL G. BLAKNEY, B.S., P.T.
Practicing Physical Therapist
Gig Harbor, Washington

DANIEL JONES, B.S., P.T.
Practicing Physical Therapist
Portland, Oregon

MAUREEN K. LYNCH, M.D., P.T.
School of Medicine
University of Washington
Seattle, Washington

Preface

The previous edition of *Management of Common Musculoskeletal Disorders: Physical Therapy Principles and Methods*, published in 1983, was the product of changing trends in medical education during the late 1970s and early 1980s with respect to nonsurgical management of musculoskeletal pathology. It was one of the first textbooks to integrate all aspects of the musculoskeletal system for physical and manual therapists and other health care professionals. The integrated approach was met with enthusiasm by students, teachers, and practicing clinicians both in this country and abroad. The need for a more current presentation became evident as a few years went by and the "growing pains" of clinical investigation and the development of new techniques intensified. It is evident that these trends are likely to continue.

In this edition the chapters on the joints of the extremities have been revised and expanded. The chapter on the wrist (Chapter 12) has been expanded to include the hand proper. Other sections of the book have also been altered. The chapter on the functional anatomy of the spine (Chapter 17) and the information on clinical applications of materials as they relate to selective conditions affecting the cervical and lumbar spine (Chapters 18 and 20) have been added. As in the chapters on the extremities, the chapters on the spine in these sections are organized to include functional anatomy, biomechanics, and specific regional evaluation of common lesions and their management.

Management of disorders of the low back remains a challenge. It is startling to realize how meager and rudimentary our knowledge is on this subject. The conservative treatment of low-back problems remains, with rare exceptions, empirical. Identification of treatment most likely to succeed has greatly improved during the past 3 decades, emphasizing either "hands on" procedures (Grieves 1986, Maitland 1987) or the "hands off" approach (McKenzie 1979). Significant clinical contributions have been made by Robin McKenzie, a New Zealand physiotherapist of international renown who has expanded on an original contribution with his lateral shift treatment technique for patients with lumbar discogenic disorders, and by Brian Edwards of Australia, who has formalized combined movements in examination and treatment of the spine.

The works of Lewit, Fryette, Mitchell, Grieves, Janda, and others have resulted in new methods of post-isometric relaxation techniques. Lewit (1985), having worked for about 30 years in the field of painful disorders stemming from impaired locomotor function, has observed that movement restrictions are not necessarily due to an articular lesion. Post-isometric relaxation techniques (which employ the patient's active participation during manual treatment techniques) rest on the prime importance of soft tissues, particularly the muscles as opposed to the skeletal elements of joint structures, in producing various abnormal states of joint pain and movement limitation.

A major contributor to this edition and author of the chapter on the cervical spine (Chapter 18) is Mitchell Blakney, P.T., who is well known for his participation in and development of numerous postgraduate courses on manual therapy and as an annual visiting lecturer in the physical therapy curriculum at the University of Washington.

The book is a practical and useful guide for evaluation and conservative management of the various common musculoskeletal dysfunctions of the extremities and spine encountered in practice. Most of the techniques described here are widely accepted, and no claim is made for an original method of treatment.

Darlene Hertling, B.S., R.P.T.

Preface to the First Edition

Management of Common Musculoskeletal Disorders: Physical Therapy Principles and Methods was written to fill a void in the rapidly expanding area of musculoskeletal medicine. The trend toward increased physical activity in a population living close to the limits of life expectancy has significantly increased the number of patients suffering musculoskeletal pain or dysfunction: more individuals are troubled with athletic injuries during their active years, and more are living long enough to experience one or more "degenerative" musculoskeletal ailments.

Patients presenting with musculoskeletal disorders which are not severely disabling and for which surgical intervention is not warranted have been among the most ignored and are perhaps the most mismanaged in modern medicine. Such patients have generated little interest among our highly trained specialists, the orthopaedist tending to be more concerned with surgically correctable problems, the rehabilitation team with permanent disabilities, and the family practitioner with "medical" disorders.

There are certainly excellent books available that deal with managing surgical orthopaedic disorders, with rehabilitating the severely disabled, and with specific areas of musculoskeletal medicine. However, few, if any, cover pertinent background material, principles of examination, concepts of management, and techniques of treatment as they relate to nonsurgical musculoskeletal medicine. *Management of Common Musculoskeletal Disorders* is a first and, we feel, very important step in developing a multifaceted approach to the musculoskeletal system.

This book was written for the student in the advanced stages of training and for the practicing clinician. Originally it was directed toward physical therapists, but we soon recognized that its cross-sectional appeal should be much broader. Patients with musculoskeletal disorders are likely to consult any one of a wide variety of practitioners, and

we trust that orthopaedists, physiatrists, rheumatologists, family practitioners, orthopaedic assistants, physical therapy assistants, athletic trainers, orthopaedic nurses, and chiropractors will also find it useful.

The book is comprised of three sections: Basic Concepts, Selected Techniques, and Clinical Applications. Part One, dealing with background material, is not meant to be a comprehensive discussion of the musculoskeletal system, which is well covered in other texts. Our purpose is to expand the traditional taxonomies of joint structure and function so as to provide a conceptual model of the musculoskeletal system that can serve as a basis for the discussions of evaluation and treatment procedures which follow. The reader is led from the notion of a joint as the junction of two bones to a concept of the synovial joint as the basic unit of the musculoskeletal system. This approach is developed by considering the functional and structural joint components in detail, under both normal and pathological conditions. Included is a discussion of pain of deep somatic origin, a topic not extensively covered in current literature. Various phenomena associated with the perception of pain arising from the musculoskeletal tissues are discussed from a neurophysiological standpoint and related to various pain theories, including the currently popular "gate control" model. The key chapter in this first section, from a clinical standpoint, is on assessment of musculoskeletal disorders. A comprehensive system of patient evaluation is a crucial component of the clinician's overall approach to management. Ways to elicit subjective and objective data are presented, along with guides to the interpretation of findings. The whole section on background material is included to provide a scientific rationale for some of the physical therapy modalities and procedures used in the management of patients with common musculoskeletal disorders. This approach is much needed in an area of medicine in which treatment programs often incorporate remedies which are not well supported by experimental or empirical evidence of their efficacy.

Part Two, which concerns techniques, is not intended to include all the procedures that might be used in the management of patients with common musculoskeletal disorders. Rather, it introduces those techniques that are not traditionally included in most professional training programs. The most important of these are the specific joint mobilization techniques which, while not widely accepted by the medical profession, have been used for many years by a few medical practitioners and other types of health-care personnel. Because over the past century considerable misunderstanding and confusion have been associated with the use of joint mobilization techniques, a chapter dealing with the history of their use and misuse is included. (A considerable portion of the chapter on Arthrology in the section on Basic Concepts is devoted to providing a rationale and indications for the use of these techniques.) We consider this a major contribution of this book. A satisfactory rationale for using these techniques has not previously been presented in the literature, and this fact has contributed considerably to the confusion and misunderstanding just mentioned.

Part Three encompasses the clinical applications of the preceding material as it relates to selected conditions affecting the extremities, with reference to some common spinal disorders. Each of the regional chapters in this section is organized to include functional anatomy and biomechanics, specific regional evaluation, and common lesions and their management.

We believe that the distinguishing strong point of this work is the integration of well established principles of human structure, mechanics, physiology, and pathology, from numerous sources, to form a rational basis for the clinician's approach to managing patients with common musculoskeletal disorders. Growing consumerism and increasing governmental regulation of the health-care industry are placing heavier demands upon accountability. These demands must be met by increased emphasis on experimental and clinical research. An organized and scientifically based rationale for commonly used therapeutic procedures is essential in providing direction and guidance to research efforts. The material contained in this book, having evolved through descriptive research, provides just such a framework for further clinical and experimental investigations.

Randolph M. Kessler, B.S., R.P.T.
Darlene Hertling, B.S., R.P.T.

Acknowledgments

On behalf of Randolph Kessler and myself, I would like to express our gratitude both to our expert contributors and to our colleagues in the field. I am grateful to Jenny Cole and Merike Muld, who provided secretarial assistance and gave their time and support to the completion of this project. Special thanks must go to the physical therapy students and graduates of the University of Washington for their ideas, which lead to the development of this second edition over the past few years. They have challenged, criticized, encouraged and supported us in this endeavor. I would like to particularly acknowledge Elizabeth Kessler for her expert illustration of this and the previous edition. She has created the artwork for the new text with patience, diligence and illustrative perfection. Finally, this book could not have been written without the help and encouragement provided by the following members of the staff of the J.B. Lippincott Company: Patti Cleary, Delois Patterson, and Kathy Crown. They have my deep thanks for their support and efforts.

Contents

Management of Common Musculoskeletal Disorders

Part One
BASIC CONCEPTS AND TECHNIQUES

1 Embryology of the Musculoskeletal System

Randolph M. Kessler

Knowledge of the development of the musculoskeletal tissues is of particular value to clinicians, whether they deal mainly with patients with developmental disabilities, long-term rehabilitation problems, or common musculoskeletal disorders, because it yields insight into the phenomenon of pain perception, segmental innervation, repair processes, and general body organization. Surely every clinician must at some time have wondered, "Why does my patient with a neck problem feel pain in the scapula?" "Why do my patients with shoulder problems not feel pain in the shoulder but in the upper arm?" "Why do some muscles receive innervation from all of the segments that they cross, whereas some muscles crossing many segments, such as the latissimus dorsi, receive innervation from relatively few segments?" Or, "What is the explanation for the 'spiraling' nature of the dermatomes, especially in the lower limb?" The answers to some of these questions are not essential for competent clinical performance. However, some concepts, such as patterns of pain referral, are of the utmost importance in patient evaluation and treatment and should be pursued in depth. The study of embryology adds to our understanding of these concepts and deserves consideration here.

AXIAL COMPONENTS

The early developing embryo is composed of three primary, or germinal, layers: ectoderm, endoderm, and mesoderm. By the fourth week of development, the neural plate lying centrally in the ectoderm begins to invaginate into the underlying mesoderm. As this occurs, the peripheral margins of the neural plate gradually become more prominent and begin to approximate one another. Eventually they meet, forming the neural tube, which pinches off from the ectoderm and ends up lying within the mesoderm (Fig. 1–1). A similar phenomenon occurs ventrally; the notochordal process migrates and pinches off to form the notochord, which lies free in the ventral mesodermal layer.

The intrusion of the notochord and neural tube results in compaction of the mesodermal cells lying lateral to them. The compaction of the paraxial mesoderm forms the somites, of which there are originally 42 to 44 pairs: 4 occipital, 8 cervical, 12 thoracic, 5 lumbar, 5 sacral, and 8 to 10 coccygeal. These roughly coincide with what are to become the craniovertebral segments. The ventromedial cells of the vertebral somites, the sclerotomes, migrate medially to surround the notochord and neural tube (Fig. 1–2). Looking longitudinally (Fig. 1–3), each sclerotome is divided by a layer of cells called the *perichordal disk*. The cranial half of one sclerotome then unites with the caudal half of the adjacent sclerotome, causing a shift in the relationship between sclerotomes and the remaining somites. The sclerotomes eventually chondrify, or become cartilaginous, then ossify to become the vertebrae. They also form cartilage, capsules, ligaments, and blood vessels. The perichordal disk becomes the annulus fibrosis, while the notochord becomes the original nucleus pulposus. The neural tube gradually differentiates into nerve tissue, becoming the spinal cord and sending out peripheral nerves to the adjacent mesoderm.

The more dorsomedial somite cells are the myotomes. These cells divide into the hypomere, which migrates around to form the ventrolateral trunk muscles, and the epimere, which forms the segmental muscles of the back. As this occurs, the spinal nerve divides to form the anterior primary ramus, which invades the hypomere, and the posterior primary ramus, which innervates the segmental back

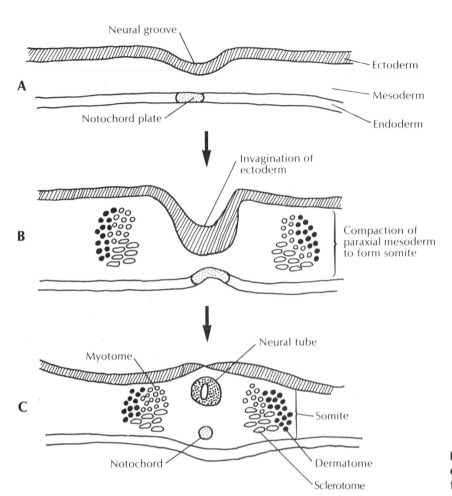

Fig. 1–1. Germinal layers of the early embryo. Invagination of the ectoderm forms the neural tube.

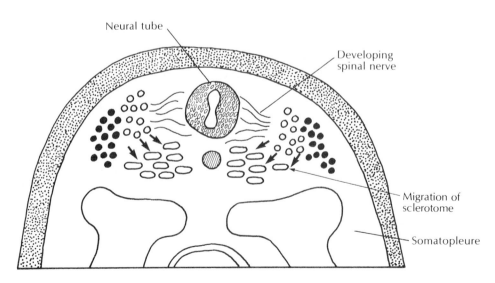

Fig. 1–2. Ventromedial migration of sclerotomic cells.

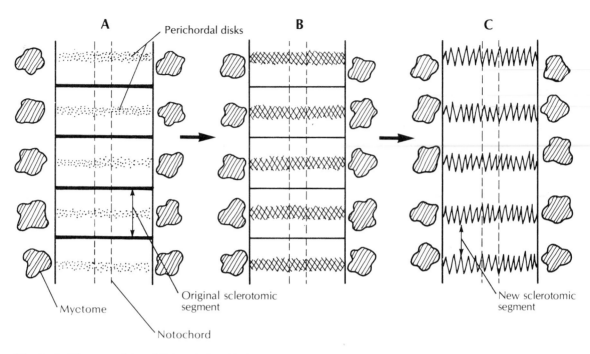

Fig. 1–3. Diagram of the shift in relationship between a sclerotome and remaining somatic segments.

muscles. Because of the segmental shift in relationship between the sclerotomes and myotomes, the segmental back muscles each cross at least one segment.

The remaining somatic cells are the dermatomes. These cells migrate out around the body wall, beneath the ectoderm, to form the dermal layer of skin. The dermis becomes innervated by sensory branches of the division (ramus) of the spinal nerve that innervates the muscles underlying it. The epidermal layer of skin is derived from the ectoderm.

LIMBS

The limb buds appear during the fourth week in the developing embryo. The forelimb, which appears a few days before the hindlimb, develops at the lateral body wall level with the C4–T2 segments. The hindlimb appears at an area level with the L1–S2 segments (Fig. 1–4). The early limb bud is a mass of mesenchymal cells arising from the laterally located somatopleure and covered by an ectodermal layer. The mesenchymal cells are pluripotential in that some will develop into osteoblasts, some into fibroblasts, some into myoblasts, and some into chondroblasts. The muscles of the limb buds develop *in situ* rather than from an invasion of cells from the myotome of the somite; this occurs as a result of differen-

tiation of primitive mesenchymal cells into myoblasts, which become multinucleated muscle cells or fibers. The anterior primary divisions of the spinal nerve invade the developing limb buds to innervate the early muscle masses. Because of the intertwining of segmental nerves throughout the regional plexus and because the early muscle masses tend to divide or fuse with one another, each muscle typically receives innervation from more than one segment, and each segmental nerve tends to innervate more than one muscle. The intertwining of segments through the plexus also explains the overlapping, somewhat unpatterned skin innervation of the limbs.

The original orientation of the limb buds is such that the upper limb is positioned laterally, lying in the frontal plane at about 90° abduction, with the palm facing forward. The lower limb is positioned similarly, with the hip externally rotated, the patella facing posteriorly, and the sole facing forward. Gradually the limbs rotate down into the fetal position. This rotation and abduction of the limb buds explains the spiraling nature of the limb segments (dermatomes, myotomes, and sclerotomes), especially in the lower limb, which undergoes more rotation. It also explains the anteversion and varus angle of the normal femoral neck in relation to the shaft of the femur and the external torsion of the tibial shaft, which compensates for the internal torsion of the femur.

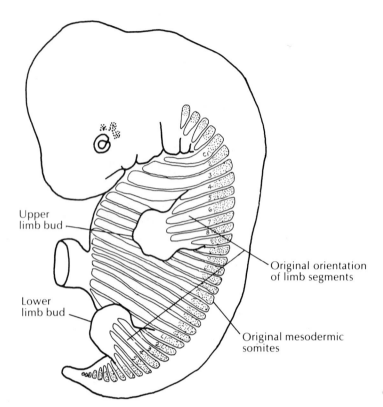

Upper
limb bud

Lower
limb bud

Original orientation
of limb segments

Original mesodermic
somites

Fig. 1-4. Diagram of embryo at about 5 weeks' gestation.

A guide to determining approximate segmental innervation of a limb is to imagine the limb in the original embryologic position. In this position, the more cranial aspects of the limb are innervated by cranial segments, the more caudal aspects by caudal segments. Thus the inner thigh, which was originally located cranially, is innervated by L2, while the outer lower leg, which was positioned caudally, is innervated by S1. Also worth noting is the fact that the scapula originates as part of the developing limb bud. As the limb develops, the scapula migrates to become "folded back" on the posterior body wall. This explains why the scapula, although it lies level with thoracic segments, is innervated primarily by cervical segments. Thus, pain of cervical origin is often referred to the scapulae, as well as to the arms. While most limb muscles split or fuse as they develop, some migrate. The latissimus is the most obvious example; it migrates so far as to attain a pelvic attachment. However, like other limb muscles it is innervated by the anterior primary divisions of mostly cervical segments, in spite of the fact that it lies over the back and extends over thoracic and lumbar segments.

The bones of the limbs also develop *in situ*. A condensation of mesenchymal cells first appears in the axial region of the limb bud. These differentiate into chondrocytes that form a "cartilage model" of the developing bone. Through the process of endochon-dral ossification, the cartilage model is gradually replaced by bone tissue. This occurs first in the diaphyseal regions of the long bones, extending toward both ends. Secondary centers of ossification appear at both ends, or epiphyses, and are separated from the primary area of ossification by the epiphyseal plates. The epiphyseal plate of cartilage tissue continues to develop cartilage cells that continue to undergo ossification, adding to the bone formed by the primary ossification site. In this way, the bone continues to grow in length until the epiphyseal plate closes in response to hormonal influence during the second decade of postpartum life (Fig. 1-5). The outer layer of the cartilage model remains as mesenchymal tissue that continually produces chondroblasts and osteoblasts that form bone tissue. This perichondrium, which later becomes the periosteum, is responsible for the growth in width of the bones. It becomes highly innervated and highly vascularized, whereas the underlying layers of bone receive blood supply but little if any innervation.

The axial regions of the developing limb bud, which later become the joints, remain as condensations of mesenchymal tissue. In the case of synovial joints, the layers of "interzonal" mesenchyma adjacent to the developing bone ends differentiate into chondrocytes that secrete cartilage matrix, thus forming articular cartilage. The intervening middle zone undergoes cavitation to form the joint cavities,

Fig. 1-5. Development of bone.

or discongruities, between joint surfaces. The surrounding layers of cells, which are continuous with the perichondrium, differentiate into fibrous capsule and synovium. The innervation of synovial joints is discussed in Chapter 2, Arthrology.

The development of the cartilage models and joint spaces and the subsequent rotation and abduction of the limb buds occurs by the seventh to eighth week of fetal life. By 8 weeks, often before the mother realizes she is pregnant, the status and form of the fetal musculoskeletal system has largely been determined and any significant teratogenic influences will have taken effect. The development of the musculoskeletal system may be summarized as follows:

1. The musculoskeletal system is largely derived from the mesoderm.
2. The ectoderm forms the epidermal layer of skin and, though its invagination into the mesoderm, the nervous system.
3. Somites form in the paraxial mesoderm. These are (a) sclerotomes, which form bones, capsules, ligaments, cartilage, and blood vessels; (b) myotomes, which form muscles; and (c) dermatomes, which form the dermal layer of skin.
4. Because of the division of sclerotomes and subsequent fusion of caudal and cranial divisions of adjacent segments, a shift occurs that offsets the relationship between axial sclerotomes and myotomes.
5. The limbs are not formed from somatic myotomes, sclerotomes, or dermatomes but from the lateral somatic mesoderm, the somatopleure. The musculoskeletal structures of the limbs develop *in situ* from differentiation of primitive mesenchymal cells.

TERMINOLOGY

Although the limbs do not form from invasion of cells from the somatic myotomes, dermatomes, and sclerotomes, these segments are often referred to as existing in the limbs. Clinicians speak of pain being referred to a particular sclerotome, weakness occurring within a particular myotome, or sensory changes in a dermatome. It is important to understand that these terms are useful in clinical description but that they refer only to the source of innervation for a particular type of tissue and not the embryologic origin of the tissue, unless the terms are applied to the axial tissues. Thus, for example, the C5 myotome refers to those muscles in the limb receiving a significant innervation from the C5 anterior primary division or those muscles of the trunk innervated by the posterior primary division of C5. The C5 sclerotome in the limb refers to those structures

(*e.g.,* capsules, ligaments, periosteum) receiving innervation from C5. A particular joint is often said to be largely derived from a particular segment. In this manner it is implied that innervation to the structures forming the joint has its source in that spinal segment. More discussion concerning the clinical importance of segmental innervation is found in Chapter 3, Pain.

RECOMMENDED READINGS

Arey LB: Developmental Anatomy, 7th ed. Philadelphia, WB Saunders, 1974
Baume LJ, Holz J: Ontogenesis of the temporomandibular joint. II. Development of the temporal components. J Dent Res 49:864–875, 1970
Falkner F (ed): Human Development. Philadelphia, WB Saunders, 1966
Fitzgerald MJT: Human Embryology, A Regional Approach. New York, Harper & Row, 1978
Hollinshead H: Anatomy for Surgeons: Back and Limbs, 3rd ed. New York, Harper & Row, 1982
Lewis WH: The development of the arm in man. Am J Anat 1:145–183, 1902
Lewis WH, Bardeen CF: The development of the limbs, body wall and back in man. Am J Anat 1:1–35, 1901
Moore KL: Before We Are Born, 2nd ed. Philadelphia, WB Saunders, 1983
Moore KL: The Developing Human, 2nd ed. Philadelphia, WB Saunders, 1977
Netter FH, Crelin ES: Embryology. In Netter FH: The Ciba Collection of Medical Illustrations. Vol 8, Musculoskeletal System. Summit, NJ, Ciba-Geigy Co, 1987
O'Rahilly R: Developmental Stage of Human Embryos, publication No. 631. Washington, DC, Carnegie Institution, 1973
O'Rahilly R, Gardner E: The embryology of the movable joints. In Sokoloff L (ed): The Joints and Synovial Fluid, vol 1. San Francisco, Academic Press, 1978
Snell RS: Clinical Embryology for Medical Students, 3rd ed. Boston, Little, Brown & Co, 1983
Thorogood P, Tickel (eds): Craniofacial development. Development (Suppl) 103:1–254, 1988
Verboat AJ: The development of the vertebral column. Adv Anat Embryol Cell Biol 90:1–118, 1985
Warwick R, Williams P (eds): Gray's Anatomy, 35th ed, pp 81–90, 110–115, 126–132. Philadelphia, WB Saunders, 1973
Wendall Smith CP, Williams PL: Basic Human Embryology, 3rd ed. London, Pitman, 1984

SELECTED PERIODICALS DEVOTED TO EMBRYOLOGY

Advances in Anatomy, Embryology and Cell Biology
Development
Journal of Cell Science
Journal of Comparative Neurology
Journal of Developmental Physiology

2 *Arthrology*

Randolph M. Kessler

A complete study of human joints would include synchondroses, syndesmoses, symphyses, gomphoses, sutures, and synovial joints. For the sake of simplicity, and because the emphasis of clinical application is on joint mobilization techniques, the discussion in this chapter will be restricted to that of the synovial joints, which are the most numerous and most freely movable of the various types of human joints. However, each of the above classifications of human joints includes joints capable of movement. Movement definitely takes place at most syndesmoses, such as the distal tibiofibular joint. The symphysis pubis moves, especially during pregnancy. There is some movement of the teeth in their sockets (gomphoses). In fact, even the sutures of the skull are movable, at least through the third decade of life. Some investigators have claimed that they move spontaneously, with a rhythm independent of heart rate or respiratory rate.[21] Based on this claim, a few practitioners actually apply therapeutic mobilization to the sutures of the cranium.[21,40]

The mutual influences of structure and function are emphasized in this discussion because the two cannot be dealt with adequately or understood when considered independently. The traditional "anatomical" concept of synovial joints must be expanded to a "physiological" concept. In addition to those structures that anatomically define a joint, those structures responsible for normal movement at the joint must also be included (Fig. 2–1). With this approach the synovial joint can be considered the basic unit of the musculoskeletal system and used as a reference for discussing normal function and disorders of this system.

KINEMATICS

CLASSIFICATION OF JOINT SURFACES AND MOVEMENTS

The nature of movement at any joint is largely determined by the joint structure, especially the shapes of the joint surfaces. The traditional classification of synovial joints by structure includes the categories of spheroid, trochoid, condyloid, ginglymoid, ellipsoid, and planar joints.[51] It should be apparent even to someone with only a basic knowledge of human anatomy and kinesiology that this classification does not accurately define the shapes of joint surfaces or the movements that occur at each type of joint. The heads of the femur and humerus do not form true spheres or even parts of true spheres. A ginglymus, such as the humeroulnar joint, does not allow a true hinge motion on flexion and extension but rather a helical movement involving considerable rotation. The humeroradial joint, which is a trochoid joint, does not move about a single axis, or pivot, because the head of the radius is oval, having a longer diameter anteroposteriorly than mediolaterally. The interphalangeal joints, the carpometacarpal joint of the thumb, the humeroulnar joint, and the calcaneocuboid joints can be considered as sellar. However, the movements occurring at these joints vary greatly, as do the shapes of the joint surfaces. Therefore, although this classification of joint structures may serve a purpose for the anatomist, in itself it is not adequate for the clinician, such as the physical therapist, who must be concerned with the finer details of joint mechanics.

A similar problem exists with classifying joint movement. The traditional classification of joint movement includes the following[51]:

Angular — Indicating an increase or decrease in the angle formed between two bones, for example, flexion–extension at the elbow

Circumduction — Movement of a bone circum-

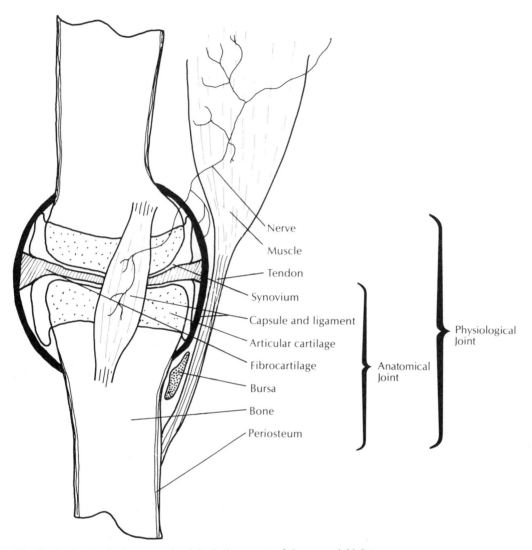

Nerve

Muscle

Tendon

Synovium

Capsule and ligament

Articular cartilage

Fibrocartilage

Bursa

Bone

Periosteum

Anatomical Joint

Physiological Joint

Fig. 2–1. Anatomical versus physiological concept of the synovial joint.

scribing a cone, for example, circumduction at the hip or shoulder

Rotation — Movement occurring about the longitudinal axis of a bone, for example, internal-external rotation at the shoulder

Sliding — One bone slides over another with little or no appreciable rotation or angular movement, for example, movement between carpals

There are two problems with this classification that make it inadequate for those clinicians concerned with joint mechanics. First, it describes movement occurring between bones but ignores movement occurring between joint surfaces. Movement takes place at joints, but often when movement is defined what happens *at the joint* is ignored. An analogy would be to consider the movement of a door but to ignore the hinge. Second, angular move-

ments almost never occur without some rotation, rotation nearly always occurs with some angular movement, gliding usually involves angular and rotary movement, and so on. Again, the classification needs to be expanded to take into consideration the specifics of joint movement.

Movements occurring between bones must be defined in such a way that they can easily be related to movements occurring between respective joint surfaces. Therefore, it is helpful to define the *mechanical axis* of any joint as a line that passes through the moving bone, touching the center of the relatively stationary joint surface and perpendicular to it (Fig. 2–2). *Osteokinematic* movement (movement occurring between two bones) can now be defined according to the mechanical axis rather than according to the long axis of the moving bone, as has been done in the past.[28,51] By relating osteokinematic movement

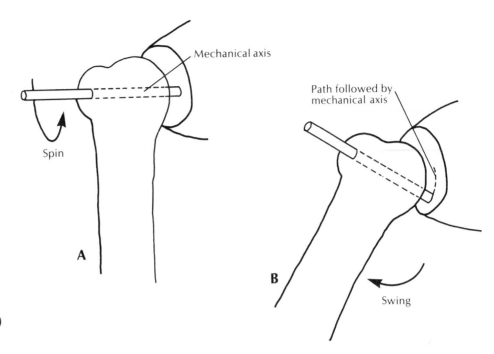

Fig. 2–2. Osteokinematic movements may be defined by the mechanical axis. These movements are *(A)* spin and *(B)* swing.

to *arthrokinematic* movement (movement occurring between joint surfaces) the movement of the mechanical axis of the moving bone relative to the stationary joint surface can be considered. In other words, one joint surface can be considered as stationary and its opposing joint surface as moving relative to it. This relative movement is defined according to the path traced by the line representing the mechanical axis of the joint on the stationary surface. The mechanical axis is determined at the starting point of a movement; once movement has begun, it maintains the same relationship to the moving bone, while moving relative to the stationary bone.

Joint Surfaces

Before discussing types of movement, it is necessary to define the shapes of joint surfaces since they largely determine the types of movements that may occur at the joint. No joint surface resembles a true geometric form; joint surfaces are neither spheres, ovals, or ellipses, nor are they true parts of these. However, any joint surface can be thought of as being part of an ovoid surface, that is, resembling the surface of an egg (Fig. 2–3A). If a cross section of an ovoid surface is examined, it is clear that the radius of the joint surface changes constantly, forming a cardioid curve (Fig. 2–4). A typical example would be a sagittal section of a femoral condyle. Some joint surfaces, rather than representing part of a simple ovoid, might be considered a complex ovoid, or sellar, surface (Fig. 2–3B). A sellar surface is convex in

one cross-sectional plane and concave in the plane perpendicular to it, although the surfaces of each of these cross sections may be represented by a cardioid curve.

Referring again to a simple ovoid (Fig. 2–5), the shortest distance between any two points on the surface is termed a *chord*, and any other line of continuous concavity toward the chord is an *arc*. A three-sided figure made up of three chords is a *triangle*. A three-sided figure in which at least one side is formed by an arc is a *trigone*.

Joint Movements

Any movement in which the bone moves but the mechanical axis remains stationary is termed a *spin* (see Fig. 2–2A). True spin of the humerus, then, would be a movement of flexion combined with some abduction, since the glenoid cavity faces slightly forward. The bone, during true spin, would rotate about its mechanical axis. Note that when the mechanical axis of the joint and the long axis of the moving bone coincide, such as at the metacarpophalangeal and the femorotibial joints, the spin is what is traditionally termed *rotation* at the joint. Where axes do not necessarily coincide, such as at the hip and shoulder, spin does not always occur when the joint "rotates." For example, spin occurs during internal and external rotation at the shoulder when the humerus is in a position of 90° of abduction; the mechanical axis (defined according to the starting position of movement) coincides with the long axis of the humerus.

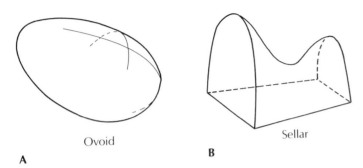

Ovoid

A

Sellar

B

Fig. 2–3. Joint surfaces may be *(A)* ovoid or *(B)* sellar.

However, internal and external rotations, performed with the arm to the side, do not involve spin at the joint surfaces; in this position, the mechanical axis does not coincide with the long axis of the humerus. A movement in which the mechanical axis follows the path of a chord is termed a *chordate*, or *pure*, swing. If the end of the mechanical axis should trace the path of an arc during movement of the bone, the bone has undergone an *arcuate*, or *impure*, swing (see Fig. 2–2*B*).

Note that with flexion or abduction of the humerus, the movement is an impure swing. Pure swing of the humerus occurs during elevation in a plane somewhat midway between the planes of flexion and abduction (because the glenoid cavity faces about 40° forward). Also note that internal and external rotation with the arm at the side is a movement of swing. An impure swing can be thought of as a pure swing with an element of spin, or rotation, about the mechanical axis. This element of rotation, which accompanies every impure swing, is termed *conjunct* rotation. Habitual movements at any joint

are usually impure swings. It follows that most habitual movements, or those movements that occur most frequently at any joint, involve some conjunct rotation. It is well known, for example, that the tibia rotates during flexion–extension at the knee. If one carefully watches the ulna flexing and extending on the humerus, a similar rotation is seen; the ulna pronates at the limits of extension and supinates at the extremes of flexion. The interphalangeal joints rotate considerably during flexion and extension. This is easily observed by holding the extended small fingers together, then flexing them simultaneously. The distal phalanges, especially, can be seen to supinate during flexion. Although such conjunct rotation occurs at every joint, it occurs to a much greater degree at joints with sellar surfaces than at those with simple ovoid surfaces. By now it should be evident that most of what have been traditionally considered "angular" movements are actually helical movements because of this element of conjunct rotation that accompanies them. This rotary component is an essential feature of normal joint mechanics.

ARTHROKINEMATICS

The study of what happens between joint surfaces on joint movement is known as arthrokinematics. When a bone swings relative to another bone, one of two types of movement may occur between joint surfaces.[28,51] If points at certain intervals on the moving surface contact points at the same intervals on the opposing surface, one surface is said to *roll* on the opposing surface (Fig. 2–6*A*). This is analogous to a tire on a car contacting the road surface as the car rolls down the street—various points on the tire contact various points on the road, the distance between contact points on the tire and road being the same. If, however, only one point on the moving joint surface contacts various points on the opposing surface, *slide* is taking place (Fig. 2–6*B*). This is analogous to a tire on a car that is skidding on ice. The tire

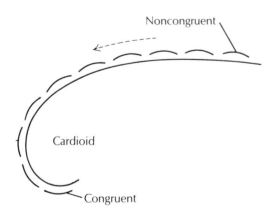

Noncongruent

Cardioid

Congruent

Fig. 2–4. A cardioid curve is representative of the cross-sectional shape of synovial joint surfaces. Because of the constantly changing radius there is one position at which the radius of the opposing joint surface attains maximal congruency.

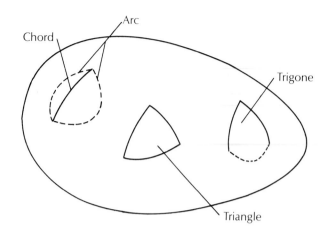

Fig. 2–5. Chords, arcs, a triangle, and a trigone are depicted on an ovoid surface.

is not turning but is moving relative to the road surface—it is sliding.

Actually, in most movements at human synovial joints, both slide and roll take place simultaneously. If only roll were to take place, the moving bone would tend to dislocate before much movement could occur; if only slide were to occur, impingement of joint surfaces would prevent full movement (Fig. 2–7). Stated in another way, the moving bone must rotate about a particular center of motion (or

centers of motion) in order for normal gliding to occur at the joint surfaces. If the bone should move about any other centroid of movement than what is normal for that joint, abnormal movement will occur between joint surfaces. Conversely, if normal movement does not or cannot occur between joint surfaces, the moving bone cannot move about its normal centroid of movement. This will be discussed later, in the section on analysis of accessory joint motions. Clinically, a meniscus tear, which causes

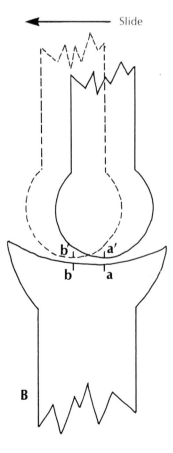

Fig. 2–6. Arthrokinematic movements showing (A) roll and (B) slide. The letters indicate points on the opposing joint surfaces which come in contact with one another. Points a' and b' are points on the moving joint surface; a and b are points on the stationary joint surface. Note that during (A) roll, points a and b contact various points on the opposing moving joint surface and during (B) slide, points a and b contact one point on the moving surface.

Fig. 2-7. Joint movements occurring in the absence of normal arthrokinematic movement cause *(A)* inpingement or *(B)* dislocation.

Fig. 2-8. Relationship between arthrokinematic movements and osteokinematic movements for the "concave-convex rule."*(A)* Represents a concave surface moving on a convex surface. *(B)* Represents a convex surface moving on a concave surface.

abnormal movement between joint surfaces, alters the normal centroid of movement at a joint.[15] This often results in abnormal stresses to the joint capsule, which are manifested as pain and muscle guarding. A tight joint capsule, which causes alteration in the normal centroid of movement, will result in abnormal movement between joint surfaces, usually with premature cartilaginous compression before the movement is completed. Physiologically, the fact that slide and roll take place together allows for economy of articular cartilage with respect to the size of the joint surface necessary for movement. It also prevents undue wearing of isolated points on joint surfaces, which would occur if, for example, only slide took place.

The Concave-Convex Rule

Obviously, roll always occurs in the same direction as the swing of the bone. However, the direction of joint slide can be determined only if the shapes of the joint surfaces are known. This is an important rule for anyone concerned with joint mechanics to know and will be referred to as the *concave-convex rule:* If a concave surface moves on a convex surface, roll and slide must occur in the same direction; if a convex surface moves on a concave surface, roll and slide occur in opposite directions (Fig. 2–8). Therefore, if the tibia extends on the stationary femur, the tibial joint surfaces must roll forward and slide forward on the femoral condyles in order for full movement to take place. However, if the femur extends on the stationary tibia, the femoral condyles must roll forward but slide backward on the tibia. If the humerus is elevated, the humeral head rolls upward but must slide inferiorly. During external rotation, with the arm at the side (a movement of swing), the head of the humerus must slide forward, whereas during internal rotation it must slide backward.

Clinicians must apply these concepts in the approach to restoration of restricted joint motion. Traditionally, in attempts to restore joint movement clinicians have tended to work only on osteokinematic movements. For example, if flexion of the humerus is restricted, active or passive motion into flexion is used in an attempt to increase this movement. However, one must also consider that inferior slide of the head of the humerus on the glenoid cavity may be restricted as well. The manual therapist may use passive joint mobilization techniques to restore inferior slide in order to facilitate the restoration of upward swing of the humerus. Thus, by knowing the concave-convex rule, the therapist knows in which direction to apply joint slide mobilizations in order to increase any restricted swing of a bone.

The type of joint surface motion that occurs with a spin of a bone about its mechanical axis is actually a form of slide. However, it should be apparent that while slide occurs in one direction at one half of the joint, it occurs in the opposite direction at the other half of the joint surface. This type of slide is referred to as *spin*, as is the osteokinematic movement it accompanies.

The Close-Packed Position

Separation of joint surfaces is termed *distraction*; approximation of opposing surfaces is *compression*. While some bone movements are accompanied by a relative compression of joint surfaces, other movements involve distraction. By knowing the close-packed position at a joint, one can determine which movements involve compression and which involve distraction.

As mentioned, ovoid surfaces are irregular in that in any one cross-sectional plane the ovoid surface is of constantly changing radius, defining a cardioid curve. If one imagines an opposing joint surface moving along this curve, it is clear that in most positions the two surfaces do not fit, or are noncongruent. However, one position exists in which the joint surfaces become relatively congruent because their contracting radii are approximately the same (see Fig. 2–4). Thus, while synovial joint surfaces tend to be noncongruent, at least one position exists for each joint in which the surfaces becomes maximally congruent. This position is termed the *close-packed position* of a joint. (The close-packed position for each extremity joint is listed in Appendix A.) At any joint, movement into the close-packed position involves an impure swing and so necessarily involves a conjunct rotation. The rotary component of movement into this position causes the joint capsule and major ligaments supporting the joint to twist, which in turn causes an approximation of joint surfaces. Once the close-packed position is reached, no further movement in that direction is possible.

Therefore, movement toward the close-packed position involves an element of compression, whereas movement out of this position involves distraction. MacConnaill and Basjaian point out that habitual movements at any joint involve movements directed into and out of the close-packed position.[28] It is likely that the resultant intermittent compression of joint surfaces has a bearing on nutrition and lubrication of articular cartilage. The squeezing out of synovial fluid with each compression phase facilitates exchange of nutrients and helps to maintain a lubricant film between surfaces (see sections on joint nutrition and lubrication).

Interestingly, moving the upper extremity in a reciprocating pattern, such that every joint is first moved simultaneously toward its close-packed position and then directly out of the close-packed position, resembles one of the basic patterns used by Knott in her proprioceptive neuromuscular facilitation techniques.[26] Considering the twisting and untwisting of the capsules and ligaments that occurs, and considering what is known of joint neurology with respect to joint–muscle reflexes (see the section on neurology later in this chapter), it seems likely that the facilitatory effect of the pattern may be related to joint position as well as muscle position.

The close-packed position also has important implications with respect to pathomechanics of many injuries. For instance, many upper extremity injuries occur from falling on the outstretched hand; Colles' fracture at the wrist, supracondylar elbow fractures, posterior dislocation of the elbow, and anterior dislocation of the shoulder are but a few. This is not surprising if one realizes that falling on the outstretched hand, in such a way that the body rolls away from the arm on impact, throws every major upper extremity joint (except the metacarpophalangeal and acromioclavicular joints) into close-packing. As mentioned, once the close-packed position is reached, the joint becomes locked and no further movement is possible in that direction. If further force is added, a joint must dislocate, a bone must give, or both. The weak link tends to be determined by age; the child is likely to fracture the humerus above the elbow, the adolescent or teenager may dislocate the shoulder, and the middle-aged or elderly person invariably sustains a Colles' fracture. In general, most fractures and dislocations occur when a joint is in the close-packed position. Most capsular or ligamentous sprains occur when the joint is in a loose-packed position. This is simply because the tight fit of the adjoining bones in the close-packed position causes forces applied to the joint to be taken up by the bones rather than by the supporting structures; there is more "intrinsic stability" at the joint.

Joint Play

In a loose-packed position, or in any position of the joint other than the close-packed position, the joint surfaces are incongruent. An obvious example is the knee joint in some position of flexion, although the menisci help to make up for the marked incongruence. In the loose-packed position, the capsule and major supporting ligaments remain relatively lax. This must be so in order to allow a normal range of movement. Thus, in most joint positions a joint has some "play" in it because joint surfaces do not fit tightly and because the capsule and ligaments remain somewhat lax.

This joint play is essential for normal joint function. First, the small spaces that exist because of joint incongruence are necessary to the hydrodynamic component of joint lubrication (see section on lubrication later in this chapter). Second, because the joint surfaces are of varying radii, movement cannot occur around a rigid axis, and so the joint capsule must allow some play in order for full movement to occur. Related to this is the fact that if normal joint distraction (one form of joint play) is lost, then joint surfaces will become prematurely approximated when moving toward the close-packed position, and movement in this direction will, therefore, be restricted. Human synovial joints cannot be compared to a door hinge, except in a limited sense, since a door moves about a single axis at its hinge and requires little or no play. Third, most joint movements are helical, involving movement about more than one axis simultaneously. In order for this type of movement to occur, a certain amount of joint play must exist, unless the movement is track-bound, which is usually not the case. One may, therefore, presume that loss of joint play from some pathology, such as a tight joint capsule, will lead to alteration in joint function, usually involving restriction of motion, pain, or both. Mennell uses the term *joint dysfunction* for loss of joint play.[38] This term is useful in a general discussion of joint mechanics but in clinical use should be avoided in favor of terms that more precisely identify the responsible pathology, since there are many possible causes of loss of joint play.

Conjunct Rotation

Conjunct rotation is the component of spin, or rotation, that accompanies any impure swing of a bone (Fig. 2–9). It is easily observed when the tibia extends on the femur, the distal phalanges of the fingers flex when held together, or the ulna flexes and extends on the humerus; such movements are helical. This rotation causes the joint capsule to twist when moving toward the close-packed position. At the shoulder, where a particularly large range of movement is possible, some rotation opposite the direction of normal conjunct rotation must occur at the later stages of movement. Thus, pure abduction in the frontal plane involves an impure swing with a medial conjunct rotation at the early phase, the first 90° to 120° of movement. This is because the glenoid cavity faces somewhat forward and the humerus on abduction swings out of the plane of the scapula. If

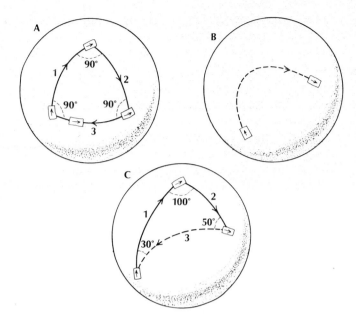

Fig. 2–9. Conjunct rotation occurring *(A)* with a succession of pure swings with return to the starting position (diadochokinetic movement), *(B)* with a single impure swing, and *(C)* with a completed cycle of pure and impure swings (also a diadochokinetic movement).

this impure swing were left to continue, at full elevation the joint capsule would be completely twisted on itself. This, however, is impossible, since the twisting of the joint capsule would cause a premature approximation of joint surfaces before full elevation could be attained. To prevent this premature locking of the joint on abduction, the humerus must rotate laterally on its long axis during the final phase of movement, bringing the humeral head back toward the plane of the scapula. Similarly, sagittal flexion involves a lateral conjunct rotation, but a medial longitudinal rotation during the final phase. This is best appreciated by observing it on a skeleton, noting the end position of the humerus on abduction or flexion without rotation and comparing it with elevation in the plane of the scapula, that is, about midway between flexion and abduction.

In addition to accompanying any impure swing, conjunct rotation may occur with a succession of swings, even if each of the swings is a pure swing. In a triangle drawn on a curved surface, such as an ovoid surface, the sum of the interior angles of the triangle may exceed 180° if the surface is convex, or the sum may be less than 180° if the surface is concave. During a succession of movements, in which the mechanical axis follows the path of a triangle or trigone, the amount of conjunct rotation that accompanies the completed cycle will be equal to the difference between the sum of the interior angles of the triangle or trigone and 180° (see Fig. 2–9). This type of conjunct rotation can be visualized by moving the humerus through a succession of movements: starting with the arm at the side, elbow bent, fingers facing forward, flex the humerus 90°, abduct 90° horizon-

tally, then adduct 90°. The fingers are now directed laterally, indicating that the humerus, during this succession of movements, rotated outward 90°. The succession may only be carried out once or twice without derotating the humerus medially because of the twisting of the capsule that results from the lateral conjunct rotation.

SUMMARY OF JOINT FUNCTION

The terminology of joint function has been expanded to accommodate the more specific features of joint kinematics, including the relationships between joint structure and function and the types of movements occurring between joint surfaces. In doing so the following osteokinematic terms, or those terms defining movement between two bones, have been defined:

Mechanical axis—Line drawn through the moving bone, at the starting position of a movement, that passes through the center of the opposing joint surface and is perpendicular to it

Spin—Movement of a bone about the mechanical axis

Pure swing—Movement of a bone in which an end of the mechanical axis traces the path of a chord with respect to the ovoid formed by the opposing joint surface; also called *chordate swing*

Impure swing—Movement in which the mechanical axis follows the path of an arc with respect to the opposing ovoid surface

Conjunct rotation—Element of spin that accompanies impure swing; also the rotation that may occur with a succession of swings

The following arthrokinematic terms, or those that define the types of movement occurring between joint surfaces, have also been defined:

Roll— Movement in which points at intervals on the moving joint surface contact points at the same intervals on the opposing surface
Slide— Movement in which a single contact point on the moving surface contacts various points on the opposing surface
Spin— Type of slide that accompanies spin of a bone; one half on the joint surface slides in one direction while the other half slides in the opposite direction, that is, the moving joint surface rotates about some point on the opposing joint surface.
Distraction— Separation of joint surfaces
Compression— Approximation of joint surfaces; always occurs when moving toward the close-packed position

The *close-packed position* was defined for a joint in which the following three conditions exist:

1. The joint surfaces become maximally congruent.
2. The joint capsule and major ligaments become twisted, causing joint surfaces to approximate.
3. The joint becomes locked so that no further movement is possible in that direction.

CLINICAL APPLICATION

Terminology

A rationale for the approach to management of joint dysfunction, including the use of specific joint mobilization techniques, can now be discussed based on the previous analysis of joint movement. However, some additional terms must first be presented. Unfortunately, a jargon has evolved relating to the clinical application of those concepts and is often the source of confusion since the terms are used inconsistently. Therefore, the most common and useful definitions of important terms are presented.

Accessory joint movements are simply those arthrokinematic movements that must occur in order for normal osteokinematic movement to take place. These might include slides, rolls, distractions, compressions, or conjunct rotations. Consider the osteokinematic movement of the humerus moving from the resting position with the arm at the side to the close-packed position. The joint is convex on concave. The head of the humerus must roll in the same direction in which the bone swings. It must slide opposite this direction or somewhat inferiorly and inward. Because the close-packed position is

being approached, the joint surfaces are becoming approximated. It is a movement of impure swing, so a conjunct rotation, in this case a lateral rotation, must occur. If any one of these accessory movements does not or cannot occur, then this particular swing of the humerus cannot be performed painlessly or harmlessly through the full range. If full osteokinematic movement does occur, it does so at the expense of the capsule or ligaments, which must be abnormally stretched, or of the articular cartilage, which must be abnormally compressed.

The term *component motions* can be used synonymously with *accessory movements*. For example, lateral rotation of the tibia is referred to as a component of knee extension. Likewise, spreading of the distal tibia and fibula is a component of dorsiflexion at the ankle. The clinician must be aware of the component motions necessary for each osteokinematic movement at a joint. Many of these are listed in Appendix A.

Joint-play movements are those accessory movements that can be produced passively at a joint but cannot be isolated actively. They might include distractions, compressions, slides, rolls, or spins at a joint in a particular position. Joint-play movements are used when applying specific mobilization techniques to restore accessory movements so that full and painless osteokinematic movement may be restored. For example, inferior glide occurs at the shoulder during active elevation. It can be performed passively, but in itself cannot be performed actively by voluntary muscle contraction; inferior glide is a joint-play movement at the glenohumeral joint.

Joint mobilization is a very general term that may be applied to any active or passive attempt to increase movement at a joint. In addition to traditional methods of increasing joint movement, such as active, passive, and active-assisted range of motion techniques, joint mobilization includes specific passive mobilization techniques. These techniques are aimed at restoring those component movements that permit pain-free or harmless osteokinematic movement. They are used especially to restore those joint-play movements that cannot be isolated actively. Specific passive mobilization techniques are graded (Fig. 2–10). Grades 1 through 4 are often referred to as *articulation* techniques, which are passive rhythmic oscillations. Grade 5 is a *manipulation* technique that is a high-velocity, low-amplitude passive thrust. These grades are relative to the pathologic amplitude of joint-play movement that exists at the joint and *not* to the normal amplitude that should exist. There are two main criteria for the selection of

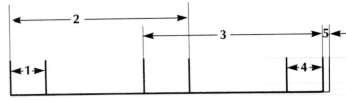

Fig. 2-10. Grades of joint-play movement.   Pathologic amplitude

the particular grade to be used: (1) the degree of pain or protective muscle spasm during passive joint-play movement (irritability) and (2) the degree or restriction of joint-play movement. The greater the irritability, the lower the numerical grade of movement used. Pain and spasm must be avoided. Manipulation is used primarily when a very slight, minimally painful restriction exists. A third criterion of selection might apply here, namely the skill and experience of the operator, since manipulative maneuvers should only be attempted after articulation techniques have been mastered and after much practice. The terms of joint movement are presented schematically in Figure 2-11.

Specific accessory joint motions that are limited may be restored by manual oscillations or thrusts. The primary goal of using specific joint mobilization techniques is restoration of normal, pain-free use of the joint. The emphasis is not on forcing a particular anatomical (osteokinematic) movement at a joint, as has been done in the past with traditional methods of mobilization; rather, it is on restoring normal joint mechanics in order to allow full, pain-free osteokinematic movement to occur. In this way, range of motion is restored to the joint with less risk of damaging the joint by compressing isolated portions of articular cartilage, and with less pain and muscle guarding from overstretching isolated capsuloligamentous structures, as may well occur if an osteokinematic movement is forced in the absence of necessary component movements. This is to say that specific passive mobilization, correctly applied, is a safer, more efficient, and less painful method of increasing range of motion at a joint. Mennell, in his

lectures, often uses the analogy of a door having lost movement because of a faulty hinge. Efforts to restore motion by pushing hard on the door are likely to result in further damage to the hinge. The logical method to remedy the situation is to direct one's attention to the hinge—to restore normal mechanics to the hinge, thereby restoring normal movement of the door.[38]

Note that this discussion ignores the physiological concept of the joint. This is done solely for the sake of simplicity. Obviously when restoring normal joint mechanics is considered, attention must be given to the anatomical joint along with those structures responsible for active movement of the joint. For example, active abduction at the shoulder is often lost because of the absence of inferior glide. Relative to the anatomical joint, the joint-play movement of inferior glide may be limited. However, the problem may also be physiological, in that inferior glide may not be occurring due to weakness of the supraspinatus muscle. These are very different problems leading to similar results. The nature of the problem must be brought out by a thorough evaluation.

Analysis of Accessory Joint Motions

Clinical Assessment. Many of the means of determining which accessory movements are components of specific osteokinematic movements have already been discussed. For instance, the direction of roll is always the same as that for the swing of the bone. If a convex surface moves on a concave surface, slide will occur in the direction opposite to the roll; if a concave surface moves on a convex surface,

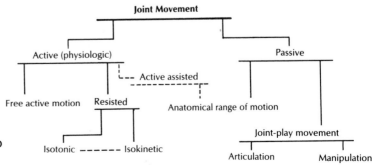

Fig. 2-11. Scheme illustrating terms related to joint movement.

slide occurs in the same direction as the roll. Distraction occurs when moving out of the close-packed position; compression occurs when moving into the close-packed position. These components can all be determined for any joint moving in any direction. Some of the other component motions, as listed for each joint in Appendix A, must be memorized or deduced anatomically.

One way of assessing the state of a particular accessory movement (its amplitude and irritability) is clinically, by evaluating the joint-play movements. These examination maneuvers are essentially the same as the specific mobilization techniques. Rather than being performed as a graded, therapeutic technique, they are used to determine the amplitude of a joint-play movement and whether the movement causes pain or spasm. The amplitude of movement and possible restriction must be compared with the operator's concept of "normal" for that movement, at that joint, for that body type. This requires experience in evaluating normal as well as pathologic joints. Whenever possible, the pathologic joint must be compared with a healthy contralateral joint. The degree of irritability is determined by the patient's subjective response, as well as by the presence of protective muscle spasm when performing the examination movement. (Refer to regional chapters for the joint-play techniques at each joint. These are performed using the same handholds as those for the therapeutic techniques included in Chapter 6, Peripheral Joint Mobilization Techniques.) Proficiency in clinically evaluating joint-play movements and correlating findings to knowledge of accessory movements at the joint, as well as other symptoms and signs presenting on examination, is essential to the effective application of joint mobilization techniques and management of musculoskeletal disorders.

Instant Center Analysis. The more scientific method of analyzing arthrokinematic movement has been described by Sammarco and co-workers.[45] This involves a determination of the centroid of movement, or instant center of movement, at various points throughout a joint movement. For any joint, the axis about which motion takes place changes constantly during a particular movement. This is because joint surfaces are irregular. The instant centers of motion can be plotted for a movement through the use of careful roentgenographic studies of a joint that record the relative position of the bones at various points throughout the movement. This is done by choosing two reference points on the moving bone; in Figure 2–12 the points lie on the central axis of the bone, point a on the joint surface, point b 7 cm

up on the shaft of the bone. A second roentgenogram taken after the bone has moved is superimposed over the original. In the new position, points a' and b' are determined along the central axis; a' is on the joint surface, b' is 7 cm up on the shaft. Now lines aa' and bb' are constructed, and perpendicular bisectors for each of these lines are drawn. The intersection of these bisectors is the instant center of motion, or the point of zero velocity, for this particular motion of the bone. Using this instant center of motion, point c, a velocity vector can be constructed showing the direction of surface motion that occurred for the particular movement. This is done by drawing a radius from the instant center to the point of contact between bones at the time for which the instant center was determined. In this case, the point of contact—the point at which the center axis of the bone crosses the joint surface—is called point p (Fig. 2–13). A perpendicular line drawn to this radius, at the joint surface, will indicate the direction of surface motion, with the arrow directed toward the movement of the bone.

Once the instant center and surface-velocity vector are determined, an interpretation can be made. An instant center lying on the joint surface at the point of contact between the bones indicates that pure roll is taking place. An instant center lying far from the joint surface point of contact indicates that pure sliding is taking place. A velocity vector pointed away from the opposing (stationary) surface indicates a distraction of the surfaces. A velocity vector aimed into the stationary surface indicates a compression of the surfaces. A velocity vector tangential to the joint surface suggests a smooth gliding motion is occurring.

The above analysis might seem somewhat complex at first but is actually quite simple. The difficult step is obtaining reliable roentgenograms that can be superimposed on each other. Plotting instant centers and surface velocity vectors for a particular movement throughout the range of motion can yield some very specific information about that motion. It reveals the relative amounts of roll and slide for various points throughout the range and how these values change during the complete motion: the closer the instant center comes to the point of contact, the more roll is taking place; the further it moves away, the more slide is occurring. Perhaps more importantly it reveals possible abnormal compression or distraction of joint surfaces throughout the range (*e.g.*, by comparison to what the operator considers "normal"). This type of scientific analysis of arthrokinematics is not practical for routine diagnostic purposes. However, it offers clinicians an op-

Fig. 2-12. Determination of instant centers of motion (C_1, C_2). *(A)* Selection of 2 reference points on the moving bone are chosen; point *a* on the central axis of the joint surface and point *b*, 7 cm up the shaft of the bone (position 1); the same points, a′ and b′ are chosen in position 2. *(B)* Lines a–a′ and b–b′ are constructed and perpendicular bisections are drawn for these lines *(C,D).* The intersection of the bisectors C1 and C2 are the instant centers of motion for movement from position 1 to 2 *(C)* and from position 2 to 3 *(D).*

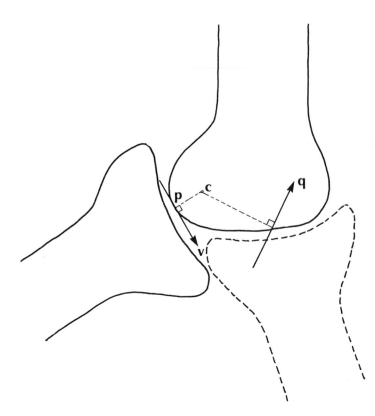

Fig. 2–13. Determination of surface velocity vectors: *p* is the point of contact during the arc of motion for which *c* applies; *v* is the calculated velocity vector indicating tangential surface motion. If *q* were the vector for the arc of motion for which *c* applies, one could conclude that joint compression took place during this motion.

portunity to demonstrate the value of specific therapeutic interventions in improving abnormal joint mechanics. It has been used already to show the value of certain surgeries, for example, meniscectomy at the knee, in restoring normal joint mechanics.[15]

Because the information is obtained from roentgenograms, which are two dimensional, arthrokinematic movements in only two dimensions can be studied. This analysis will not yield information concerning the amount of spin or conjunct rotation that is occurring.

NEUROLOGY

The neuroanatomy and, especially, the neurophysiology of joints are subjects not well covered in the current literature. Following the original works of Sherrington on neuromuscular physiology, a vast amount of information was collected concerning the role of muscle and tendon receptors in influencing posture, movement, muscle tone, and various reflex phenomena.[47] Little has been done until recently to identify specific joint receptors, and even less has been done to determine their clinical significance.[48,55] Since the subject of joint neurology is directly relevant to the management of common mus-

culoskeletal disorders, an overview is presented here.

INNERVATION

Joints tend to receive innervation from two sources: (1) articular nerves that are branches of adjacent peripheral nerves and (2) branches from nerves that supply muscles controlling the joint. Each joint is usually supplied by several nerves, and their distributions tend to overlap considerably. In general, a particular aspect of a joint capsule is innervated by branches of the nerve supplying the muscle or muscles that would, when contracting, prevent overstretching of that part of the capsule. One notable exception is the anteroinferior aspect of the glenohumeral capsule, which is innervated by a branch from the axillary nerve. The nerve fibers of an articular nerve are purely afferent, with the exception of small vasomotor efferents to the blood vessels. The fiber sizes range from large myelinated fibers to small myelinated and unmyelinated fibers.

RECEPTORS

Four types of joint receptors have been identified, each serving a relatively specific role in the sensorimotor integration of joint function.[48,51,55]

Type I

Description—Encapsulated ending, similar to Ruffini corpuscle

Location—Numerous in the superficial joint capsule; usually found in clusters of six

Related fibers—Small (6–9 μm) myelinated (relatively slow conduction)

Action—Slowly adapting, low threshold; mechanoreceptor

Function—Provides information concerning the static position of the joint; is constantly firing; contributes to regulation of postural muscle tone; contributes to kinesthetic (movement) sense; senses direction and speed of movement; contributes to regulation of muscle tone during movement of the joint

Type II

Description—Thickly encapsulated, similar to pacinian corpuscle

Location—Sparse (relative to type I), in joint capsule (deeper layers) and fat pads

Related fiber—Medium (9–12 μm) myelinated

Action—Rapidly adapting, low threshold; dynamic mechanoreceptor

Function—Fires only on quick changes in movement; provides information concerning acceleration and deceleration of joint movement; acts at initiation of movement as "booster" to help overcome inertia of body parts

Type III

Description—Thinly encapsulated, similar to Golgi end organ

Location—Intrinsic and extrinsic joint ligaments

Related fiber—Large (13–17 μm) myelinated (fast conduction)

Action—Very slowly adapting, high threshold; dynamic mechanoreceptor

Function—Monitors direction of movement; has reflex effect on muscle tone to provide a "braking" mechanism against movement tending to overdisplace the joint (movement too fast or too far)

Type IV

Description—Free nerve endings and plexus

Location—Fibrous capsule, intrinsic and extrinsic ligaments, fat pads, periosteum (*absent* in articular cartilage, intra-articular fibrocartilage, and synovium)

Fiber—Small (2–5 μm) myelinated and unmyelinated (2 μm) (slow conduction)

Action—Nonadapting, high threshold; pain receptors

Function—Inactive under normal conditions; active when related tissue is subject to marked deformation or other noxious mechanical or chemical stimulation

CLINICAL CONSIDERATIONS

It is apparent from the previous descriptions that stimulation of joint receptors contributes to sense of static position (type I), sense of speed of movement (type I), sense of change in speed of movement (type II), sense of direction of movement (types I and III), regulation of postural muscle tone (type I), regulation of muscle tone at the initiation of movement (type II), regulation of muscle tone during movement (coordination) (type II), and regulation of muscle tone during potentially harmful movements (type III). Of course, skin receptors, connective tissue receptors, and muscle receptors also contribute to many of these same functions. Some of the clinical problems that remain unresolved, or only partially resolved, include the following:

1. How important are these joint receptors, relative to muscle and skin receptors, for example, in the regulation of muscle tone, posture, and movement?
2. Are some of the persistent problems, such as chronic limp, residual incoordination, chronic instability ("giving way"), and chronic muscle atrophy, encountered in patients following some joint injuries the result of damage to these receptors?
3. How might treatment techniques, such as joint mobilization, neuromuscular facilitation, and inhibition, be refined to accommodate the functions of these joint receptors?

One particularly interesting study demonstrates a case in which malocclusion of dentures, causing abnormal afferent discharge from the temperomandibular joint capsules, resulted in an almost total reflex inhibition of the temporal muscles during active occlusion by the patient.[25] Restoration of normal joint mechanics, by remodeling of the dentures, restored normal muscular activity. A study by Wyke showed marked postural changes in a boy with apparent alteration of afferent impulses from the ankle capsule following injury to the lateral aspect of the capsule.[55] The postural deficit persisted in spite of an otherwise complete recovery, with restoration of normal strength and range of motion and with no residual pain. The boy's only complaint was that of occasional "giving way" of the ankle. Freeman advocates the use of coordination exercises on a balance board for patients with chronic ankle "instability" in the absence of demonstrable structural instability.[20] He reports good results with such a program, attributing such giving way at the ankle to alteration of normal joint afferent flow following injury to the joint, such as from an ankle sprain. Most physical therapists have encountered the common phenomenon of gross quadriceps atrophy following knee injury in spite of preventive efforts to maintain muscle function. Although there is little current literature on the subject, it seems reasonable to attribute this problem to reflex muscle inhibition by abnormal joint receptor stimulation.[9]

As far as techniques of treatment are concerned, it is interesting to relate what is known about the function of these joint receptors, and what is known of arthrokinematics, to techniques that have already evolved. Consider the diagonal pattern commonly used in proprioceptive neuromuscular facilitation techniques—moving the arm through flexion, abduction, external rotation to extension, adduction, and internal rotation. Part of the explanation of this pattern refers to moving from a position of maximum elongation and unspiraling of functionally related muscles to a position of spiraling and shortening of these same muscles.[50] In addition, this pattern involves moving all joints simultaneously from a close-packed to a loose-packed position. In doing so, the joint capsule of each joint moves from a position of maximum shortening and spiraling to a position of lengthening and unspiraling. Studies thus far on animals have indicated that maximum afferent stimulation occurs when approaching the close-packed position of a joint; this is to be expected since it is the position of maximum tightening of the capsule and ligaments in which the receptors lie. The techniques of proprioceptive neuromuscular facilitation evolved with primary consideration of the neurophysiology of muscles, using movement patterns that combine actions of functionally related muscles to bring about a mutual facilitation of each muscle in the chain. It is now suggested that these patterns also combine functionally related joint movements that add to the facilitative effect of the patterns on the muscles involved through joint receptor stimulation. It also seems probable that the joint receptors play a significant role in other techniques of facilitation, such as "quick stretch," that tend to stimulate the type II receptor.

It is important to consider the function of joint receptors when using joint mobilization or other treatment techniques involving joint movement. The effectiveness of efforts to increase movement at a joint will naturally be compromised by any muscle contraction tending to restrict joint movement. Emphasis, then, must be made on avoiding reflex muscle contractions that would tend to prevent or restrict a desired joint movement. For this reason—and for other obvious reasons—pain must be avoided during joint mobilization, since it is well known that pain at a joint tends to elicit a reflex muscle response to restrict movement at the joint. Sudden joint movement tends to stimulate firing of the type III receptors, which sets up a reflex muscle contraction to restrict further movement. Gradual initiation of movement tends to stimulate the type II receptor, which affects a small facilitative muscular response. Passive and active mobilization techniques are best performed rhythmically, without sudden changes in speed or direction of movement. A manipulation must be performed so quickly that it is completed before the reflex muscular response produced by stimulation of the type III receptor can act to interfere with the movement. Similarly, it must be performed through a very small amplitude to minimize the number of type III receptors stimulated.

With respect to the type IV pain receptors, it is worth emphasizing that articular cartilage, fibrocartilage (*e.g.*, menisci), synovium, and compact bone are essentially aneural. This is well documented in anatomical studies as well as clinically.[24,48,55] In the anatomical joints the major pain-sensitive structures are the fibrous capsule, ligaments, and periosteum. This carries some important clinical implications. It suggests that pathologic conditions that might alter joint mechanics, such that the articular cartilage undergoes undue compression stress, may go unnoticed by the patient in their initial stages. In fact, the patient may notice nothing until either joint mechanics are altered sufficiently to place an abnormal stress on the joint capsule or until the joint cartilage undergoes sufficient degeneration, causing a low-grade synovitis with resultant pressure on the capsule from effusion. This may explain why persons with "frozen shoulders" or osteoarthrosis of other joints often do not present to a physician until the disease has progressed considerably. It also suggests that clinicians must learn to routinely examine for subtle changes in joint mechanics rather than considering only gross range of motion, strength, and complaints of pain by the patient. Patients presenting with very early symptoms or signs of osteoarthrosis could enjoy complete arrest or reversal of the joint problem if properly managed, rather than resigning themselves to future joint replacement.

As is discussed in more detail in Chapter 3, *Pain*, small oscillatory articulations may, in themselves, be useful in reducing pain at the joint being moved or at other joints derived from the same segment. The added proprioceptive input may inhibit the perception of pain through modulation at the substantia gelatinosa in the dorsal horn of the spinal cord.

JOINT NUTRITION

In addition to being aneural, articular cartilage is for the most part avascular. This is also true of intra-articular fibrocartilage. Since, in general, body tissues depend on blood supply for nutrition, these structures would seem to be at a disadvantage. It is generally believed that the articular margins do receive some nutrients from the highly vascularized synovium and periosteum adjacent to them.[17] The menisci at the knee also receive nutrients at their peripheral capsular attachments, and it is suggested that the deep layers of articular cartilage are fed by the blood supply to the subchondral bone. However, the problem of nutrition to the more superficial, centrally located portions of the articular cartilage and to the more centrally located parts of the intra-articular fibrocartilage remains. These cartilaginous areas are primary articulating surfaces, not the more peripheral areas or deeper layers. It is generally agreed that nutrition to these regions occurs by diffusion and inhibition of synovial fluid. This is a unique situation because nutrients must cross at least two barriers in order to reach the chondrocytes embedded within the cartilage. First, they must pass from the capillary bed of the highly vascularized synovium. They must then diffuse through the superficial matrix layers of the cartilaginous surface, before reaching the cell wall of the chondrocyte. Thus, synovial fluid serves a major function as a source of nutrition for articular cartilage and intra-articular fibrocartilage.[17,30-32]

Intermittent compression and distraction of joint surfaces must occur in order for an adequate exchange of nutrients and waste products to take place. A joint that is immobilized undergoes atrophy of articular cartilage, just as a joint in which there is prolonged compression of joint surface undergoes similar atrophic changes.[2,12,13,53] The three primary mechanisms by which synovial joints undergo normal compression and distraction are the following: (1) weight-bearing in lower extremity and spinal joints; (2) intermittent contraction of muscles cross-

ing a joint; and (3) twisting and untwisting of the joint capsule as the joint moves toward and away from the close-packed position during habitual movements. With respect to the last mechanism, it is necessary to recall that as the joint approaches the close-packed position, its joint surfaces not only become compressed but also approach a position of maximal congruency. Thus, compression normally occurs in a position in which greater areas of the opposing joint surfaces are in contact. This ensures that relatively large portions of the joint surfaces undergo adequate exchange of nutrients. From a pathologic standpoint, a joint that has lost movement, as from a tight joint capsule, does not receive a normal exchange of nutrients over the parts of the joint surfaces that no longer come into contact. This is especially true in the case of a tight joint capsule, since movements toward the close-packed position in which there is maximal joint surface contact are usually the movements that are most restricted.

Attritional changes in articular cartilage related to aging are observed in the relatively noncontacting portions of the joint surfaces.[4,35-37] Several reasons for this may be postulated. First, these are the areas of articular cartilage that undergo less deformation with use of the joint over time; as a result, the rate and degree of exchange of nutrient fluids is less in these areas. Also, with age there is a reduction of the chondroitin sulfate component of cartilaginous tissue. Since the fluid-binding capacity of articular cartilage is largely dependent on its chondroitin sulfate content, a decrease in this constituent might interfere with normal nutrition to the tissue. Furthermore, because loss of joint range of motion occurs with advancing age, the exchange of nutrients to portions of the articular cartilage is reduced.

LUBRICATION

Synovial fluid, in addition to serving as a nutritional source for articular cartilage, also acts as a lubricant to prevent undue wear of joint surfaces from friction.[11,16,34,54] In studying lubrication of human joints, however, not just the properties of synovial fluid and how they affect movement and friction between two surfaces are considered. In addition there are the shape and consistency of the joint surfaces as well as the types of movement that occur between joint surfaces. Many models have been proposed for human joint lubrication. Some of the earlier models tend to ignore many of the unique properties of human joints. The more recent models evolved with the sophistication of engineering principles, which are better able to deal with some of the complex factors involved in human joint lubrication. However, it is generally agreed that no one model of joint lubrication applies to all joints under all circumstances. The major mode of lubrication in a particular joint may change, depending on factors such as loading and speed of movement.

Synovial fluid has essentially the same composition as blood plasma, except for the addition of mucin. Mucin is the mucopolysaccharide hyaluronic acid, which is a long-chain polymer. The viscous properties of synovial fluid are attributed to hyaluronic acid. The most important property to be considered in this respect is the *thixotropic* or nonnewtonian quality of synovial fluid; the viscosity decreases with increased shear rate (increased speed of joint movement).

MODELS OF JOINT LUBRICATION

An analogy cannot accurately be drawn between a machine model of lubrication and the lubrication of synovial joints. One of the major reasons for this is that the physical properties of articular cartilage differ considerably from the physical properties of most machine components. Articular cartilage is porous and relatively spongelike in that it has the capacity to absorb and bind synovial fluid. Articular cartilage is also viscoelastic; the deformation rate is high on initial application of the load and levels off with time. When the load is removed, the initial "reformation" rate is high and decreases over time (Fig. 2–14). Although macroscopically articular cartilage appears quite smooth and shiny, it is, in fact, relatively rough microscopically. Articular cartilage also has the tendency to absorb large molecules, such as hyaluronic acid in synovial fluid, to its surface. The significance of this is discussed later in this section.

The early model of joint lubrication described a hydrodynamic, or fluid film, situation (Fig. 2–15A).[27] In this case, synovial fluid fills in the wedges of space left by the joint surface incongruencies. On movement between surfaces the synovial fluid is attracted to the area of contact between the surfaces. This occurs because of (1) the pressure gradient produced by the movement and (2) the fact that relative movement tends to pull the viscous fluid in the direction of the moving surface. The result of this is the maintenance of a layer of fluids between joint surfaces during movement. Any friction occurring as a result of movement occurs within the fluid rather than between joint surfaces. This meets the requirements of a good lubrication system because it allows free movement and prevents wear to the joint surfaces. This system works well during movement; however, it would tend to fail under very slow velocity or under heavy loading. It would also fail under reciprocal motion, since it would not adapt well to changes in direction of motion, at which time the velocity of movement is zero. Since human joints often move slowly, under heavy loads, and reciprocally, by itself it seems an unsatisfactory model for human joint lubrication.

The hydrodynamic model, however, cannot be completely repudiated because the previous description does not consider the viscoelasticity of joint surfaces. This model can be modified to an elastohydrodynamic system (Fig. 2–15B). Because of the nature of articular cartilage to deform, not all of the energy of heavy loading goes to decreasing the thickness of the layer of film between the surfaces, thus increasing friction between the surfaces. Instead, deformation of the joint surfaces occurs, increasing the effective contact area between surfaces and thus reducing the effective compression stress (force per unit area) to the lubrication fluid. This allows the protective layer of fluid to remain at about the same thickness. Thus, the elastohydrodynamic

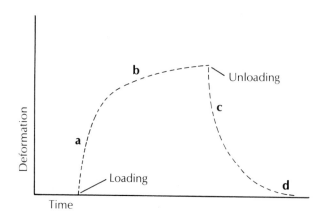

Fig. 2–14. Viscoelastic response of articular cartilage. Parts **a** and **c** of the curve are due to elastic properties, while parts **b** and **d** show viscous behavior.

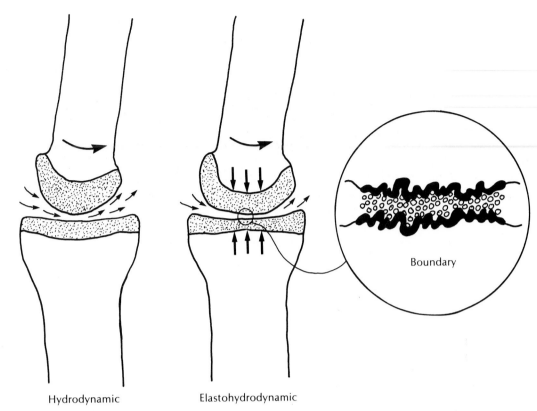

Hydrodynamic   Elastohydrodynamic   Boundary

Fig. 2–15. Hydrodynamic, elastohydrodynamic, and boundary models of joint lubrication.

model describes a system that withstands loading in the presence of movement. It lacks an explanation, however, for the means of lubrication at the initiation of movement or at the period of relative zero velocity during reciprocating movements or during very heavy loading with very little movement.

This model of joint lubrication can be expanded by including the concepts of boundary lubrication and weeping lubrication.[34,42,49,54] With any materials undergoing relative shear between two surfaces, friction is the result of the irregularities of the surfaces; the greater the irregularities, the greater the friction. Effective lubrication must reduce this friction to a minimum, thus reducing wear of the surfaces to a minimum. In the case of boundary lubrication, the lubricant is adsorbed to the surface of the material, in effect reducing the roughness of the surfaces by filling in the irregularities. Because articular cartilage is able to adsorb long-chain molecules of hyaluronic acid, these molecules are able to fill in the irregularities as well as to coat the surface. Any friction occurring as the result of shear movement occurs between molecules of the lubricant rather than between the joint surfaces themselves. This probably serves as an adjunct to the elastohydrodynamic system, especially in cases of extreme loading

sufficient to decrease significantly the thickness of the layer of fluid maintained by the elastohydrodynamic model under lighter loads. It may also play a role at the initiation of movement or periods of zero velocity, since a layer of fluid would not be present because of its dependence on movement under an elastohydrodynamic system. The concept of weeping lubrication is actually an expansion of the elastohydrodynamic model. Because of the porosity and elastic qualities of articular cartilage, loading sufficient to cause a deformation of the articular surfaces also causes a "squeezing out" of the synovial fluid absorbed by the cartilage. The fluid that is squeezed out further serves to maintain a protective layer of lubricant between joint surfaces.

By the use of this "mixed lubrication" model, which combines elastohydrodynamic concepts with boundary lubrication concepts, the demands of human synovial joints are met.[11,43] The system allows movement, change in direction of movement, loading, and variations in congruencies of joint surfaces. It takes into consideration, at least in general terms, the properties of the lubricant (synovial fluid) and the surface materials. There is still considerable controversy over the relative importance of each of the lubrication models under various conditions, but most authors agree with the general concepts presented previously. Since it is still unknown how each model contributes to normal joint lubrication, very little investigation into the mutual effects of pathologic joint conditions and joint lubrication has taken place. A breakdown in some aspect of the lubrication system is likely to cause or add to the progression of joint disease, such as degenerative joint disease. On the other hand, certain joint diseases result in changes in structure and function of joint constituents. For instance, there is a loss of joint cartilage in degenerative joint disease and changes in synovial fluid viscosity in rheumatoid arthritis. It is probable that in such cases the disease will, in turn, alter the function of the lubrication system, thus contributing to a progressive degenerative cycle.

RESOLVING PROBLEMS OF JOINT-SURFACE WEAR

It has been emphasized that synovial joint surfaces are incongruent. Because of the incongruency that exists in most positions of movement, a relatively small contact area exists between joint surfaces. The wedges of space that surround this contact area are necessary in order for a hydrodynamic lubrication system to operate effectively; without these spaces the lubricant could not be drawn, or forced, between the contacting surfaces. One may wonder if such a small area of contact might increase the likelihood of wear between joint surfaces, since loading forces from weight-bearing and muscle contraction would be distributed over a small surface area, thus increasing the compressive stress to the joint. This would, in fact, be the case if the area of contact on one or both surfaces was consistently the same throughout habitual movements. In this respect the clinician might be concerned about joints that are relatively track-bound, such as the humeroulnar, patellofemoral, ankle mortise, and interphalangeal joints. In each of these joints movement tends to be restricted to one arc of movement that is determined almost entirely by the shapes of the joint surfaces. It would seem that during movement at these joints, the contacting area on one joint surface would consistently "follow a rut" on the opposing surface, increasing the likelihood of excessive wear in the rut or at the area of the surface contacting the rut. In these joints the problem of excessive wear is resolved in a number of ways. First, these joint surfaces are, relatively speaking, the most congruent in the body, so that forces are distributed over a somewhat larger area. Consider, for example, the close fit between the ulna and the trochlear surface of the humerus. Second, the contact area on each surface is constantly

changing throughout an arc of movement. A change in contact areas occurs in one sense because a combination of roll and slide takes place between joint surfaces. In another sense, the contact area changes because contact alternates from the "bottom of the valley to the sides of the slopes" on one surface and correspondingly on the opposing surface. For instance, with the knee in full extension, the articular surface of the patella makes contact with the femur at a strip extending mediolaterally across the middle of the patellar surface. In flexion, however, only the medial and lateral margins of the patella make contact with the femoral condyles while the ridge in the middle of the patellar facets lies freely in the intercondylar notch.[22] A comparable situation occurs at the elbow, ankle, and finger joints mentioned throughout their respective movements. Note that at the ankle mortise, which undergoes intermittent heavy loading in habitual use, maximal loading (stance) takes place with the joint closer to its close-packed position, dorsiflexion. This is the position of maximal congruence and, therefore, the position in which the compressive force per unit area would tend to be smallest.

But at joints such as the knee, a more complex situation exists. The knee is markedly incongruent compared with the joints discussed previously; it must be in order to allow some degree of rotation to occur independently of flexion or extension or in conjunction with them. The knee must also withstand heavier loading from weight-bearing in a wide variety of positions. Thus, the knee is often required to undergo heavy loading in positions of flexion, in which the surfaces are very incongruent—a small area of contact withstands relatively large compressive forces. Thus there might be concern that in a situation of heavy loading, relatively low velocity, and small contact area between surfaces, the lubrication system would not be sufficient to prevent excessive friction (shear) and wear between joint surfaces. This might very well be the case in a joint such as the knee that must undergo such conditions during normal daily activities, such as climbing stairs, squatting, and lifting. There might also be concern about the tendency for the femur to slip forward on the tibia under such conditions, again because of the incongruency of joint surfaces and the lack of intrinsic stability. Are the posterior cruciate and popliteus and other intrinsic stabilizers sufficient to prevent this problem?

The knee, then, is a joint that must allow movement of spin between the tibia and the femur and swing between the tibia and femur because of the functional demands placed on it. In order for this to be possible, the joint surfaces must be sufficiently noncongruent. But because of this noncongruence and because of normal heavy loading in a variety of positions, the knee appears susceptible to excessive shear forces between contacting joint surfaces during movement, excessive compressive forces between contacting surfaces on static loading, and intrinsic instability when loaded in flexion. It is probable that the intra-articular menisci serve to compensate for what would otherwise be unsatisfactory engineering at the knee joint—unsatisfactory in that the joint would not withstand the normal forces applied to it without giving way or undergoing premature wearing of joint surfaces.[27] Under heavy static loading, the menisci act to increase the effective load-bearing surface area at the joint, thus reducing the force per unit area. Being firmly attached to the joint capsule and tibia but mobile enough to conform to the shape of the articulating segments of the femoral condyles, they serve to increase the intrinsic stability of the joint by increasing the effective congruency between joint surfaces. During movement with heavy loading, they again act to increase the load-bearing surface area, but also to maintain a wedge-shaped interval surrounding the area of contact into which the lubricant fluid can be drawn.[27] Since the menisci are semicartilaginous, they can also absorb synovial fluid. With increased loading, fluid can be squeezed out from the menisci as well as the articular load-bearing surface, contributing to a weeping lubrication phenomenon. Also, as the menisci recede before the advancing condyles during movement, they can act to spread a layer of lubricant over the joint surfaces just prior to contact. This, incidentally, may also be a function of the rather large infrapatellar fat pad at the knee.[5] The menisci, because they are semimobile, allow the knee to act as though it were maximally congruent with respect to the requirements of lubrication and intrinsic stability, but to actually function as though it were very incongruent with respect to the types of movement that occur at the joint.

One should also take note of the considerable slide of the femoral condyles along the tibial surface during the complete range of flexion–extension. This feature also reduces the likelihood of excessive wear on the tibial surfaces by distributing the load-bearing surface over a larger area. The degree of slide could not occur normally without the extrinsic control provided by the cruciates, nor without the intrinsic stability provided by the menisci. This type of motion, in which the area of contact of a particular joint surface constantly changes with movement at the joint, is necessary to allow for the intermittent com-

pression of articular cartilage essential to normal nutrition and lubrication. Loss of a constantly changing area of contact during use of a joint is likely to increase the probability of degeneration of articular cartilage by interfering with normal nutrition and normal lubrication, and by increasing the compressive forces over time per unit area per unit time. Unused areas of articular cartilage would not undergo necessary exchanges of nutrients; areas of cartilage in which loading occurs would eventually fail from fatigue (see section on arthrosis later in this chapter).

It is worth mentioning that fibrillation of articular cartilage in normal hip and shoulder joints occurs first in non–weight-bearing surfaces.[36] Also, a marked acceleration of degenerative changes is shown to occur in weight-bearing animal joints in which a joint is immobilized but full use of the limb is allowed.[12] These are both examples of the effects on articular cartilage of the load-bearing contact area not being distributed over a large area of the opposing surfaces. This is perhaps a partial explanation for the frequency of degenerative arthritis occurring in human hip joints; a relatively small surface area is used for weight-bearing, while much of the articular cartilage receives little or no compression. As will be discussed later in the section on arthrosis, it also contributes to the explanation of how abnormal joint arthrokinematics may lead to joint pathology.

APPROACH TO MANAGEMENT OF JOINT DYSFUNCTION

The rationale for specific joint mobilization requires the restoration of normal joint play in order that full, pain-free motion may occur at the joint. The term joint dysfunction is used by Mennell to indicate loss of normal joint play.[38] There are many explanations for the causes of joint dysfunction, some of which are specific for certain joints and some of which may be applied to all joints. In the spine, entrapment of "meniscoid inclusions" is postulated by some as a cause of joint dysfunction. Frankel and co-workers have demonstrated through instant center analysis the presence of joint dysfunction at the knee from meniscus tears (confirmed later by surgery) and dysfunction in ankle joints that had been classified as unstable, postfracture, or having degenerative disease.[15,45] It has also been shown that joint dysfunction in "frozen shoulders" is often caused by adherence of the anteroinferior aspect of the joint capsule to the humeral head.[39] A loose body in a joint may be a cause of dysfunction, as may joint effusion causing some distention of the capsule. The list goes on, the point being that *there is no single cause of joint dysfunction.*

The use of specific mobilization is not indicated in all cases of dysfunction. For this reason, a thorough evaluation performed in an attempt to clarify the nature and extent of the lesion is a necessary step in the management of joint problems. Those cases in which a physical therapist must play a major role in treatment of joint dysfunction are those dysfunctions occurring as a result of isolated or generalized capsular tightness or adhesion. These typically follow traumatic sprains to the capsule or immobilization. In some cases, they occur for no *apparent* reason, for example, "adhesive capsulitis" at the shoulder.

The traditional approach to management of patients presenting with loss of pain-free movement at a joint usually involves various modes of pain relief, active and passive measures to improve osteokinematic movement, and encouragement of normal use of the part. It should be clear that this approach is inadequate and perhaps dangerous. First, it ignores the basic problem, which is often loss of normal arthrokinematics. Second, it involves considerable forcing of osteokinematic movements in the absence of normal arthrokinematic movement, which may only occur at the expense of the articular cartilage. This is to say that the resiliency of the cartilage may allow a certain amount of osteokinematic movement to occur without the normal accompanying arthrokinematic movements. Frankel and co-workers describe the case of a boy who continued to use his knee in the absence of normal external rotation of the tibia on the femur during knee extension.[14] One and a half years later, at surgery, dimpling of the articular cartilage of the medial femoral condyle was observable with the naked eye, presumably owing to continued abnormal compression of this portion of the articular surface from loss of normal arthrokinematic movement.

A more logical approach to the management of these patients emphasizes the restoration of joint play to allow free movement between bones. This can be achieved only by (1) evaluating to determine the nature and extent of the lesion, (2) deciding if joint mobilization is indicated based on the evaluation, (3) choosing the appropriate techniques based on the direction and extent of restrictions, and (4) skillfully applying techniques of specific mobilization. Efforts to relieve pain and reduce muscle guarding are, of course, important adjuncts to treatment but do not in themselves constitute a treatment program. Also, some movement should be encour-

aged in the cardinal planes, but only as normal kinematics are restored. To a certain extent, functional use of the part should be restricted through careful instructions to the patient until normal joint mechanics are restored. This approach minimizes the possible danger of undue stresses to the articular cartilage during attempts to restore movement. It also minimizes the possibility of discharging a patient who has relatively pain-free functional use of the joint, but who may have some residual kinematic disturbance sufficient to cause cartilage fatigue over time and perhaps osteoarthrosis in later years.

PATHOLOGIC CONSIDERATIONS

A high percentage of the chronic musculoskeletal problems seen clinically are fatigue disorders. These are disorders in which abnormal stresses imposed on a structure over a prolonged period result in a tendency toward an increased rate of tissue breakdown. All tissues, including those with low metabolic activity such as articular cartilage, undergo a necessary process of repair to continuously replace the microdamage resulting from normal use. In bone, such microdamage would involve fracturing of bony trabeculae, whereas in other connective tissues there is disruption of individual collagen fibers. As long as the rate of microtrauma does not exceed normal limits, and the rate at which the tissue is able to repair itself is not compromised, the tissue remains "normal." The tendency to maintain an equilibrium against opposing, unbalancing factors is a homeostatic mechanism; a shift in the nature of one factor will cause a compensatory reaction by the body to correspondingly alter the other factor in order to maintain balance.

In general, the nature of the various pathologies affecting the musculoskeletal tissues can be considered according to this homeostatic model. The two factors that the body is attempting to balance are (1) the process of tissue breakdown and (2) the process of tissue production or repair. In discussing abnormal, or pathologic, situations then, attention must be paid to the causes of, and homeostatic responses to, a tendency toward increased tissue breakdown and a tendency toward a decreased rate of breakdown. Factors that might disturb the body's ability to maintain an appropriate balance, such as those that might cause an abnormal degree of tissue production and those that might compromise the body's ability to produce enough tissue, must also be considered.

INCREASED RATE OF TISSUE BREAKDOWN

Increased tissue breakdown results when the frequency or magnitude of stresses to the part increases, when the capacity of the tissue to repair itself is reduced, or both. Under conditions of significantly increased stress over time, the body attempts to compensate by laying down more tissue in order to increase the capacity of the tissue to withstand the higher stress levels. The result is tissue hypertrophy. In well-vascularized tissues, this occurs in conjunction with a low-grade inflammatory process incited by the increased rate of tissue damage. A new equilibrium is reached in favor of a more massive structure, better able to withstand higher stress levels without failing. Typical examples include muscle hypertrophy in response to increased loading of a muscle over time; subchondral bony sclerosis in response to increased compressive forces over a joint; and fibrosis of a joint capsule receiving increased stresses from faulty joint movement occurring over a prolonged period of time.

Such tissue hypertrophy, especially when affecting bone and capsuloligamentous structures, causes tissue to gain in strength at the expense of extensibility; the tissue becomes better able to withstand loads without undergoing gross failure but does not deform as readily when loaded. An increase in the ratio of collagen (mineralized collagen in the case of bone) and the remaining extracellular ground substance (mucopolysaccharide) reduces extensibility. This is believed to allow increased interfiber bond formation, with a subsequent reduced mobility, or gliding capacity, of individual elements. The added stiffness reduces the energy-attenuating capacity of the structure. Less of the energy of loading is attenuated as work, and more of the energy must be absorbed internally by the structure or attenuated by increased deformation of other structures that are in series with the hypertrophic tissues. Thus, with sclerosis of subchondral bone, the overlying articular cartilage is made to undergo greater strain per unit of load because of the reduced deformability of the subjacent bone. This is believed to be an important factor in the progressive degeneration of cartilage occurring with degenerative joint disease.[43] With fibrosis of tendon tissue, such as the extensor carpi radialis brevis origin at the elbow, the reduced extensibility of the tendon fibers results in greater strain to the tenoperiosteal junction of the tendon at the lateral humeral epicondyle. The ensuing inflammatory process is responsible for the symptoms and signs of the "tennis elbow" syndrome.

Although in such situations the hypertrophic structure is more massive and less likely to fail when loaded, the rate of microdamage may remain elevated. Although the stress to the structure tends to be reduced because of the increased cross-sectional area resulting from the hypertrophy, the internal energy within the structure may be increased because of the reduced extensibility. An increase in internal energy must be dissipated as heat or microfracturing of individual structural components. Clinically, a painful, low-grade inflammatory reaction may result from the added mechanical and thermal stimulation.

Thus, when a tissue hypertrophies in response to increased stress levels, the rate of microdamage tends to remain elevated—there is simply more tissue present to ensure that the structure, as a whole, does not fail. Pain may arise from the increased internal stresses on the involved tissue or from increased strain on connected tissues.

For any tissue there is a critical point past which the rate of breakdown may exceed the rate at which the tissue is able to repair or strengthen itself. Under normal metabolic conditions, this critical point is reached soonest in tissues with limited capacity for regeneration and repair. These are tissues that are poorly vascularized and have a low metabolic turnover. The typical example of such a tissue is articular cartilage. With increased compressive stress levels to a joint, the well-vascularized bone will tend to hypertrophy, while the cartilage degenerates. Even bone, however, can be stressed at a frequency or magnitude at which it can no longer repair itself fast enough to prevent progressive breakdown. A common clinical disorder in which this occurs is the stress fractures affecting athletes or other persons who habitually engage in high-stress-level activities.

REDUCED RATE OF TISSUE BREAKDOWN

Decreased stress levels on tissue over time will reduce the rate of breakdown. Thus, with relative inactivity the rate of microdamage is less and the body takes the opportunity to economize by reducing the rate of tissue production. The tissue no longer needs to be as strong because of the reduction in the everyday stresses it must withstand. The typical condition in which this occurs is disuse atrophy. When a part is immobilized, the bone becomes less dense, and capsules, ligaments, and muscles atrophy. The important clinical consideration in such situations is to gradually increase the stress levels on the tissue in order to promote strengthening of the structure by stimulating increased tissue production, but without causing the weakened structures to fail. This is especially true following healing of a structure such as bone or ligament; not only must new tissue be produced, but it must also mature. Maturation involves reorientation of major structural elements along the lines of stress that the structure will normally undergo. The process of maturation takes time, and the necessary stimulus is the judiciously applied loading of the part in ways that simulate the loads the part will need to withstand with normal use.

INCREASED RATE OF TISSUE PRODUCTION

The rate of tissue production increases in conjunction with any inflammatory process. The reparative phase that follows acute inflammation usually involves a proliferation of collagen tissue. This is especially true in certain virulent inflammatory processes associated with bacterial infections. Chronic, low-grade inflammation, such as that mentioned previously in conjunction with increased stress levels, is also accompanied by increased collagen production. Regardless of the cause, the result is a relatively fibrosed, less extensible structure. Loss of extensibility will be especially marked if the part is immobilized during the period of increased collagen production. The new collagen will not be laid down along the appropriate lines of stress, and abnormal interfiber cross-links develop that do not accommodate normal deformation. If, on the other hand, some movement of the part occurs during the period of increased collagen production, the loss of extensibility will not be so great. Appropriate orientation of the newly laid fibers is stimulated by the stresses imposed on the tissue by movement. Loss of extensibility in the immobilized part is due to the increased density of the structure, as well as abnormal orientation of the structured elements, whereas in the part in which some movement occurs, reduced extensibility is primarily a result of the change in density.

Clinically, then, a part that is strictly immobilized during an acute inflammatory process, such as that induced by surgery, trauma, infection, or rheumatoid arthritis, is likely to lose more movement, and the loss of movement is likely to be more persistent than in the case of a part in which some movement continues in the presence of a chronic, low-grade inflammation, such as degenerative joint disease.

Restoration of normal extensibility of the tissue requires (1) removing the stimulus of increased tissue production (*e.g.*, stress, infection, trauma); (2) gradually stretching the structure to break down abnormal interfiber cross-links; and (3) restoring normal use of the part to induce normal orientation of structural elements.

REDUCED RATE OF TISSUE PRODUCTION AND REPAIR

Reduced rate of tissue production and repair occurs with reduced stress levels to the tissue, but it may also occur with some change in the metabolic status of the tissue. Examples of the latter include nutritional deficiencies, reduced vascularity, and abnormal hormone levels. When the cause is related to reduced stress levels, amelioration simply involves a gradual return to normal stress conditions. However, when the cause is metabolic, treatment is more complex and will vary with the type of disturbance. In these cases, stress levels must be reduced, since the body is unable to keep up with the normal rate of tissue breakdown. Continued use of the part will result in fatigue failure of the involved tissues.

Typical examples of common musculoskeletal disorders that are related to such an alteration in the metabolic status of the involved tissues include the following:

Supraspinatus tendinitis at the shoulder—The tendon begins to fatigue from reduced vascularity in an area of the tendon close to its insertion. Occasionally the body attempts to compensate for its inability to produce new tendon tissue by laying down calculus deposits. These lesions often progress to complete tendon ruptures because the rate of breakdown continues to exceed the capacity of the tissue to repair itself.

Reflex sympathetic dystrophy—Generalized hypovascularity to a part, caused by increased sympathetic activity, results in atrophy of bone, nails, muscle, and skin—in short, all musculoskeletal components.

Senile and postmenopausal osteoporosis—Bone metabolism is compromised as a result of alteration in hormone levels and other age-related influences. The bone atrophy is most marked in cancellous bone, such as that of the vertebral bodies. Roentgenograms often show collapsed vertebrae, resulting from progressive trabecular buckling.

Age-related tissue changes—Aging, in itself, does not seem to result in changes in the collagen content of musculoskeletal tissues. However, with advancing age, the protein–polysaccharide (glycosaminoglycan) content of most somatic tissues is reduced. There is also an associated reduction in water content, since the protein–polysaccharide component of the tissue matrices is responsible for the fluid binding capacity of the tissues. The result is a relative fibrosis of the involved tissues, since the ratio of collagen to ground substance is increased. It is postulated that the protein–polysaccharide ground substance normally acts as a lubricating spacer between collagen fibers. As its content is reduced, the collagen fibers approximate one another and form increased numbers of inter-fiber cross-links (intermolecular bonds), and the fibers no longer glide easily with respect to each other. Thus, the stiffness of the structure increases. Because of the increased stiffness, the tissue as a whole looses its deformability and therefore looses its ability to attenuate the energy of loading. With loading more stress is imposed on individual structural elements, and the rate of tissue breakdown subsequently increases. For many elderly persons this does not pose a problem since activity levels, and therefore stress levels, decrease with advancing age.

The reduced fluid-binding capacity of the tissue, associated with protein–polysaccharide depletion, may alter the nutritional status of the tissue. This is especially important in structures, such as articular cartilage and intervertebral disks, that depend on fluid inhibition for normal exchange of nutrients. Thus, the capacity of the tissue to repair itself will also be reduced. This is a likely explanation for the degeneration of intervertebral disks and articular cartilage that occurs with advancing age.

INTERVENTION AND COMMUNICATION

From a clinical standpoint, the clinician should be prepared to estimate the nature of a pathologic process according to this scheme. This is necessary in order to plan a treatment program specific for the type of pathologic process present. Awareness of the various ways the clinician can effectively intervene so as to appropriately alter the pathologic state is also important.

The terms used to refer to common musculoskeletal pathologies usually provide little information relating to the nature of the disorder. The same term may be applied to different conditions in which the cause and nature of the pathologic process are quite distinct. *Tendinitis* at the shoulder is an atrophic, degenerative condition resulting from reduced vascularity to an area of the rotator cuff tendons; *tendinitis* at the elbow is a hypertrophic, fibrotic condition often related to increased stress levels. Also, many

terms, such as *degenerative joint disease*, refer to situations in which a number of tissues may be involved, and the nature of the changes affecting the involved tissues may differ. In the case of degenerative joint disease, for example, the subchondral bone and the joint capsule tend to hypertrophy while the articular cartilage atrophies and degenerates.

Therapeutically, there are many physical agents and procedures that may be used in order to influence various types of pathologic processes. Perhaps the most important form of intervention is well-planned instructions to the patient regarding the performance of specific activities. In order to give appropriate instructions the clinician must gear the patient's activity level to the nature of the disorder. This requires a knowledge of the response of tissues to various loading conditions under normal and abnormal circumstances. A careful examination must be carried out, including a biomechanical assessment. It also requires that the clinician be aware of the types of stresses imposed on a part by various activities. The patient must understand the instructions and be able and willing to carry them out.

ARTHROSIS

When considering a diseased joint one usually thinks in terms of the physiological changes that have occurred at the joint. There is much information concerning the histologic and biochemical changes in periarticular tissues, changes in hemodynamics, and synovial fluid changes that accompany some of the more common joint diseases.[3,7,29–31,33,35] Although mechanical changes also occur, these are usually not dealt with until advanced structural changes have resulted. The treatment then is usually surgical. The earlier, conservative treatment in joint disease typically involves measures to counter the physiological changes taking place. This seems the logical approach in arthropathies in which the etiology is apparently some physiological change and in which the primary joint changes are physiological. Thus, in rheumatoid arthritis, gout, and spondylitis, the primary treatments are those aimed at control of inflammation and metabolic disturbances. The mechanical changes in joint function are generally agreed to be secondary and often left to improve (or degenerate) along with the primary physiological changes.

Although our knowledge of normal joint mechanics is becoming more sophisticated, little has been written concerning the mechanical changes that occur with, or possibly lead to, joint disease. It is well accepted, however, that joint disease may result from some mechanical disturbance. These cases are usually referred to as *secondary osteoarthritis*, in which some past joint trauma can be cited as a precipitating factor. This is distinguished by many researchers from *primary osteoarthritis*, in which several joints may be involved with no known causative factor. However, the pathologies of primary and secondary osteoarthritis are essentially identical, and since these disorders are for the most part noninflammatory, they are best referred to as *osteoarthroses*. As the probable etiologies of osteoarthroses are investigated, the more it appears that the classifications of primary and secondary are often arbitrary. Although it has been postulated by some that primary osteoarthrosis has a physiological or metabolic etiology, it appears that in many cases it is due to mechanical changes, the onset of which are much more subtle than those causing secondary osteoarthrosis.[18,19,46]

It is generally agreed that changes in the articular cartilage trigger a cycle leading to the progression of degenerative joint disease. Cartilage damage may occur following a single traumatic incident causing a tension or compression strain sufficient to interfere with the structural integrity of the cartilage. This is relatively rare and usually accompanies a fracture of the adjacent bone. More common is cartilage wearing from fatigue, or the cumulative effects of abnormal stresses, neither of which is sufficient in itself to cause structural damage.[52] Cartilage may be susceptible to fatigue in part because it is aneural; any other musculoskeletal tissue is relatively immune to fatigue because protective reflex inhibition occurs with abnormal stress. This inhibitory response requires, of course, intact innervation. Cartilage is also susceptible to damage because it is avascular. It lacks the normal inflammation and repair response that would replace damaged parts of the tissue. In fact, when cartilage is lacerated without involvement of the vascularized subchondral bone, there is a brief proliferation of chondrocytes but no repair of the defect ensues. If the lesion is sufficient to penetrate the subchondral bone, it immediately fills with blood and a clot is formed. This clot is invaded with new blood vessels that apparently bring in undifferentiated mesenchymal cells. These cells proceed to fill the defect with fibrocartilage (not hyaline cartilage).[10,23]

Hyaline cartilage in part makes up for the fact that it is aneural and avascular by its considerable ability to deform when loaded in compression. Much of the substance of articular cartilage is a mucopolysaccharide ground substance, a chief component of which is chondroitin sulfate. Chondroitin sulfate is highly hydrophilic with the ability to bind large quantities of water. Cartilage is 70% to 80% water and depends on this water content for its resiliency—its ability to withstand compression stresses without structural damage. The energy of compressive loading is dissipated as cartilage undergoes strain, or deformation. This strain results in tension stresses that are absorbed by the collagen fibers embedded within the ground substance (Fig. 2–16). Thus, the extracellular cartilage matrix normally withstands compression stresses, through the mucopolysaccharide gel, and tension stresses, through the collagen fibers. Interspersed throughout this matrix are the chondrocytes, or cartilage cells, that are responsible for production of the matrix components. It must be added that a considerable proportion of compressive forces is attenuated by the cancellous subchondral bone that, although stiffer than the articular cartilage, is thicker and has more volume for energy attenuation.[43]

Although cartilage was once believed to be inert metabolically, studies now indicate that turnover of cartilage does occur.[31] Chondrocytes apparently secrete some matrix material continuously to replace that lost by normal attrition. It has also been shown that in response to mild or moderate osteoarthrosis in which cartilage degradation has increased, proliferation and metabolic activity of chondrocytes also increase. At least for a while the chondrocytes are able to keep pace with the disease. For some reason as yet unknown, this process shuts down in later stages of the disease. It is also poorly understood why lacerations of cartilage do not undergo repair, whereas some repair does take place in the earlier stages of osteoarthrosis.

The Degenerative Cycle

The initial changes that occur in the cartilage when abnormal stresses leading to acute damage or chronic fatigue are applied are (1) fibrillation, or fracturing of collagen fibers, and (2) depletion of ground substance, primarily a loss of chondroitin sulfate.[7,29,33,35–37,52] There remains some dispute over which change takes place first; however, it seems to be agreed that once initiated, a vicious cycle of degeneration will follow. This cycle is countered up to a point by the proliferation of chondrocytes and the increased secretion of cartilage matrix by the chondrocytes. A cycle, such as shown in Figure 2–17 is likely to develop. Loss of chondroitin sulfate leaves the collagen fibers more susceptible to fracture; fracturing of these fibers causes a "softening" of the

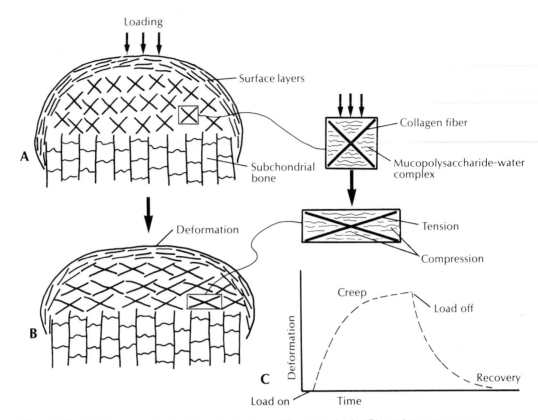

Fig. 2-16. *(A)* Compressive loading of articular cartilage results in *(B)* tension stresses to the collagenous elements and compression stresses to the mucopolysaccharide–water complex. *(C)* The total response is viscoelastic. The viscous creep with sustained loading is largely the result of a time-dependent squeezing out of fluid.

surface layers of the cartilage; the cartilage becomes less able to withstand stresses in this region, with the resultant death of local chondrocytes; the death of chondrocytes is believed to allow the release of proteolytic enzymes that have a further degradatory effect on chondroitin sulfate. The adjacent areas of cartilage, peripheral and deep to this damaged area, must now absorb increased stresses, so the process of cartilage degeneration tends to spread. Added to this mechanical factor in spreading is the chemical factor due to destructive enzyme release.[44]

Because of the absence of pain receptors in articular cartilage, considerable degeneration may take place before symptoms bring the problem to the attention of the patient. Pain or stiffness may not occur until synovial effusion causes sufficient pressure to

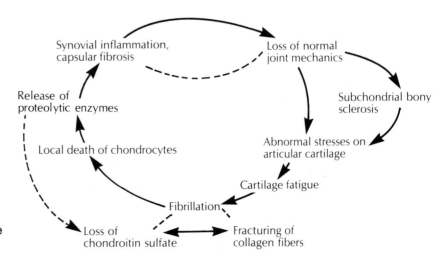

Fig. 2-17. Cycle of degenerative changes in a joint.

the joint capsule to fire pain- or pressure-sensitive receptors. The effusion is a result of synovial irritation caused by the release of proteolytic enzymes and other cartilaginous debris. Further irritation may result from abnormal stresses to the joint capsule from altered joint mechanics. In the case of low-grade, chronic inflammation of the synovial lining, the patient may be aware of only transient symptoms. Such a low-grade inflammation, if chronic, will result in capsular fibrosis, or thickening, which will further alter joint mechanics. Fibrosis of the joint capsule may be thought of as a relative increase in the collagen–mucopolysaccharide ratio. The result is that which occurs with any scarring process—reduced extensibility from loss of elasticity, gradual contracture, and adherence to adjacent tissues. The loss of capsular mobility often goes unnoticed by the patient until it causes sufficient limitation of motion to interfere with daily activities. In joints such as the shoulder, which in the inactive person may be used only through a small range of motion to perform daily activities, a rather marked limitation of movement may occur before the patient realizes that a problem exists. Such a lack of mobility of the joint capsule will, of course, contribute significantly to the cycle of degeneration shown in Figure 2–17 because of the resultant alteration of normal joint mechanics. Other reactive joint tissue changes will also occur if the process is allowed to continue, including osteophyte formation, subchondral sclerosis, subchondral cyst formation, and eburnation of exposed bone. It should be realized that subchondral bone changes are likely to lead to an alteration in the forces that must be absorbed by the articular cartilage since normally subchondral bone takes up much of the force of compressive loading.[54] In fact, some researchers believe that subchondral bone changes, such as sclerotic changes due to altered blood flow, are often the first changes to take place in the degenerative cycle.[7]

Changes in composition and structure of the articular surface, caused by fibrillation and chondroitin sulfate depletion, are also likely to compromise the lubrication system of the joint. Large irregularities would gradually make boundary lubrication less effective; loss of cartilage resiliency from chondroitin sulfate loss would interfere with weeping lubrication. These potential changes in lubrication efficiency would also seem to contribute further to the progression of degeneration.

CAPSULAR TIGHTNESS

As indicated in the section on clinical application, specific joint mobilization techniques are primarily used in cases of capsuloligamentous tightness or adherence. There are, of course, cases in which an isolated portion of a joint capsule or supporting ligament is injured and heals in a state of relative shortening or becomes adhered to adjacent tissues during the healing process. Such pathologies are usually of traumatic origin, with a well-defined mechanism of injury and subsequent course. More often, however, the therapist is confronted with cases in which the entire joint capsule is "tight," as suggested by the presence of a capsular pattern of restriction at the joint. Conditions that cause a capsular pattern of restriction at a joint can be classified into two general categories: (1) conditions in which there is considerable joint effusion or synovial inflammation, and (2) conditions in which there is a relative capsular fibrosis. It is important to make this distinction since the implications for management will vary according to the cause of the restriction.

Joint Effusion

Joint effusion causes a capsular pattern of restriction because of the distention of the joint capsule by the excessive intra-articular synovial fluid. Portions of the capsule that are normally lax in order to allow a certain range of movement become taut because of capsular distention. The joint tends to assume a position in which the joint cavity—the space enclosed by the joint capsule—is of maximum volume. The continuous pressure applied to the capsule by the joint fluid may effect abnormal firing of joint receptors, which results in an alteration in function of the muscles controlling the joint.[54] The rapid wasting of the quadriceps in the presence of knee joint effusion is believed to be a result of reflex muscle inhibition from abnormal receptor firing.[9] There may also be reflex facilitation of muscle activity, observed as muscle spasm or guarding, when the joint is moved. Those conditions that cause limited movement because of articular effusion may be broadly classified as inflammatory arthritis. These may, of course, include traumatic arthritis, in which some portion of the joint capsule is torn or stretched, rheumatoid arthritis, in which the synovial layer of the capsule is inflamed, infectious arthritis, gout, and others. In the acute stage of each of these conditions, the capsular restriction is primarily a result of the increased secretion of synovial fluid accompanying the acute stage of the inflammatory process or one result of reflex muscle guarding from abnormal firing of joint receptors. The cause of the restriction must be appreciated since, in such cases, clinicians do not wish to stretch the joint capsule to restore movement but rather to assist in the resolution of the acute inflammatory process.

Relative Capsular Fibrosis

Relative capsular fibrosis most commonly accompanies one, or some combination, of the three following situations: (1) resolution of an acute articular inflammatory process; (2) a chronic, low-grade articular inflammatory process; and (3) immobilization of a joint.[2,12,13] The term *relative capsular fibrosis* has been used, up to this point, since histologically the capsular changes do not necessarily involve an increase in collagen content. It seems, instead, that inextensibility of capsular tissue may come about from either an increase in collagen content with respect to mucopolysaccharide content or by internal changes in the nature of the collagen tissue, such as changes in intermolecular cross-linking. The former might arise from an increased laying down of collagen, such as takes place during the repair phase of any inflammatory process.[1,8] It might also occur from a net loss of mucopolysaccharide content, with the total collagen content remaining constant. This typically occurs with prolonged immobilization of a joint.[12,41,53] One might consider the mucopolysaccharide content of connective tissue as serving as a lubricant for the collagen fibers; loss of the lubricant permits collagen fibers to approximate each other and to form abnormal interfiber cross-links. This inhibits their ability to glide against each other and thus reduces extensibility of the tissue.[1]

Clinically, it seems that conditions in which there is an actual increase in collagen content are more resistant to efforts to restore motion than are those cases of capsular restriction in which there is a net loss of mucopolysaccharide caused simply by immobilization. Also, inflammatory arthritis from infection resolves with a much greater degree of fibrosis (increase in collagen) than the capsular fibrosis that accompanies low-grade, noninfectious joint inflammation such as degenerative joint disease. Thus, the rate of improvement in range of motion might be expected to be more rapid in conditions at the top of the following list and slower when dealing with the capsular fibrosis, which follows conditions near the bottom of this list:

Simple immobilization
Traumatic arthritis
Degenerative arthrosis
Rheumatoid arthritis
Infectious arthritis

Several explanations might be offered to account for the differences in rates of improvement noted above. First, relatively destructive processes, such as infectious arthritis or rheumatoid arthritis, might be met with a more vigorous repair response and, therefore, more collagen production during the resolution of the acute inflammatory process. Second, the period of immobilization, either prescribed or due to pain, is usually greater in acute inflammatory conditions, such as infectious or rheumatoid arthritis, than in relatively chronic conditions such as degenerative joint disease. The tendency, then, is for them to heal with less mobility. Third, during the mobilization period, the tissues may adapt more readily to increased mobility by laying down more mucopolysaccharide ground substance than they could by remodeling collagen. The maturation of the highly collagenous "scar tissue" is a longer, more involved process, involving reabsorption of excess collagen, realignment of collagen fiber orientation, and changes in the intermolecular cross-links within the collagen tissue.[1] In this way, capsular restriction from immobilization only, in which there is no increase in collagen content, is more easily resolved than conditions that lead to an actual increase in the collagen content of the joint capsules. It should be clear from this discussion that in order to accurately set treatment goals, the therapist should understand the nature of the pathologic process and its implications.

CLINICAL CONSIDERATIONS

Considering what is now known of the pathogenesis of osteoarthrosis, the accompanying biochemical responses, the pathologic tissue changes, and the clinical manifestations, some important conclusions and correlations are worth considering in the management of patients with arthrosis.

Subtle changes in joint kinematics, persisting over a period of time, may cause abnormal stresses sufficient to result in gradual cartilage fatigue, which may, in turn, trigger a progression of changes leading to osteoarthrosis. Perhaps the most convincing evidence of this process is found in studies by Frankel and co-workers that show changes in the normal instant centers of motion in knee joints with minimal clinical signs or symptoms.[14,15] These changes suggested premature compression of joint surfaces accompanying knee extension. On careful clinical testing, loss of longitudinal external rotation of the tibia, with respect to the normal side, was found during extension on the involved side. Subsequent surgery revealed obvious "dimpling" of the cartilaginous joint surface, in the area of the cartilage compressed at full knee extension. In these cases internal derangement of the knee, while not sufficient to cause significant symptoms or signs, was responsible for altering normal knee mechanics enough to cause early cartilaginous changes, observable with the naked eye.

Up to a point in the progression of the disease, the cartilaginous destruction is repaired by increased proliferation and metabolic activity of chondrocytes, with laying down of new cartilage. The suggestion here is that osteoarthrosis is indeed somewhat reversible if managed correctly before severe progression has taken place. It is well known that osteotomy in the case of hip osteoarthrosis will cause the femoral head to become covered with fibrocartilage, with resultant restoration of the joint space on roentgenography. Studies suggest that it is partly a biologic phenomenon, perhaps from the hyperemia induced by the surgical procedure, as well as a mechanical phenomenon from the redistribution of stresses over the joint.[6]

If it is accepted that subtle changes in joint kinematics can lead to osteoarthrosis or, taken one step further, if this is the etiology in many of the cases that are considered primary or secondary osteoarthrosis, then evaluation techniques that can detect these changes are valuable. Instant center analysis is probably the best technique for detection of altered joint kinematics. However, because of the extra number of roentgenograms necessary, this technique is not practical for routine evaluation. In view of this, it seems that testing of joint-play movements is the most valuable technique, clinically, for detecting subtle joint changes that may be causing only minor signs or symptoms but may eventually lead to more serious joint changes in the form of osteoarthrosis. Joint-play techniques are important not only in evaluation of the patient presenting with obscure musculoskeletal complaints but also in evaluating the patient recovering from more serious trauma. Simply because a patient has regained full range of motion and strength does not guarantee that normal joint kinematics have been restored.

If osteoarthrosis may be caused by loss of normal joint mechanics, then primary treatments should be aimed at restoration of normal mechanics. This may entail surgery in cases such as meniscal tears and malalignment of bony structures. In cases of capsular tightness or capsular adhesion, treatment must consist of specific mobilization aimed at restoration of normal accessory movements at the joint. The approach to treatment of joint problems that appear to be mechanical should have a biomechanical basis. At the present time, treatment is too often "supportive" until obvious physiological changes occur. Currently, treatment tends to be directed at those physiological changes, including various modalities for pain relief and pharmaceutical agents for controlling inflammation. Efforts to restore joint mechanics too often consist only of range of motion exercises

and muscle strengthening, carried out without regard for the possible deleterious effects to the joint and without regard for abnormal reflex activity accompanying joint movement in the absence of normal arthrokinematics.

I believe that we, as clinicians, have yet to realize our full potential in the management of patients with mechanical joint disturbances. Knowledge of normal kinematics, ability to detect changes in joint mechanics through joint-play movements, and ability to restore normal component movements to a joint are necessary in successful management of patients with joint problems that are of a mechanical etiology or in which mechanical dysfunction is a prime factor.

REFERENCES

1. Akeson WH: An experimental study of joint stiffness. J Bone Joint Surg 43(A):1022–1034, 1961
2. Akeson WH, Amiel D, LaViolette D: The connective tissue response to immobility. Clin Orthop 51:183–197, 1967
3. Akeson WH, Woo SL, Amiel D: Biomechanical and biochemical changes in periarticular connective tissues during contracture development in the immobilized rabbit knee. Connect Tissue Res 2:315–323, 1974
4. Barnett CH, Cochrane W, Palfray AJ: Age changes in articular cartilage of rabbits. Ann Rheum Dis 22:389–400, 1963
5. Barnett CH, Davies DV, MacConnaill MA: Synovial Joints, Their Structure and Function. Springfield, IL, Charles C Thomas, 1961
6. Bentley G: Articular cartilage studies and osteoarthrosis. Ann R Coll Surg Engl 57:86–100, 1975
7. Bollet AJ: Connective tissue polysaccharide metabolism and the pathogenesis of osteoarthritis. Adv Intern Med 13:33–60, 1967
8. Clayton ML, James SM, Abdulla M: Experimental investigations of ligamentous healing. Clin Orthop 61:146, 1968
9. de Andrade JR, Grant C, Dixon A: Joint distention and reflex muscle inhibition in the knee. J Bone Joint Surg 47(A):313–322, 1965
10. de Palma A, McKeever LD, Subin DK: Process of repair of articular cartilage demonstrated by histology and autoradiography with tritiated thymidine. Clin Orthop 48:229–242, 1966
11. Dowson D: Modes of lubrication in human joints. In Lubrication and Wear in Living and Artificial Joints, Vol 181. London, Institute of Mechanical Engineers, 1967
12. Ely LW, Mensor MC: Studies on the immobilization of the normal joints. Surg Gynecol Obstet 57:212–215, 1963
13. Evans EB, Eggers GW, Butler JK, Blumel J: Experi-

mental immobilization and remobilization of rat knee joints. J Bone Joint Surg [Am] 42:737–758, 1960

14. Frankel VH: Biomechanics of the knee. In Ingwersen O (ed): The Knee Joint. New York, Elsevier-Dutton, 1973

15. Frankel VH, Burstein AH, Brooks DB: Biomechanics of internal derangement of the knee: Pathomechanics as determined by analysis of the instant centers of motion. J Bone Joint Surg [Am] 53:945–962, 1971

16. Frankel VH, Nordin M: Basic Biomechanics of the Skeletal System. Philadelphia, Lea & Febiger, 1980

17. Freeman MAR (ed): Adult Articular Cartilage. London, Pitman and Sons, 1973

18. Freeman MAR: The fatigue of cartilage in the pathogenesis of osteoarthrosis. Acta Orthop Scand 46:323, 1975

19. Freeman MAR: The pathogenesis of primary osteoarthrosis. Mod Trends Orthop 6:40–90, 1972

20. Freeman MAR: Treatment of ruptures of the lateral ligament of the ankle. J Bone Joint Surg 47(B):661–668, 1965

21. Frymann VM: A study of the rhythmic motions of the living cranium. J Am Osteopath Assoc 70:928–945, 1971

22. Goodfellow J, Hungerford DS, Woods C: Patellofemoral joint mechanics and pathology, I and II. J Bone Joint Surg [Br] 58:287, 1976

23. Johnell O, Telhag H: The effect of osteotomy and cartilage damage and mitotic activity: An experimental study in rabbits. Acta Orthop Scand 48:263–265, 1977

24. Kellgren JH: On the distribution of pain arising from deep somatic structures, with charts of segmental pain areas. Clin Sci 4:35, 1939

25. Klineberg IJ, Greenfield BE, Wyke B: Contribution to the reflex control of mastication from mechanoreceptors in the temperomandibular joint capsule. Dent Pract 21:73, 1970

26. Knott M, Voss D: Proprioceptive Neuromuscular Facilitation: Patterns and Techniques. New York, Harper & Row, 1968

27. MacConnaill MA: The function of intra-articular fibrocartilage with special references to the knee and inferior radioulnar joints. J Anat 66:210–227, 1932

28. MacConnaill MA, Basjaian JV: Muscles and Movements: A Basis for Human Kinesiology. Baltimore, Williams & Wilkins, 1969

29. Mankin HJ: Biochemical and metabolic aspects of osteoarthritis. Orthop Clin North Am 2:19–31, 1971

30. Mankin HJ: The reaction of articular cartilage to injury and osteoarthrosis: I. N Engl J Med 291:1284, 1974

31. Mankin HJ: The reaction of articular cartilage to injury and osteoarthrosis: II. N Engl J Med 291:1335, 1974

32. Mankin HJ, Thrasher AZ, Hall D: Characteristics of articular cartilage from osteonecrotic femoral heads. J Bone Joint Surg 59(A):724–728, 1977

33. Mankin HJ, Dorfman H, Lipiello L et al: Biochemical and metabolic abnormalities in articular cartilage from osteoarthritic human hips. J Bone Joint Surg 53(A):523–537, 1971

34. McCutcheon CW: Lubrication of joints. Br Med J 1:384–385, 1964

35. Meachim G: Articular cartilage lesions in osteoarthritis of the femoral head. J Pathol 107:199–210, 1972

36. Meachim G, Emergy IA: Cartilage fibrillation in shoulder and hip joints in Liverpool necropsies. J Anat 116:161–197, 1973

37. Meachim G, Emergy IH: Quantitative aspects of patellofemoral fibrillation in Liverpool necropsies. Ann Rheum Dis 33:39–47, 1974

38. Mennell J: Joint Pain. Boston, Little, Brown & Co, 1964

39. Neviaser JS: Adhesive capsulitis of the shoulder: A study of pathological findings in periarthritis of the shoulder. J Bone Joint Surg 27(A):211–222, 1945

40. Paris SV: Cranial manipulation. Fysioterapeuten 39:310, 1972

41. Peacock EE: Comparison of collaginous tissue surrounding normal and immobilized joints. Surg Forum 14:440, 1963

42. Radin EL, Paul IL: A consolidated concept of joint lubrication. J Bone Joint Surg 54(A):607–616, 1972

43. Radin EL, Paul IL: Does cartilage compliance reduce skeletal impact loads? Arthritis Rheum 13:138, 1970

44. Roach JE, Tomblin W, Eyring EJ: Comparison of the effects of aspirin, steroids and sodium salicylate on articular cartilage. Clin Orthop 106:350–356, 1975

45. Sammarco GJ, Burstein AH, Frankel VH: Biomechanics of the ankle: A kinematic study. Orthop Clin North Am 4:75–95, 1973

46. Seileg AJ, Gerath M: An *in vivo* investigation of wear in animal joints. J Biomech 8:169–172, 1975

47. Sherrington C: The Integrative Action of the Nervous System. New Haven, CT, Yale University Press, 1906

48. Skogland S: Anatomical and physiological studies of knee joint innervation in the cat. Acta Physiol Scand (Suppl) 124:1–100, 1956

49. Swanson SA: Lubrication of synovial joints. J Physiol 223:22, 1972

50. Voss D, Ionta MK, Myers BJ: Proprioceptive Neuromuscular Facilitation, 3rd ed. Philadelphia, Harper & Row, 1985

51. Warwick R, Williams P (eds): Gray's Anatomy, 35th ed. Philadelphia, WB Saunders, 1973

52. Weightman BO, Freeman MAR, Swanson SAV: Fatigue of articular cartilage. Nature 244:303–304, 1973

53. Woo SL, Mathews JV, Akeson WH et al: Connective tissue response to immobility. Arthritis Rheum 18:257–264, 1975

54. Wright V (ed): Lubrication and Wear in Joints. Philadelphia, JB Lippincott, 1969

55. Wyke B: The neurology of joints. Ann R Coll Surg Engl 41:25–50, 1967

3 Pain

Maureen K. Lynch and Randolph M. Kessler

It is not a fixed response to a noxious stimulus, its perception is modified by past experiences, expectations and even by culture. It has a protective function, warning us that something biologically harmful is happening, but anyone who has suffered prolonged severe pain would regard it as an evil, a punishing affliction that is harmful in its own right.

—Ronald Melzack

There are many reasons why the clinician should understand mechanisms of pain perception. Patients are often seen whose primary complaint is pain, which often leads to a loss of function. Usually, a careful assessment of pain behavior is invaluable in determining the nature and extent of the underlying pathologic process. Development of an appropriate treatment program and evaluation of progress may depend largely on pain assessment. Therefore, it is important for the clinician who sees patients with pain complaints to have a basic understanding of the neurophysiology of pain, including mechanisms of pain perception and the phenomena of referred and projected pain. The clinician should understand how specific treatment modalities influence the nature of pain and how knowledge of pain mechanisms can be applied to its management.

PAIN OF DEEP SOMATIC ORIGIN

When examining a patient with pain of musculoskeletal origin, the clinician often finds that the site that the patient indicates as the most painful does not correspond well with the site of the lesion. The patient often gives a history of proximal or distal radiation of pain and may describe it as moving from one place to another. In addition, cutaneous hyperalgesia or hypalgesia and tenderness to palpation at sites distant from — or at least not directly over — the site of the pathologic process are often evident. For example, patients with shoulder problems often describe pain over the lateral brachial region, radiating to the elbow or hand. This type of radiation eliminates muscle spasm as a possible cause of pain since no muscle traverses the extent of this distribution. Similarly, the patient with a low-back problem often describes more pain in the buttock than in the lumbar region. In the past, a discrepancy between the site of the pathologic process and the site where pain is perceived was often attributed to muscle spasm or sciatic nerve inflammation. These possibilities are unlikely, however, since the pain is often described as traveling distally down the leg and spiraling around the thigh to the front of the lower leg, a distribution that does not correspond to any nerve or muscle. Pain patterns that are associated with deep somatic lesions relate to the embryological development of the musculoskeletal system (see Chapter 1, Embryology of the Musculoskeletal System). Kellgren and other researchers have clarified and supported this association by mapping areas of pain reference from stimulation of deep somatic structures, by determining the relative sensitivities of the various structures, and by describing the general qualities of pain of somatic origin.[27,30]

EXPERIMENTAL DATA

In their series of studies, Kellgren and co-workers injected saline into various joint tissues, including the fibrous capsule, ligaments, tendons, muscle, fascia, menisci, synovia, and articular cartilage.[30,31] They also stimulated the periosteum with a Kirschner wire. These studies revealed several significant findings on the nature of musculoskeletal pain that, unfortunately, are still widely ignored clinically.

> The structures most sensitive to noxious stimulation are the periosteum and joint capsule. Subchondral bone, tendons, and ligaments are moderately pain sensitive, while muscle and cortical bone are somewhat less sensitive. Synovium, articular cartilage, and fibrocartilage are essentially insensitive to nociceptive stimulation.

Thus, cartilaginous erosion accompanying degenerative joint disease, synovitis, meniscal tears, and disk protrusions are not painful. Secondary or concomitant involvement of other tissues must occur in order for the patient to be aware of the problem. These, then, are pathologic conditions that can be "silent" for a period, leading to insidious, and often significant, progression before being seen by the clinician.

Tendon and ligament injuries are likely to be most painful when their junction with the periosteum is affected. Too often, muscle is implicated as the source of pain in patients with somatic pain complaints.

> Pain of musculoskeletal origin is usually delocalized; the site at which pain is perceived rarely corresponds exactly with the site of stimulation. Generally, the closer the tissue is to the body surface, the better the site of pain corresponds to the site of stimulation.

This finding deviates markedly from the way we are accustomed to thinking of pain, or sensation in general. Most common sensations affect the skin and are well localized to the site of stimulation. This, however, is not true of subcutaneous sensations, whether somatic or visceral. Thus, for example, pain from lesions about the glenohumeral joint is felt in the lateral brachial region, pain from cervical joints is felt in the scapular area, and pain from the hip joint is felt anywhere from the groin to the knee. These are common cases of deeply situated pathologic processes that cause delocalized sensations. On the other hand, pain from ligament sprains at the knee, ankle, or wrist, all of which are relatively superficial lesions, is well localized to the site of involvement.

Although documented years ago, this characteristic of pain of deep-tissue origin still goes widely unrecognized by clinicians. Patients continue to re-

ceive injections, ultrasound, or massage about the scapulae for disorders arising from the neck; the sacroiliac joint or sciatic nerve is often blamed for pain originating in the lumbar spine; and on occasion, an adolescent presenting with slipped capital femoral epiphysis may receive treatment for "knee pain."

> With increased stimulation, pain of deep somatic origin may radiate into a characteristic distribution. The pattern of distribution is always the same for a particular site of stimulation, and tends to follow a segmental, or sclerotomic, pathway. The extent of radiation is dependent upon the intensity of stimulation, and pain tends to radiate distally rather than proximally.

Recall that a sclerotome is defined as those deep somatic tissues that are innervated by the same segmental spinal nerve. These areas have been mapped by Inman and Saunders and are shown in Figure 3-1. Note that they do not correspond exactly to dermatomes (Figs. 3-2 and 3-3). When a tissue of a particular sclerotome is irritated, the patient may perceive the resulting pain as arising from any or all of the tissues innervated by the same segmental nerve. This is a result of the lack of precision in central neural connections and is not related to abnormal impulses "spreading down a nerve;" in other words, the "problem" is central, not peripheral, and there is nothing wrong with most of the area from which pain seems to arise. Furthermore, it is crucial to realize that *radiating pain does not necessarily imply nerve irritation.*

Thus, patients with supraspinatus tendinitis often have pain referred down the lateral aspect of the arm and forearm to the wrist; disk protrusions may cause pain to radiate into a limb without nerve-root pressure; and trochanteric bursitis is often mistaken for L5 nerve-root irritation or is diagnosed as fascitis of the iliotibial band. Again, the clinical implications of referred pain cannot be overemphasized and must be appreciated by the clinician seeing patients with musculoskeletal disorders.

> Pain of deep somatic origin is of a deep, aching, generalized quality as opposed to the sharp, well-localized pain that may arise from stimulation of the skin. In addition, deep somatic pain is often associated with autonomic phenomena such as increased sweating, pallor, and reduced blood pressure, and is commonly accompanied by a subjective feeling of nausea and faintness.

Fig. 3–1. Sclerotomes.

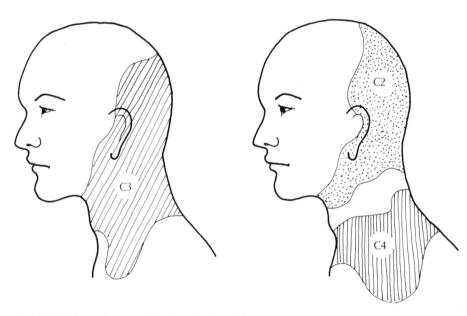

Fig. 3–2. Dermatomes of the head and neck.

The terms *sclerotomic* and *dermatomic* are often used to distinguish between pain arising from deep somatic tissues and from the skin. Sclerotomic pain is typically deep, aching, and poorly localized, whereas dermatomic pain is sharp, sometimes shooting, and well localized. In most clinical settings, pain arising from the surface of the skin is not commonly encountered and therefore is insignificant. However, a very important source of both dermatomic and sclerotomic pain is direct irritation of nerve pathways projecting afferent input from a particular area. This is properly referred to as *projected* pain, rather than *referred* pain, and the most common site of irritation is the nerve root. Thus, an intervertebral disk protrusion or bony osteophyte may directly excite nerve fibers subserving sensory or motor functions, producing symptoms or signs confined to the relevant dermatome, myotome, or sclerotome. The symptoms or signs will vary, depending on the fibers affected.

The largest myelinated nerve fibers are most sensitive to pressure, whereas small-diameter, unmyelinated fibers are least sensitive. It is generally agreed that eventual dissociation of the quality of sensation is, in part, related to fiber size, and that sensations may be arranged in order of decreasing fiber size, as follows:

Vibration sense, proprioception—Large, myelinated (A-alpha) fiber
"Fast" (dermatomic) pain, temperature—Small, myelinated (A-delta) fiber
"Slow" (sclerotomic) pain—Unmyelinated (C) fiber

Touch and pressure travel over fibers spanning the entire range of diameters. Consistent with the above scheme is the clinical observation that patients presenting with nerve root irritation may complain of paresthesia (A-alpha stimulation); pain of a sharp, well-localized, dermatomic quality (A-delta irritation); or deep, aching, sclerotomic pain (C-fiber involvement). In any case, the sensation is perceived as arising from any or all of the tissues innervated by the involved nerve.

It should be mentioned that projected pain rarely occurs clinically from nerve irritation at sites other than the nerve root. Pressure on nerves farther out in the periphery, as in the case of carpal tunnel syndrome, thoracic outlet syndrome, or ulnar nerve palsy, are subjectively manifested primarily by paresthesia—a "pins and needles" sensation.

Differences in central projections between large-fiber afferent input and small-fiber input are responsible for observed differences in associated motor and sensory phenomena. Small-fiber afferent nerves transmitting sclerotomic and visceral pain follow a multisynaptic pathway with diffuse projections to areas such as the hypothalamus, limbic system, and reticular formation. These projections may mediate autonomic changes, such as changes in vasomotor tone, blood pressure, and sweat gland activity, that may accompany the pain experience. They may also be responsible for associated affective phenomena, such as depression, anxiety, fear, and anger. Sensory modalities transmitted over large fibers, such as dermatomic pain and non-noxious sensations, project largely to the thalamus and cortex and skip areas of the brain involved with affective and autonomic mediation. They are thus less likely to be associated with emotional and behavioral changes.

HISTORY AND DEVELOPMENT OF PAIN THEORIES AND MECHANISMS

Inconsistencies in interpreting the experiential and behavioral aspects of pain complicate any discussion of the physiology of a nociceptive system. Although some researchers attempt to discuss pain as a sensory experience, others define pain in terms of associated behavioral responses, both somatic and autonomic. One might argue that extreme pain may affect a person as a sensory experience without being recognized by an observer. Another would counter that even if this were possible, pain is insignificant unless it somehow alters the victim's body functions, behavior, or life-style.

Still another concern of those interested in the phenomenon of pain is the affective component—the suffering, hopelessness, despair, or depression that may accompany pain, especially long-standing pain. On the basis of experience, most would agree that a "painful event" might comprise any combination of sensory, behavioral, or affective components. A person may prick a finger with a pin without significant despair or depression, and in the absence of subsequent shouting, sweating, or shaking of the part. However, smashing the thumb with a hammer is frequently followed by some verbal display of displeasure and significant motor activity, including flailing of the injured part as well as generalized increased sympathetic tone. But this event is not usually associated with depression or sorrow because the person realizes that the swelling will soon subside. On the other hand, loss of a loved one may lead to excruciating "pain" manifested as grieving and sorrow but without a painful sensation. It is often accompanied by diminished motor activity, loss of appetite, and weeping. Interestingly, the sufferer of chronic pain behaves similarly. While persons in each of the above situations may well complain of pain, psychosocial rewards may condition a person to complain of pain and manifest other pain-associated behaviors in the absence of prior nociceptive events. There seem to be areas in which the neural pathways involved with pain sensation, with certain affective phenomena, and with stereotyped skeletal and smooth muscle activation intersect. Activation of all or part of these pathways results in the experiential or behavioral events generally classified as pain. Which components of the system will be activated depends on the nature of the stimulus as well as central modulation of information reaching the central nervous system (CNS). A given stimulus may or may not result in pain, and pain behavior may occur in the absence of nociception. Everyone has heard stories about soldiers wounded in war who deny pain at the time of severe tissue damage. On the other hand, persons with no demonstrable tissue damage may complain of pain and display disabling pain behaviors. In summary, nociception may occur without pain and pain may occur without nociception. Theories dealing with the neurophysiology of pain must explain these facts in terms of known mechanisms and their anatomical correlates.

Knowledge of the evolution of pain theory is interesting on a historical level and contributes to an appreciation of present pain research. Today's understanding of the nociceptive system is a composite of past and present research, hypotheses, and theories, each of which has emphasized different components of the nociceptive system. Therefore, one approach to understanding pain mechanisms would be to follow the evolution of pain theory and select and combine important contributions.

One of the first recorded pain theories was proposed by Aristotle, who postulated that pain occurs with every kind of stimulation whenever that stimulation becomes excessive. Therefore, anything too hot, too sharp, or abnormally loud causes pain. Excessive stimulation was carried from the periphery by blood vessels to the heart where it was perceived as a negative passion or absence of pleasure. Aristotle's proposal implied that the pain experience has emotional, psychological, and physiological dimensions. The proposed anatomical pathway for nociceptive input is of course, incorrect. Aristotle chose the heart — the center of emotion — as the organ receiving and interpreting painful stimulation, which suggests that he considered the affective or emotional component of pain to be of critical importance. The affective dimension of pain was not em-

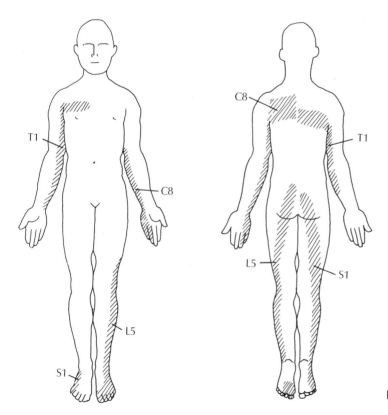

Fig. 3-3. Dermatomes of the body.

Fig. 3-3 *(Continued).*

phasized again until the development of modern theories.

SPECIFICITY THEORY

With the advent of the microscope, scientists became greatly preoccupied with morphologic detail. Investigators in the early 1800s searched for precise anatomical evidence to support hypothesized pain mechanisms. Mueller and others found minute structures in the skin, viscera, and muscles that they believed were receptor end organs for various modalities of sensation.[41,51,52] The primary theory based on microscopic evidence was Von Frey's specificity theory proposed in 1895.[45,57] Von Frey proposed a specific relationship between the type of end organ stimulated and the nature of the resulting sensation. For example, pressure is perceived when the pacinian corpuscles are stimulated, whereas stimulation of free nerve endings causes pain.

It has since been found that such a precise one-to-one relationship between type of receptor and sensation does not exist. Weddell found, for example, that the cornea, which contains only free nerve endings, is sensitive to many types of sensory stimuli.[13,45,55] The specificity theory proponents demonstrated, however, that there are peripheral receptors that must be excited in order for pain sensation to be perceived. Unfortunately, the theory paid little attention to central pain modulation (the influence of spinal cord or brain on input) and considered only the sensory experience of pain. It ignored the associated emotional, psychological, and motor responses.

PATTERN THEORY

Several years later, investigators became interested in peripheral nerves. Head cut a peripheral nerve in his own arm, knowing that smaller nerve fibers regenerate before larger ones. With regeneration of the small nerve fibers, Head noted spontaneous tingling, dysesthesia, and other abnormal nociceptive sensations.[13,18,45] Not until the large nerve fibers regenerated, and light pressure, touch, and vibration sense returned, were the painful sensations abolished. From this information and from insight gained through their own research (including research on cornea sensation), Weddell and Sinclair proposed a pattern theory of pain.[13,18,45,51,55] The pattern theory emphasized that it is the anatomical variation in fiber size over which afferent impulses travel that leads to temporal and spatial summation of input in central receiving areas. The pattern theory suggested that variation in fiber size was related to both the site of central connections and the pattern of central excitation. For example, input traveling over small fibers ascends multisynaptically in the contralateral anterolateral tract with little cortical input, whereas large-fiber input ascends in the ipsilateral dorsal column to the thalamus, with subsequent projections to the cortex. Weddell also noted that signals traveling over larger fibers reach the spinal cord before small-fiber input. Weddell and Sinclair combined this information in a theory that stated that patterns of input over various fiber sizes are a major determinant of sensation and pain perception. Thus, large fiber stimulation may be felt as light touch or pressure, whereas small-fiber stimulation tends to cause noxious sensations. A mixture may result in a combination or cancellation of sensory input.

The pattern theory postulates that a specialized system exists that combines and modifies all peripheral sensory input before it ascends to higher brain centers, thus modifying the nature of the resultant sensation. The theory also proposes that all stimulus information from the periphery must summate in the CNS to allow determination and execution of a proper response. Weddell and Sinclair stated that major determinants of intensity and quality of experienced sensations are the discharge characteristics of afferent fibers and the sites of central connections. The weaknesses in the pattern theory are (1) that pain is again considered to be largely a sensory phenomenon, and little reference is made to associated affective phenomena; (2) that knowledge of the role of receptors was ignored or denied; and (3) that the influence of central modulation of input was not considered.

NEUROANATOMY

Before discussing the gate theory of pain, it is important to compare the pathways taken by large as opposed to small, or nociceptive, afferent nerve fibers. On entering the dorsal horn of the spinal cord, nociceptive afferents from both somatic and visceral tissues travel in the dorsolateral fasciculus (Lissauer's tract) a few segments rostrally and caudally before entering the gray matter of the dorsal horn.[13,35,57] They then relay with cells in the substantia gelatinosa (SG) (lamina II and III) and proceed to synapse ipsilaterally in the dorsal funicular gray matter (lamina V), a nuclear mass that lies at the base of the dorsal horn (Fig. 3–4). The second- or third-order fiber crosses by way of the anterior white commissure to ascend contralaterally in the anterolateral tract. This

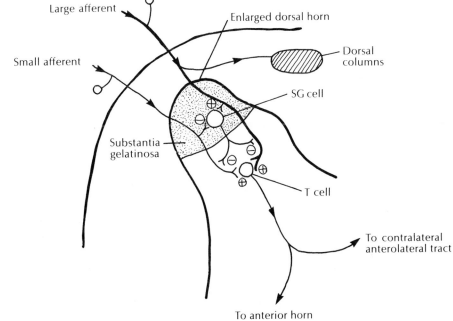

Fig. 3–4. Modulation of afferent input as proposed by the gate theory. Activation of the T cells results in ascending nociceptive input and reflex motor changes. The T cell is inhibited by substantia gelatinosa (SG) cell input, which is, in turn, inhibited by small-fiber input and facilitated by large-fiber input.

fiber tract continues rostrally to synapse in the ventroposterolateral and ventroposteromedial nuclei of the thalamus; collaterals also project to the medullary reticular formation, limbic system, and hypothalamus. The nociceptive afferents are small myelinated and unmyelinated, slowly transmitting nerve fibers, and the receptors for this system adapt slowly to the application or removal of the irritating stimulus. The final synapses are in regions where past experience, motivation, and emotion may influence the ultimate response to noxious stimulation.[13,35,57]

Large fiber afferents from proprioceptors and mechanoreceptors transmitting information concerning light touch, vibration, and joint and muscle position enter the dorsolateral fasciculus and send collaterals to segments several spinal levels above and below the level of entry. The collateral branches enter the dorsal horn and synapse on interneurons in the SG (see Fig. 3–4). The large myelinated fibers then enter the dorsal columns ipsilaterally and ascend to the medulla where they synapse, decussate, and ascend as the medial lemniscus to the ventroposterolateral nuclei of the thalamus. The third-order neuron leaves the thalamus and projects to the postcentral gyrus, the sensory cortex.[13,35,57]

Both large- and small-fiber systems send collaterals to the anterior horn of the spinal cord before entering ascending tracts. These projections mediate reflex motor activity associated with noxious and non-noxious stimulation.

GATE THEORY

In 1965 Melzack and Wall proposed the gate theory of pain.[41,42,45,54,57] Several investigators studying the SG measured electrical potentials in some of the interneuron synapses. They found that with small-fiber input (C fibers mediating pain and temperature), hyperpolarization was recorded, and when large fibers were stimulated, depolarization was recorded. Melzack and Wall postulated that interneurons in the SG act as a "gate" to modulate sensory input (Fig. 3–5). They proposed that the SG interneuron projected to the second order neuron of the pain–temperature pathway located in the dorsal funicular gray matter (lamina V), which they called the *transmission cell* or *T cell*.[41,42] If the SG interneuron were depolarized it would inhibit T-cell firing and thus decrease further transmission of input ascending in the spinothalamic tract. For example, nociceptive fibers enter the dorsal horn and send a collateral fiber into the SG, which hyperpolarizes the interneuron. The nociceptive afferent continues to lamina V where it synapses with the T-cell. On reaching threshold levels of excitation, the T-cell sends nociceptive input rostrally in the anterolateral spinal tract. Large-fiber input (joint movement, pressure, vibration) enters the dorsal horn, sending a collateral into the SG, which depolarizes the SG interneuron. This interneuron projects to lamina V and presynaptically inhibits the T cell, preventing or decreasing ascending

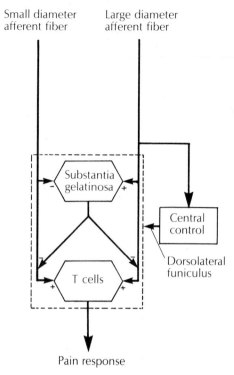

Small diameter afferent fiber

Large diameter afferent fiber

Substantia gelatinosa

Central control

Dorsolateral funiculus

T cells

Pain response

Fig. 3-5. Scheme of dorsal horn pain-modulating system.

nociceptive input.[41,42,45,57] Melzack and Wall thus used concepts presented in the pattern theory and described a specific anatomical pathway by which modulation of peripheral stimuli could occur. Essentially, the theory proposed an analogy to a gate that allows ongoing transmission of painful input when opened. The position of the gate is determined by the balance between large-fiber and small-fiber input to the system and is regulated by interneurons in the SG of the dorsal horn.

The gate theory was, and is, supported by both practical and experimental evidence. When one hits one's skin on a coffee-table corner, the immediate response is to rub the injured area, thus increasing the large-fiber input that decreases the pain. Physical therapists use a large number of modalities to decrease pain by increasing large-fiber input. Hot packs, whirlpools, massage, vibrators, and joint mobilization all act to increase large-fiber input and, therefore, to decrease nociceptive transmission. There are also certain clinical pain states, such as alcoholic neuropathy, in which preferential destruction of large fibers leads to chronic, relatively spontaneous pain.

Melzack and Wall also suggested that the gate could be modified by a descending inhibitory pathway from the brain or brain stem.[41,42,45,57] This was originally proposed largely on the basis of everyday

experience. For example, it has been noted that persons injured during stressful, life-threatening, or athletic events often do not realize the seriousness of the injury. Following frontal lobotomy or while on morphine, a patient knows when noxious stimulation is occurring but it is no longer painful or worrisome. Melzack and Wall postulated that these observations could be explained by central inhibitory input descending to the spinal cord to decrease T-cell firing. Sometimes patients experience more pain than expected following a certain amount of noxious input. In this case it was speculated that learned or affective behavior prevented or decreased inhibition of T-cell activity.

Since the proposal of the gate theory, researchers have identified many clinical pain states that cannot be fully explained by the gate mechanism.[45,57] However, the theory has made several significant contributions to current pain research. First, it directed the attention of researchers to the importance of pain modulation by higher CNS centers. Second, it accommodated most past research findings dealing with receptors, peripheral nerves, the dorsal horn, and ascending sensory pathways. Third, clinical applications of this theory are still useful, and many effective clinical procedures are based on the model provided by the gate theory. Transcutaneous nerve stimulation increases large-fiber input and abolishes or decreases pain to acceptable levels for many patients living with chronic pain. Clinics specializing in treatment for patients with chronic pain use behavior modification techniques to increase a patient's activity level. These techniques may act to increase large-fiber input and decrease pain or they may activate a central descending pathway that inhibits nociceptive input at the spinal cord level.[12,13,17]

CENTRAL MODULATION OF NOCICEPTIVE INPUT

During the last decade there has been a wealth of research and discovery related to central pain modulation. Current research continues to explore the relationship between the anatomical and physiological components of central pain pathways. The spark for this research was provided by technical advancements that provide a better understanding of biochemical and neurohistological features of the nociceptive system. After years of studying morphine and other opiate derivatives, researchers discovered "endogenous opiates," peptides native to the CNS that are now believed to be involved in nociceptive modulation. More recently the role of other neurotrans-

Fig. 3–6. Scheme of large- and small-fiber afferent systems and the ascending-descending inhibitory loop. The small fiber system is often referred to as the paleospinothalamic tract and the large-fiber system as the neospinothalamic tract.

mitters in the nociceptive system has begun to be elucidated. Additionally, there is much more interest in the affective and behavioral components of the nociceptive system—a return to Aristotle's emphasis. It is becoming generally agreed that any comprehensive pain theory must explain pain as a sensory experience as well as its associated affective and motor (autonomic and somatic) phenomena.

OPIATES AND ENKEPHALINS

Research leading to the discovery of endogenous opiates, the enkephalins, began with studies of morphine and its mechanism of action. For years researchers and the medical community have searched for a nonaddictive opiate agonist. Because morphine exerts analgesic effects with very small doses, it was generally agreed that morphine might act as a neurotransmitter in the CNS. The subsequent prediction was that receptors for morphine must exist in the CNS.[52,53] Pert and Snyder, using advanced neurohistological and neurochemical techniques, were able to trace morphine receptor sites in the CNS. Kumar, Pert, and Snyder demonstrated the distribution of opiate receptors in many brain regions using direct receptor-binding techniques and autoradiography of brain sections containing radioactive morphine.[26,52] The receptor distribution pathway strikingly parallels the paleospinothalamic pathway (Fig. 3–6), which ascends along the midline of the brain, synapsing in the central gray matter of the brain stem, the reticular formation, and the central thalamus. This pathway mediates duller, more chronic, and less localized pain; it is the phylogenically older pain pathway and contains many synapses and small-diameter, unmyelinated nerves.[13,32,52] Consistent with this is the observation that morphine exerts its analgesic effects on dull pain, whereas sharp, well-localized pain is poorly relieved by opiates.

Other brain areas with opiate receptors are the amygdala, the corpus striatum, and the hypothalamus, all of which are parts of the limbic system—a group of brain regions that largely mediate emotional phenomena.[52,58] These brain regions seem to be concerned with the affective components of pain, such as rage, anger, and depression, and perhaps the euphoric effects of morphine. Hypothalamic connections may mediate associated autonomic activity, such as sweating, pallor, or blood pressure changes. Opiate receptors are also localized in lamina II in the SG of the dorsal horn of the spinal cord—an important synapse area for the upward conduction of nociceptive information—as well as in lamina II of the caudal trigeminal nucleus, which receives nociceptive input from the face.[52,58]

With the discovery of morphine receptors, the search began for an endogenous substance with opiate activity. Several researchers simultaneously identified a morphine-like brain factor consisting of two closely related pentapeptides, which were named *enkephalins*.[26,52,57] It was found that naloxone, a morphine antagonist, also inhibited the analgesic effects of enkephalins.[5,15,16,38,57] Research in morphine addiction revealed that an increase in the presence of morphine is accompanied by a decrease in enkephalin production and release. It was speculated that opiate withdrawal symptoms occur from enkephalin depletion and subside as soon as enkephalin concentrations return to normal.[37,52] Several studies have also described decreased enkephalin levels associated with chronic pain.[6,7,33,34]

The mechanism of enkephalin action as a neurotransmitter is both interesting and speculative. Enkephalin is an excitatory transmitter believed to presynaptically inhibit the dorsal horn T cell of lamina V, and thus modulate input to ascending pain pathways in the spinal cord and the brain.[38,52,57] This has special significance for the gate theory, which 24 years ago suggested that descending inhibition occurred at the level of the dorsal horn in the spinal cord and that perhaps the mechanism was presynaptic inhibition of the T cell in lamina V.[53]

STIMULUS-PRODUCED ANALGESIA

Following the discovery of enkephalins, researchers began to investigate possible mechanisms by which enkephalin-mediated circuits might be activated. Therefore, they have attempted to define the role of enkephalins in the nociceptive system. Opiate receptor sites (and synaptic vescicles of enkephalin) are located in the periventricular, periaqueductal, and mesencephalic central gray matter, in the dorsal horn, and in some limbic regions (*e.g.*, amygdala, corpus striatum) of the CNS.[38,52,57] It was found that electrical stimulation of the periaqueductal gray matter (PAG) in rats, cats, monkeys, and humans produced profound analgesia.[8,10,13,19,32,36–39,47,49,52,57] Subsequently, researchers noted that this stimulus-produced analgesia (SPA) was partially reversed by administering naloxone.[1,4,37,38] Because SPA is only partially reversed by naloxone, it was concluded that SPA was the result of the release of both enkephalin and another unknown neurotransmitter. Investigators have measured in the cerebrospinal fluid a significant increase in enkephalin content following stimulation of the PAG in rats and have found that injections of enkephalin into the central gray matter increase the animal's pain tolerance and produce a long-lasting analgesia to electrically evoked pain.[5,38,49,52,57] It was subsequently postulated that enkephalins were released in the PAG following noxious input. Researchers then administered radioactively labeled amino acids to experimental animals in order to label enkephalins, which incorporate the amino acids. Following stimulation of A-delta nerve fibers (which mediate thermal and nociceptive input), the animals' brains were sectioned and analyzed for labeling. It was found that the areas where enkephalins were released overlapped the anatomical substrate for SPA.[52] This area appears to be concentrated in medial brain-stem structures extending from the diencephalon (periventricular gray matter and PAG) caudally to the medullary raphe nuclei, which is part of the midbrain reticular formation.[7,8,19,21,36,38,39,48,58] It was subsequently noted that stimulation of A-delta nerve fibers also caused increased firing of nerve cells located in the medullary raphe nuclei.[7,38]

In humans, stimulation of periventricular structures was effective in relieving diverse pain syndromes.[36,38] Electrical stimulation of the PAG was also shown to increase experimental pain tolerance to both painful heat and electrical shock.[38,57,58] Morphine injections into and electrical stimulation of the periventricular gray matter and PAG in cats clearly depress the discharge of neurons in lamina V of the dorsal horn (site of the first synapse in the afferent pain pathway) evoked by strong cutaneous and thermal stimulation.[19] Non-noxious stimulation was not affected by PAG stimulation or morphine injection. Finally, experiments have revealed that morphine injected into the amygdala produces analgesia as well as the characteristic euphoric behavior.[38,52]

The implications are fascinating. There are specific brain sites that when stimulated block pain; these areas mediate the response to morphine; a natural morphine-like substance exists exerting its influence in the same brain site as morphine; and finally, stimulation of these brain areas can prevent transmission of nociception at the level of the spinal cord.

CENTRAL DESCENDING INHIBITORY PATHWAY

The findings discussed previously strongly suggest that endogenous opiates are neurotransmitters in a nociceptive modulating system.[38,50,53] The physiological mechanism proposed is an "endogenous pain inhibitory system" or negative feedback loop[21,38] (see Fig. 3–6). Specifically, peripheral nociception leads to activation of the PAG and nuclei of the midbrain and medullary reticular formation. These nuclei then send descending inhibitory signals to the dorsal horn to reduce ongoing transmission of nociceptive input. The descending inhibitory system includes the rostral and caudal PAG, the medullary nuclei of the reticular formation, and connections in the dorsal horn. The descending limb of this feedback loop begins with neurons in the rostral PAG, an important area for SPA that is known to be rich in enkephalins.[8,38,58] The PAG neuron makes an excitatory synapse with the nucleus raphe magnus (NRM) of the medulla, near the caudal PAG, and with the adjacent nucleus reticularis magnocellularis (Rmc), perhaps using dopamine or enkephalin as a neurotransmittor. These two nuclei send fibers to the spinal cord by way of the dorsolateral funiculus that terminate among pain-transmission cells concentrated in laminae II and V of the dorsal horn.[11,12,38] Both the NRM and the nucleus Rmc exert an inhibitory effect spe-cifically on pain-transmission neurons. The NRM uses serotonin as a transmittor; the Rmc transmittor is speculated to be enkephalin. The pain-transmission neurons (activated by substance P following peripheral nociceptive stimulation) cross and project cranially in the anterolateral spinal tract.[14,25,39] As the anterolateral tract continues cranially, it contacts the cells of the descending analgesia system in the PAG through the nucleus reticularis gigantocellularis (RgC) of the medulla, thus establishing a negative feedback loop.[21,36,38,49] Norepinephrine-containing neurons of the locus ceruleus (LC) may also contribute to pain-modulating systems through the dorsolateral funiculus (DLF).

There is ample evidence supporting the existence of such a negative feedback loop. It has been shown that SPA readily suppresses spinal cord nociceptive reflexes.[38] Morphine injected into PAG can clearly depress the discharge of pain-transmission neurons in lamina V.[57] Stimulation of caudal PAG in the cat markedly inhibits the responses of most dorsal horn lamina V cells to noxious skin stimuli.[19] Furthermore, the analgesia due to PAG stimulation or systemic opiate administration is markedly reduced caudal to transection of the spinal DLF.[11,12] Central gray matter stimulation, while inhibiting nociceptive input, does not affect responses to gentle tactile stimulation.

The NRM's critical link in the descending nociceptive inhibitory system is also well supported experimentally. Stimulation of the NRM in cats results in analgesia.[47] Several investigators found that after PAG stimulation or morphine administration, they noted a significant increase in neuronal activity in NRM neurons.[46] Lesions of the NRM block opiate analgesia, while electrical stimulation of the NRM produces a potent analgesia reversed by the opiate antagonist naloxone.[7,48] Studies have demonstrated a population of neurons in the NRM projecting to the spinal cord.[38] It was further found that this population of NRM neurons was excited by electrical stimulation of the PAG as well as by opiates administered systemically or by local injection into midbrain PAG. The PAG and NRM receive a large amount of input from the nucleus RgC, which in turn receives input from spinal cord pain-transmission neurons.[21,38] PAG stimulation in the rat has been shown to suppress the nociceptive responses of neurons in the nucleus RgC.[49] This could have been the result of supraspinal descending inhibition of the nucleus RgC or inhibition of incoming nociceptive input at the spinal cord level.

Bilateral lesions of the DLF in rats reverse the analgesic effects of systemically administered morphine.[11,12,38] Lesions of the DLF also abolish the analgesic effects of morphine injected into the PAG in rats.[11,12,36,38] Other researchers have documented that lesions of the DLF reverse both SPA and morphine-induced analgesia. This evidence implies that a descending pathway inhibits nociceptive input at the level of the spinal cord and that this inhibition functions as part of a negative feedback loop.

MONOAMINERGIC NEUROTRANSMITTERS

It is interesting that naloxone administration only partially blocks SPA. From recent studies it now appears clear that monoaminergic neurotransmitters also play important roles in SPA and morphine analgesia.[2,20,29,42] These transmitters are serotonin, dopamine, and norepinephrine. Depletion of serotonin with *p*-chlorophenylalanine (*p*-CPA) has been shown to reduce SPA, but the analgesia can be restored by administration of the serotonin precursor 5-hydroxytryptamine.[2,3] *p*-CPA is most effective in reducing SPA when the electrode stimulating sites are in the region of the NRM or dorsal raphe magnus (DRM). Both of these reticular nuclei contain serotoninergic neurons.[14,38] The NRM descends through the DLF to the dorsal horn. The DRM is part of the ascending nociceptive pathway that involves complex multisynaptic pathways first ascending to forebrain structures and then descending to the spinal cord in an as yet unknown circuit.[14] An inhibitor of serotoninergic neurons, LSD-25, has been shown to reduce the inhibitory effect that SPA has on dorsal horn lamina V neurons. Animals treated with *p*-CPA were found to be more reactive to electroshock presentations. Humans with migraine headaches who were treated with *p*-CPA experienced superficial and muscular algesias and pain with facial movement or with clothing friction — in short, fairly spontaneous pain.[38] In animals, injections of a serotonin uptake-blocking drug produces analgesia and will antagonize the hyperalgesia associated with injections of *p*-CPA.[29,43] Lesions of the NRM, DRM, medial forebrain bundle, or the septum produce large reductions in serotonin concentrations, leading to increased pain sensitivity.[38,57] Destruction of the DRM or of the NRM and resultant loss of serotoninergic activity blocks the analgesic effect of systemically administered morphine, while increased serotonin levels potentiates morphine analgesia.[38,43] Another method of disrupting the pain inhibition pathway involves blocking the action of NRM fibers, as they synapse in the dorsal horn. Research has documented that morphine-induced analgesia could be antagonized by administration of antiserotonin drugs to the dorsal horn. Other studies have shown that serotonin has an inhibitory effect on neurons located in the superficial laminae of the dorsal horn that respond to noxious stimuli.[28,29,43] These are also the laminae where NRM fibers terminate. In summary, it has been found that with increased serotonin levels, morphine and stimulus-produced analgesia are potentiated, while depletion of serotonin causes hyperalgesia and spontaneous pain and blocks morphine analgesia and SPA.

Catecholaminergic neurotransmitters (*e.g.*, norepinephrine, dopamine) also appear to be involved in both SPA and morphine analgesia.[2,38,57] Compounds that deplete all monoamines almost completely abolish SPA. When compounds that deplete only catecholamines are used, a smaller reduction in SPA is found.[20] Increasing catecholamine levels with L-dopa, which leads to increased dopamine levels, potentiates SPA.[38] Researchers have found that blocking dopamine receptors inhibits SPA and morphine analgesia, whereas stimulation of dopamine receptors potentiates both. The reverse is true for norepinephrine.[20,38] Depletion of norepinephrine increases the effect of morphine and stimulus-produced analgesia; injections of excess norepinephrine block morphine and SPA.

The evidence for dopaminergic involvement in the nociceptive inhibitory pathway is less extensive than that for serotonin involvement. The only known dopamine systems ascend from the brain stem to forebrain structures, so that dopamine involvement necessitates complex ascending and descending pathways.[20,38,43] Even though the location of the dopamine pathway operating in the descending nociceptive inhibitory pathway is not known, it has been shown that dopamine plays some role. Norepinephrine-containing neurons of the LC in rats and of the subceruleus parabrachialis in cats may contribute to pain modulating systems by sending fibers in the dorsolateral funiculus to lamina V of the dorsal horn.[38]

CENTRAL STRUCTURES MODULATING DESCENDING INHIBITION

Other CNS structures may play a role in nociceptive modulation. The PAG region of the midbrain receives diverse inputs from numerous brain areas and is involved in various emotional, motivational, and sensory systems.[38,49] The rostral PAG neurons integrate input from many brain areas, and the resulting output determines the level of nociceptive modulation at the midbrain and spinal cord. The PAG receives nociceptive input from the spinal cord by way of the RgC while simultaneously receiving thalamic, limbic, and cortical input. In this way, memory, learned responses, and affective components may all contribute to modulation and perception of ascending nociceptive input.

The reticular formation contains the NRM and DRM and a number of other ascending and descending pathways.[14,38] The major descending pathway concerned with nociception is that of the NRM and nucleus Rmc, which both send fibers to the dorsal horn. The ascending pathways include reticular formation (1) to the cortex—a direct pathway; (2) to several thalamic nuclei (posterior, ventral, and intralaminar); and (3) to the hypothalamus, limbic forebrain, and frontal cortex.[14] The pathway also includes a catecholamine system that arises in parts of the brain-stem reticular formation and passes through the medial forebrain bundle and septum to reach the neocortex.[14,38] This last pathway may be part of an ascending serotoninergic fiber tract.

These ascending pathways, activated by nociceptive input, excite regions of the brain involved in behavioral, affective, and motor responses to nociception. Output from these higher centers (frontal cortex, limbic regions, and thalamus) may in turn descend to the PAG to modulate ongoing nociception through the previously mentioned descending loop.[9,14,23,38] The higher cortical centers and PAG integration of input appear to determine each person's response to nociceptive input. This explains why some persons perceive intense pain, others a mild discomfort, and some no noxious sensation at all in response to the same nociceptive stimulus.

There are several other brain areas that produce analgesia when electrically stimulated. One well-studied region is the medial forebrain bundle–lateral hypothalamic region.[38] Stimulation of this region in the rat has produced analgesia to pin prick, hot plate, and electric shock. For several reasons it appears that the medial forebrain bundle must produce analgesia by a pathway other than PAG → NRM → dorsal horn. Some evidence indicates that stimulation of the medial forebrain bundle can reduce clinical pain in humans.

Stimulation of the septal region also produces analgesia, again by a seemingly different pathway than the medial brain-stem system. Septal region stimulation has been reported to be effective in relieving clinical pain syndromes in humans.[38]

ENDORPHINS

Another class of polypeptides with endogenous opiate activity are the endorphins.[24,49] Beta-endorphin, with a chain of 30 amino acids, is among the most potent endogenous analgesics known. It has been found that a sequence of five amino acids on the amino terminal of the beta-endorphin molecule corresponds to the sequence of enkephalin. This may account for their similar analgesic properties. In fact, beta-endorphins have been shown to bind to some of the same sites in the brain, such as the PAG, as the enkephalins. Endorphins do not appear to bind in the spinal cord, however. There is no evidence that enkephalins are products of endorphins; it is probable that enkephalins are primarily produced within neurons, to be used as neurotransmitters.

Immunochemical studies have demonstrated endorphins in the pituitary, brain, and intestinal tract. They seem to be released from the pituitary as part of a much larger polypeptide molecule, beta-lipotropin (Fig. 3–7), which may in turn be a product of a still larger "prohormone." Beta-lipotropin is also a precursor of adrenocorticotropic hormone (ACTH), and there is evidence that endorphins are released in response to the same stimuli that trigger ACTH release, for example, stress.[44]

The role of endorphins in pain modulation has not yet been elucidated. Intracerebral injections of endorphins produce profound and prolonged analgesia, but large doses administered into the peripheral bloodstream have no analgesic effects. There is a tendency to want to attribute apparent cases of relative analgesia under stress, such as in the case of the war-injured or shark-bite victim, to massive endorphin release. However, there is no experimental evidence to demonstrate analgesia from endorphins released from the pituitary, and it is unlikely that they cross the blood–brain barrier. While speculation on the role of endorphins in mediating such phenomena as the "runner's high" is interesting, corroboration awaits further study. It is likely, however, that the endorphins do influence the maintenance of behavioral homeostasis, perhaps affecting the central nociceptive modulating system.[24]

SUMMARY OF SENSORY PATHWAYS

Nociceptive stimulation of free nerve endings is usually associated with concomitant stimulation of non-nociceptive receptors, such as mechanoreceptors. Touch and pressure input travels to the cord over large myelinated fibers and to the cortex by a dorsal column–medial lemniscus–thalamus–cortex pathway (see Fig. 3–6). It serves to localize the stimulus, including associated nociceptive input. Nociceptive signals travel by A-delta and unmyelinated C fibers to Lissauer's tract in the apex of the dorsal horn. There they bifurcate into short neurons and ascend or descend one to two segments before synapsing in the

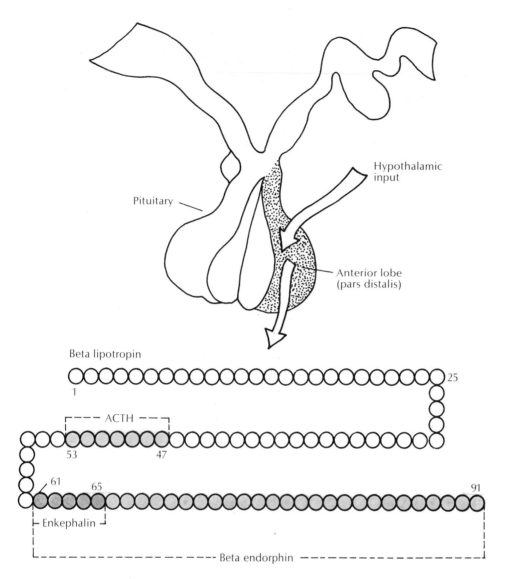

Beta lipotropin

Fig. 3-7. The beta-lipotropin hormone complex released from the anterior pituitary contains amino acid sequences corresponding to ACTH and beta-endorphin. Beta-endorphin, in turn, contains the sequence for enkephalin.

SG (lamina II). Cells of laminae I, IV, V, and perhaps VI respond to nociceptive stimulation. Neurons in laminae V and VI project axons to the contralateral cord, which ascend as the anterolateral tract. Some lamina V cells send axons to the ipsilateral anterolateral tract.

Evidence suggests that the spinothalamic system is composed of two divisions, the neospinothalamic tract and the paleospinothalamic tract. The neospinothalamic tract is located laterally and is a more recent evolutionary development. It is composed of myelinated fibers that project directly to the ventrolateral and posterior thalamus, where they synapse. The third-order neuron then projects to the somatosensory cortex. Nociceptive input traveling over this pathway is perceived as sharp, well-localized pain with little or no accompanying affective component and a short latency between stimulus and perception. It travels over larger pain fibers (*e.g.*, A-delta fibers). The paleospinothalamic tract, on the other hand, is located medially and is an evolutionarily older pathway. It is composed of more unmyelinated fibers that make many synapses, so that input travels more slowly than in the neospinothalamic tract. The paleospinothalamic tract projects to the reticular formation (especially the nucleus RgC), to the lateral pons, to the limbic midbrain area, and then to the intralaminar thalamic nuclei. Fibers then continue rostrally and synapse ultimately with neurons in the hypothalamus, in the limbic forebrain structures, and with diffuse projections to many other parts of the brain. Nociceptive input traveling over this pathway is perceived as diffuse, poorly localized pain, with a strong affective component and a long latency between stimulus and perception. The paleospino-thalamic tract mediates suprasegmental reflex responses, such as autonomic responses, as well as affective phenomena associated with pain. It is the more important system with respect to clinical pain states.

Nociceptive input to the medullary reticular formation, thalamus, cortex, and limbic regions activates neurons that feed back to the PAG integration center. The PAG in turn provides input to the NRM and the adjacent nucleus Rmc (see Fig. 3–6). Each sends nerve fibers to the dorsal horn through the dorsal lateral funiculus fiber tract. These fibers presynaptically inhibit the nociceptive T cells in laminae I and V of the dorsal horn. As the paleospinothalamic tract ascends rostrally, it synapses and activates the nucleus Rgc in the medulla. The Rgc sends projections to the PAG and to the NRM. In some manner it also activates the DRM. The DRM (another reticular formation nucleus) forms a portion of the ascending serotoninergic pathway that eventually excites neurons in the hypothalamus, limbic forebrain areas, frontal cortex, and septum. Presumably, the DRM contributes to affective, memory, sensory, autonomic, and somatic motor responses to pain. Descending output from these areas impinges on the PAG, thus modulating nociceptive input originating at spinal cord levels. The nature of modulation depends on the integration of ongoing activity in these areas.

CLINICAL APPLICATIONS

Because of the knowledge of the gate theory and the central modulation of pain clinical applications can be made with variable success. It has been known for centuries that counterirritants such as heat and massage reduce pain. More modern counterirritant techniques, such as transcutaneous nerve stimulation and dorsal column stimulation, may also relieve pain in patients with certain pain problems. All of these techniques stimulate pressure and touch receptors that send information to the dorsal horn through large, myelinated fibers. This large-fiber input leads to partial or complete inhibition of nociceptive T-cell firing, and therefore to less transmission of nociceptive input to higher brain centers by way of segmental modulation.[40]

Some reports suggest that acupuncture-induced analgesia may be reversed by naloxone.[39,56] Generally, it is speculated that the opiate-system activation is involved in acupuncture analgesia, although some studies cast doubt on this.[38,39] It should be noted that

acupuncture points, "trigger points," and motor points coincide closely; perhaps they are simply convenient sites for eventual activation of PAG and descending inhibition of nociceptive input by peripheral stimulation.

Behavior modification approaches to management of chronic pain patients often result in decreased pain behavior (fewer complaints, reduced drug dependency), increased activity level, and often a return to a more acceptable life-style.[22,50] Increasing activity, ignoring pain complaints, and replacing old behaviors with new ones may all lead to stimulation of the PAG and, therefore, activate the central descending pathway that inhibits nociceptive input at the spinal cord level. Increasing activity also increases large-fiber input. This may balance small fiber nociceptive input and lead to inhibition of the nociceptive T cell in lamina V of the dorsal horn. However, many patients with chronic pain have symptoms with apparently minimal somatic contribution but excessive affective components. After behavior modification, many patients claim that their pain is the same even though they are now able to engage in more activities and lead a more normal life. It is likely that more complex pathways are involved than have yet been described.

As more research is done, the evidence becomes highly suggestive that little difference exists between the biologic substrate and clinical manifestations of chronic pain and depression. Researchers have measured serotonin levels in severely depressed and suicidal patients and have found them to be markedly reduced. Remember that serotonin inhibitors administered to human subjects lead to hyperalgesia and spontaneous pain syndromes.[3,38] Decreased serotonin levels block morphine effects and SPA in laboratory animals.[20] Patients with chronic pain and depression often behave similarly. Both are generally less active, have altered appetite and sleep patterns, lose motivational and sexual drives, and may become self-abusive.[22] Perhaps the same component of the nociceptive system is involved in both kinds of patients. This may explain why patients with chronic pain exhibit "depressive behaviors," and why depressed patients frequently complain of pain. Interestingly, tricyclic drugs, which inhibit serotonin depletion, have been found to be useful in treating depression as well as chronic pain. This suggests that serotoninergic pathways may be important in both disorders.

Of primary importance clinically is the understanding that pain involves much more than a simple relay of sensory input. Culture, past experience, emotional state, personality, motivation, role expectations, and learned behavior can all contribute to modulation of nociceptive stimuli and can influence the final pain experience. Persons with a strong will to complete a task (*e.g.*, athlete, soldier) undoubtedly receive a barrage of nociceptive input, but pain, suffering, or pain behavior may not accompany nociceptive input, presumably because segmental or central modulation creates a relatively analgesic state. On the other hand, pain can occur without nociceptive input, just as suffering, depression, grief, or other affective phenomena associated with pain can occur without pain or nociception. Many patients exhibit pain behaviors when nociception is no longer present. For clinicians treating patients with pain problems, it is essential to understand the nociceptive process and to consider possible contributing factors affecting nociceptive input. For this purpose, patient history and evaluation are invaluable. The patient with musculoskeletal pain may also be depressed, lonely, have a drug or alcohol problem, or be going through a difficult adjustment period. The clinician must consider these possibilities when the treatment program is established, as well as provide the appropriate treatment and all other necessary resources to enable the patient to deal with the pain problem most effectively.

REFERENCES

1. Adams JE: Naloxone reversal of analgesia produced by brain stimulation in the human. Pain 2:161–166, 1976
2. Akil H, Liebeskind JC: Monoaminergic mechanisms of stimulation-produced analgesia. Brain Res 94:279–296, 1975
3. Akil H, Mayer DJ: Antagonisms of stimulation-produced analgesia by p-CPA, a serotonin synthesis inhibitor. Brain Res 44:692–697, 1972
4. Akil H, Mayer DJ, Liebeskind JC: Antagonism of stimulation-produced analgesia by naloxone, a narcotic antagonist. Science 191:961–962, 1976
5. Akil H, Richardson DE, Hughes J, Barchas JD: Enkephalin-like material elevated in ventricular cerebrospinal fluid of pain patients after analgetic focal stimulation. Science 201:463–465, 1978
6. Almay BG, Johansson F, Von Knorring L, Terenius L, Wahlstrom A: Endorphins in chronic pain: Differences in CSF endorphin levels between organic and psychogenic pain syndromes. Pain 5:153–162, 1978
7. Anderson SD, Bausbaum AI, Fields HL: Responses of medullary raphe neurons to peripheral stimulation and to systemic opiates. Brain Res 123:363–368, 1977
8. Balagura S, Ralph T: The analgesic effect of electrical stimulation of the diencephalon and mesencephalon. Brain Res 60:369–381, 1973
9. Barnes DC, Fung SJ, Adams WL: Inhibitory effects of substantia nigra on impulse transmission from nociceptors. Pain 6:207–215, 1979
10. Basbaum AI, Marley N, O'Keefe J: Effects of spinal cord lesions on the analgesic properties of electrical brain stimulation. Presented at a symposium held at the First World Congress on Pain. Advances in Pain Research, p. 268, 1975
11. Basbaum AI, Marley N, O'Keefe J, Clanton C: Reversal of morphine and stimulus-produced analgesia by subtotal spinal cord lesions. Pain 3:43–56, 1977
12. Black RG: The chronic pain syndrome. Surg Clin North Am 55:999–1011, 1975
13. Bonica JJ: Neurophysiologic and pathologic aspects of acute and chronic pain. Arch Surg 112:750–761, 1977
14. Bowsher D: Role of the reticular formation in responses to noxious stimulation. Pain 2:361–378, 1976
15. Buchsbaum MS, Davis GC, Bunney WE: Naloxone alters pain perception and somatosensory evoked potentials in normal subjects. Nature 270:620–622, 1977
16. Buscher HH, Hill RC, Romer D, Cardinaux F, Closse A, Hauser D, Pless J: Evidence for analgesic activity of enkephalin in the mouse. Nature 261:423–425, 1976
17. Callaghan M, Sternbach RA, Nyquist JK, Timmermans G: Changes in somatic sensitivity during transcutaneous electrical analgesia. Pain 5:115–127, 1978
18. Clark WC, Hunt HF: Pain. In Downey J, Darling R (eds): Physiological Basis of Rehabilitation Medicine, pp 373–401. Philadelphia, WB Saunders, 1971
19. Duggan AW, Griersmith BT: Inhibition of spinal transmission of nociceptive information by supraspinal stimulation in the cat. Pain 6:149–161, 1979
20. Fennessy MR, Lee JR: Modification of morphine analgesia by drugs affecting adrenergic and tryptaminergic mechanisms. J Pharm Pharmacol 22:930–935, 1978
21. Fields HL, Anderson SD: Evidence that raphe-spinal neurons mediate opiate and midbrain stimulation-produced analgesias. Pain 5:333–349, 1978
22. Fordyce WE: Behavioral Methods for Chronic Pain and Illness. St Louis, CV Mosby, 1976
23. Guilbaud G, Peschanski M, Gautron M, Binder D: Neurons responding to noxious stimulation in VB complex and caudal adjacent regions in the thalamus of the rat. Pain 8:303–318, 1980
24. Guillemin R: Beta-lipotropin and endorphins: Implications of current knowledge. Hosp Pract 13(11)53–60, 1978
25. Henry JL, Sessle BJ, Lucier GE, Hu JW: Effects of substance P on nociceptive and non-nociceptive trigeminal brain stem neurons. Pain 8:33–45, 1980
26. Hughes J, Smith TW, Kosterlitz HW, Fothergill LA, Morgan BA, Morris HR: Identification of two related pentapeptides from the brain with potent opiate agonist activity. Nature 258:577–579, 1975
27. Inman VT, Saunders JB: Referred pain from skeletal structures. J Nerv Ment Dis 99:660–667, 1944
28. Johansson F, Von Knorring L: A double-blind controlled study of a serotonin uptake inhibitor (Zimeli-

dine) versus placebo in chronic pain patients. Pain 7:69–78, 1979

29. Jordan LM, Kenshalo DR, Martin RF, Haber LH, Willis WD: Depression of primate spinothalamic tract neurons by iontophoretic application of 5-hydroxytryptamine. Pain 5:135–142, 1978

30. Kellgren JH: On the distribution of pain arising from deep somatic structures with charts of segmental pain areas. Clin Sci 4:35–46, 1939

31. Kellgren JH, Samuel EP: The sensitivity and innervation of the articular capsule. J Bone Joint Surg 32(B):84–92, 1950

32. Kerr FW, Wilson PR: Pain. Annu Rev Neurosci 1:83–102, 1978

33. Leavitt F, Garron DC: Psychological disturbance and pain report differences in both organic and non-organic low back pain patients. Pain 7:187–195, 1979

34. Lindblom U, Tegner R: Are the endorphins active in clinical pain states? Narcotic antagonism in chronic pain patients. Pain 7:65–68, 1979

35. Loeser JD, Black RG: A taxonomy of pain. Pain 1:81–84, 1975

36. Mayer DJ, Liebeskind JC: Pain reduction by focal electrical stimulation of the brain: An anatomical and behavioral analysis. Brain Res 68:73–93, 1974

37. Mayer DJ, Murphin R: Stimulation-produced analgesia (SPA) and morphine analgesia: Cross tolerance from application at the same brain site. Fed Proc 35:385, 1976

38. Mayer DJ, Price DD: Central nervous system mechanisms of analgesia. Pain 2:379–404, 1976

39. Mayer DJ, Price DD, Rafii A, Barber J: Acupuncture hypalgesia: Evidence for activation of a central control system as a mechanism of action. In Proceedings of the First World Congress on Pain. New York, Raven Press, 1976

40. Mayer DJ, Wolfe TL, Akil H, Carder B, Liebeskind JC: Analgesia from electrical stimulation in the brain stem of the rat. Science 174:1351–1354, 1971

41. Melzack R: The gate theory revisited. In LeRoy PL (ed): Current Concepts in the Management of Chronic Pain. Miami, Symposia Specialists, 1977

42. Melzack R, Wall PD: On the nature of cutaneous sensory mechanisms. Brain 85:331–356, 1962

43. Messing RB, Lytle LD: Serotonin-containing neurons: Their possible role in pain and analgesia. Pain 4:1–21, 1977

44. Millan MJ, Przewlocki R, Herz A: A non-β-endorphin adenohypophyseal mechanism is essential for an analgetic response to stress. Pain 8:343–353, 1980

45. Nathan PW: The gate-control theory of pain—A critical review. Brain 99:123–158, 1976

46. Oleson TD, Twombly DA, Liebeskind JC: Effects of pain-attenuating brain stimulation and morphine on electrical activity in the raphe nuclei of the awake rat. Pain 4:211–230, 1978

47. Oliveras JL, Woda A, Guilbaud G, Besson JM: Analgesia induced by electrical stimulation of the inferior centralis of the raphe in the cat. Pain 1:139–145, 1975

48. Proudfit HK, Anderson ED: Morphine analgesia: Blockade by raphe magnus lesions. Brain Res 98:612–618, 1975

49. Rhodes DL: Periventricular system lesions and stimulation-produced analgesia. Pain 7:51–63, 1979

50. Roberts AH, Reinhardt L: The behavioral management of chronic pain: Long-term follow-up with comparison groups. Pain 8:151–162, 1980

51. Sinclair DC, Weddell G, Feindel WH: Referred pain and associated phenomena. Brain 7:184–211, 1948

52. Snyder SH: Opiate receptors and internal opiates. Sci Am 240(3):44–56, 1977

53. Stacher G, Bauer P, Steinringer A, Schreiber E, Schmierer G: Effects of the synthetic enkephalin analogue FK 33-824 on pain threshold and pain tolerance in man. Pain 7:159–172, 1979

54. Wall PD: The gate control theory of pain mechanisms—A re-examination and restatement. Brain 101:1–18, 1978

55. Weddell G, Palmer E, Pallie W: Nerve endings in mammalian skin. Biol Rev 30:159–193, 1954

56. Wyke B: Neurological mechanisms in the experience of pain. Acupuncture and Electro-Therapeutical Research International Journal 4:27–35, 1979

57. Yaksh TL, Rudy TA: Narcotic analgetics: CNS sites and mechanisms of action as revealed by intracerebral injection techniques. Pain 4:299–359, 1978

58. Yeung JC, Yaksh TL, Rudy TA: Concurrent mapping of brain sites for sensitivity to the direct application of morphine and focal electrical stimulation in the production of antinociception in the rat. Pain 4:23–40, 1977

RECOMMENDED READINGS

Adler M: Endorphins, enkephalins and neurotransmitters. Medical Times 110:32–37, 1982

Aronoff GM (ed): Evaluation and Treatment of Chronic Pain. Baltimore, Urban & Schwarzenberg, 1985

Basbaum AI, Fields HL: Endogenous pain control systems: Brain-stem spinal pathways and endorphin circuitry. Ann Rev Neurosci 7:309–338, 1984

Biedenbach MA, Van Hassel HJ, Brown AC: Tooth pulp–driven neurons in somatosensory cortex of primates: Role in pain mechanisms including a review of the literature. Pain 7:31–50, 1979

Bond MR: Pain: Its Nature, Analysis and Treatment. New York, Churchill Livingstone, 1984

Booker J: Pain: It's all in your patient's head (or is it?). Nursing 82:47–51, 1982

Browne RB, Segal DS: Alterations in beta-endorphin–induced locomotor activity in morphine-tolerant rats. Neuropharmacology 197:619–621, 1980

Burrows GD, Elton D, Stanley GV (eds): Handbook of Chronic Pain Management. Amsterdam, Elsevier, 1987

Chapman CR, Turner JA: Psychological control of acute pain in medical setting. J Pain Symptom Management 1:9–20, 1986

Clelland J, Savinar E, Shepard KF: The role of the physical therapist in chronic pain management. In Burrows GD, Elton D, Stanley GV: Handbook of Chronic Pain. Amsterdam, Elsevier, 1987

Cousins MJ, Bridenbaugh PO: Neural Blockade in Clinical Anesthesia and Management of Pain, 2nd ed. Philadelphia, JB Lippincott, 1988

Dubner R, Bennett GJ: Spinal and trigeminal mechanisms of nociception. Ann Rev Neurosci 6:381–418, 1983

Echtenach JL (ed): Pain. New York, Churchill Livingstone, 1987

Edmeads J: The physiology of pain: A review. Prog Neuropsychopharmacol Biol Psychiatry 7:413–419, 1983

Feinstein B, Langton NJ, Jameson RM, Schiller F: Experiments on pain referred from deep somatic tissues. J Bone Joint Surg 36(A):981–997, 1954

Fields HL: Pain. New York, McGraw-Hill, 1987

Fields HL, Dubner FC, Jones LE (eds): Advances in Pain Research and Therapy, vol 9. New York, Raven Press, 1984

Fields HL, Heinricher MM: Anatomy and physiology of a nociceptive modulatory system. Philos Trans R Soc Lond [Biol] 13:361–374, 1985

Fordyce WE: Evaluating and managing chronic pain. Geriatrics 33:59–62, 1978

France RD, Krishnam KRR: Chronic pain. Washington, DC, American Psychiatric Press, 1988

Gerhart KD, Yezierski RP, Giesler GJ, Willis WD: Inhibitory receptive fields of primate spinothalamic tract cells. J Neurophysiol 46:1309–1325, 1981

Grieves GP: Referred pain and other clinical features. In Grieves GP (ed): Modern Manual Therapy of the Vertebral Column. New York, Churchill Livingstone, 1986

Grieves GP: The autonomic nervous system in vertebral pain syndromes. In Grieves GP (ed): Modern Manual Therapy of the Vertebral Column. New York, Churchill Livingstone, 1986

Hendler N, Long DM, Wise TN: Diagnosis and Treatment of Chronic Pain. Boston, John Wright and PSG Inc, 1982

Herbert W. Placebo: Killing pain without opiates. Sci News 124:359–364, 1983

Hokfelt T, Ljundahl A, Ternius L et al: Immunohistochemical analysis of peptide pathways possibly related to pain analgesia: Enkephalin and substance P. Proc Natl Acad Sci USA 74:3081–3085, 1977

Howe JF: A neurophysiological basis for the radicular pain of nerve root compression. In Bonica JJ (ed): Advances in Pain Research and Therapy. New York, Raven Press, 1979

International Association on the Study of Pain: Abstracts of the Fifth World Congress. Amsterdam, Elsevier, 1987

Jassell TM: The role of substance P in sensory transmission and pain perception. In Martin JB, Reichlin S, Bick KL (eds): Neurosecretion and Brain Peptides. New York, Raven Press, 1981

Jensen TS: Endogenous antinociceptive systems: Studies on spinal and supraspinal modulating mechanisms with particular reference to monoaminergic and opioid systems. Acta Neurol Psychol (Suppl) 108:1–51, 1986

Kruger L, Liegeskind JC (eds): Advances in Pain Research and Therapy, vol 6. New York, Raven Press, 1981

Lembeck F, Folkers K, Donnerer J: Analgesic effect of antagonists of substance P. Biochem Biophys Res Commun 103:1318–1321, 1981

Lewis T: Suggestions relating to the study of somatic pain. Br Med J 1:321–327, 1938

Lewis T, Kellgran JH: Observation relating to referred pain, visceromotor reflexes and other associated phenomena. Clin Sci 49:470–471, 1939

Lundberg TCM: Vibratory stimulation for the alleviation of chronic pain. Acta Physiol Scand (suppl 523), 1983

Mannheimer JS: Clinical Transcutaneous Electrical Nerve Stimulation. Philadelphia, FA Davis, 1984

Marx J: Analgesia: How the body inhibits pain perception. Science 195:471–473, 1977

Mayer D, Price D, Rahi T: Antagonism of acupuncture analgesia in man by the narcotic antagonist naloxone. Brain Res 21:368–372, 1977

McCormack GL: Pain management by occupational therapists. Am J Occup Ther 42:582–590, 1988

Melzack R: Myofascial trigger points: Relation to acupuncture and mechanisms of pain. Arch Phys Med Rehab 62:114–117, 1981

Melzack R: Pain Measurement and Assessment. New York, Raven Press, 1983

Melzack R, Loeser JD: Phantom body pain in paraplegia: Evidence for a central pattern generating mechanism for pain. Pain 4:195–210, 1978

Melzack R, Wall PD: Pain mechanisms: A new theory. Science 150:971–979, 1965

Mense S: Sensitization of group IV muscle receptors to bradykinin by 5-hydroxytryptamine and prostaglandin E2. Brain Res 225:95–105, 1981

Merskey H: Classification of Chronic Pain: Description of Chronic Pain Syndromes and Definitions of Pain Terms. Amsterdam, Elsevier, 1986

Nathan PW: The gate-control theory of pain: A critical review. Brain 99:123–158, 1976

Newburger P, Sallan S: Chronic pain: Principles of management. J Pediatr 98:180–186, 1981

Nigl AJ: Biofeedback and Behavioral Strategies in Pain Treatment. New York, SP Medical and Scientific Books, 1984

Paklovitz M: Distributions of neuropeptides in central nervous system: Biochemical mapping studies. Prog Neurobiol 23:151–189, 1984

Pertovarra A: Modification of human pain threshold by specific tactile receptors. Acta Physiol Scand 107:339–341, 1979

Piercey MF, Folkers K: Sensory and motor function of spinal cord substance P. Science 214:1361–1365, 1981

Procacci P, Maresca M, Zoppi M: Visceral and deep somatic pain. Acupunct Electrother Res Int J 3:135–160, 1978

Porter R, O'Connor M (eds): Substance P in the nervous system. Ciba Foundation Symposium 91. London, Pitman, 1982

Prithvi Raj P: Practical Management of Pain: With Special

Emphasis on Physiology of Pain Management. Chicago, Year Book Medical Publishers, 1986

Ruda MA, Bennett GJ, Dubner R: Neurochemistry and neural circuitry in the dorsal horn. Prog Brain Res 66:219–268, 1986

Snyder S: Neurosciences: An integrative discipline. Science 225:1255–1257, 1984

Swendlow M: The Therapy of Pain. Philadelphia, JB Lippincott, 1981

Terman G, Shavit Y, Lewis J, Cannon T, Liebeskind M: Intrinsic mechanisms of pain inhibition: Activated by stress. Science 226:1270–1278, 1984

Tiengo M et al (eds): Pain and mobility. In Advances in Pain Research and Therapy, vol 10. New York, Raven Press, 1987

Vallbo A, Hagbarth H, Torebjork H: Somatosensory, proprioception, sympathetic activity in human peripheral nerves. Physiol Rev 59:919–957, 1979

Wall PD: On the relation of injury to pain. Pain 6:253–264, 1979

Wall PD, Melzack R (eds): The Textbook of Pain. Edinburgh, Churchill Livingstone, 1984

Watson J: Pain and nociception—mechanism and modulation. In Grieve GP (ed): Modern Manual Therapy of the Vertebral Column. New York, Churchill Livingstone, 1986

Weddell G, Sinclair DC: "Pins and needles": Observations on some of the sensations aroused in a limb by the application of pressure. J Neurol Neurosurg Psychiatry 10:26–46, 1947

Well PE, Frampton V, Bowster D (eds): Pain Management in Physical Therapy. Norwalk, CT, Appleton and Lange, 1988

West A: Understanding endorphins: Our natural pain relief system. Nursing 81:50–53, 1981

Willis WD: The pain system: The neural basis of nociceptive transmission in the mammalian nervous system. Pain Headache 8:1–346, 1985

Yiannikas C, Shahani BE, Phil D: Painful sequelae of injuries to peripheral nerves. Am J Phys Med 63:53–83, 1984

4 Assessment of Musculoskeletal Disorders

Randolph M. Kessler and Darlene Hertling

RATIONALE

A comprehensive examination is, without question, the most important step in the physical therapist's management of patients with common musculoskeletal disorders. The physical therapist's role is to clarify the nature and extent of the lesion, to assess the extent of the resulting disability, and to record significant data in order to establish a basis against which to judge progress. These activities must not be confused with or mistaken for the physician's diagnosis. A diagnosis, in addition to clinical evaluation, often requires the use and interpretation of laboratory tests, roentgenograms, and other data employing skills and knowledge not included in the physical therapist's training. A diagnosis must *differentiate* a particular disease state from other possible causes of the symptoms and signs. The therapist, in performing a *clarifying* examination, is not concerned with such differentiation but with collecting qualitative and quantitative data on the existing lesion, so as to judge how best to apply certain treatment procedures and to assess their effectiveness.

Consider the case of a patient referred to a therapist with the diagnosis of "shoulder tendinitis." This is a condition easily managed by physical therapy over a relatively short period of time. However, in order for an effective program to be instituted, several features of the problem must be clarified. The therapist must determine which tendon is at fault in order to know where to direct treatment and at what site on the tendon the lesion exists. Assessment of the lesion's chronicity will influence the choice of treatment procedures and their application. It is important to know whether secondary problems such as stiffness or weakness exist; if so, they must be dealt

with as well. The therapist must obtain information concerning the possible behavioral effects of the lesion. Are the conditions accompanying the problem reinforcing in any way to the patient's disease behaviors or is the patient "highly motivated"? Daily activities must be assessed, not only to determine the existence of any functional deficit but also to judge whether any present activity will aggravate or prolong the condition. Generally, such information does not accompany the referral, but it is precisely this information that is required in order to institute an effective treatment program. The physical therapist must perform a thorough initial examination on every patient to be treated.

As mentioned, information collected as part of the initial examination is used to set a baseline against which to judge progress and to assess the effectiveness of treatment. Therefore, the therapist not only must perform a complete initial examination but also must assess certain key signs before, during, and after each treatment session. In this way the clinician can determine whether, in fact, a particular procedure is effective and can quantitatively document the patient's progress. Progress must be judged on objective evidence. The patient's subjective report of the degree of pain must be considered but not dwelt on; in itself, it is not a valid measurement of progress. Instead, the therapist should be able to inform the patient as to whether the condition has improved. Treatment sessions should begin less often with, "Hello, Mrs. Jones. How is your back today?" but rather with, "Hello, Mrs. Jones. Let's take a look at your back to see how it's doing." This approach is possible only after complete initial examination and continued assessment of objective signs.

There are, of course, several approaches to patient examination. It is most important that the examination of musculoskeletal disorders be systematized. This avoids the possibility of omitting a crucial test or step, which may prevent accurate interpretation. Perhaps no one has contributed more to systematization of soft-tissue examination than James Cyriax. (His approach is well described in his book *Textbook of Orthopaedic Medicine* and should be reviewed by anyone dealing with patients with common musculoskeletal disorders.)[1] The format set out here is fashioned after Cyriax's approach. It consists of the history, physical examination, and correlation interpretation.

HISTORY

To help determine the nature and extent of the lesion and the resultant degree of disability, the clinician must gather data from the patient that cannot be determined by physical examination. These subjective findings are correlated with the findings of the physical examination.

In the case of common musculoskeletal disorders the lesion is usually manifested primarily by pain. Some of the routine questions suggested here as part of every history are directed at obtaining a complete account of the history of the pain and the present status of the pain as perceived by the patient. However, the clinician must also inquire about other symptoms, such as paresthesias, feelings of weakness, feelings of instability, and autonomic disturbances. It is important to keep in mind that the patient's perception of pain and other symptoms offers valuable clues to the nature and extent of the lesion but does not alone serve as an indicator of progress. Instead assessment of objective signs and examination of the patient's functional status must be relied on.

Determination of the degree of disability does offer some data by which to legitimately judge progress. It also yields information concerning the nature and extent of the lesion. This is an important part of the history and is too often omitted. To determine the degree of disability the patient's "health-state" behaviors and activity level (occupation, recreation, and other activities of daily life) can be assessed, as well as the patient's "disease-state" behaviors and activity level. Documentation of the disease-state behaviors will set a baseline against which to judge progress; comparison with the patient's health-state behaviors may provide clues to the nature and extent of the problem. For example, the patient with a shoulder problem who has been able to comb her hair all her life but since the onset of the problem is unable to do so lacks full, pain-free active elevation and external rotation. This is very suggestive of a capsular restriction. In this example there are some data to compare with the physical findings that may

help determine the nature and extent of the lesion. One treatment goal will naturally be restoring the patient's ability to comb her hair. A criterion by which to judge progress has also been established. Consequently, when judging progress, the clinician must be less concerned with whether Mrs. Jones had shoulder pain that morning and its extent or duration and more concerned with whether Mrs. Jones was able to comb her hair or fasten her bra.

Disability assessment and disease-state behavior assessment become especially important in evaluating patients with a chronic-pain state but no physical findings or pain that is out of proportion to physical findings and in evaluating patients with a permanent functional deficit from some serious pathologic process. In the first situation, it is often necessary to change from a "medical model," in which treatment is aimed at the lesion in order to change behavior, to an "operant model," in which treatment is aimed at altering the consequences to the disease state behaviors.[2-4] In the second situation, treatment is no longer directed at the primary lesion, such as a spinal cord lesion but rather at improving residual function. There are some relatively common disorders in which pain complaints and functional disability are out of proportion to the extent of the pathologic process. Some of these abnormal pain states, such as reflex sympathetic dystrophy (see Chapter 12, The Wrist and Hand Complex), have a physiological basis. Other cases, such as those involving pending litigation, substantial monetary compensation, or welcomed time away from activities the patient finds undesirable, may have a psychosocial basis. The patient's pain or disability may promise rewards, which may in turn reinforce disease-state behaviors. It is essential that the presence of such abnormal behavior states be determined on examination. In these cases, treatment aimed primarily at some physical pathologic process may only serve to maintain the patient's disability. Primary emphasis must be placed on improved function by altering the consequences of the disabled state (Fig. 4–1).

Although this text emphasizes the assessment and treatment of the lesion itself, clinicians must not lose sight of the fact that they are treating patients and that the ultimate goal in any treatment program is rehabilitation of the patient. Even when treatment is aimed largely at the lesion, care must be taken not to reinforce the disease-state, especially pain behavior. Similarly, clinicians must also be concerned with functional deficits associated with the disease state and see that they are resolved, when possible, along with the primary pathologic process. Thus, whether patient management is approached through a "medi-

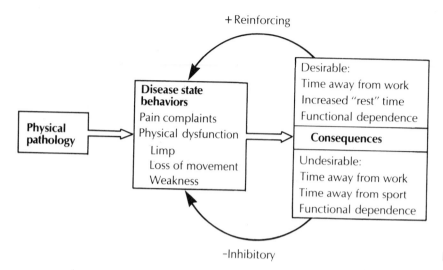

Fig. 4–1. Disability scheme.

cal model" or through an "operant model," the primary goal is to restore health-state behaviors. When a well-defined lesion exists, and the consequences of the resulting disability appear to have a negative effect on the patient's attitude toward the disability, it can be reasonably expected that resolving the pathologic process will restore health-state behavior. However, when the consequences of disability are rewarding to the patient, treatment of the pathologic process may have little or no effect.

The specific inquiries during the initial history naturally vary according to the site of the lesion, the nature of the lesion, and other factors. Questions that are particularly important for specific anatomical regions will be discussed in the respective chapters dealing with those regions. There are, however, certain routine inquiries that should be included in virtually every case.

The most efficient method of obtaining subjective information is to direct a list of specific, predetermined questions to the patient. However, this is not always the *best* method for eliciting certain important pieces of information, and it is certainly not the best method for developing the most effective patient–health care professional relationship. The direct-question approach is close-ended; it assumes that the relevant information will fall into predetermined categories, and it does not encourage consideration of factors outside these categories. It leads or directs the line of inquiry to specific categories. The patient often attempts to please the examiner by providing information related to these categories but not necessarily pertinent to the problem at hand. Alternatively, a more open-ended approach guides the discussion but does not restrict information to

certain categories. Furthermore, it allows the patient the freedom to relate what the patient feels is important, in addition to what the examiner may feel is important. The open-ended patient interview is structured to be a discussion session rather than a question-and-answer period. The examiner structures the discussion carefully, however, to elicit the necessary information.

A close-ended, direct-question method of interviewing creates a patient–therapist relationship in which the therapist assumes the authoritarian role of "healer" while the patient assumes a passive role. Within this relationship the patient need only provide the requested information, after which the examiner will perform the appropriate tests, decide what the problem is, and correct it. Such an approach favors the assumption that there is a specific pathologic process that the therapist will treat while the patient assumes a relatively passive role in the treatment program. This is consistent with a medical model of patient management and excludes from the outset the possibility of an operant disease-state or an operant approach to management.

In an open-ended interview, the therapist and patient discuss the patient's problem on a one-to-one basis. The therapist maintains a position as an expert in the field by virtue of the professional atmosphere in which the interview takes place. The patient is the expert with respect to the particular problem, being more familiar with it than anyone else. The interview serves as a forum in which the patient is encouraged to offer information and insight concerning the problem in return for advice and help in overcoming it. Both patient and therapist maintain distinct roles but remain equals. They establish an understanding that mutual cooperation and effort are required to execute an effective treatment program.

There are appropriate uses for both the open-ended and closed-ended approaches to history taking. In all situations, it is important to begin the interview open-endedly to establish an effective professional relationship and to get a feeling for the patient's problem. But as the nature of the problem becomes more obvious, it is necessary to seek more detailed information by directing specific questions to the patient. However, even during a close line of questioning, examiners must avoid asking leading questions that may elicit irrelevant or inaccurate information. For example, instead of asking, "Does the pain travel down the arm?" the examiner should ask, "Is the pain felt in any other parts?" Instead of, "Do you have a lot of pain in the morning?" one might ask, "When do you typically feel the pain?" The same is true when inquiring about disability. Rather than asking if a particular activity is painful or difficult, one should ask, "Which activities are particularly painful or difficult to perform?" In this way the patient is responsible for judging what information in a particular category is important and is less likely to provide information primarily for the purpose of satisfying the examiner.

The following list of questions is presented to indicate the type of information one should attempt to elicit. As much of the information as possible should be obtained through an open-ended discussion in an environment in which the patient feels free to discuss his problem and provide related information. The setting should be quiet, private, and free from disturbances. The examiner should be seated, and the patient should still be in street clothes. Following a well-structured discussion, any information that has not come out should be sought through specific questions. The discussion should end with a fairly open-ended question, as indicated below, to reestablish an appropriate working relationship.

1. Tell me about your problem.
The patient referred for a back problem may be more concerned with his prostatic neoplasm; some valuable information may be elicited by letting the patient discuss freely whatever he feels is most important. On the other hand, the patient is likely to go on for as long as the examiner allows. One should be prepared to interrupt politely by saying, for example, "I'm beginning to get an idea of the nature of your problem. Now I would like to obtain some specific information pertaining to it." The patient, having been allowed the opportunity to talk freely, is assured that the examiner is interested in him as a person and has begun to involve him in the therapeutic process by listening to his opinion.

2. Where, exactly, is your pain?
The patient is asked to indicate with one hand or one finger the primary area of pain and then any areas to which it might spread. It is important to determine whether in fact it does or does not spread.

— If the patient points to one, small, localized area and claims that the pain does not spread from it, the lesion is probably not severe or it is relatively superficial or both.
— If a diffuse area is indicated as the primary site, it suggests that the lesion is more severe or more deeply situated or both.
— If the pain spreads, determine if it is confined to a segment. If so, determine if it follows a well-delineated pathway, as in dermatomic radiation, or if it is more diffuse, as in sclerotomic reference of pain. Well-delineated, radiating pain suggests pressure on a nerve root in which the A-delta fibers are irritated but still transmitting. Diffuse, segmental referred pain may have its origin in the viscera, a deep somatic structure, or a nerve root in which the large myelinated fibers are no longer conducting but the small C fibers are. Cyriax proposes that some structures such as the dura mater and viscera will refer pain extrasegmentally.[1]
— In general, reference of pain is favored by a strong stimulus (a severe lesion), a lesion of deep somatic structures or nerve tissues, and a lesion lying fairly proximally (since pain is more often referred distally than proximally).

3. When did the present pain arise? Was the onset gradual or sudden? Was an injury or unusual activity involved?
An insidious onset unrelated to injury or unusual activity should always be viewed with suspicion since this history is typical of a neoplasm. However, degenerative lesions or lesions due to tissue fatigue are common and may also arise in this manner. If the patient blames some injury or activity, keep in mind that he may or may not be correct. The exact nature of the event or mechanism of injury should be determined so that correlation can be made to symptoms and signs for interpretation. Determining the direction and

nature of forces producing the injury may give some clues as to which tissues may have been stressed.

4. *What is the quality of the pain (sharp, dull, burning, tingling, aching, constant, boring, excruciating, etc.)? Has it changed at all in quality or intensity since its onset?*
   —Sharp, well-localized pain suggests a superficial lesion.
   —Sharp, lancinating, shooting pain suggests a nerve lesion, usually at a nerve root, presumably affecting the A-delta fibers.
   —Tingling suggests stimulation of nerve tissue affecting A-alpha fibers. A segmental distribution suggests a nerve root; a peripheral nerve distribution implicates that nerve. Tingling in both hands, both feet, or all four extremities suggests spinal cord involvement or some other more serious pathologic process.
   —Dull, aching pain is typical of pain of deep somatic origin.
   —Excruciating pain, unrelenting pain, intolerable pain, and deep, boring pain all suggest a serious lesion.
   —Change in intensity of the pain may offer some clue as to the progression of the problem. This must be considered when treatment begins. If the patient's condition was getting worse prior to treatment and continues to worsen once treatment has begun, then the treatment has probably not been effective. However it is probably not the cause of the worsening following initiation of treatment. On the other hand, if the patient's condition had been improving but stops getting better or gets worse once treatment has begun, the treatment is probably at fault.
   —Change in quality of the pain may offer many clues as to the nature and extent of the lesion. Progression of nerve-root pressure, such as from a disk protrusion, typically leads to rather marked changes in symptoms (see Chapter 3, Pain).

5. *What aggravates the pain? What relieves it? Is it any better or worse in the morning or evening? When do you typically feel pain?*
   —Pain *not* aggravated by activity or relieved by rest should be suspected as arising from some pathologic process other than a common musculoskeletal disorder. The exception is a disk problem that may be aggravated by sitting and relieved by getting up and walking.
   —Morning *pain* is suggestive of arthritis, espe-

cially the inflammatory varieties. Morning *stiffness* is suggestive of degenerative joint disease or chronic arthritis.
   —Pain awakening the patient at night is typical of shoulder or hip problems that may be aggravated by lying on the affected side. Otherwise, a more serious problem should be suspected, particularly if the patient is kept awake and especially if he must get up and walk about.
   —Arthritis in weight-bearing joints leads to pain on fatigue (long walks, etc.) in its early stages. In later stages, the pain is felt when beginning a walk, somewhat relieved once going, and returns after walking too far.

6. *Have you had this problem in the past? If so, how was it resolved? Did you seek help? Was there any treatment? Is the pain the same this time?*
   Should the examiner elicit a history of recurrence, the patient might be asked in depth about the first episode and the most recent episode, with an estimate of the number of intervening episodes. Recurrences are typical of spinal cord lesions, but many common extremity lesions such as ankle sprains, minor meniscus lesions or other internal derangements, minor degenerative joint problems, tendinitis, and frozen shoulder also may tend to recur.

   By inquiring about previous management, some helpful information may also be obtained for treatment planning. However, the patient's judgment of the effectiveness or value of previous treatment must not be weighed too heavily. If an injection helped before, for example in the case of supraspinatus tendinitis, it does not necessarily follow that another injection is necessary or indicated. If physical therapy (perhaps inadequately instituted) was unsuccessful in the past, do not assume that it will not be helpful on this occasion.

7. *Are there any other symptoms that you have or have had that you associate with the problem, such as grinding, popping, giving way, numbness, tingling, weakness, dizziness, or nausea?*
   By concentrating on the patient's account of pain, the examiner may well overlook some other important symptoms. A wide variety of responses may be elicited with this question, each of which must be carefully weighed and considered. A patient's description of "numbness" is very often not true hypesthesia but is actually

referred pain. In most cases, considerable weakness must be present before the patient can accurately perceive it as such, and very often what the patient describes as "weakness" is actually instability or giving way. Symptoms inconsistent with musculoskeletal dysfunction must be viewed with some suspicion and medical consultation sought for interpretation.

8. *How has this problem affected your dressing, grooming, or other daily activities? Has it affected your ability to work at your job or around the house? Has it affected or altered your recreational activities? Is there anything that it difficult or impossible for you to do since the onset of this problem?*

The patient's normal occupation and daily activity level is determined. The existence of a functional deficit often contributes to interpretation of the problem by considering the demands placed on various musculoskeletal structures in performing the task. Later quantification of the deficit or residual function during physical examination will set a baseline against which to assess progress.

Any functional deficit must be correlated later with the apparent nature of the lesion, and any inconsistencies must be considered. In cases involving compensation or litigation, the disease-state may be reinforced in such a way that a functional deficit is no longer the result of the problem but rather its cause.

9. *What treatment are you having or have you had for the present problem? Are you taking any medications for this problem or for any other reason?*

Here again, it may or may not be helpful to determine whether certain attempts at treatment have had any good or bad effects, especially treatments involving physical agents.

The examiner must determine whether pain medications, anti-inflammatory agents, or muscle relaxants are being taken. Symptoms or signs may be masked accordingly. Certain medications may produce rather marked musculoskeletal changes (in addition to effects on other tissues and functions). Most important, perhaps, is the long-term use of corticosteroids, which produces osteoporosis; proximal muscle weakness; generalized tissue edema; thin, fragile skin; collagen tissue weakening; and increased pain threshold. These factors, of course, will affect findings on examination. More importantly,

however, they must be considered when planning treatment.

10. *How is your general health?*

It is necessary to determine whether the patient has or has had any disease process or health problem that may have contributed to the present problem or that may influence the choice of treatment procedures.

11. *Do you have any opinions of your own as to what the problem is?*

Some useful information may be elicited concerning what the patient has learned from others, what his insight is into the problem, and so on. If nothing else, the patient can be reassured that the examiner is interested in him and his opinions and that he is to be involved in the therapeutic program.

PHYSICAL EXAMINATION

A complete history performed by the experienced clinician will often be sufficient to determine the extent and nature of the lesion. Even so, the physical examination must not be excluded or cut short. Objective data are needed to facilitate or confirm the interpretation of subjective findings. It is equally important that every effort be made to quantify objective data to allow documentation of a baseline and, therefore, accurate assessment of progress.

Specific tests and measurements will vary, of course, depending on the area to be examined and to a certain extent on the information obtained from the history. In this chapter we present a systematic approach that can be applied to any region to be evaluated; tests specific to particular regions will be discussed in the chapters on those regions. This discussion will include general guidelines and statements meant to assist in interpretation of findings. It should be noted that the order of testing procedures presented here is for the sake of conceptual organization. Clinically, tests must be organized according to patient positioning. This point will be elaborated in the chapters on specific regions.

Having discussed the phenomenon of referred pain, it should be apparent that at times clinicians may be at a loss as to which region should be singled out as the primary area to be examined. For example, elbow pain may have its origin locally or at the neck or shoulder, but surely it is not necessary that each of these areas be examined in depth. Fortunately, the physician's referral, the history, or both, will often implicate the involved area. However, this is not always the case. When such a difficulty arises, it is often helpful to perform a brief *scan examination.* This is done by asking the patient to actively move each joint within the suspected areas and by applying some passive overpressure to the extremes of each motion. If pain or dysfunction is noted at a particular area, it may be examined in depth. In general, every structure derived embryologically from the same segment must be considered as the segment or portion of a segment in which the patient indicates the pain exists.

The physical examination is organized as follows:

Observation
Inspection
Selective tissue tension
  Active movements
  Passive movements
  Resisted movements
Neuromuscular tests
Palpation

OBSERVATION

The patient's general appearance and functional status can be observed when he walks in, during dressing activities, during the examination and treatment session, and as he leaves. If specific functional disabilities are related during the history, the examiner may ask the patient to attempt to perform the involved activity in order to assess the exact degree and nature of the disability.

The patient's general appearance and body build —slim, obese, muscular, emaciated, short, tall— are noted and recorded. Obvious postural deviations as well as abnormalities in positionings of body parts are reported.

All functional abnormalities or deficits noted during the patient's visit are described as precisely as possible. These might typically include observations relating to gait, guarding of particular movements, use of compensatory or substitution movements, or use of certain aids or assistive devices.

INSPECTION

The inspection part of the examination entails a closer assessment of the patient's physical status. It is usually performed in conjunction with palpation, which is discussed later in this section. To avoid excluding crucial assessments, it is convenient and helpful to organize inspection of body parts according to the following three layers: bony structure and alignment, subcutaneous soft tissue, and skin.

Bony Structure and Alignment

Inspection of the bony structure and alignment is a critical component of the biomechanical examination, especially when correlated with specific functional abnormalities such as gait deviancies and altered range of motion. For example, a person with increased femoral anteversion is likely to present with a loss of external rotation at the hip, but with respect to his structure, a decrease in average external rotation is normal. If a careful assessment of static alignment were not made, one might make the mistake of attempting to restore external rotation in this case. Similarly, a common gait abnormality seen clinically is increased pronation of the hindfoot during stance phase. This often occurs secondary to structural malalignments elsewhere in the extremity, such as increased internal tibial torsion, increased femoral anteversion, or adduction of the first metatarsal. The ultimate cause of the pronation can only be determined through a careful structural examination. Assessment of structural alignment is likewise of utmost importance following the healing of fractures. A person who has sustained a Colles' fracture invariably ends up with some residual angulation dorsally and radially; restoration of full wrist flexion and ulnar deviation should never be expected. Thus, structural assessment becomes important in planning treatment as well as in setting treatment goals.

Assessment of a particular part in which some pathologic lesion may exist should often include structural assessment of biomechanically related parts. In the case of a patient with a low back disorder, the clinician should examine the alignment of the lower extremities and vice versa. The same is true for the cervical spine and upper extremities. Each part should be assessed with respect to frontal, sagittal, and transverse planes. Key bony landmarks are identified, and their relationships to fixed points of reference (*e.g.*, ground, wall, plumb-bob) as well as their relationships to each other are determined. In judging whether malalignments exist, clinicians must often rely on their experience of what is normal, as well as on comparison to a normal side in cases of unilateral problems. Malalignments should be documented through careful measurements when possible.

Specific assessments related to particular regions of the body will be discussed in the chapters on those body regions. The following list includes some key bony landmarks that must often be identified when testing structural alignment, and with which the clinician must become familiar:

Navicular tubercles
Talar heads
Malleoli
Fibular heads
Tibular heads
Patellar borders
Adductor tubercles
Greater trochanters
Ischial tuberosities
Posterior and anterior iliac spines
Iliac crests
Spinous processes
Scapular borders
Mastoid processes
Clavicles
Acromial processes
Greater tubercles
Olecranons
Humeral epicondyles
Radial and ulnar styloid processes
Lister's tubercles
Carpal bones

Subcutaneous Soft Tissues

The soft tissue is inspected and palpated for abnormalities. The examiner should look for swelling or increase in the size of an area, wasting or atrophy of the part, and alterations in the general contours of the region. When an increase in size is noted, an attempt should be made to distinguish the cause, whether generalized edema, articular effusion, muscle hypertrophy, or hypertrophic changes in other tissues. The area is examined for localized cysts, nodules, or ganglia. In the presence of wasting, the examiner should determine whether localized or generalized muscle atrophy exists or whether there is perhaps some loss of continuity of soft tissues.

Measurements should be taken to carefully document soft-tissue changes and to use as baseline measurements. Volumetric measurements of small parts, such as fingers, hands, and feet, can be made by measuring the displacement of water in a tub. Swelling or wasting elsewhere in an extremity can often be documented with circumferential measurements using a tape measure.

Skin and Nails

Local or generalized changes in the status of the skin are noted and recorded. These changes might include

—Changes in color either from vascular changes ac-

companying inflammation (erythema) or vascular deficiency (pallor or cyanosis).
—Changes in texture and moisture. These commonly accompany reflex sympathetic dystrophies, in which the sympathetic activity of the part becomes altered. Increased activity results in hyperhidrosis; smooth, glossy skin; cyanosis; atrophy of skin; and splitting of the nails. Decreased sympathetic activity may result in pink, dry, scaly skin.
—Local scars, distinct blemishes, abnormal hair patterns, calluses, blisters, open wounds, and other localized skin abnormalities. When a scar exists, whether surgical or traumatic, the type of surgery or injury should be determined because it may have some bearing on the present problem. Blemishes such as large, brownish, pigmented areas (*café au lait* spots) and localized hairy regions often accompany underlying bony defects, such as spina bifida. Calluses develop with increased shear or compressive stresses; blisters occur with increased shear between the skin and subcutaneous tissue. When an open wound is observed, the clinician should determine whether it is of traumatic origin or of insidious origin, as often accompanies diabetes.

Local skin changes are described according to size and location. Size can be most precisely documented by outlining the borders of the defect on a piece of acetate, such as old x-ray film.

SELECTIVE TISSUE TENSION TESTS

This portion of the examination consists of specific active-, passive-, and resisted-movement tests designed to assess the status of each of the component tissues of the physiological joint. When properly interpreted, findings from these tests can yield very specific information relating to both the nature and extent of the pathologic process. The organization and interpretation of these tests is largely the work of Cyriax and is certainly a significant contribution to the field.[1]

  I. **Active movements.** These yield very general information, relating primarily to the patient's functional status. They provide information concerning the patient's general willingness and ability to use the part. They offer no true indication of the range of motion or strength of a part. If a patient is asked to lift an arm overhead and only lifts it to horizontal, it cannot be determined at that point whether the loss of function is due to pain, weakness, or stiffness.

Therefore, active movement tests are used primarily to assess the patient's ability to perform common functional activities related to the part being evaluated. For lower extremity and spinal regions, then, active movements should be performed while bearing weight. Upper extremity parts should be moved in functional directions. At the shoulder, for example, internal and external rotation are performed by asking the patient to reach behind and to touch the back of the neck rather than rotating the humerus with the arm to the side.

The following should be noted and documented for the active movements tested:

A. *The patient's account of the onset of, or increase in, pain associated with the movement, and at what point or points in the range of movement the pain occurs.* The existence of a painful arc of movement is best detected on active, weight-bearing, or antigravity movements. A painful arc of movement, in which pain is felt throughout a small arc of movement in the midrange of motion, suggests an irritable structure being (1) pulled across a protuberance or (2) pinched between two structures. An example of the former is a nerve root pulled across a disk protrusion during straight-leg raises. An example of the latter is an inflamed supraspinatus tendon squeezed between the greater tubercle and the acromial arch during abduction of the arm.

B. *The range of motion through which the patient is able to move the part.* This should be measured by some easily reproducible method.

C. *The presence of crepitus.* This can usually be best detected on active movement, with the forces of weight-bearing or muscle contraction maintaining compression of joint surfaces. Crepitus usually indicates roughening of joint surfaces or increased friction between a tendon and its sheath due to swelling or roughening of either the tendon or the sheath. Fine crepitus at a joint suggests early wearing of articular cartilage or tendinous problems, whereas more course crepitus implies considerable cartilaginous degeneration. A creaking sound, not unlike that which a large tree makes when swaying in the wind, often occurs when bones articulate in the late stages of joint-surface degeneration.

II. Passive movements

A. *Passive range of motion testing.* The part is passively put through the major motions in the frontal, sagittal, and transverse planes that normally occur at the joint being moved. Very specific information concerning both the nature and extent of a disorder may be obtained by making the following assessments:

1. Range of movement. The examiner should determine whether movement is normal, restricted, or hypermobile. The degree of any abnormal movements is measured carefully. If there is restriction of movement at a joint, the first and foremost determination that should be made is whether the restriction is in a capsular or noncapsular pattern. (See Appendix A for a description of the capsular pattern of restriction at each joint.)

   a. Capsular patterns of restriction indicate loss of mobility of the entire joint capsule from fibrosis, effusion, or inflammation. Differentiation can be made by assessing the "end feel" at the extremes of movement (see below). Capsular restrictions typically accompany arthritis or degenerative joint disease (fibrosis, inflammation, or effusion), prolonged immobilization of a joint (fibrosis), or acute trauma to a joint (effusion).

   b. Noncapsular patterns of joint restrictions typically occur with intra-articular mechanical blockage or extra-articular lesions. Common causes include

      i. Isolated ligamentous or capsular adhesion. A common example of isolated ligamentous adhesion is that of adherence of the medial collateral ligament at the knee to the medial femoral condyle during healing of a sprain. This results in restriction of knee flexion to about 90°, with extension being of full range. Isolated anterior capsular tightness at the shoulder often occurs following an anterior dislocation, resulting in a disproportionate loss of external rotation.

      ii. Internal derangements, such as displacement of pieces of torn menisci and cartilaginous loose bodies. These typically produce a mechanical block to movement in a noncapsular pattern. The most common example is a "bucket handle" medial meniscus tear, resulting in blockage of knee extension, with flexion remaining relatively free in the absence of significant effusion.

    iii. Extra-articular tissue tightness, such as reduced lengthening of muscles from contracture (fibrosis) or myositis ossificans.

    iv. Extra-articular inflammation or swellings, such as those accompanying acute bursitis and neoplasms.

2. End feel at extremes of painful or restricted movements. This is the quality of the resistance to movement that the examiner feels when coming to the end point of a particular movement. Some end feels may be normal or pathologic, depending on the movement they accompany at a particular joint and the point in the range of movement at which they are felt. Other end feels are strictly pathologic.

  a. End feels that may be normal or pathologic include

    i. Capsular end feel. This is a firm, "leathery" feeling felt, for example, when forcing the normal shoulder into full external rotation. When felt in conjunction with a capsular pattern of restriction, and in the absence of significant inflammation or effusion, it indicates capsular fibrosis.

    ii. Bony end feel. This feels abrupt as when moving the normal elbow into full extension. When accompanying a restriction of movement, it may suggest hypertrophic bony changes, such as those that occur with degenerative joint disease, or possible malunion of bony segments following healing of a fracture.

    iii. Soft-tissue–approximation end feel. This is a soft end feel, as when fully flexing the normal elbow or knee. It may accompany joint restriction in the presence of significant muscular hypertrophy.

    iv. Muscular end feel. This more rubbery feel resembles what is felt at the extremes of straight-leg raising from tension on the hamstrings. It is less abrupt than a capsular end feel.

  b. End feels that are strictly pathologic include

    i. Muscle-spasm end feel. Movement is stopped fairly abruptly, perhaps with some "rebound," due to muscles contracting reflexively to prevent further movement. It usually accompanies pain felt at the point of restriction. When occurring with a capsular restriction, it indicates some degree of synovial inflammation of the portion of the joint capsule being stretched during the movement.

    ii. Boggy end feel. This is a very soft, mushy end feel that typically accompanies joint effusion in the absence of significant synovial inflammation. It will usually occur together with a capsular pattern of restriction.

    iii. Internal derangement end feel. This is often a pronounced, springy rebound at the end point of movement. It typically accompanies a noncapsular restriction from a mechanical block produced by a loose body or displaced meniscus.

    iv. Empty end feel. The examiner feels no restriction to movement, but movement is stopped at the insistence of the patient because of severe pain. This end feel is relatively rare except with acute bursitis at the shoulder or a few other painful extra-articular lesions such as neoplasms. The muscles do not contract to prevent movement since this would cause compression at the painful site and further pain.

3. Pain on movement and the point in the range in which it is felt

  a. Pain at the extremes of a movement indicates

    i. A painful structure is being stretched. In this case, one should consider first a lesion of the joint capsule or a ligament and second a lesion of a muscle or tendon. For biarticular muscles, the constant-length phenomenon can be used to differentiate the location. Otherwise one must correlate this finding with findings of resisted movement tests (see below) in order to differentiate between capsuloligamentous and musculotendinous lesions. If the lesion lies in a muscle or tendon, resistance to the movement opposite the direction of the painful passive movement will be painful, whereas resisted movements are painless with capsuloligamentous lesions.

    ii. A painful structure is being squeezed. This usually occurs with extra-articular lesions such as tendinitis and bursitis. An inflamed subdeltoid bursa is susceptible to impingement beneath the acromial arch; the trochanteric bursa is squeezed on abduction of the hip; the semimembranosus bursa, when swollen, is squeezed on full knee flexion. With supraspinatus tendinitis, pain will be felt on elevation of the arm from squeezing of the involved part of the tendon between the greater tuberosity and the posterior rim of the glenoid cavity.

  b. A painful arc may occur with passive movement tests. (See section on active movements for a discussion of its significance.)

4. Crepitus on movement. This is best detected by active movement testing but may be noted on passive movements as well. (See section on active movements for discussion.)

B. *Passive joint play movement tests (capsuloligamentous stress tests)* are designed to stress various portions of the joint capsule and major ligaments to detect the presence of painful lesions affecting these structures or loss of continuity of these structures. The method of performing the movements and the various movements performed at each joint are the same as the movements included in the section on specific joint mobilization techniques. Instead of being performed therapeutically as rhythmic oscillations, the movements are performed as examination procedures. In doing so, one can assess

1. The degree of mobility (amplitude). The possibilities include

  a. Hypermobility, suggesting a loss of continuity (partial tear or complete rupture) of the structure being tested

  b. Hypomobility, suggesting fibrosis, as from increased laying down of collagen in the presence of chronic stresses and low-grade inflammation, or suggesting adhesion to adjacent structures, as may occur during healing of a sprain. Hypomobility may be due to protective muscle spasm, in which case some degree of inflammation of the structure or synovial lining is implied.

  c. Normal mobility, implying normal status of the structure being tested.

2. Presence of pain or muscle guarding (irritability) at extremes of movement. Pain on joint-play movement testing suggests the presence of a sprain or actual tear of the structure being stressed.

3. One must consider, then, six possible findings on joint-play movement testing and their probable interpretations.

  a. Normal mobility—painless. There is no lesion of the structure tested.

  b. Normal mobility—painful. There is a minor sprain of the structure tested.

  c. Hypomobility—painless. A contracture or adhesion involves the tested structure.

  d. Hypomobility—painful. A more acute sprain of the structure may be accompanied by guarding. If the hypomobility is due to muscle guarding, one cannot, at this point, know whether an actual tear or rupture exists.

  e. Hypermobility—painless. A complete rupture of the structure is suggested; there are no longer intact fibers from which pain can be elicited.

  f. Hypermobility—painful. A partial tear is present in which some fibers of the structure are still intact and being stressed.

III. Resisted isometric tests. These are tests designed to assess the status of musculotendinous tissue. Traditional muscle testing procedures that are included in the following section on neuromuscular tests are used primarily to evaluate neurologic function, while here the intention is to determine whether there is some lesion, or loss of continuity, of the musculotendinous tissue itself. In order to do so, ideally the clinician needs to stress the muscle and tendon that is to be tested without stressing other joint tissues. These tests are performed, then, as maximal, isometric contractions, disallowing any movement of the joint. Realistically, in most cases other tissues are going to be squeezed or compressed by the contracting muscles, but this seldom poses a problem when the test is done correctly. A particular muscle and tendon are tested in the position that best isolates them, and in a position in which they are at an optimal length for maximal contraction (usually a midposition). Maximal stabilization is required to prevent substitution and to minimize joint movement.

When performing resisted isometric tests, one must determine whether the contraction is strong or weak and whether it is painful or painless. Weakness may be due to a neurologic deficit or to actual loss of continuity of muscle or tendon tissue; appropriate neurologic testing may be performed to determine which is the case. Few neurologic disorders result in isolated weakness of a single muscle. A painful contraction signifies the presence of some painful lesion involving the muscle or tendon tissues being tested. In the majority of cases the problem will be in the tendon, since muscle strains are rare except in sports-related injuries. Very often the patient feels the most pain as the contraction is released rather than during maximal contraction. When this occurs, it should be considered a positive test; the lengthening that occurs as a muscle relaxes apparently stresses the involved fibers sufficiently to cause more pain than does the shortening that occurs during contraction. Practically speaking, these resisted tests are often performed in conjunction with standard neuromuscular strength tests.

There are four possible findings on resisted tests:
A. *Strong and painless.* There is no lesion or neurologic deficit involving the muscle or tendon tested.
B. *Strong and painful.* A minor lesion of the tested tendon or muscle exists; usually the tendon is at fault. Occasionally auxiliary resisted tests must be performed to differentiate the involved structure from synergists.
C. *Weak and painless*
 1. There may be some interruption of the nerve supply to the muscle tested. The

findings must be correlated with those of other muscle tests and neurologic tests.
 2. There may be a complete rupture of tendon or muscle; there are no longer fibers intact from which pain can be elicited.
D. *Weak and painful*
 1. There may be a partial rupture of muscle or tendon in which there are still some intact fibers that are being stressed.
 2. This may be the result of painful inhibition in association with some serious pathologic condition, such as a fracture or neoplasm or an acute inflammatory process.

NEUROMUSCULAR TESTS

If, at this point in the examination, one suspects that there may be a lesion interfering with neural conduction, the appropriate clinical tests should be performed in an attempt to detect loss of neurologic function. The common nerve lesions are extrinsic. Loss of conduction usually results from pressure on a nerve from some adjacent structure or structures. In the common nerve disorders, the pressure is usually minor, intermittent, or both and usually involves a single nerve or segment. For this reason, the manifestations of the disorder are often quite subtle; findings on evaluation are largely subjective, and some objective signs may be detected only with more sophisticated electrotesting procedures.

When neurologic function is assessed clinically, if a deficit is detected, the approximate site of the lesion can be estimated by correlating the extent of the deficit with peripheral nerve and segmental distributions. More central or serious lesions must be suspected when the extent of the deficit exceeds the distribution of a single segment or a single peripheral nerve. Peripheral nerve and segmental innervations are indicated in Table 4–1 and Figure 4–2. Key segmental distributions, both myotomal and dermatomal, are listed in Table 4–2. These are the muscles and skin areas that are most likely to be affected by involvement of a particular segment. These are important to know, since segmental deficits, such as those that occur with disk protrusions, are very common neural disorders seen clinically. Because of the overlapping of dermatomes and myotomes in the extremities, lesions involving a single segment, even when conduction is completely interrupted, result in only subtle deficits.

The tests described below may be used when performing clinical neurologic assessment.

Table 4–1. Peripheral Nerves and Segmental Innervation

ACTION TO BE TESTED	MUSCLES	CORD SEGMENT	NERVES	PLEXUS
Shoulder Girdle and Upper Extremity				
Flexion of neck Extension of neck Rotation of neck Lateral bending of neck	Deep neck muscles (sternomas-toid and trapezius also participate)	C1–C4	Cervical	Cervical
Elevation of upper thorax	Scaleni	C3–C5	Phrenic	
Inspiration	Diaphragm	C3–C5		
Adduction of arm from behind to front	Pectoralis major and minor	C5–C8 T1	Medial and lateral pectoral (from medial and lateral cords of plexus)	Brachial
Forward thrust of shoulder	Serratus anterior	C5–C7	Long thoracic	
Elevation of scapula	Levator scapulae	C5 (C3–C4)	Dorsal scapular	
Medial adduction and elevation of scapula	Rhomboids	C4–C5		
Abduction of arm	Supraspinatus	C4–C6	Suprascapular	
Lateral rotation of arm	Infraspinatus	C4–C6		
Medial rotation of arm Adduction of arm front to back	Latissimus dorsi, teres major, and subscapularis	C5–C8	Subscapular (from posterior cord of plexus)	
Abduction of arm	Deltoid	C5–C6	Axillary (from posterior cord of plexus)	Brachial
Lateral rotation of arm	Teres minor	C4–C5		
Flexion of forearm Supination of forearm	Biceps brachii	C5–C6	Musculocutaneous (from lateral cord of plexus)	
Adduction of arm Flexion of forearm	Coracobrachialis	C5–C7		
Flexion of forearm	Brachialis	C5–C6		Brachial
Ulnar flexion of hand	Flexor carpi ulnaris	C7–T1	Ulnar (from medial cord of plexus)	
Flexion of terminal phalanx of ring finger and little finger Flexion of hand	Flexor digitorum profundus (ulnar portion)	C7–T1		
Adduction of metacarpal of thumb	Adductor pollicis	C8–T1	Ulnar	Brachial
Abduction of little finger	Abductor digiti quinti	C8–T1		
Opposition of little finger	Opponens digiti quinti	C7–T1		
Flexion of little finger	Flexor digiti quinti brevis	C7–T1		
Flexion of proximal phalanx; extension of two distal phalanges; adduction and abduction of fingers	Interossei	C8–T1		
Pronation of forearm	Pronator teres	C6–C7	Median (C6,C7 from lateral cord of plexus; C8, T1 from medial cord of plexus)	Brachial
Radial flexion of hand	Flexor carpi radialis	C6–C7		
Flexion of hand	Palmaris longus	C7–T1		
Flexion of middle phalanx of index, middle, ring, little fingers Flexion of hand	Flexor digitorum sublimis	C7–T1		
Flexion of terminal phalanx of thumb	Flexor pollicis longus	C7–T1	Median	Brachial
Flexion of terminal phalanx of index finger, and middle finger Flexion of hand	Flexor digitorum profundus (radial portion)	C7–T1		
Abduction of metacarpal of thumb	Abductor pollicis brevis	C7–T1	Median	Brachial
Flexion of proximal phalanx of thumb	Flexor pollicis brevis	C7–T1		
Opposition of metacarpal of thumb	Opponens pollicis	C8–T1		
Flexion of proximal phalanx and extension of 2 distal phalanges of all fingers	Lumbricals (the two lateral) Lumbricals (the two medial)	C8–T1	Median Ulnar	Brachial
Extension of forearm	Triceps brachii and anconeus	C6–C8	Radial (from posterior cord of plexus)	Brachial
Flexion of forearm	Brachioradialis	C5–C6		
Radial extension of hand	Extensor carpi radialis	C6–C8		
Extension of phalanges of fingers Extension of hand	Extensor digitorum communis	C6–C8		
Extension of phalanges of little finger Extension of hand	Extensor digiti quinti proprius	C6–C8		

Table 4–1. *(Continued)*

ACTION TO BE TESTED	MUSCLES	CORD SEGMENT	NERVES	PLEXUS
Shoulder Girdle and Upper Extremity				
Ulnar extension of hand	Extensor carpi ulnaris	C6–C8	Radial	Brachial
Supination of forearm	Supinator	C5–C7		
Abduction of metacarpal of thumb	Abductor pollicis longus	C7–C8		
Radial extension of hand				
Extension of thumb	Extensor pollicis brevis and longus	C6–C8		
Radial extension of hand				
Extension of index finger	Extensor indicis proprius	C6–C8		
Extension of hand				
Trunk and Thorax				
Elevation of ribs	Thoracic, abdominal, and back		Thoracic and posterior lumbro-sacral branches	
Depression of ribs				
Contraction of abdomen				
Anteroflexion of trunk				
Lateral flexion of trunk				
Hip Girdle and Lower Extremity				
Flexion of hip	Iliopsoas	L1–L3	Femoral	Lumbar
Flexion of hip and eversion of thigh	Sartorius	L2–L3		
Extension of leg	Quadriceps femoris	L2–L4		
Adduction of thigh	Pectineus	L2–L3	Obturator	Lumbar
	Adductor longus	L2–L3		
	Adductor brevis	L2–L4		
	Adductor magnus	L3–L4		
	Gracilis	L2–L4		
Adduction of thigh	Obturator externus	L3–L4		
Lateral rotation of thigh				
Abduction of thigh	Gluteus medius and minimus	L4–S1	Superior gluteal	Sacral
Medial rotation of thigh				
Flexion of thigh	Tensor fasciae latae	L4–L5		
Lateral rotation of thigh	Piriformis	L5–S1		
Abduction of thigh	Gluteus maximus	L4–S2	Inferior gluteal	
Lateral rotation of thigh	Obturator internus	L5–S1	Muscular branches from sacral plexus	
	Gemelli	L4–S1		
	Quadratus femoris	L4–S1		
Flexion of leg (assist in extension of thigh)	Biceps femoris	L4–S2	Sciatic (trunk)	Sacral
	Semitendinosus	L4–S1		
	Semimembranosus	L4–S1		
Dorsiflexion of foot	Tibialis anterior	L4–L5	Deep peroneal	Sacral
Supination of foot				
Extension of toes II–V	Extensor digitorum longus	L4–S1		
Dorsiflexion of foot				
Extension of great toe	Extensor hallucis longus	L4–S1		
Dorsiflexion of foot				
Extension of great toe and the three medial toes	Extensor digitorum bevis	L4–S1		
Plantar flexion of foot in pronation	Peronei	L5–S1	Superficial peroneal	Sacral
Plantar flexion of foot in supination	Tibialis posterior and triceps surae	L5–S2	Tibial	Sacral
Plantar flexion of foot in supination	Flexor digitorum longus	L5–S2		
Flexion of terminal phalanx of toes II–V				
Plantar flexion of foot in supination	Flexor hallucis longus	L5–S2		
Flexion of terminal phalanx of great toe				
Flexion of middle phalanx of toes II–V	Flexor digitorum brevis	L5–S1		
Flexion of proximal phalanx of great toe	Flexor hallucis brevis	L5–S2		
Spreading and closing of toes	Small muscles of foot	S1–S2		
Flexion of proximal phalanx of toes				
Voluntary control of pelvic floor	Perineal and sphincters	S2–S4	Pudendal	Sacral

(Chusid JG: Correlative Neuroanatomy and Functional Neurology. Los Altos, CA. Lange Medical Publications, 1970)

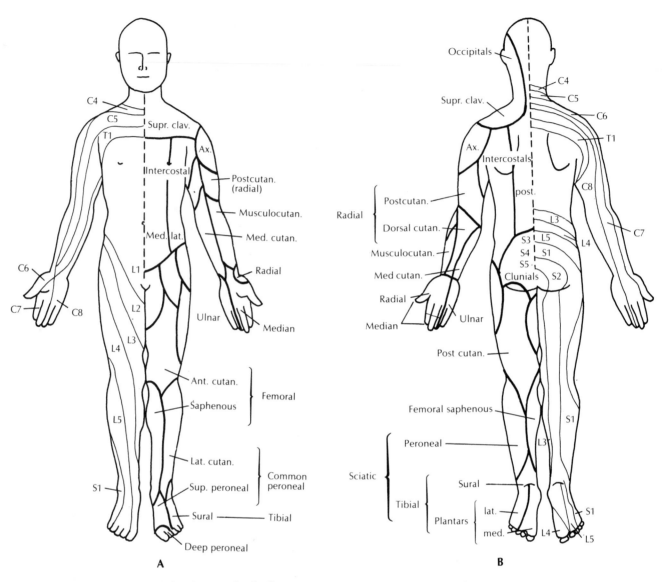

Fig. 4–2. Segmental and peripheral nerve distributions.

Strength Tests

Traditional muscle testing procedures should be employed. It is often necessary to repeat a test, comparing the strength carefully to the normal side if possible, since weaknesses resulting from common nerve lesions are usually subtle. Weaknesses and asymmetries in strength are noted.

Sensory Tests

A pin, wisp of cotton, and tuning fork may be used to assess conduction along sensory pathways. Pressure on a nerve will usually result in loss of conduction along the large myelinated fibers first and the small

unmyelinated fibers last. Therefore, minor deficits will often be manifested first by loss of vibration sense, with sensation to touch and noxious stimulation being reduced with more severe or long-lasting pressure.

When performing sensory tests, a particular area on the normal side is tested and the patient is asked if the sensation is perceived. Then the involved side is retested and the patient again asked if the sensation is felt. If sensation is intact on both sides, the patient is asked if it felt the same on both sides. This procedure is followed when testing each key segmental sensory area and each peripheral nerve distribution. Sensory deficits and asymmetries in perception are noted.

Table 4–2. Key Segmental Distributions (Myotomal and Dermotomic)

SEGMENTS	KEY MOVEMENTS TO TEST
C4	Shoulder shrug, diaphragmatic function
C5	Shoulder abduction, external rotation
C6	Elbow flexion, wrist extension
C7	Elbow extension, wrist flexion
C8	Ulnar deviation, thumb abduction, small finger abduction
T1	Approximation of fingers
L2	Hip flexion
L3	Knee extension, hip flexion
L4	Knee extension, ankle dorsiflexion
L5	Ankle/large toe dorsiflexion, eversion of ankle
S1	Plantar flexion, eversion, knee flexion
S2	Knee flexion, ankle plantar flexion

	REFLEXES TO TEST
Cranial nerve V	Jaw jerk[5,7]
C5,C6	Biceps, brachioradialis
(C7),C8	Triceps
(L3–L4)	Patellar tendon (quadriceps)
L5	Great toe jerk[6,8]
S1–S2	Achilles tendon

	KEY SEGMENTAL SENSORY AREAS TO TEST (distal part of segment)
C6	Thumb and index finger, radial border of hand
C7	Middle three fingers
C8	Ring and small finger, ulnar border of hand
L2	Medial thigh
L3	Anteromedial, distal thigh
L4	Medial aspect of large toe
L5	Web space between large and second toes
S1	Below lateral maleolus
S2	Back of heel
S3–S4	Saddle, anal region

Note: Others (*e.g.*, upper cervical, thoracic, and lumbar) are less definite due to overlapping.

(Chusid JG: Correlative Neuroanatomy and Functional Neurology. Los Altos, CA, Lange Medical Publications, 1970)

Deep Tendon Reflexes

Lower motor neuron lesions, such as segmental or peripheral nerve disorders, may result in diminution of certain deep-tendon reflexes, while more central, upper motor neuron lesions may cause hyperreflexia. The important assessments to make when testing deep tendon reflexes are whether the responses at homologous tendons are symmetrical and whether any responses are clonic. The presence of hyporeflexia is difficult to judge since some persons normally have reflexes that are difficult to elicit. In general, if it is equally difficult to elicit responses at corresponding tendons, no significance can be attributed. However, if upper extremity responses are difficult to elicit but lower extremity responses are strong, a myelopathy or some other more serious pathologic process should be considered.

Coordination, Tone, and Pathologic Reflexes

Coordination, tone, and pathologic reflexes should be assessed if myelopathy or other upper motor neuron disturbances are suspected. For example, myelopathy resulting from cervical spondylosis may result in a mildly spastic gait, increased lower extremity tone, lower extremity hyperreflexia, and perhaps a positive Babinski response (dorsiflexion of big toe in response to noxious stimulation along the sole of the foot).

PALPATION

Palpation tests are usually conveniently performed at the same time as the inspection tests discussed previously. As in inspection, palpation tests should be organized according to layers, assessing the status of the skin, subcutaneous soft tissues, and bony structures (including tendon and ligament attachments). Significant findings are documented.

Skin

The back of the examiner's hand is moved lightly across the area of skin to be examined. The following should be noted:

Tenderness. Minor pressure on a nerve supplying a particular area of skin may result in dysesthesia that may be perceived as a painful burning sensation to normally non-noxious stimulation, such as light touch. A similar phenomenon may also occur in the presence of lesions involving other tissues innervated by the same segment. This is believed to be the result of summation of otherwise subthreshold afferent input to a segment of the spinal cord.

Moisture and Texture. Moisture and texture may be altered with changes in vascularity or changes in sympathetic activity to the part. In the presence of increased sympathetic activity, such as that which commonly occurs in the chronic stages of reflex sympathetic dystrophy, the skin will be abnormally moist and very smooth. With reduced sympathetic activity, sometimes preceding a reflex sympathetic dystrophy, the skin may be dry and scaly.

Temperature. Skin temperature will be elevated in the presence of an underlying inflammatory process or with reduced sympathetic activity. A reduction in skin temperature may accompany vascular deficiency or increased sympathetic activity.

Mobility. The skin should be moved relative to the underlying tissues to examine for the presence of skin adhesions. This is especially important following healing of surgical and other traumatic wounds.

Subcutaneous Soft Tissues

The soft tissues are palpated deep to the skin—fat, fascia, muscles, tendons, joint capsules and ligaments, nerves, and blood vessels. No more pressure than what is necessary is used. A common mistake is to press harder and harder in an attempt to distinguish deep structures. This only serves to desensitize the palpating fingertips and does not assist in determining the nature of the tissues being palpated. Soft-tissue palpation may offer information concerning the following:

Tenderness. Tenderness to deep palpation is a very unreliable finding. In itself it is never indicative of the site of a pathologic process because of the prevalence of referred tenderness associated with lesions of deep somatic tissues. The phenomenon is similar in all respects to that of referred pain. In many common lesions, the area of primary tenderness does not correspond well to the site of the lesion. Thus, patients with low back disorders are often most tender in the buttock, those with supraspinatus tendinitis are most tender over the lateral brachial region, and persons with trochanteric bursitis are most tender over the lateral aspect of the thigh. These "trigger points," or referred areas of tenderness, are found in some area of the segment corresponding to the segment in which the lesion exists. Generally, tenderness associated with more superficial lesions, such as medial ligament sprains at the knee, corresponds more closely with the site of the lesion than does tenderness occurring with more deeply situated pathologic processes.

Edema and Swelling. The size and location of localized soft-tissue swellings are noted. Abnormal fluid accumulations should be differentiated as intra- or extra-articular. Articular effusion will be restricted to the confines of the joint capsule; pressure applied over one side of the joint may, therefore, cause increased distention observed over the opposite side. This type of "ballottement" test can be used with more superficial joints. Often articular effusion is distinguished by its characteristic distribution at a particular joint; these distributions are discussed in the chapters on specific regions. Extra-articular swelling may accompany acute inflammatory processes, such as abscesses and those following acute trauma, because of protein and plasma leaking from capillary walls. Generalized tissue edema may accompany vascular disorders, lymphatic obstructions, and electrolyte imbalances.

Consistency, Continuity, and Mobility. Normal soft tissue is supple and easily moved against underlying tissue. Palpation for abnormalities such as indurated areas, loss of mobility, stringiness, doughiness, nodules, and gaps is done and results noted.

Pulse. Palpating for the pulse of various major arteries can assist in assessing the status of blood supply to the part. Heart rate may also be determined.

Bony Structures

Bony structures also include ligaments and tendon attachments. When palpating bony structures, the following should be noted:

Tenderness. As with deep, soft-tissue tenderness, tenderness at various bony sites may be referred and is therefore often misleading. Lesions involving both ligaments and tendons commonly occur at the site where these structures join the periosteum. Typically, these are highly innervated regions and may be tender to palpation in the presence of tenoperiosteal or periosteoligamentous strains and sprains. Periosteal tenderness will also accompany specific bony lesions, such as stress fractures or other fractures.

Enlargements. Bony hypertrophy often accompanies healing of a fracture and degenerative joint disease. In the latter, the bony changes will be noted at the joint margins in more superficial joints.

Bony Relationships. Structural malalignments, as discussed in the section on inspection, may be detected clinically by assessing the relationships, in the various planes of reference, of one bony structure to another. This is especially important following healing of fractures and in cases of vague, subtle insidious disorders that may have a pathomechanical basis.

GUIDES TO CORRELATION AND INTERPRETATION

Judgments relating to the nature and extent of the disorder and the resultant degree of disability can be made by correlating the information obtained during a comprehensive initial patient examination. With respect to the nature of the problem, it is important to judge whether the disease state is a "medical" disorder or if perhaps operant behavior patterns have developed that may account for a significant part of the disability. The clinician should consider whether the degree of disability is consistent with the apparent nature and extent of the physical lesion or whether the patient is exhibiting disability behaviors that are out of proportion to clinical findings. If the latter is the case, the possibility that the disease state is being maintained by external consequences that have a reinforcing effect should be considered. It is essential that such determinations be made, since treatment directed at some physical pathologic process in the presence of an operant disease state will be futile and can further reinforce "learned" disability behaviors.

THE NATURE OF THE LESION

If it appears that some physical pathologic process is primarily responsible for the patient's disorder, the nature of the lesion should be estimated as precisely as possible. To do so, the information obtained on examination must be correlated with knowledge of anatomy, physiology, kinesiology, and pathology in order to identify the involved tissue or tissues. Some estimate should also be made concerning the extent to which these tissues are involved. A few common lesions make up the majority of disorders affecting each musculoskeletal tissue. For each of these lesions, there are also consistent key clinical findings. In developing judgments concerning the nature of common clinical disorders, it is helpful to be aware of the lesions common to each tissue and how they are manifested clinically. The following descriptions are meant to guide the clinician in this respect but are not meant to be all-inclusive.

Bone

Fractures are best identified in the physician's examination through the use of roentgenograms. When examining a patient following healing of a fracture, it is important to determine the malunion of bone on inspection of bone structure and alignment. This may affect eventual functioning of the part. Dislocations are also best detected through the physician's interpretation of roentgenograms, although dislocations are often obvious on inspection.

Articular Cartilage

Degeneration from wearing due to fatigue is the most common lesion affecting this tissue. It causes roughening of the normally smooth surface layers of cartilage. Clinically this is manifested as crepitus on movements when opposition of joint surfaces is maintained by weight-bearing or other compressive forces. However, considerable degeneration must usually take place before crepitus is detected clinically.

A loose body is a fragment of articular cartilage that has broken away and lies free in the joint. This may occur in the late stages of cartilage degeneration or as a result of avascular necrosis of an area of subchondral bone (osteochondrosis). A loose body becomes symptomatic when it alters the mechanical functioning of the joint, usually causing a restriction of movement in a noncapsular pattern (joint block).

Intra-articular Fibrocartilage

The common disorder affecting intra-articular fibrocartilaginous disks and menisci is tearing, usually from traumatic injury. Forces sufficient to tear a meniscus or disk in the extremities will usually also cause some strain on the joint capsule to which these structures attach. This causes synovial inflammation in the acute stage. Thus, movement is likely to be restricted in a capsular pattern.

Minor displacement of a torn fragment of fibrocartilage may simply result in "clicking" of the joint on specific movements. Lower extremity joints, namely the knee, may give way when a tag of a torn meniscus is caught between the articular surfaces, suddenly interfering with the normal mechanics of the joint.

A major displacement of a torn fragment may grossly interfere with normal mechanics and block joint movement in a noncapsular pattern. The classic example is a "bucket-handle" tear of a medial meniscus.

When the annular ring of a vertebral disk is torn, secondary neurologic symptoms or signs may result from bulging of the nucleus against adjacent nerve tissue.

Joint Capsule

Fibrosis (see section on capsular tightness) typically occurs with prolonged immobilization of a joint, in association with a chronic, low-grade inflammatory process such as occurs with degenerative joint disease, and with resolution of acute inflammation of the synovium. Joint motion is limited in a capsular pattern, and there is a capsular end feel at the extremes of movement.

Synovial inflammation is commonly caused by rheumatoid arthritis, acute trauma to the joint, joint infection, and arthrotomy. Joint motion is limited in a capsular pattern. There is a painful, muscle spasm end feel at the points of restriction of movements.

Inflammation of the synovium results in an increased production of synovial fluid, causing capsular distention and loss of the capsular laxity necessary for full movement. In the more superficial joints, the articular swelling can be observed and palpated. If the effusion persists following resolution of the synovial inflammation, motion will continue to be limited in a capsular fashion, with a boggy end feel to movement.

Patients with capsular pathology typically have some combination of fibrosis, synovial inflammation, and effusion. Therefore, end feels are not always distinct.

Forces sufficient to sprain a ligament usually cause some capsular disruption as well. Occasionally in traumatic injuries, a particular portion of a joint capsule is ruptured, such as the anterior capsule of the shoulder when the humerus dislocates anteriorly. Synovial inflammation and joint effusion usually follow capsular sprains.

In the case of a sprain, the joint play movement that stresses the involved portion of the capsule will be of normal amplitude. In more severe sprains, the joint may be slightly hypermobile, with a painful muscle-guarding end feel.

Ligaments

The history of a sprain invariably includes a traumatic onset. In the case of a mild sprain, the joint-play movement that stresses the ligament is of normal amplitude and is painful. More severe sprains (partial ruptures) will present as somewhat hypermobile and painful on the associated joint-play test. The synovial lining of the adjacent aspect of the joint capsule will often become inflamed, resulting in capsular effusion in the acute stage. There is usually tenderness over the site of the lesion.

The onset of a rupture is also usually traumatic. The associated joint-play movement test will be *hypermobile* and *painless* in the chronic stages. Even in the acute stage it is usually painless, since there are no fibers intact from which to elicit pain. If adjacent capsular tissue is also sprained, there may be some pain on stress testing in the acute stage. Capsular effusion often does not occur because fluid leaks through the defect. In the chronic stages the patient may give a history of instability. The joint gives way during activities that stress it in the direction that the ruptured ligament is supposed to check.

Bursae

The common disorder is inflammation, secondary to chronic irritation, infection, gout, or, rarely, acute trauma. Movement of the nearby joint will cause pain, restriction of motion, or both in a noncapsular pattern. There may be a painful arc of movement as well.

In acute bursitis, such as at the shoulder, the end feel to movement is often empty and painful; protective muscle spasm would only serve to squeeze the inflamed structure, increasing the pain. There is usually tenderness over the site of the lesion.

Tendons

Tendinitis is a minor lesion of tendon tissue involving microscopic tearing and a chronic, low-grade inflammatory process. In most cases it is degenerative; the lesion results from tissue fatigue rather than from acute injury. Since progression of the pathologic process will result in a partial tear (macroscopic) or rupture of the tendon, tendinitis should be considered on a continuum with more serious lesions.

The key clinical sign associated with tendinitis is a strong but painful resisted test of the involved musculotendinous structure. There may be pain at the extremes of the passive movement or movements that stretch the tendon. Seldom is there limitation of movement. There may be palpable tenderness at the site of the lesion, referred tenderness into the related segment, or both.

When the involved part of a tendon is that which passes through a sheath, two other terms are often used: *tenosynovitis* and *tenovaginitis*. Tenosynovitis is an inflammation of the synovial lining of a sheath resulting from friction of a roughened tendon gliding within the sheath. This will present similarly to tendinitis, but there is often pain on active movements that produce movement of the tendon within the sheath. Thus, active movement in the direction or opposite the direction of pull of the tendon may be painful. In tenovaginitis, a tendon gliding within a swollen, thickened sheath causes pain. The classic example occurs with rheumatoid arthritis. The clinical signs are essentially the same as those for tenosynovitis. There may be palpable and visible swelling of the tendon sheath.

In the case of a partial tendon tear, actual loss of continuity of tendon tissue will cause the resisted test for the musculotendinous complex to be weak and painful. The passive movement that stretches the tendon may be painful.

When the tendon has torn completely, the findings of the related resisted test will be weak and painless. In some cases, for example, rupture of the Achilles tendon, there may be a palpable gap at the site of the rupture.

Muscles

Muscle strains and ruptures are relatively rare. When they do occur they are invariably the result of acute trauma, and are therefore most prevalent in sports-medicine settings. Muscles, being well vascularized and resilient, do not commonly undergo fatigue degeneration as do tendons.

In the case of a strain, a minor tear of muscle fibers will result in a strong and painful finding on the resisted test that stresses the involved muscle. There may be pain on full passive stretch of the muscle, as well as palpable tenderness. In the case of a rupture, the associated resisted test will be weak and painless. A gap may be palpable, or occasionally visible, at the site of the defect.

Nerves

The common conditions affecting nerves are those in which some extrinsic source of pressure results in altered conduction along some or all of the nerve fibers—the so-called *entrapment syndromes.* The most common sites of pressure are the points of exit of the lower cervical and lower lumbar spinal nerves from the intervertebral foramina. Here pressure is usually from a protruding disk or projecting osteophyte. There are other common sites of pressure further out in the periphery that affect the nerves to the extremities. As indicated in Chapter 3, Pain, pressure tends to alter conduction first along the largest fibers and last along the smallest. Altered nerve conduction is usually manifested subjectively before any objective clinical evidence of neurologic dysfunction can be detected. In fact, in the case of the common entrapment syndromes, objective clinical findings are rare, and when present they are usually quite subtle. Often more sophisticated electrodiagnostic tests are required to objectively detect changes in nerve conduction.

The subjective complaints associated with common entrapment disorders can generally be classified as paresthesia (pins-and-needles), dysesthesia (altered sensation in response to some external stimulus), and pain. Although some patients may describe paresthesia and dysesthesia as painful, pain is usually not a primary complaint when there is pressure on a nerve farther out in the periphery rather than at the nerve-root level. Thus, patients with thoracic outlet syndrome, ulnar nerve palsy, and carpal tunnel syndrome, as well as those who have sat too long with the legs crossed, do not complain of pain but of a pins-and-needles sensation. Pain is a common complaint, however, in cases in which there is pressure on a nerve at nerve-root level. With initial pressure, when the larger, myelinated, "fast pain" fibers are stimulated, patients describe a sharp, shooting dermatomic quality of pain. With prolonged or increased pressure, when the larger fibers cease to conduct and the small, unmyelinated, C

fibers are stimulated, a dull, aching sclerotomic type of pain will be perceived.

Paresthesia, the primary subjective complaint with pressure farther out in the periphery, may occur with the onset of pressure, when the pressure is released, or both. For example, a person usually feels little or nothing when sitting with legs crossed, applying pressure to the tibial or peroneal nerve. It is not until the person uncrosses the legs, releasing the pressure, that the pins-and-needles sensation of the foot being "asleep" is felt. A similar situation holds true for pressure on the lower cord of the brachial plexus from depression of the shoulder girdle; the patient invariably describes the onset of pins-and-needles in the early morning hours (1 or 2 AM) some time after the pressure is released. It seems that the interval between the release of pressure and the onset of paresthesia is in some way proportional to the length of time during which the pressure was applied. In other common nerve problems, the onset of symptoms occurs when the pressure is applied. For example, many patients with carpal tunnel syndrome describe paresthesia felt primarily during fine finger movements; the tension on the finger flexor tendons produces pressure on the median nerve sufficient to cause symptoms. Similarly, when a person sits or lies with pressure over the ulnar groove, pins-and-needles are usually felt in the ulnar side of the hand while the pressure is applied and relieved after the pressure is released.

As mentioned, more objective findings associated with common nerve-pressure disorders are usually very subtle when present. They are more common with nerve-root pressure from a disk protrusion than with more peripheral entrapment syndromes. The earliest evidence of decreased conduction will be related to those functions mediated by the largest myelinated fibers, since these fibers are most sensitive to pressure. Therefore, reduced vibration sense is often the earliest deficit detected by clinical testing. With increased or prolonged pressure, diminished deep-tendon reflexes may be noted, followed by reduced muscle strength. Finally, there is reduced sensation, first to light touch, then to noxious stimulation. Because of overlapping dermatomes and myotomes, and because each muscle and skin area typically receives innervation from more than one segment, even completely severing a nerve root will usually cause only a minor deficit.

EXTENT OF THE LESION

When clinicians speak of "acute" and "chronic" lesions, it is often unclear whether they are referring to the length of time that the pathologic process has existed, the severity of the disorder, or the nature of the inflammatory process. There are relatively few consistent clinical findings related to either the duration or the severity of common musculoskeletal problems. However, there are certain symptoms and signs that are consistently present with acute inflammatory processes and others that are pathognomonic of lesions in which a more chronic inflammatory state exists. *Acute inflammation* is that stage or type of inflammatory process in which hyperemia, increased capillary permeability with protein and plasma leakage, and an influx of granulocytes and other defense cells take place. *Chronic inflammation* is characterized by an attempt at repair, with increased numbers of fibrocytes and other "tissue building" cells, and the presence of granulation tissue. An acute lesion is characterized by the following clinical findings:

1. Pain is relatively constant.
2. On passive range of motion of the related joint, there is a muscle spasm end feel or an empty end feel to movement.
3. Pain is likely to be referred over a relatively diffuse area of the related segment.
4. There may be a measurable increase in skin temperature over the site of the lesion.
5. There is often difficulty in falling asleep, difficulty in remaining asleep, or both.

In the presence of chronic lesions, the patient is likely to present with the following symptoms or signs:

1. Pain is increased by specific activities and relieved by rest.
2. On passive movement of the related joint, there is no muscle spasm or empty end feel.
3. Pain is likely to be felt over a relatively localized area, close to the site of the lesion, though often not directly over the site of the lesion.
4. There is little or no temperature elevation over the involved part.
5. Unless the lesion involves the shoulder or hip, there is little or no difficulty in sleeping.

REFERENCES

1. Cyriax J: Textbook of Orthopaedic Medicine, Vol I, 8th ed. London, Ballière-Tindall, 1983
2. Fordyce WE: Behavioral Methods for Chronic Pain and Illness. St Louis, CV Mosby, 1976
3. Fordyce WE: Evaluating and managing chronic pain. Geriatrics 33:59–62, 1978
4. Fordyce W, Fowler RS, Lehmann JF, DeLateur BJ, Sands PL, Trieschmann RB: Operant conditioning in the treatment of chronic clinical pain. Arch Phys Med Rehabil 54:399–408, 1973
5. Goldie IF, Reichman S: The biomechanical influence of traction on the cervical spine. Scand J Rehab Med 9:31–34, 1977
6. Grieve GP: Mobilisation of the Spine. Notes on Examination, Assessment and Clinical Method. New York, Churchill Livingstone, 1984
7. Ongerboer De Visser BW, Goor C: Jaw reflexes and masseter electromyograms in mesencephalic and pontine lesions: An electrodiagnostic study. J Neurol Neurosurg Psychiatry 39:90–92, 1976
8. Taylor TKF, Weinir M: Great-toe extensor reflexes in the diagnosis of lumbar disc disorders. Br Med J 2:487–489, 1969

RECOMMENDED READINGS

Corrigan B, Maitland GD: Practical Orthopaedic Medicine. Boston, Buttersworths, 1985
Cyriax J: Textbook of Orthopaedic Medicine, Vol I, The Diagnosis of Soft Tissue Lesions, 8th ed. London, Baillière-Tindall, 1982
Cyriax JH, Cyriax PJ: Illustrated Manual of Orthopaedic Medicine. London, Butterworths, 1985
Endow AJ, Swisher SN: Interviewing and patient care. New York, Oxford University Press, 1972
Hoppenfeld S: Physical Examination of the Spine and Extremities. New York, Appleton-Century-Crofts, 1976
Magee DJ: Orthopedic Physical Assessment. Philadelphia, WB Saunders, 1987
Maitland GD: Musculoskeletal Examination and Recording Guide, 3rd ed. Adelaide, Lauderdale Press, 1981
McRae R: Clinical Orthopaedic Examination, 2nd ed. Edinburgh, Churchill Livingstone, 1983
Stolov WC: Evaluation of the patient. In Krusen FH, Stillwell GK, Lehmann FJ (eds): Krusen's Handbook of Physical Medicine and Rehabilitation, 3rd ed. Philadelphia, WB Saunders, 1982

5 *Concepts of Management*

Randolph M. Kessler

Only those procedures that may not be well understood or are new to most professional training programs are discussed in this section. It is assumed that the reader is familiar with many basic therapeutic procedures and modalities, such as therapeutic exercise, use of assistive devices, massage, and electrotherapy. The application of these forms of treatment, in conjunction with traditional therapies, to specific pathologic processes affecting the various extremity regions is discussed in Parts Two and Three.

REHABILITATION

The correlation and interpretation of findings from a comprehensive initial patient examination is the basis for developing a treatment plan. As mentioned in Chapter 4, Assessment of Musculoskeletal Disorders, during the initial examination clinicians seek to elicit information that relates to the nature and extent of the pathologic process as well as to the degree of disability. The choice of therapeutic procedures depends on this information.

The primary considerations are the site of the lesion and the type of tissue involved. Once the nature of the lesion has been determined, there is often a tendency to direct treatment primarily at the site of the lesion with the expectation that resolving the pathologic process will alleviate any resultant physical dysfunction, and will in turn restore the patient to a normal "health state." There are many potential fallacies to this approach that make it unsuitable as a reliable treatment model.

First, such an approach ignores the secondary effects that a lesion involving a particular structure may have on the normal functioning of other related structures. It calls for treatment of "anatomical structures" rather than "physiological units." By considering the synovial joints as the basic physiological — rather than anatomical — unit of the musculoskeletal system, one is better prepared to respect the interactions of the various components of this system under normal and abnormal conditions. This is essential, since an alteration in one component of a functional unit often leads to dysfunction of other components of the same or neighboring units, which may act to maintain the primary pathologic condition, predispose to recurrence, or result in secondary disease. Thus, even in the case of relatively localized lesions, clinicians must respect such interactions and be prepared to deal with them therapeutically.

For example, a painful lesion of the supraspinatus tendon tends to result in reflex inhibition of the supraspinatus and other rotator cuff muscles. This will predispose to subacromial impingement from abnormal movement of the head of the humerus during elevation activities, which may further traumatize the supraspinatus tendon as well as the subdeltoid bursa. Also, muscles such as the deltoid and the trapezius may reflexively contract abnormally during movement of the arm, secondary to abnormal afferent input from the site of the lesion to the lower cervical segments. This may further interfere with normal joint mechanics at the shoulder as well as at the neck, to which the trapezius attaches. It should be clear that effective treatment of this problem involves more than resolution of the pathologic process affecting the tendon. The rotator cuff muscles must, at some time, be strengthened; excessive elevation of the arm must be temporarily avoided; and relaxation of abnormally contracting muscles should be promoted. If one were to treat only the lesion of the tendon, it is likely that treatment would be ineffective or take much longer than necessary to be effective. Continued subacromial impingement would enhance the chance of recurrence. The patient would also be predisposed to the development of a coexistent cervical lesion from increased stresses to the neck due to abnormal muscle activity.

Second, an approach in which treatment is aimed exclusively at some discrete pathologic process tends to ignore etiologic considerations. Temporary amelioration may ensue without true resolution of the problem. Unless underlying causes, such as biomechanical abnormalities, are recognized and dealt with, chronic recurrent problems can be expected. Thus, a patient with chondromalacia patellae resulting from abnormal foot pronation may temporarily do very well on a program of reduced activity and strengthening of the vastus medialis muscle. However, the patient is likely to experience similar problems with the resumption of normal activity levels unless the alignment of the foot and leg is corrected. Similarly, the patient with trochanteric bursitis caused by a tight iliotibial band usually responds well to ultrasound over the site of the lesion, but if extensibility of the iliotibial band is not increased, relief will be short-lived. The clinician should implement the concept that prevention is the ultimate cure by attempting to identify etiologic factors and by employing appropriate measures to deal with them. This should be a major consideration in fatigue disorders that are chronic, since they tend to be self-resolving once the cause of the abnormal stresses is corrected. (See the discussion of treatment of chronic disorders in this chapter.)

Third, and most important, when treatment is directed only at a physical disorder, the psychosocial implications of the problem are not given due respect. Comprehensive rehabilitation requires restoration of an optimal level of function. Although a physical disorder may have been the original cause of physical dysfunction or other "disease behaviors," such as complaints of pain, there are often other factors that may serve to maintain or inhibit the disability behaviors. Such "motivational factors" may eventually assume a greater influence on the disability state than the original pathology (see Fig. 4–1). These factors must be recognized since they often determine whether treatment is successful, whether an optimal level of function is restored, and whether disability behaviors (pain complaints, physical dysfunction, and functional dependence) are resolved. If being disabled carries excessively negative consequences for the patient, such as often occurs in sports-medicine settings, these consequences will strongly inhibit the disability state. As a result, the patient often attempts to do more than is appropriate and imposes deleterious effects on the lesion. This may counteract any beneficial effects of other treatment procedures. On the other hand, if the patient stands to gain in some way from being disabled, such

as time away from work, financial compensation, or welcomed dependence, the potential for gain may have a significant reinforcing effect on the disability state. The patient is not likely to improve in spite of otherwise effective treatment of the pathologic condition. In both of these situations, the psychosocial motivational influences are likely to have a greater effect on the disease state than the physical process itself. Unless these influences are dealt with, the patient cannot be truly rehabilitated. To estimate the relative influence of such factors, the clinician must determine whether the degree of disability is consistent with the symptoms and signs manifested by the disease. If there are inconsistencies, significant psychosocial influences affecting the nature of the disability state should be suspected.

TREATMENT OF PATIENTS WITH PHYSICAL DISORDERS

Although the principle of "treating the patient, not the disease" has become somewhat of a cliché, its application to patients with common musculoskeletal disorders is too often overlooked. The first and foremost consideration when devising a therapeutic program should always be how the patient's ability to function normally has been compromised. One must ask, what conditions are responsible for the dysfunction and are these conditions reversible? If they are reversible, what would be the most appropriate means of intervening therapeutically so as to affect these conditions? If the conditions at fault appear irreversible, what can be done to optimize residual function? And finally, what can be done to prevent recurrences, secondary problems, and progression of the existing disorder? With such an approach, therapy is disability-oriented rather than pathology-oriented. The primary goal of management becomes restoration of an optimal level of functioning rather than simply resolution of some pathologic process. Resolution of a physical disorder does not necessarily lead to restoration of function, reduction in pain behavior, or other necessary signs of improvement.

In the case of many common musculoskeletal disorders, in which the degree of disability appears to be consistent with the nature and extent of the lesion, physical treatment will constitute a major component of the therapeutic program. When this is the case, clinicians must choose, among the various forms of intervention at their disposal, the procedures and modalities most appropriate for the management of the specific disorder. Treatment must be individualized for each patient and according to the nature and extent of the pathologic process. The tendency to incorporate "standardized" programs of exercises and other treatments, usually for the sake of efficiency, should be avoided. The controversies over and misconceptions about so many forms of treatment (*e.g.*, massage, manipulation, traction, and certain exercises) stem largely from their having been advocated or misconstrued as panaceas for disorders affecting certain regions.

CLASSIFYING PATHOLOGIES: ACUTE VS. CHRONIC

As a preface to discussing specific types of treatments and their respective applications, some general concepts that are related to the overall approach to physical treatment are considered. As mentioned previously, approaches to treating a physical disorder should depend on its nature and extent. The two common terms used clinically to classify pathologic processes according to their nature and extent are *acute* and *chronic*. As suggested in Chapter 4, these terms should not be used to refer to the severity or duration of a disorder, since when used in these contexts they have little relationship to symptoms and signs. A patient with a relatively severe lesion such as a ligamentous rupture, for example, may present with much less pain and dysfunction than one who has sustained a minor sprain. It is well known, even to those outside the health care professions, that a sprained ankle may be more painful and disabling shortly after injury than a fractured ankle. With respect to duration, disorders of fairly recent onset often present with subtle symptoms and signs when compared with certain long-standing problems. If a clinician has two patients, one with recent onset of aching in the shoulder but no gross loss of function and the other with long-standing severe pain and dysfunction, which condition is acute and which is chronic?

The terms *acute* and *chronic* do have some significance when used to refer to the nature of the symptoms and signs with which a patient presents, as differentiated in Chapter 4. This is because symptoms and signs reflect the nature of various disorders and, more specifically, they tend to reflect the nature of the inflammation or repair process that accompanies any physical lesion. Because these symptom–sign complexes do relate to the nature of pathologic processes, they are used here as a basis for a discussion of general approaches to management. The fol-

lowing scheme is based on the definitions of *acute* and *chronic*.

TREATMENT OF ACUTE AND CHRONIC DISORDERS

I. **General concepts**
A. *Consider the nature and extent of the disorder, whether* acute *or* chronic.
1. The terms are sometimes used to refer to duration of the problem and not to symptoms and signs.
2. They should be used to refer to the nature of the inflammatory process
a. Acute hyperemic phase
i. Pain is felt at rest and aggravated by activity.
ii. Pain is felt over a relatively diffuse area and may be referred into any or all of the related segment (sclerotome).
iii. Passive movement of related joints when limited is restricted by pain, muscle guarding, or both.
iv. The skin temperature over the site of the lesion is often elevated.
b. Chronic/reparative phase
i. There is no pain at rest and pain is felt only with specific activities.
ii. Pain is felt over a fairly localized area, close to the site of the lesion (often not directly over the site of the lesion, however).
iii. Movement of related joints, when limited, is restricted by soft-tissue tightness; pain is felt only at the extremes of movement or through a small arc of movement.
3. The terms are not useful in describing the severity of the lesion. For example, a patient with a complete rupture of a ligament may present with less pain and disability and with fewer cardinal inflammatory signs than a person with only a partial tear of a ligament.
B. *Assess, control, and monitor the patient's functional status.*
1. Assessment of disability. Determine by history and physical examination the degree of disability. Compare disease (injury) status with health (normal) status, and compare with other symptoms and signs.
a. Is the degree of disability consistent

with the apparent nature and extent of the disorder? This yields important information relating to the patient's "motivational" status and is a major consideration in treatment planning.

   i. The "well-motivated" patient is one for whom the consequences of injury (disability) are punishing. For example, they imply time away from desirable situations or possibility of financial loss. It can be presumed that resolution of the disease will lead to resolution of the disability state. A medical approach to treatment is appropriate.

   ii. The "poorly motivated" patient is one for whom the consequences of disability are *reinforcing*. For example, they offer time away from undesirable situations or the possibility of financial gain. It cannot be presumed that treatment of the disease will result in resolution of the disability state. Rehabilitation must include attempts to alter the consequences to disability. An operant approach must be incorporated into the treatment program.

   b. Record and use information as a baseline by which to judge progress.

2. Control functional status (see below under techniques of management).

   a. Inappropriate activities must be restricted to prevent prolongation or recurrence of the disorder.

   b. Appropriate activities must be resumed as the pathologic process resolves. *This is the ultimate goal of management.*

3. Monitor functional status to judge improvement. The patient is not rehabilitated until an optimal level of function is restored, regardless of the state of the lesion.

II. **Treatment of acute inflammatory disorders (traumatic).** The primary goal is to promote progression to a chronic state while minimizing dysfunction.

   A. *Physiological intervention to control the acute inflammatory response*
      1. Ice — to reduce blood flow
      2. Compression — to prevent and reduce swelling
      3. Elevation — to prevent and reduce swelling and hyperemia
      4. Relaxation — to reduce pain and muscle spasm

   B. *Avoidance and prevention of continued trauma and irritation by reducing loading of the part*
      1. Braces, slings, splints, assistive devices, strapping
         a. Lower extremity — Crutches or canes to reduce forces of weight-bearing; splints, braces, or strapping to reduce forces of movement
         b. Upper extremity — Slings to reduce forces of gravity and, therefore, postural muscle tone; splints, braces, or strapping to reduce the forces imposed by movement
         c. Spine — Passive support with collar or corset if indicated
      2. Control of activities causing undesirable loading of the part. This requires careful, well-understood instructions to the patient. With respect to the spine:
         a. Rest is interspersed with periods of controlled activity.
         b. Positions that increase intradiskal pressure should be avoided (*e.g.*, acute disk protrusions).

   C. *Maintaining optimal levels of function and preventing unnecessary dysfunction.*
      1. Isometric resistive exercises to maintain muscle function but avoid undesirable movement of the part
      2. In acute nuclear prolapse — isometric activities (*e.g.*, pelvic tilt exercises, straining, and Valsalva maneuvers) must be avoided.
      3. With respect to the spine:
         a. Rest is interspersed with periods of controlled activity.
         b. Positions that increase intradiskal pressure should be avoided (*e.g.*, acute disk protrusions)
      4. Gentle active or passive movement (when appropriate according to the nature of the disorder) to avoid pain and muscle guarding

III. **Treatment of chronic disorders**
   A. *Causative factors.* The majority of disorders seen in most clinical settings have two primary causes:
      1. Abnormal modeling of tissue during reso-

lution of an acute disorder. The following are examples:

a. Malunion of fractures resulting in a change in the direction or magnitude of forces acting on the part during use (increased stress)

b. Abnormalities in collagen maturation or production (scarring, fibrosis, adhesions). An excess amount of collagen may be produced, and that which is produced may not be oriented along the normal lines of stress. Abnormal collagen cross-links are formed, and the tissue may adhere to adjacent structures. The net result is reduced extensibility, and therefore reduced capacity to attenuate energy by deforming when stressed.

2. Fatigue response of tissues. The two types of response are

a. Tissue breakdown—the rate of attrition exceeds the rate of repair (*e.g.,* stress fractures, cartilage degeneration). The tissue becomes "weaker" and begins to yield under loading conditions. It occurs with mild to moderately increased stress levels in tissues with low regenerative capacity (*e.g.,* articular cartilage); with higher stress levels in other tissues (*e.g.,* tendon, bone); under conditions of altered tissue metabolism (*e.g.,* hypovascularity).

b. Tissue hypertrophy (*e.g.,* fibrosis and sclerosis) occurs with mild to moderately increased stress levels in tissues with good regenerative/repair capacity, acting over a prolonged period of time. Tissue becomes stiffer, with reduced energy attenuation capacity. Individual fibers or trabeculae begin to yield under loading conditions, resulting in low-grade inflammation, pain, increased tissue production, and so on.

B. *Treatment planning*

1. Reduce stresses to involved tissue over time.

a. Reduce magnitude of loading (control of activities).

b. Reduce magnitude of stresses by altering direction or magnitude of forces acting on the part through control of activities, use of protective/assistive devices, and use of orthotic devices to control position or the part.

c. Increase surface area of loading (*e.g.,* foot orthosis).

d. Provide for external energy attenuation (*e.g.,* pads, helmets, cushioned heels).

2. Increase energy-attenuating capacity of the part.

a. Increase compensatory muscle strength/activity with strengthening exercises; increase neuromuscular facilitative (afferent) input (*e.g.,* taping, coordination training).

b. Increase tissue extensibility (ability to deform without loss of structural integrity):

i. Active stretching

ii. Passive stretching, using passive range of motion stretching for musculotendinous tightness and specific joint mobilization for capsuloligamentous tightness

iii. Use of ultrasound in conjunction with stretch

iv. Use of transverse friction massage to increase interfiber mobility and to prevent or reduce fibrous adhesion without longitudinally stressing the tissue

c. Promote increase in structural integrity of the part (increased "strength"). This requires tissue hypertrophy, without loss of extensibility from overproduction of immature collagenous tissue, and so on, and maturation of collagen fiber orientation along normal lines of stress and development of appropriate cross-links.

The necessary stimulus is stress to the part. This means gradual, controlled participation in high-stress-level activities (training).

3. Resumption of optimal activity levels and prevention of recurrence. Judgments are based on

a. Clinical evidence of having accomplished above objectives

b. Awareness of the nature of stresses imposed by various activities and an estimate of the capacity of the part to withstand those stresses. This requires biomechanical assessment and analysis and familiarity with research related to biomechanical properties of musculoskeletal tissues under various conditions of loading and healing.

   c. Extrinsic "motivational" factors — the consequences of disability for the patient

RECOMMENDED READINGS

Abraham WM: Heat vs. cold therapy for the treatment of muscle injuries. Athletic Training 9:4, 1974

Adams A: Effects of exercise upon ligament strength. Res Q 37:163–167, 1965

Akeson WH, Amiel D, LaViolette D, Secrist D: The connective tissue response to immobility: An accelerated aging response? Exp Gerontol 3:289–300, 1968

Clayton ML, James SM, Abdulla M: Experimental investigations of ligamentous healing. Clin Orthop 61:146, 1968

Darling RC: Exercise. In Dawney JA, Darling RC (eds): Physiological Basic of Rehabilitation Medicine. Philadelphia, WB Saunders, 1971

DeLateur BJ, Lehmann JF, Fordyce WE: A test of the De-Lorme axiom. Arch Phys Med Rehabil 49:245–248, 1968

DeLateur BJ, Lehmann JF, Giaconi R: Mechanical work and fatigue: Their roles in the development of muscle work capacity. Arch Phys Med Rehabil 57:321–324, 1976

DeLateur BJ, Lehmann J, Stonebridge J, Warren CG: Isotonic vs. isometric exercise: A double-shift transfer-of-training study. Arch Phys Med Rehabil 53:212–217, 1972

Fordyce WE: Behavioral Methods for Chronic Pain and Illness. St Louis, CV Mosby, 1976

Fordyce WE, Fowler RS, Lehmann JF, DeLateur BJ, Sands PL, Trieschmann RB: Operant conditioning in the treatment of chronic clinical pain. Arch Phys Med Rehabil 54:399–408, 1973

Frankel VH, Hang Y: Recent advances in the biomechanics of sport injuries. Acta Orthop Scand 46:484–497, 1975

Gradosar IA: Fracture stabilization and healing. In Gould JA, Davies GJ (eds): Orthopaedic and Sports Physical Therapy. St Louis, CV Mosby, 1985

Hettinga DL: Inflammatory response of synovial joint structures. In Gould JA, Davies GL (eds): Orthopaedic and Sports Physical Therapy. St Louis, CV Mosby, 1985

Keene JS: Ligament and muscle-tendon unit injuries. In Gould JA, Davies GL (eds): Orthopaedic and Sports Physical Therapy. St Louis, CV Mosby, 1985

Kennedy JD, Hawkins RJ, Willis RB, Danylchuk KD: Tension studies in human knee ligaments. J Bone Joint Surg 58(A):350–355, 1976

Knight K: The effects of hypothermia on inflammation and swelling. Athletic Training 11:1, 1976

Lehmann JF, DeLateur BJ, Stonebridge JB, Warren CB: Therapeutic temperature distribution produced by ultrasound as modified by dosage and volume of tissue exposed. Arch Phys Med Rehabil 48:12:662–666, 1967

Lehmann JF, Warren CG: Therapeutic heat and cold. Clin Orthop 99:207–245, 1974

Mannheimer JS, Lampe GN: Clinical Transcutaneous Electrical Nerve Stimulation. Philadelphia, FA Davis, 1984

Noyes FR, Edward SG: The strength of the anterior cruciate ligament in humans and rhesus monkeys. J Bone Joint Surg 58(A):1074–1082, 1976

Noyes FR, Grood ES, Nussbaum NS, Cooper SM: Effects of intra-articular corticosteroids on ligament properties. Clin Orthop 123:197–209, 1977

Noyes FR, Torvik DJ, Hyde WB, Delucas JL: Biomechanics of ligament failure: An analysis of immobilization, exercise and reconditioning effects in primates. J Bone Joint Surg 56(A):1406–1418, 1974

Radin EL, Paul IL: A comparison of the dynamic force transmitting properties of subchondral bone and articular cartilage. J Bone Joint Surg 52(A):444–456, 1970

Santiesteban JA: Physical agents and musculoskeletal pain. In Gould JA, Davies GJ (eds): Orthopaedic and Sports Physical Therapy. St Louis, CV Mosby, 1985

Stolow WC: Evaluation of the patient. In Kottke FJ, Stillwell K, Lehmann JF (eds): Krusen's Handbook of Physical Medicine and Rehabilitation, 3rd ed. Philadelphia, WB Saunders, 1982

Warren CG, Lehmann JF, Koflanski JN: Heat and stretch procedures: An evaluation using rat tail tendons. Arch Phys Med Rehabil 57:122–126, 1976

6 *Peripheral Joint Mobilization Techniques*

Randolph M. Kessler and Darlene Hertling

HISTORY

Although specific mobilization techniques are just being introduced in physical therapy curricula in this country, their use in the management of patients with musculoskeletal disorders is certainly not new. It seems somewhat odd that physical therapists have been so slow in adopting joint mobilization techniques. After all, therapists have been delegated the duty of passive movement for years, and joint mobilization is simply a form of passive movement. Some time in the past this important method of treatment was lost from medical practice and is just beginning to emerge again. The explanation for its disappearance probably lies in the fact that early users of mobilization techniques based their value on purely empirical evidence of their effectiveness; there was no scientific basis for their use. Later, specific joint mobilization was practiced only by more esoteric "professions" that claimed beneficial effects on all disease processes, usually from manipulations of the spine. This tended to further alienate orthodox medical practitioners, with the result that the use of any and all forms of joint mobilization, other than movement in the cardinal planes, became somewhat taboo. Our approach to the management of many joint conditions is still largely influenced by the teachings of the early orthopaedic surgeons, who advocated strict rest in the management of all joint conditions. While scientific proof of the effectiveness of specific joint mobilization is still largely lacking, our expanded knowledge of joint kinematics at least provides a scientific *basis* for its use. It is becoming evident that in order to deal with mechanical joint dysfunctions effectively and safely, a knowledge of joint kinematics as well as skill in the use of joint examination and mobilization techniques are required.

EARLY PRACTITIONERS

The use of specific mobilization techniques did not arise with the emergence of osteopathy and chiropractic. Some of the earliest recorded accounts of the use of joint manipulation and spinal traction are from Hippocrates, a physician in the fourth century B.C. In fact, Hippocrates proposed refinements in some of the techniques used in his time. For example, one traction technique required that the patient be tied to a ladder and dropped 30 feet, upside down, to the ground. Hippocrates suggested that ropes be tied to the ladder so that two people could shake it up and down, thus affecting an "intermittent" traction. Hippocrates also developed many of the methods of reducing dislocations that are still in use today. Accounts of the use of manipulation by Cato, Galen, and other physicians during the time of the Roman Empire also exist.[1]

Little is known of the practice of joint manipulation during the disintegration of the Roman Empire and the beginning of the Middle Ages. During this time most hospitals were attached to monasteries, and treatment was carried out by members of the religious orders. Friar Moulton, of the order of St. Augustine, wrote *The Complete Bonesetter*. The text, which was revised by John Turner in 1656, suggests that manipulation was practiced in medical settings throughout the Middle Ages and early Renaissance. With the reign of Henry VIII in England and the subsequent dissolution of the monasteries, medicine lost its previous "mystic" influences and became the practice of "art and science." The English orthopaedic surgeons of the late 1700s and early 1800s, such as John Hunter and John Hilton, advocated strict rest in the early management of joint trauma.[5] This view was emphasized by Hugh Owen Thomas in the late 1800s. For two centuries this influence prevailed, and joint manipulation remained in the hands of "bonesetters." Bonesetting was practiced by lay people, and the art was passed down over the centuries within bonesetting families. The bonesetters had no basis for the use of their manipulations other than past experience. The successful bonesetters were those who remembered details of cases in which ill effects had resulted and avoided making the same mistakes over again. Bonesetters tended to guard their techniques, keeping them secret among family members. A few bonesetters, because of their success, became quite famous. One such bonesetter, a Mrs. Mapp, was called upon to treat nobility and royalty.

Bonesetters vs. Physicians

During this particular period there was extreme rivalry and animosity between physicians and bonesetters. Physicians were well aware of disastrous effects that bonesetting had at times on tuberculous joints or other serious pathologies. It is interesting that Thomas, who was particularly outspoken against bonesetters, was the son and grandson of bonesetters. Thomas, who gave his name to the *Thomas splint*, was the originator of many of the orthopaedic principles concerning immobilization of fractures and joint injuries still adhered to today. It goes without saying that medical opinion of joint manipulation has changed very little since his time.

Despite medical opinion, Sir James Paget, a famous surgeon and contemporary of Thomas in England, recognized the value of judiciously applied bonesetting techniques. His lecture entitled "Cases that Bonesetters Cure," which appeared in the *British Medical Journal* in 1867, spoke of the rivalry between bonesetters and physicians. He described types of lesions for which manipulation may be of value and advised that physicians "imitate what is good and avoid what is bad in the practice of bonesetters." Unfortunately, the medical profession at the time, and for years to come, ignored this advice.

The first medical book on manipulation since Friar Moulton's work was published in the 1870s. It was written by Dr. Wharton Hood, whose father, Dr. Peter Hood, treated a bonesetter, a Mr. Hutton, for a serious illness. Dr. Hood did not charge Hutton since he was aware of Hutton's free services to many poor people. In repayment, however, Hutton offered to teach Hood all he knew of bonesetting. The elder Hood was too busy to accept the offer, but his son Wharton did. In his paper on the subject, published in *Lancet* in 1871, Hood describes Hutton's techniques of spinal and peripheral manipulation.[6] He

lists the conditions that Hutton was willing to treat as primarily postimmobilization stiffness, displaced cartilage and tendons, carpal and tarsal subluxations, and ganglionic swellings; he also states that Hutton avoided working on acutely inflamed joints. Hutton usually applied heat before manipulating, especially to the larger joints. Hood describes Hutton's manipulations as being very precise as to the direction and amplitude of motion. They were always of a high-velocity thrust. The illustrated descriptions of some of the common manipulations used by Hutton show them to be essentially identical to the manipulations used by manual therapists and even some orthopaedists and physiatrists today. Hutton admitted to knowing nothing of anatomy and felt that in all of his cases a bone was "out." Of his techniques he says that forced pushing and pulling are useless; "the twist is the thing."

Osteopathy and Chiropractic

Meanwhile in the United States, Dr. Andrew Taylor Still was practicing medicine in Kansas.[19] It happened that Still's children contracted meningitis and all three died. Still, being frustrated and angered by the failure of current medical practices to save his children, set out to find a solution. For a time he spent his days studying the anatomy of exhumed Indian remains, paying special attention to the relationships among bones, nerves, and arteries. In 1874, through a "divine revelation," Still claimed he had discovered the cause of all bodily disease. His "law of the artery" claimed that all disease processes were a direct result of interference with blood flow through arteries that carried vital nutrients to a part. If normal blood flow to the part could be restored, then the body's natural substances would resolve the disease process. In 1892, Still founded the first school of osteopathy in Kirksville, Missouri, offering a 20-month course. By 1916 the osteopathic course was extended to 3 years, and by 1920 the United States Congress granted equal rights to osteopaths and M.D.s.[15] In the early 1900s, the osteopathic profession gradually became aware that some of Still's original proposals were incorrect. Over the years they incorporated traditional medical thought with the practice of joint manipulation. Especially during the last decade, osteopathic schools have de-emphasized the practice of manipulation, and have attained essentially the same standards as medical schools. Osteopaths now qualify for residency programs in all medical and surgical fields.

In 1895 a grocer named D. D. Palmer, who had been a patient of Still, founded the Palmer College of

Chiropractics in Davenport, Iowa. No prior education was required, and one of the first graduates was Palmer's 12-year-old son, B. J. Chiropractic theory evolved around the "law of the nerve," which stated that "vital life forces" could be cut off from any body part by small vertebral subluxations placing pressure on nerves. Since this could cause disease in the part to which the nerve ran, most, if not all, disease could be prevented or cured by maintaining proper spinal alignment through manipulation. Chiropractic was a "drugless" remedy that often supplemented manipulative treatment with various herbs, vitamins, and so forth. The chiropractic profession was fraught with internal turmoil from the outset.[16] (B. J. apparently grew up hating his father, and later bought him out. When the father died, he stipulated that B. J. was not to attend his funeral.) Unlike osteopathy, most chiropractors adhered to their original concept, the law of the nerve, although the profession has always been divided into two or more schools of thought. They have received bitter opposition from the medical profession, which views them as charlatans and quacks. Today there remains some division in chiropractic philosophy. The "straights" continue to follow the law of the nerve, claiming to treat most disease by manipulating the spine or other body parts. The "mixers" tend to accept the limitations of this practice and use local application of ultrasound, massage, exercises, and so on, to supplement their manipulative treatment. It is significant that due to a strong lobbying force and the realization by chiropractors that, in order to survive, professional standards and education must be upgraded, chiropractors are rapidly gaining acceptance by governing bodies, the public, and even some physicians. It will be interesting to see if the profession of physical therapy keeps abreast of this trend.

CURRENT SCHOOLS OF THOUGHT

In spite of efforts by Paget and Hood to emphasize the value of bonesetting techniques, manipulation was not readopted as a method of treatment by medical doctors until this century. The earliest physicians to practice manipulation were Englishmen. Books on the subject were published by A. G. Timbrell Fisher, an orthopaedic surgeon, in 1925, and by James Mennell in 1939.[5,11] Mennell was a doctor of physical medicine at St. Thomas' Hospital. Both he and Fisher often performed their manipulations with the patient anesthetized. In 1934 Mixter and Barr published an article in the *New England Journal of Medicine*, and T. Marlin published *Manipulative*

Treatment for Medical Practitioners.[10,13,14] These works have had a powerful effect on medical thought, stimulating much interest and leading to a series of excellent publications since then. Later in the century books advocating manipulative treatment were published by Alan Stoddard and James Cyriax.[3,17] Cyriax was to succeed Mennell at St. Thomas' Hospital. Cyriax advocated manipulations performed without anesthesia. Most of allopathic medicine's knowledge of manipulations can be traced to Mennell and Cyriax; the former made contributions in the field of synovial joints, the latter in the area of the intervertebral disk. Cyriax's examination approach is considered superb and contains a wealth of medical logic.

Currently, a school of thought that has attracted some attention (especially in Europe) is being led by Robert Maigne, who has postulated the "concept of painless and opposite motion."[8] This concept states that a manipulative maneuver should be administered in the direction opposite to the movement that is restricted and causing pain. Maigne, like Cyriax, has worked hard to focus medical attention on manipulative therapy as an effective modality in the relief of pain.

The driving force behind a school of thought that has flourished in Scandinavia is F. M. Kaltenborn.[7] Under his leadership, a systematic postgraduate education program that requires passage of practical and written exams leads to certification in the specialty of manual therapy. The philosophy behind Kaltenborn's technique is a fusion of what he has considered the best in chiropractic, osteopathy, and physical medicine. He uses Cyriax's methods to evaluate the patient and employs mainly specific osteopathic techniques for treatment. Disk degeneration and facet joint pathologies are the two main spinal pathologies that the Scandinavians theorize are amenable to physical therapy.

Maitland, an Australian physical therapist whose approach is currently being taught in Australia, has a nonpathologic orientation to the treatment of all joints.[2,9] His techniques are fairly similar to the "articulatory" techniques used by osteopaths, involving oscillatory movements performed on a chosen joint. To increase movement of a restricted joint, movement is induced within the patient's available range of movement tolerance. He distinguishes between mobilizations and manipulations, but puts heavy emphasis on mobilization. A meticulous examination is essential to this method because examination provides the guideline to treatment.

A prominent figure in the United States has been Dr. John Mennell, the son of the late James Mennell, who came to practice in this country. His work on the spine and extremities has been described in several publications and is particularly well known in this country. He has made a significant contribution to a better understanding of joint pain and its treatment by placing stress on the function of small involuntary movements within a joint. He refers to these small movements as *joint play;* a disturbance of these movements is termed *joint dysfunction.* He states that full, painless, voluntary range of motion is not possible without restoration of all joint-play motions.[12]

In spite of their efforts, Mennell, Cyriax, Stoddard, and Maigne remain among the very few medical physicians to practice joint manipulation. As a result, manipulative treatment was not — and still is not — available to most patients seeking help from the medical profession. The original reasons for avoiding the practice of manipulation stemmed from the teachings of Hilton, Thomas, and Hunter, and the occasional disasters that occurred at the hands of bonesetters and other manipulators. Today many more medical physicians accept the value of judiciously applied manipulative treatment. However, to be effective, this treatment requires considerable evaluative and therapeutic management, and most physicians simply do not have the time to learn or practice manipulative technique.

THE ROLE OF THE PHYSICAL THERAPIST

Physical therapists are the logical practitioners to assume the responsibility for manipulative treatment. They work closely with physicians, who are capable of ruling out serious pathology. They tend to develop close and ongoing rapport with patients because the nature of their work requires close patient contact. They are taught to evaluate and treat by use of the hands. The advantages of the physician/physical therapist team in orthopaedic manual therapy are perhaps best described by Cyriax: "Between them they have every facility: informed selection of cases, a wide range of different types of treatment, alternative approaches when it is clear that manual methods cannot avail."[4]

The United States, which has lagged far behind other countries in the development of orthopaedic manual therapy, is gradually catching up. Thanks to the efforts of Mennell and Stanley Paris, a therapist originally from New Zealand, American therapists have at least had the opportunity to take postgraduate courses and to gain some competency in manual therapy and the management of orthopaedic patients. It is hoped that the formation of the Orthopae-

dic Section of the American Physical Therapy Association in 1974 and increased education will improve this situation. Undergraduate courses in the physical therapy schools, clinically oriented long-term courses, postgraduate apprenticeships, and orthopaedic specialization in master's degree programs are still needed.

INTRODUCTION TO JOINT MOBILIZATION TECHNIQUES

GENERAL RULES

The following rules and considerations should guide the therapist when performing joint mobilization techniques:

1. *The patient must be relaxed.*
   This requires that the patient be properly draped, and that the room be of comfortable temperature without distracting noises, and so on. Joints, other than the joint to be mobilized, must be at rest and well supported.
   The operator's handholds must be firm but comfortable. He or she must remove watches, jewelry, and so forth, and be sure buttons and belt buckles are not in contact with the patient.

2. *The operator must be relaxed.*
   This requires good body mechanics, especially with regard to the spine. The operator should attempt to create a situation in which his body and the part to be treated "act as one." This requires close body contact between the operator and patient for optimal control and mobilization.

3. *Do not move into or through the point of pain.*
   One must be able to determine the difference between the discomfort of soft tissue stretch, which is at times desirable, and the pain and muscle guarding that are a signal to ease up lest damage be done.
   The advanced manual therapist at times will move into or through the point of pain, but only in highly selective circumstances. These techniques are not to be taught, nor are they expected to be learned in a basic-level course.

4. *When performing any of the joint mobilization techniques, one hand will usually stabilize while the other hand performs the movement.*
   At times the plinth, the patient's body weight, and so on, are used for external stabilization. This allows both hands to assist in the movement. The therapist uses his hand or a belt to fix or stabilize

one joint partner against a firm support. The fixation is maintained close to the joint space without causing pain. The mobilizing hand grips the joint structure to be moved as close to the joint space as possible.

5. *The operator must consider*
   — Direction of movement — almost always parallel to or perpendicular to a tangent across adjoining joint surfaces
   — Velocity of movement — slow stretching for large capsular restrictions; faster oscillations for minor restrictions
   — Amplitude of movement — graded according to pain, guarding, and degree of restriction

6. *Compare accessory joint movement to the opposite side (extremity), if necessary, to determine presence or degree of restriction.*

7. *One movement is performed at a time, at one joint at a time.*

8. *Each technique can be used as*
   — An examination procedure by taking up the slack, only, to determine the existing range of accessory movement and the presence or absence of pain
   — A therapeutic technique in which a high-velocity, small-amplitude thrust or graded oscillations are applied to regain accessory joint movement and relieve pain

9. *Reassessment*
   This should be done at the beginning of each treatment session, as well as during the treatment session. A selection of a few important "markers" for assessment enables a quick estimate of progress to be made without repeatedly going through the whole examination procedure.

INDICATIONS

Joint mobilization techniques are indicated in cases of joint dysfunction, due to restriction of accessory joint motion causing pain or restriction of motion during normal physiological movement. However, as discussed in Chapter 2, Arthrology, there may be numerous causes of loss of accessory joint movement. The most common of these include capsuloligamentous tightening or adherence; internal derangement, as from a cartilaginous loose body or meniscus displacement; reflex muscle guarding; and bony blockage, as from hypertrophic degenerative changes. From this it should be clear that the proper indication for using specific mobilization techniques

is loss of accessory joint motion (joint-play movement) secondary to capsular or ligamentous tightness or adherence. Other causes of joint dysfunction are relative contraindications. Refer to the section on capsular tightness in Chapter 3, Pain.

CONTRAINDICATIONS

1. *Absolute*
   — Bacterial infection, neoplasm, recent fracture
2. *Relative*
   — Joint effusion or inflammation
   — Arthrosis (*e.g.*, degenerative joint disease) if acute, or if causing a bony block to movement to be restored
   — Rheumatoid arthritis
   — Osteoporosis
   — Internal derangement
   — General debilitation (*e.g.*, influenza, pregnancy, chronic disease)

GRADING OF MOVEMENT

Gaining a feel for the appropriate rate, rhythm, and intensity of movement is perhaps the most difficult aspect of learning to administer specific joint mobilization. Generally, rate, rhythm, and intensity must be adjusted according to how the patient presents — whether acute or chronic — and according to the response of the patient to the technique. When significant pain or muscle spasm is elicited, the rate of movement must be adjusted, or the intensity reduced, or both.

The type of movement performed ultimately depends upon the immediate effect desired. These techniques, in the majority of cases, are used to provide relief of pain and muscle guarding, to stretch a tight joint capsule or ligament, and, rarely, to reduce an intra-articular derangement that may be blocking movement.

1. *Relief of pain and muscle guarding*
   This is desirable in relatively acute conditions, as a treatment in and of itself, and in chronic conditions to prepare for more vigorous stretching. The techniques in this case are performed to increase proprioceptive input to the spinal cord so as to inhibit ongoing nociceptive input to anterior horn cells and central receiving areas (see Chapter 3, Pain). They are what Maitland refers to as Grade I and II techniques.[9] Movement is performed at the beginning or midpoint of the available joint-play amplitude, avoiding tension to joint capsules and ligaments. A rhythmic oscilla-

tion of the joint is produced at a rate of perhaps two to three cycles per second.

In the case of acute joint conditions, these may constitute the only passive mobilization techniques used until the acute manifestations subside. In more chronic cases, these techniques should be used at the initiation of a treatment session, between stretching techniques, and at the end of a session in order to promote relaxation of muscles controlling the joint. Here they are used on a continuum with stretching techniques, gradually increasing in intensity as the patient relaxes.

2. Stretching techniques

Since clinicians use these techniques primarily in cases of capsular tightness or adherence, the goal is ultimately to apply an intermittent stretch to the particular aspect of the capsule that is to be mobilized. In doing so, the clinician must move the joint up to the limit of the pathologic amplitude of a particular joint-play movement and attempt to increase the amplitude of movement. These techniques must be applied rhythmically —no abrupt changes in speed or direction—to prevent reflex contractions of muscles about the joint that might occur from overfiring of joint receptors. They must also be applied slowly in order to allow for the viscous nature—resistance to quick change in length—of connective tissue. The slack that is taken up in the joint-play movement is not released as the movement is performed. In effect, one is applying a prolonged stretch with superimposed rhythmic oscillations of small amplitude. The rationale is twofold. A prolonged stretch is the safest, most effective means of increasing the extensibility of collagenous tissue. Rhythmic oscillations reduce the amount of discomfort and facilitate maximal relaxation during the procedure, presumably by increasing large-fiber input to the "gate."

STOPS

When stretching at the limits of a particular osteokinematic movement in the presence of a tight capsule, it is usually helpful to provide a rigid "stop" against which the oscillation is made. It is best for the practitioner to arrange one of his or her body parts (*e.g.*, thigh, forearm, or trunk) as a stop. In this way the stop is easily moved to allow progressively increased range of movement. Such a stop also gives the patient an indication of exactly how far the therapist is going to move the part during a particular series of oscillations. This will reduce anticipatory

muscle guarding to a minimum. If a greater range of movement is desired, the patient is informed where the stop will be made. The therapist rearranges the stop so as to allow a small increase in motion, and the oscillations are resumed. Such a technique seems to be most effective if the patient's part is brought up rather firmly against the stop with each oscillation. (See Figure 6–3B for the shoulder, in which the therapist's thigh is brought up onto the plinth to act as a stop for external rotation, while the therapist simultaneously applies a posterior glide at the glenohumeral joint.)

Note: For the sake of simplicity, the operator will be referred to as the male, and the patient as the female. All of the techniques described apply to the patient's left extremities, except where indicated. (P—patient; O—operator; M—movement)

TECHNIQUES FOR THE UPPER EXTREMITY

THE SHOULDER

Techniques performed with the arm at the side of the body are primarily used to promote relaxation of the muscles controlling the joint, to relieve pain, and to prepare for more vigorous stretching techniques. In relatively acute cases of adhesive capsulitis, they may constitute the primary techniques used until resolution of the acute state allows more aggressive mobilization. In more chronic cases, they are typically used at the initiation of the mobilization session, between techniques, and at the end of the session to prevent and reduce reflex muscle cramping. As these techniques are performed, the arm may be gradually moved from the side of the body toward positions in which more vigorous techniques may be applied. For chronic conditions, these techniques should be used on a continuing basis in conjunction with the stretching techniques described.

1. *The Shoulder Joint*—Elevation and relaxation
   a. *Inferior Glide*—with the arm at the side of the body (Fig. 6–1A)
      P—Supine, with arm resting at side of body
      O—Stabilizes the scapula with the left hand at the patient's axilla. The web of the hand contacts the inferior aspect of the neck of the glenoid. The right hand grasps the patient's forearm as proximally as possible. **Note:** The patient's arm and the operator's forearm are essentially parallel. The patient's wrist rests across the antecubital fossa of the operator's stabilizing hand.
      M—The scapula is held fixed while the humerus is moved caudally. The movement is performed initially with the patient's

arm to the side and resting on the plinth. As the patient relaxes, the arm may gradually be moved toward abduction or flexion. **Note:** This is an important technique for relaxation of spasm and relieving pain, to be used before and after a treatment session and between other techniques. For greater ranges of elevation, see Technique 1, *b–e*.

b. *Progressive Long-Axis Extension (Distal Glide)*—moving toward abduction (Fig. 6–1B)

P—Supine, with the arm resting at the side

O—Stabilizes the inferior neck of the glenoid with the web space of his left hand. The forearm is pronated and the elbow is straight. The other hand grasps the humerus just above the elbow, gaining a purchase on the humeral epicondyles. **Note:** The operator stands with his body facing away from the patient. The patient's forearm is tucked between the therapist's arm and trunk, and the therapist fixes the patient's arm against his trunk.

M—With the scapula held stable and the patient's arm fixed against the operator's trunk, the humerus is moved distally along its long axis. To perform the movement, the therapist shifts his trunk into outward rotation. As the patient relaxes, the arm may be gradually moved toward abduction. When about 60° abduction is obtained, the therapist must shift his stabilizing hand to contact the lateral border of the scapula with the heel of the supinated hand.

This technique may be performed up to about 80° abduction. For greater ranges of abduction, see Technique 1, *d* and *e*.

c. *Inferior Glide*—moving toward flexion (Fig. 6–1C)

P—Supine, with the humerus flexed 60° to 100° and the elbow bent, with the wrist resting across the clavicular region

O—Grasps the proximal humerus with both hands, the fingers interlaced. The patient's elbow region is contacted with the clavicular region of the operator's shoulder closest to the patient.

M—The operator pulls caudally with his trunk to produce a movement of combined flexion of the humerus and inferior glide at the glenohumeral joint.

The arm is gradually moved toward greater ranges of flexion up to about 110°. For greater degrees of flexion, see Technique 1, *e*.

d. *Inferior Glide*—in abduction (Fig. 6–1D)

P—Supine, elbow bent. The arm is close to the limits of abduction and external rotation, but comfortable.

O—Approaches the arm superiorly. He supports the elbow with the left hand at the distal humerus. The patient's forearm is tucked and supported between the operator's arm and trunk. The right hand contacts the superior aspect of the proximal humerus with the heel of the hand, with the forearm supinated and elbow bent.

M—Inferior glide of the humeral head is produced by the right hand. As the patient relaxes, the arm can be guided into gradually increasing degrees of abduction with the stabilizing hand.

This may be performed up to about 90°. The choice of position is guided by the ease with which a relaxed movement can be produced. This technique is used to increase abduction, allowing stretching into abduction while avoiding impingement of the greater tubercle on the acromial arch.

e. *Inferior Glide*—in more than 90° elevation (Fig. 6–1E)

P—Supine, with arm elevated comfortably, but close to the limits of full elevation in a somewhat horizontally abducted position, between flexion and abduction. The elbow is bent. **Note:** When moving into ranges past 90°, the patient's forearm may be supported on her forehead or on a pillow above her head, or the operator may support it (as shown).

O—Approaches the arm superiorly. He supports the elbow with the left hand, supporting the patient's arm on his right arm. The operator contacts the superior aspect of the proximal humerus with the right hand, with the thumb positioned ventrally just distal to the acromion.

M—Inferior glide of the humoral head is produced with the right hand. The arm can be guided into gradually increasing degrees of elevation. **Note:** The direction of movement is performed caudally and in a somewhat lateral direction in keeping with the relationship of the joint surfaces in this position.

Movements in elevation beyond 90° are particularly useful as stretching techniques and may be used even when only a few degrees of elevation are restricted; however, they have no place in the treatment of a very painful shoulder.

2. *The Shoulder Joint*—Internal rotation
   a. *Posterior Glide*—with the arm in various degrees of abduction (10° to 55°), (Fig. 6–2A)
   P—Supine, with the arm slightly abducted
   O—Stands between the patient's arm and body, and supports the patient's elbow with the right hand. The hand, wrist, and forearm are supported by tucking them between his elbow and side. The left hand contacts the anterior aspect of the upper humerus with the heel of the left hand,

with the forearm pronated and elbow straight.
   M—A posterior glide is produced by leaning forward slightly and flexing the knees, transmitting the force through the straight arm.

This technique is used to increase joint play necessary for internal rotation and flexion.
   b. *Anterior Glide*—arm close to the limits of internal rotation (Fig. 6–2B)
   P—Lies on uninvolved side with the arm behind the back so it rests comfortably, but close to the limits of internal rotation.
   O—Stands behind patient with both thumb pads over the posterior humeral head. The finger of the right hand grasps around

A

B

Fig. 6–1. Techniques for elevation and relaxation of the shoulder joint; (*A*) inferior glide, arm at side; (*B*) progressive long-axis extension moving toward abduction; (*C*) inferior glide toward flexion; (*D*) inferior glide in abduction; (*E*) inferior glide in more than 90° elevation.

C

D

E

Fig. 6–2. Techniques for internal rotation of the shoulder joint; (*A*) posterior glide, arm slightly abducted; (*B*) anterior glide, arm close to the limits of internal rotation, at side or behind back; (*C*) internal rotation, arm close to 90° abduction.

anteriorly to stabilize at the anterior aspect of the acromion and clavicle. Elbows remain almost fully extended. The left knee may be brought up onto the plinth to support the patient's arm.

M—An anterior glide is produced by leaning forward with the upper trunk, transmitting the force through the thumbs. Internal rotation is gradually increased by progressively moving the patient's hand up the back.

This technique results in a posterior capsular stretch, stretching into internal rotation while

avoiding posterior impingement of the humeral head on the glenoid labrum. A similar technique may be performed with the patient prone (see Technique 2,*c*).

c. *Anterior glide*—alternate technique (not shown)

P—Prone, with the arm abducted approximately 45° to 60°. The flexed forearm extends over the edge of the plinth. The upper arm is supported on the plinth. A towel roll or pad is placed under the anterior aspect of the shoulder girdle.

O—Stands between the patient's arm and

trunk. He supports the patient's elbow against his body with one hand, maintaining the arm in abduction and neutral rotation. The posterior aspect of the upper humerus is contacted with the heel of the opposite hand. The forearm is pronated, and the elbow is straight.

M—An anterior glide is produced by leaning forward with the trunk, transmitting the force through the straight arm and flexion of the knees. **Note:** By shifting the supporting hand to the patient's wrist, internal rotation may be gradually increased by simultaneously rotating the arm internally. The operator's body provides a stop to internal rotation. This is an oscillatory technique.

d. *Internal Rotation Technique*—arm close to 90° abduction (Fig. 6–2C)

P—Supine, with the arm resting comfortably, but as close to 90° abduction as possible, the elbow bent to 90°, and forearm pronated.

O—Supports the wrist with the left hand; supports under the elbow with the fingers of the right hand from the medial side. He positions the right upper arm in front of and just medial to the shoulder. The left knee is brought up onto the plinth to act as a stop.

M—The right upper arm provides only enough counterpressure to the shoulder to prevent lifting of the shoulder girdle; the hand maintains the arm in abduction. The left hand simultaneously rotates the arm internally. The left thigh provides a stop to internal rotation. The stop is close to the limit of movement so as to minimize anticipatory guarding by the patient. The stop is progressively moved as motion increases. This is an oscillatory movement.

Methods for internal rotation are useful for restoring necessary joint-play movements with the arm near the side, or in various degrees of abduction (see Technique 2,*a*), or as stretching techniques in functional positions (see Techniques 2,*b–d*).

3. *The Shoulder Joint*—External rotation

a. *Anterior Glide*—arm at the side (Fig. 6–3A)

P—Supine, arm at the side, elbow bent, forearm supported by operator's arm

O—Stabilizes with the right hand, grasping the distal humerus just proximal to the

elbow. He grasps around medially to the posterior aspect of the humerus with the left hand, as far proximally as possible.

M—An anterior glide is effected with the left hand, after the "slack" in the shoulder girdle has been taken up. This is oscillatory mobilization.

This technique is used to increase the joint-play movement necessary for external rotation.

b. *Posterior Glide*—arm close to 90° abduction (Fig. 6–3B)

P—Supine, with the arm resting comfortably, but as close to 90° abduction as possible; elbow bent to 90°

O—Supports the wrist with his right hand. He contacts the anterior aspect of the proximal humerus with the heel of the left hand. The right knee is brought up onto the plinth to act as a stop.

M—Posterior glide is produced with the left hand, while the right hand simultaneously rotates the arm externally. The right thigh provides a stop to external rotation close to the limit of movement. This minimizes anticipatory guarding by the patient. The stop is progressively moved as motion increases. This is an oscillatory movement, produced synchronously with posterior glide.

This method results in an anterior capsular stretch, stretching into external rotation while avoiding anterior impingement of the humerus on the glenoid labrum.

4. *The Shoulder Joint*—Horizontal adduction and general capsular stretch

a. *Lateral Glide*—arm at side (glenohumeral distraction) (Fig. 6–4A)

P—Supine, arm at the side with the elbow bent and the hand resting on her stomach or on the forearm of the operator

O—Stabilizes with the right hand at the lateral aspect of the patient's elbow. The left hand grasps the humerus medially, as far proximally as possible. The forearm is brought around over the patient's thorax, in line with the direction of movement.

M—A lateral glide is effected by moving the upper humerus laterally with the left hand. The elbow should be allowed to move laterally through the same excursion as the humeral head, avoiding a tilting maneuver, unless it is specifically in-

A

B

Fig. 6–3. Techniques for external rotation of the shoulder joint: (*A*) anterior glide, arm at side; (*B*) posterior glide, arm close to 90° of abduction.

tended to stretch the superior joint capsule.

This technique (performed at the side of the body) is used to promote relaxation, to relieve pain, to prepare for more vigorous stretching techniques, and as a general capsular stretch. As the latter, it may be useful in increasing movement toward the close-packed position by helping to prevent premature compression of the joint.

b. *Lateral Glide* — in flexion (Fig. 6–4*B*)

P — Supine, with the arm flexed comfortably to 90° and elbow bent so that the hand rests on the upper chest

O — Stabilizes distal humerus with his right hand at the elbow. The left hand is placed against the medial surface of the upper end of the humerus. By bending forward the arm is placed in a horizontal position in line with the movement.

M — The proximal humerus is moved laterally. This technique is used to restore joint play necessary for horizontal adduction. It results in separation of the joint surfaces (lateral distraction).

c. *Lateral and Backward Glide* — in flexion (Fig. 6–4*C*)

P — Supine, with the arm flexed comfortably

Fig. 6–4. Techniques for horizontal adduction and general capsular stretch of the shoulder joint: (*A*) lateral glide, arm at side (glenohumeral distraction); (*B*) lateral glide in flexion; (*C*) lateral and backward glide in flexion.

Fig. 6–5. Techniques for distraction of the humer-oulnar joint: (*A*) joint distraction in flexion (ulna moved inferiorly); (*B*) joint distraction in flexion (ulna moved superiorly); (*C*) joint distraction, moving toward extension.

to 90° and elbow bent so that the hand rests on the upper chest

O—Stabilizes distal humerus and elbow by resting them against his trapezial ridge. He grasps the medial aspect of the proximal humerus with both hands, interlacing the fingers.

M—The proximal humerus is moved backward, toward the plinth, and outward simultaneously in a rocking forward and downward movement of the operator's trunk.

The arm may be progressively moved toward increased horizontal adduction as the patient relaxes. This technique is used to increase joint play necessary for horizontal adduction by employing lateral glide with a backward glide simultaneously.

Scapulothoracic, acromioclavicular, and sternoclavicular mobilizations may also be performed in certain circumstances. However, these are rarely necessary in cases of glenohumeral capsular tightness, because these joints tend to become hypermobile by compensating for the restriction at the glenohumeral joint. They may be useful following immobilization of the entire shoulder complex or in other disorders, such as arthritis or injury in the different joints (*i.e.*, fractures and dislocations) as well as neuromuscular dysfunction.[7,8,9,18]

THE ELBOW AND FOREARM

1. *The Humeroulnar Joint* — Distraction
   a. *Joint Distraction* — in flexion (ulna moved inferiorly) (Fig. 6–5*A*)
   P—Supine with the arm at the side, elbow bent, and forearm supinated
   O—Stabilizes the wrist with the left hand. He grasps the proximal forearm high up in the antecubital space with the right hand in a pronated position, using the web of the hand for contact.
   M—The proximal ulna is moved inferiorly, affecting a joint distraction, with perhaps some inferior glide. As movement increases, the elbow can be progressively flexed.

   This technique is used as a general capsular stretch primarily to increase elbow flexion.
   b. *Joint Distraction* — in flexion (ulna moved superiorly) (Fig. 6–5*B*)
   P—Supine, with the arm at the side, forearm supinated, and the elbow flexed

O—Stabilizes the upper arm by holding the distal humerus at the elbow down against the plinth with the right hand. With the left hand, he grasps the back of the supinated wrist.

M—The proximal ulna is moved superiorly, producing joint distraction. **Note:** By holding the forearm against his body, the operator can combine distraction with increasing flexion (oscillatory movement) by a rocking motion of his body, while maintaining constant stabilization of the humerus.

This technique is also used to increase elbow flexion.
   c. *Joint Distraction* — moving toward extension (Fig. 6–5*C*)
   P—Supine, with the arm at the side, elbow bent, and forearm in neutral position
   O—Stabilizes the distal humerus against the plinth with the left hand, forearm pronated. He grasps the distal ulna with his right hand, using primarily the thumb and index finger.
   M—Ulnar distraction is effected as a distal pull and by a little outward rotation of the operator's entire body. The elbow may be gradually extended as movement increases.

This technique may be considered an inferior glide of the coronoid on the trochlea or, in a sense, a joint distraction. When used at the limit of extension it becomes an anterior capsular stretch.

2. *The Humeroulnar Joint* — Medial-lateral tilt (Fig. 6–6)
   P—Supine, with arm at the side, forearm supinated; the elbow is close to the limit of extension.
   O—Supports the wrist with the left hand; grasps the humeral epicondyles, supporting the olecranon in the palm of the hand.
   M—Keeping the patient's wrist stationary, the right hand moves medially or laterally, producing a medial or lateral (valgus or varus) tilt of the patient's humeroulnar joint. The elbow is gradually extended as movement increases.

This technique is used only when the elbow lacks a few degrees of extension. It is intended to increase a joint-play movement necessary for full elbow extension.

3. *The Proximal Radioulnar Joint* — Distal glide of radius on ulna (Fig. 6–7)

Fig. 6–6. Medial-lateral tilt of humeroulnar joint.

P—Supine, with arm resting at the side, elbow bent, and forearm in neutral position.
O—Stabilizes the distal humerus against the plinth with his left hand, forearm pronated. He grasps the distal radius with his right hand, using primarily the thumb, index, and long fingers.
M—The radius is pulled distally with the right

hand and by a little outward rotation of the operator's entire body. This elbow may be gradually extended as movement increases. This technique may also be considered distraction at the radiohumeral joint and is intended to increase joint-play movement necessary for full elbow extension.

4. *The Proximal Radioulnar Joint*—Dorsal-ventral glide (Fig. 6–8)
   P—Supine, with the arm at the side, elbow slightly flexed, and forearm in slight supination. The patient's forearm is supported by placing her hand lightly on the operator's left forearm.
   O—Supports the medial aspect of the distal humerus and proximal surface of the upper forearm with his left hand. The right hand holds the ventral surface of the proximal radius with the thumb and the dorsal surface with the crook of the flexed proximal interphalangeal (PIP) joint of the index finger.
   M—The radial head may be moved dorsally or ventrally as separate motions. These movements can be performed in varying degrees of elbow flexion, extension, supination, or pronation.

This technique may also be considered a movement at the radiohumeral joint. It is used to increase joint movement necessary for pronation and supination.

Fig. 6–7. Distal glide of radius on ulna for proximal radioulnar joint.

Fig. 6–8. Dorsal-ventral glide of proximal radioulnar joint.

5. *The Proximal Radioulnar Joint* — Technique to regain pronation (after Mennell[12]) (Fig. 6–9)

   P — Supine, with the arm in full supination and slightly abducted

   O — With his left hand, he supports the wrist with his fingers over the ventral aspect and his thumb on the dorsal aspect. He places the thenar eminence of his right hand over the anterior aspect of the head of the radius and maintains the patient's upper arm on the plinth. The position of the head of the patient's radius is maintained with his thenar eminence.

   M — The carrying angle of the patient's elbow is increased by the operator's hand at the wrist while maintaining full supination (Fig. 6–9A). Maintaining both supination and the carrying angle of the forearm, the operator flexes the patient's elbow until the head of the radius is felt to press firmly against his right thenar eminence (Fig. 6–9B). While maintaining the forearm in this position with firm pressure against the radial head, the forearm is moved into pronation (Fig. 6–9C). **Note:** This technique requires considerable practice to be effective. If supination, flexion, and pressure of the thenar eminence are not maintained throughout the technique, the proper movement will not be achieved. The angle of flexion should not be

altered while the forearm is moved from supination to pronation.

This is a most valuable technique in regaining joint-play movements necessary for pronation and supination.

6. *The Distal Radioulnar Joint* — Dorsal-ventral glide (Fig. 6–10)

   P — Supine, with arm somewhat abducted and elbow bent, so that the forearm may rest on the plinth in a neutral position with respect to pronation and supination.

   O — Stabilizes the distal radius against the plinth, grasping it between the heel of his hand and the pads of the second through fifth fingers. He grasps the distal ulna dorsally with the thumb pad and ventrally with the pads of the index and long fingers.

   M — The distal ulna may be moved dorsally or ventrally relative to the distal radius. These motions should be performed separately. **Note:** Alternatively, the distal ulna may be stabilized and the distal radius moved by reversing the handholds. The movement may also be performed with the forearm vertical.

These techniques are used to increase joint-play motions necessary for pronation and supination.

THE WRIST AND HAND

1. *The Ulnomeniscotriquetral Joint* — Dorsal glide (Fig. 6–11)

   P — Supine or sitting, with the elbow resting on the plinth or table, and the forearm vertical.

   O — Stabilizes the radial side of the wrist and hand with his left hand. The right hand contacts the dorsal aspect of the head of the ulna with the thumb, and the palmar aspect of the triquetrum and the pisiform with the radial aspect of the crook of the flexed PIP joint of his index finger.

   M — A dorsal glide of the pisiform and triquetrum on the ulna is produced by a squeezing action between the thumb and the crook of the index finger.

This technique is used to increase a joint-play movement necessary for pronation and supination.

2. *The Radiocarpal Joint (and Ulnomeniscotriquetral Joint)* — Joint distraction (Fig. 6–12)

   P — Sitting or supine, with the elbow bent and resting on the plinth, and the forearm in neutral pronation and supination

   O — Stabilizes the distal humerus and elbow against the plinth with his right hand at the

Fig. 6–9. Technique to regain pronation of proximal radioulnar joint (after Mennell): (*A*) increasing the carrying angle of the elbow; (*B*) moving the arm toward flexion; (*C*) pronation of the arm near the end of motion.

Fig. 6–10. Dorsal-ventral glide of distal radioulnar joint.

antecubital space. The left hand grasps around the proximal row of carpals, just distal to the styloid processes.

M — A distraction is produced with the left hand, paying particular attention to the radiocarpal joint.

This technique is used as a general mobilization procedure to increase joint play at the radiocarpal joint. Distraction tends to occur with palmar flexion of the wrist. By increasing the amount of joint distraction, movement toward the close-packed

Fig. 6–11. Dorsal glide of ulnomeniscotriquetral joint (right hand).

position, dorsiflexion, may be increased. This prevents premature compression of joint surfaces.

3. *The Radiocarpal Joint* — Dorsal-palmar glide (Fig. 6–13)

P — Sitting with the arm somewhat abducted, the elbow bent, and the forearm resting on the plinth in pronation. The hand extends over the edge of the table or plinth.

O — Stabilizes the distal end of the forearm with his right hand, just proximal to the styloid processes. He grasps the proximal row of carpals with his left hand using the styloid processes and pisiform for landmarks.

M — The proximal row of carpals may be moved dorsally or palmarly, paying particular attention to the radiocarpal joint. Dorsal glide and palmar glide should be performed as separate techniques. **Note:** Dorsal glide may be performed more effectively with the arm in full supination and the hand extended over the edge of the plinth or table.

Palmar glide is used to increase joint-play movements necessary for dorsal flexion. Dorsal glide is used to increase joint-play movements necessary for palmar flexion.

4. *The Radiocarpal Joint (and Ulnomeniscotriquetral Joint)* — Radial-ulnar glide (or tilt) (Fig. 6–14)

P — Sitting, with the arm near the side, the elbow bent, and the forearm resting on the plinth in neutral pronation and supination. The radial aspect of the forearm faces superiorly.

O — Stabilizes the distal end of the forearm with the left hand, just proximal to the styloid processes. He grasps the proximal row of carpals with the right hand.

M — The proximal row of carpals may be glided radially or ulnarly on the distal ends of the radius and ulna (articular disk). Alternatively, a radial tilt or ulnar tilt may be produced.

Radial glide and ulnar tilt are joint-play movements necessary for ulnar deviation. Ulnar glide and radial tilt are joint-play movements necessary for radial deviation.

5. *Midcarpal Joint* — Joint distraction (not illustrated)

This technique is produced in exactly the same way as that for the radiocarpal joint except the left handhold moves distally to grasp the distal row of carpals. (See Technique 2 and Fig. 6–12 for distraction of the radiocarpal joint.)

This technique is used for general mobilization to increase joint play at the midcarpal joint.

Fig. 6–12. Distraction of radiocarpal joint (and ulnomeniscotriquetral joint) (right arm).

6. *Midcarpal Joint*—Dorsal-palmar glide (not illustrated)

This technique is produced in exactly the same way as that for the radiocarpal joint except the left handhold moves distally to grasp the distal row of carpals (See Technique 3 and Fig. 6–13 for dorsal-palmar glide of the radiocarpal joint.)

Palmar glide is used to increase joint-play movements necessary for dorsal flexion. Dorsal glide is used to increase joint-play movements necessary for palmar flexion.

7. *The Midcarpal Joint*—Palmar glide of the distal row of carpals on the proximal row of carpals (Fig. 6–15)

P—Sitting or supine, with the elbow resting on the plinth and the forearm vertical

O—Approaches from the ulnar aspect. The thenar eminence of his left hand contacts the distal row of carpals dorsally. The thenar eminence of his right hand contacts the proximal row of carpals palmarly. The fingers are interlaced over the radial aspect of the wrist. The forearms are directed outward, perpendicular to the plane of the palm.

M—A palmar glide of the distal row of carpals on the proximal row is produced by a squeezing motion between the thenar eminences.

Note: This is a more effective method of palmar glide than that described in Technique 6 for dorsal-palmar glide. The performance of this movement depends on the accurate placement of the operator's thenar emi-

nences over the correct bones. Extension and spreading of the patient's fingers should take place when this movement is elicited correctly.[12]

This technique is used to increase joint-play motion necessary for dorsal flexion of the wrist.

Specific movements between adjacent bones of the wrist and carpal joints may be indicated. Mobility between triquetrum and lunate, lunate and radius, or capitate and lunate, for example, can be tested and mobilized. In general, one joint partner is always fixated while the other is moved. The

Fig. 6–13. Dorsal-palmar glide of radiocarpal joint.

Fig. 6–14. Radial-ulnar glide (or tilt) of radiocarpal joint (and ulnomeniscotriquetral joint).

individual carpal bones can be mobilized by placing the thumb and index finger on the volar and dorsal sides of two adjacent carpal bones (*e.g.,* lunate and capitate) respectively. The thumbs may mobilize one carpal while the index fingers stabilizes the other carpal bone, or *vice versa.* The reader is referred to detailed descriptions of these advanced techniques by Kaltenborn and others.[7,12,18] Only one example will be described.

8. *The Intercarpal Joints*—Palmar glide of the scaphoid on the radius (Fig. 6–16)

   P—Sitting or supine, with the forearm resting on the table, or with the arm held forward by the operator

O—Stands or sits facing the hand. Both hands hold the patient's thenar and hypothenar eminence. The index fingers are placed on the proximal palmar surface of radius, stabilizing it in this position. The thumbs contact the scaphoid dorsally.

M—The scaphoid is moved palmarly relative to the distal end of the radius.

This technique is used to increase joint-play motion necessary for dorsal glide of the scaphoid on the radius.

9. *The Intermetacarpal Joints*—Dorsal-palmar glide (Fig. 6–17) (These joints between the metacarpal heads are not true synovial joints, but movement must occur here during grasp and release, as described in Appendix A.)

   P—Sitting or supine, with the elbow resting on the plinth, the forearm pronated

   O—Approaches from the dorsal aspect. The left hand stabilizes the head and neck of the third metacarpal. The thumb pad contacts dorsally, and the pads of the index and long fingers palmarly. The left hand grasps the head and neck of the fourth metacarpal in a similar fashion.

   M—The head of the fourth metacarpal can be moved palmarly or dorsally with respect to the third metacarpal. Similarly, the right hand can stabilize the third metacarpal, while the left hand moves the second metacarpal. Note that the third metacarpal is the "center of movement" as the hand flattens and arches during release and grasp. It is always stabilized, while the other metacarpals are moved relative to it.

Fig. 6–15. Palmar glide of the distal row on the proximal row for midcarpal joint (right hand).

Fig. 6–16. Palmar glide of scaphoid on radius for intercarpal joints.

These techniques are used to increase joint-play movements necessary for the arching and flattening of the hand that occur with grasp and release.

THE FINGERS

1. *The Metacarpophalangeal (MP) or Interphalangeal (IP) Joints* — Distraction (Fig. 6–18)
   P — Sitting or supine
   O — Supports the forearm and elbow by tucking them between his forearm and side. To treat the more radial joints, the operator ap-

Fig. 6–17. Dorsal-palmar glide of intermetacarpal joints.

Fig. 6–18. Distraction of metacarpophalangeal or interphalangeal joints (right hand).

proaches from the ulnar side for the thumb, index, and long fingers, and from the radial side for the ring and small fingers. He grasps the head of the proximal bone dorsally with the thumb pad and palmarly with the crook of the index finger. He grasps the base of the distal bone in a similar manner.
   M — Keeping the joint in slight flexion (avoiding close-packed position), a long-axis distraction is produced with the operator's more distal hand.
These techniques are used for general joint mobilization to increase joint play. Distraction is necessary, especially during flexion at the MPs and extension at the IPs, since these are movements toward the close-packed position. Premature compression of joint surfaces will result if sufficient joint play into distraction cannot occur.

2. *The Metacarpophalangeal or Interphalangeal Joints* — Dorsal-palmar glide (Fig. 6–19)
   P — Supine or sitting
   O — The handholds are essentially the same as those for distraction, except that during dorsal glide the palmar contact of the more distal hand is with the pad of the index finger.
   M — The base of the distal bone may be moved palmarly or dorsally.
Palmar glide is necessary for flexion. Dorsal glide is a joint-play movement necessary for extension.

3. *The Metacarpophalangeal or Interphalangeal Joints* — Radioulnar glide (or tilt) (Fig. 6–20)
   P — Supine or sitting
   O — The handholds are similar to those used for distraction except that the thumbs are brought around to the aspect of the bones closest to the operator, and the crooks or pads of the index fingers are brought around to the aspect of the bone farthest from the operator. The contacts are then made on the radial and ulnar sides of the joint.

Fig. 6-19. Dorsal-palmar glide of metacarpophalangeal or interphalangeal joints (right hand).

M — Radial or ulnar glide or tilt may be produced by the thumb pad in one direction, and by the index pad in the other. While one pad is producing the movement, the other moves to the more distal part of the bone.

Ulnar glide (radial tilt) is necessary for extension at the IP joints. Radial glide (ulnar tilt) is necessary for flexion at the IP joints. The same is true, but to a lesser extent, at the MP joints.

4. *The Metacarpophalangeal or Interphalangeal Joints* — Rotation (pronation and supination) (Fig. 6-21)

 P — Supine or sitting

 O — The proximal handhold is the same as that for distraction. The distal handholds are also similar to those used for long-axis distraction, except the operator may gain some leverage by holding the more distal segment of the digit, semiflexed, in his remaining fingers. This must be performed with caution.

 M — A pronation or supination of the distal end of the bone is produced by the operator's more distal hand.

Supination is a joint-play movement (conjunct rotation) necessary for flexion, especially at the IPs. Pronation occurs during extension. **Note:** The same techniques may be used at the carpometacarpal joint of the thumb. As for their specific uses in this case, consider the convex–concave rule and how it applies to this sellar joint.

TECHNIQUES FOR THE LOWER EXTREMITY

THE HIP

Like the shoulder joint, techniques performed with the hip in a neutral position are primarily used to promote relaxation of the muscles controlling the joint, to relieve pain, and to prepare for more vigorous stretching techniques. The hip joint is, however, much more stable than the shoulder joint.

Note: All of the techniques described in this section apply to the patient's *right* extremities, except where indicated.

Fig. 6-20. Radial-ulnar glide of metacarpophalangeal or interphalangeal joints (right hand).

Fig. 6-21. Rotation (pronation and supination) of metacarpophalangeal or interphalangeal joints (right hand).

Fig. 6–22. Inferior glide of hip joint (A) in neutral and (B) in flexion.

1. *The Hip Joint* — Elevation and relaxation
   a. *Inferior Glide* — in neutral (Fig. 6–22A)
      P—Supine. A belt may be used to keep the upper body from sliding inferiorly on the plinth. The leg is in slight abduction, external rotation, and flexion.
      O—Grasps the patient's ankle just proximal to the malleoli with his left hand, behind his back. He grasps the femur distally, just proximal to the condyles and from the medial aspect, with the right hand. **Note:** If the patient has a knee disorder, both handholds may be shifted proximal to the knee or Technique 1,*b* can be used, with the hip in about 30° flexion.
      M—The operator's arms remain fixed. An inferior glide is produced by leaning backward with the trunk. This may be done through various degrees of abduction.

This technique is used as a general mobilization to increase joint play. Inferior glide is a joint-play movement necessary for hip flexion and abduction. It is also used for relaxation of spasm and pain relief and may be used before and after a treatment session and between other techniques. This procedure should be used on a continuing basis and in conjunction with the stretching techniques described in Techniques 1,*b* and *c*.

b. *Inferior Glide* — in flexion (Fig. 6–22B)
   P—Supine, with hip and knee each flexed to 90°. A belt may be used to stabilize the upper body.
   O—Supports the lower leg by letting it rest on his shoulder. He grasps the anterior aspect of the proximal femur as far proximally as possible, using both hands with the fingers interlaced.
   M—An inferior glide is imparted with the

Fig. 6–23. Anterior glide of hip joint (*A*, right hip) in supine and (*B*, left hip) in prone positions.

hands. This may be performed while simultaneously rocking the thigh into flexion.

This technique is used to increase joint-play movement necessary for hip flexion.

  c. *Inferior Glide* — in extension (not illustrated)

    P — Supine. A belt may be used to keep the upper body from sliding inferiorly on the plinth. The leg is extended over the side of the plinth and positioned in various degrees of abduction and internal rotation.

    O — Same as that for Technique 1,*a*.

    M — The operator's arms remain fixed. An inferior glide is produced by leaning backward with the trunk. The leg may be progressively moved into various degrees of abduction and internal rotation combined with extension, working toward the close-packed position of the hip joint.

This technique is particularly useful for stretching.

2. *The Hip Joint* — Anterior glide

  a. *Anterior Glide* — in supine (Fig. 6–23*A*)

    P — Supine. A belt may be used to stabilize the pelvis.

    O — Grasps around posteriorly with both hands to the posterior aspect of the proximal femur, level with the greater trochanter. The fingers are interlaced or overlapping. The operator stabilizes the distal thigh and knee against the plinth with his trunk.

    M — The slack is taken up, and an anterior glide of the proximal femur is imparted with the hands.

This technique is used to increase the joint-play movement necessary for external rotation.

  b. *Anterior Glide* — in prone (Fig. 6–23*B*)

    P — Prone, with the knee bent to 90°. A one-inch thickness of towelling may be placed under the anterior aspect of the pelvis, just proximal to the acetabulum, for extra stabilization.

    O — Supports the knee with the right hand by grasping around medially to the anterior aspect of the distal femur. He supports the lower leg by tucking it between his elbow and side. The left hand contacts the posterior aspect of the proximal femur with the heel of the hand. It is level with, and medial to, the greater trochanter.

    M — The left hand imparts an anterior glide to the proximal femur. The right hand may simultaneously guide the leg into internal rotation or abduction.

This technique is considered more progressive than Technique 2,*a*. It is used to increase joint

Fig. 6-24. Posterior glide of hip joint.

play necessary for external rotation. It also serves as a specific capsuloligamentous stretch by internally rotating the femoral head while simultaneously preventing its impingement on the acetabulum.

3. *The Hip Joint* — Posterior glide (Fig. 6-24)
   P — Supine. An inch of padding is placed beneath the pelvis just proximal and medial to the acetabulum.
   O — Supports the knee and distal thigh with the right hand by grasping around medially to the posterior aspect. He contacts the anterior aspect of the proximal femur with the heel of his left hand, with the forearm supinated.
   M — A posterior glide is imparted with the opera-

tor's left hand by leaning forward with the trunk.
This technique is used to increase a joint play movement necessary for internal rotation.

4. *The Hip Joint* — Backward glide (Fig. 6-25)
   P — Supine, with the hip flexed 90° and the lower leg supported comfortably on the crook of the operator's elbow.
   O — Both hands contact the distal end of the femur. He places one hand over the other to provide reinforcement.
   M — A backward (dorsal) glide is effected by leaning forward with the trunk, and is assisted by the operator's body weight.
This technique is used to increase joint-play movement necessary for horizontal adduction of the thigh.

THE KNEE AND LEG

1. *The Femorotibial Joint* — Distraction (Fig. 6-26)
   P — Sitting on the edge of the plinth, with several layers of towelling supporting the underside of the distal thigh
   O — Stands with his back to the patient so as to direct his forearms in the line of force. Both hands grasp the tibia proximal to the malleoli to gain a purchase on them.
   M — A long-axis distraction is produced by leaning forward with the trunk. This may be performed through varying degrees of flexion and extension.
This technique is used as a general mobilization to increase femorotibial joint play. Distraction at this joint tends to occur when moving into flexion (out of the close-packed position). As with any joint, if normal distraction does not occur, premature compression of joint surfaces will re-

Fig. 6-25. Backward glide of hip joint (left hip).

Fig. 6–26. Distraction of femorotibial joint.

A

B

Fig. 6–27. Techniques for posterior glide of the
femorotibial joint, tibia on femur: (*A*) with the right
knee flexed to about 90°; (*B*) with the knee—
here, the left knee—approaching full extension.

sult when moving toward the close-packed position.

2. *The Femorotibial Joint* — Posterior glide

   a. *Posterior Glide* — of tibia on femur with knee flexed (Fig. 6–27A)

      P — Supine, with the knee flexed about 90°, the foot flat on the plinth.

      O — Stabilizes the anterior aspect of the distal femur by contacting it with his entire left hand. The forearm is directed horizontally. The operator contacts the tibial tuberosity with his right hand so that the tuberosity lies in the groove between the thenar and hypothenar eminences. The forearm is directed horizontally.

      M — The right hand produces a posterior glide of the tibia, while the left hand stabilizes the femur.

      This technique is used to increase a joint-play movement necessary for knee flexion.

   b. *Posterior Glide* — of tibia on femur with knee approaching full extension (Fig. 6–27B)

      P — Supine, with the knee slightly flexed from the limit of extension. A one-inch thickness of towelling may be placed under the posterior aspect of the distal femur.

      O — Supports the knee with the right hand placed under the distal femur. He uses the forearm of the right extremity to support and control the femur. The left hand is placed on the proximal aspect of the tibia just distal to the joint space.

      M — A posterior glide is produced with the left hand by moving the lower leg dorsally.

This technique is used to increase joint-play movement necessary for knee flexion. Since the knee is approaching full extension (close-packed position), it is considered more vigorous than Technique 2,a.

3. *Femorotibial Joint* — Anterior glide

   a. *Anterior Glide* — of the tibia on the femur with the knee flexed about 90° (Fig. 6–28)

      P — Supine, with the knee flexed about 90° and the foot flat on the plinth.

      O — Stabilizes the foot and lower leg by partially sitting on the plinth, placing the proximal thigh over the dorsum of the patient's foot. He grasps the proximal tibia by wrapping the fingers of both hands around posteriorly and contacting the tibial tuberosity with both thumbs anteriorly.

      M — Anterior glide is produced by keeping the arms fixed and leaning backward with the trunk.

This technique is used to increase a joint-play movement necessary for knee extension.

   b. *Anterior Glide* — of tibia on femur (or posterior glide of femur on tibia) with the knee approaching full extension (not illustrated)

      This is performed in the same manner as Technique 2,b. See Fig. 6–27B for posterior glide of tibia on femur. However, the handholds are reversed. The right hand contacts the anterior surface of the distal femur, just proximal to the condyles. The operator reaches around medially with the left hand to grasp the posterior aspect of the proximal tibia. Both elbows are only slightly flexed. An anterior glide of the tibia on the femur is pro-

Fig. 6–28. Technique for anterior glide of the femorotibial joint, tibia on femur, with the knee flexed to about 90°.

Fig. 6–29. Internal rotation of femoro-tibial joint: (*A*) with the knee flexed to about 90° and (*B*) at varying degrees of flexion–extension.

duced by leaning to the left. The right hand prevents movement of the femur. **Note:** Often the operator will find it better to stabilize the tibia with the left hand (hand underneath the tibia) and to use the right hand to mobilize the femur dorsally on the tibia. This takes advantage of gravity and the concave–convex rule. With this approach the femur is moved dorsally, resulting in an anterior glide of tibia on femur.

This technique is used to increase a joint-play movement necessary for knee extension.

4. *The Femorotibial Joint* — Internal rotation

a. *Internal Rotation* — with the knee flexed about 90° (Fig. 6–29*A*)
   P — Supine, with the knee flexed 90°, the foot flat on the plinth.
   O — Stabilizes the foot by sitting on the plinth, placing the proximal thigh over the dorsum of the patient's foot. The left hand grasps the proximal tibia laterally, with the fingers wrapped around posteriorly, the thumb contacting the lateral aspect of the tibial tuberosity so as to gain a purchase against it. The right hand grasps the tibia anteriorly and medially,

just distal to the left hand, gaining a purchase on the tibial crest.

M — Both hands rotate the proximal tibia medially (internal rotation), gaining purchase on the tibial tuberosity and lateral tibial condyle with the left hand, and the tibial crest and medial tibial condyle with the right hand.

This technique is used to increase a joint-play movement necessary for knee flexion.

b. *Internal Rotation* — at varying degrees of flexion and extension (Fig. 6–29B)

P — Supine

O — Controls the distal thigh with the left hand grasping from the lateral aspect, the thumb wrapping around posteriorly and the fingers anteriorly. The right hand grasps the heel of the foot. He must place the ankle in close-packed position by fully dorsiflexing it so that the rotary

force is transmitted to the tibia rather than to the ankle joint. The operator's forearm is kept in close alignment with the patient's tibia.

M — The right hand rotates the entire foot medially, transmitting the movement to the tibia through the close-packed ankle. Starting with the knee slightly flexed, the movement can be applied at various degrees of flexion and extension. Do not, however, rotate and simultaneously flex or extend.

This technique is considered more vigorous than Technique 4,a. It increases joint-play movement necessary for flexion.

5. *The Femorotibial Joint* — External rotation

a. *External rotation* — with the knee flexed to about 90° (Fig. 6–30A)

This is performed in the same manner as Technique 4,a. The handholds are reversed,

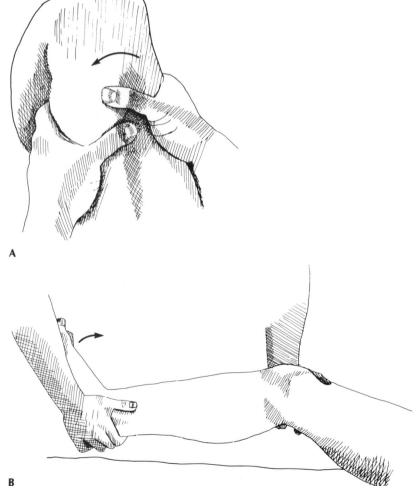

A

B

Fig. 6–30. External rotation of femorotibial joint (A) with the leg flexed to about 90° and (B) applied in various positions, approaching full extension.

however, so that the right thumb contacts the tibial tuberosity medially, while the left hand grasps the tibial crest and lateral aspect of the proximal tibia.

This technique is used to increase a joint-play movement necessary for knee extension.

b. *External Rotation* — applied in various positions approaching full extension (Fig. 6–30*B*)

P — Supine

O — Supports the knee and distal end of the thigh with his left hand from the lateral aspect, wrapping the fingers around posteriorly. The left hand primarily controls the position of the knee, keeping it from dropping into extension. He grasps the ankle and foot with the right hand, wrapping the fingers around the calcaneus and the Achilles tendon posteriorly from the medial side. The forearm contacts the entire medial border of the foot. The ankle must be kept in close-packed position so as to transmit the rotatory force to the tibia rather than to the ankle joint.

M — The right hand and forearm rotate the foot and ankle externally (lateral rotation), keeping the ankle in close-packed position. The left hand controls the position of the knee. This may be performed at various positions approaching full extension. *Do not* rotate and simultaneously flex or extend the knee.

This technique is used to increase a joint-play

movement necessary for knee extension. It is considered more vigorous than Technique 5,*a.*

6. *The Femorotibial Joint* — Valgus tilt (Fig. 6–31)

P — Supine

O — Supports the foot and lower leg by resting the ankle on his proximal thigh. His knee is placed up onto the plinth. He tucks the leg between his elbow and side. The operator supports the proximal tibia and knee with his right hand from the medial side, wrapping the fingers around posteriorly and the thumb anteriorly. The left forearm is supinated and in line with the direction of force. The heel of the left hand contacts the lateral aspect of the femoral and tibial condyles. The fingers wrap around posteriorly for additional support. The patient's knee is kept slightly flexed.

M — The left hand gently moves the knee into valgus tilt, taking care to avoid any flexion or extension of the knee. (The operator's right hand supports the knee, but yields with the valgus movement.)

This technique is used to increase joint play at the knee. As with any joint-play movement, it must not be moved past normal anatomical limits.

7. *The Femorotibial Joint* — Varus tilt (Fig. 6–32)

This is performed in a similar manner as Technique 6. The handholds are reversed so that the left hand supports the proximal tibia and the

Fig. 6–31. Valgus tilt of femorotibial joint.

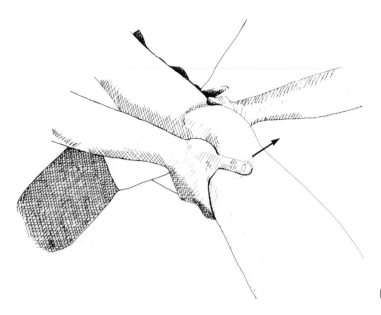

Fig. 6–32. Varus tilt of femorotibial joint.

knee. The right hand contacts the medial condyles. The right forearm comes around and is in line with the varus force to be produced.

8. *The Patellofemoral Joint*—Medial-lateral tilt (Fig. 6–33)

   P—Supine, with the knee slightly flexed over a firm support of towelling

   O—Contacts the lateral or medial patellar border with his thumb pads. The remaining

fingers rest over the anterior aspect of the patient's leg to help support the operator's hands. He keeps the elbows close to full extension.

M—A medial glide of the patella is produced by leaning forward with the trunk. The movement should *not* be performed by pushing

Fig. 6–33. Medial-lateral glide of patellofemoral joint.

Fig. 6–34. Superior-inferior glide of patellofemoral joint (left knee).

with the thumbs, radially deviating the wrists, or extending the elbows. A lateral glide is produced by using the pads of the index fingers.

This technique is used for general patellar mobilization in the presence of restricted patellar movement.

9. *The Patellofemoral Joint*—Superior-inferior glide (Fig. 6–34)

This is performed in the same manner as Technique 8. The thumb pads contact the patella superiorly or inferiorly. The fingers rest over the medial and lateral aspect of the knee joint. The forearms are in line with the direction of force.

The patella must glide superiorly during knee extension, and inferiorly on knee flexion.

10. *The Proximal Tibiofibular Joint*—Anterior-posterior glide (Fig. 6–35)

P—Supine, with knee flexed about 90°, the foot flat on the plinth

O—Stabilizes the knee with the right hand contacting the medial aspect of the knee area. He grasps the head and neck of the proximal fibula with the left hand, the thumb contacting anteriorly, the index and long finger pads contacting posteriorly. The operator must take care to avoid direct pressure to the common peroneal nerve.

M—The left hand may move the proximal fibula posteriorly or anteriorly. This should be performed through a movement of flexion and extension at the shoulder, rather than through finger or wrist movements.

This technique is used to increase joint play at the tibiofemoral joint. The fibular head must move forward on knee flexion and backward on knee extension.

11. *The Distal Tibiofibular Joint*—Anterior-posterior glide (Fig. 6–36)

P—Supine

O—Cradles the ankle in his right hand, fixing it to the plinth, so that the fingers wrap around the heel posteriorly. The medial malleolus rests over the palmar aspect of his dorsiflexed wrist. The left hand contacts the lateral malleolus anteriorly with the heel of the hand.

M—While the right hand prevents downward movement of the medial malleolus, the left hand glides the lateral malleolus posteriorly in relation to the medial malleolus. The handholds may be reversed to move the medial malleolus posteriorly on the lateral malleolus.

These techniques are used to increase joint play at the distal tibiofibular joint. This joint must spread slightly during ankle dorsiflexion, since the talus is wider anteriorly than posteriorly. Although spreading cannot be performed passively by the operator, increasing anteroposterior movement is likely to increase other joint-play movements such as spreading.

Fig. 6–35. Anterior-posterior glide of proximal tibiofibular joint.

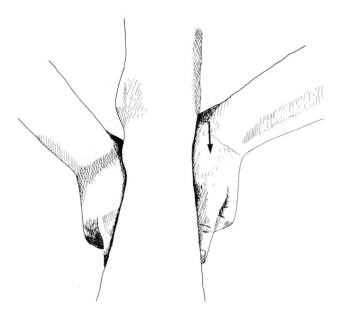

Fig. 6–36. Anterior-posterior glide of distal tibiofibular joint.

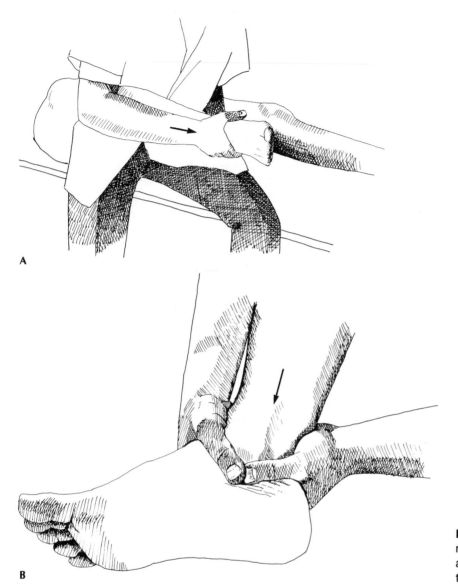

A

B

Fig. 6–37. Distraction of ankle mortise joint: (A) position of the operator; (B) view of the operator's grip at the ankle.

THE ANKLE

1. *The Ankle Mortise Joint* — Distraction (Fig. 6–37)
   P — Supine, with the knee flexed about 90°, the hip flexed and somewhat abducted
   O — Half sits on the edge of the plinth, with his back to the patient. He wraps the patient's leg around his right side to support the knee on his iliac crest, tucking the lower leg between his elbow and side (Fig. 6–37A). The operator grasps the ankle with both hands so that the thumbs wrap around medially and the fingers laterally. The web of his right hand contacts the neck of the talus dorsally, the web of his left hand contacts the calcaneus

posteriorly. The forearms are kept in line with the direction of force (Fig. 6–37B).
   M — A distraction is imparted with both hands. The ankle may be slightly everted to help lock the subtalar joint.
This technique is used to increase joint play at the ankle mortise joint. Distraction must occur here during plantar flexion, and is necessary for full movement toward the close-packed position, which is dorsiflexion.

2. *The Ankle Mortise Joint* — Posterior glide of tibia on talus (or anterior glide of talus on tibia) (Fig. 6–38)
   P — Supine
   O — Stabilizes the talus and foot by grasping

Fig. 6–38. Posterior glide of tibia on talus of ankle mortise joint (left foot).

around medially to the posterior aspect of the calcaneus with the left hand. He contacts the distal tibia by placing his right hand over the anterior distal aspect of the tibia, just proximal to the malleoli.

M—The tibia is glided posteriorly on the talus with the right hand. **Note:** An anterior glide of the talus on the tibia may be performed by stabilizing the tibia with the right hand and

moving the talus anteriorly. When this technique is used, it is important to keep the subtalar joint slightly everted to lock the calcaneus on the talus. The talus is glided anteriorly on the tibia via the calcaneus at the ankle mortise. This is a slightly more difficult technique, because the operator must work against gravity.

Both of these techniques are used to increase joint-play movements necessary for plantar flexion at the ankle mortise joint.

3. *The Ankle Mortise Joint*—Posterior glide of the talus on the tibia (Fig. 6–39)

 P—Supine, with the calcaneus hanging over the end of the plinth

 O—Stabilizes the distal tibia against the plinth by grasping it with the left hand, wrapping the fingers around posteriorly. The left forearm rests over the dorsum of the patient's lower leg to prevent it from rising up from the plinth during the movement. He contacts the neck of the talus dorsally with the web of the right hand, bringing the thumb around laterally and the index finger medially. The remaining three fingers of the right hand wrap around the sole of the foot for support and control of the degree of plantar flexion.

 M—The right hand moves the talus posteriorly on the tibia.

This technique is used to increase a joint-play movement necessary for ankle dorsiflexion.

4. *The Subtalar Joint*—distraction (not illustrated)

Fig. 6–39. Posterior glide of talus on tibia of ankle mortise joint.

Fig. 6–40. Valgus tilt (eversion) of the subtalar joint.

This is performed in the same manner as distraction at the ankle mortise (see Technique 1), except that the dorsal handhold moves distally to contact the navicular. In this way the calcaneus is distracted from the talus by the navicular and cuboid.

5. *The Subtalar Joint*—Valgus tilt (eversion) (Fig. 6–40)

   P—Supine, with the knee flexed about 90°, the hip flexed and somewhat abducted

   O—Assumes the same position as for distraction (see Fig. 6–37A) and grasps the ankle so that the thumb pads contact the medial aspect of the calcaneus and the remaining finger pads contact laterally, just proximal to the calcaneus and level with the sinus tarsi

   M—A valgus tilt of the calcaneus is produced by ulnar deviation of the wrists, transmitting the force through the thumb pads. The finger pads act as a fulcrum about which the movement occurs.

Fig. 6–41. Varus tilt (inversion) of subtalar joint.

This technique is used to increase eversion at the subtalar joint.

6. *The Subtalar Joint*—Varus tilt (inversion) (Fig. 6–41)

   This is carried out in the same manner as valgus tilt (see Technique 5). The operator's thumb pads move just proximal to the calcaneus; the finger pads move distally to contact the calcaneus laterally. The finger pads move the calcaneus into inversion about a fulcrum created by the thumb pads.

   This technique is used to increase inversion at the subtalar joint.

7. *The Subtalar Joint*—Dorsal rock of the calcaneus on the talus (Fig. 6–42)

   P—Supine, with the knee flexed about 90°, the hip flexed and somewhat abducted

   O—Assumes the same position as for distraction (see Fig. 6–37A) and stabilizes the talus dorsally with the web of the right hand, wrapping the thumb around medially and the fingers laterally. He contacts the upper border of the calcaneus posteriorly with the web of his left hand in a similar fashion.

   M—While the right hand stabilizes the talus, the left hand rocks the calcaneus forward and dorsally. **Note:** According to Mennell, a small amount of movement must occur at the subtalar joint at the extremes of plantar flexion and dorsiflexion. This technique, and the one that follows, have been developed to restore that movement.[12]

8. *The Subtalar Joint*—plantar rock of the calcaneus on the talus (Fig. 6–43)

   This is carried out in the same manner as dorsal

Fig. 6-42. Dorsal rock of the calcaneus on the talus of subtalar joint.

rock (see Technique 7), except the handholds are changed so that the right hand moves down to contact the navicular. The navicular tubercle is used as a landmark. The left hand moves just proximal to the posterior aspect of the calcaneus. The right hand rocks the calcaneus backward and plantarly via the navicular and cuboid. The web of the left hand acts as a fulcrum about which movement occurs.

THE FOOT

1. *The Mid-tarsal Joints (talonavicular and calcaneo-cuboid joints)* — Dorsal-plantar glide (Fig. 6-44)
   P—Supine, with the knee bent about 60°, the heel resting on the plinth

O—The left hand fixes the calcaneus and talus to the plinth by grasping dorsally at the level of the talar neck, the thumb wrapping around laterally and the rest of the fingers medially. The right hand grasps the navicular, using the navicular tubercle as a landmark. The web and the thumb contact dorsally, and the hand and fingers wrap around the foot medially and plantarly.

M—As the left hand stabilizes and prevents movement at the ankle, the right hand may move the navicular dorsally or plantarly on the talus.

The cuboid is moved in a similar manner, with one hand fixating the calcaneus and talus while the other hand moves the cuboid dorsally or plan-

Fig. 6-43. Plantar rock of the calcaneus on the talus of subtalar joint.

Fig. 6-44. Dorsal-plantar glide of talonavicular joint.

tarly on the calcaneus. These techniques are used to increase joint play at the forefoot.

2. *The Naviculocuneiform Joint*—Dorsal-plantar glide (Fig. 6-45)

This is performed in the same manner as dorsal-plantar glide at the talonavicular joint (see Technique 1), with the handholds moved distally. The left hand stabilizes the navicular while the right hand moves the cuneiforms.

This technique is used to increase joint play at the forefoot.

3. *The Cuneiform-Metatarsal Joints*—Dorsal-plantar glide (not illustrated)

This technique is also performed in the same manner as for the talonavicular joint, with the handholds shifted distally. The right hand grasps

the cuneiforms and provides stabilization while the left hand moves the metatarsal joints.

This technique, like Techniques 1 and 2 for the talonavicular and naviculocuneiform joints, is used to increase joint play of the forefoot.

4. *The Cuneiform-Metatarsal and Cuboid-Metatarsal Joints*—Rotation (pronation and supination) (Fig. 6-46)

P—Supine, with the knee bent about 70°, the heel resting on the plinth

O—Stabilizes the cuneiforms and cuboid with the left hand, the thumb wrapping around the foot dorsally, the fingers plantarly. For *pronation*, the operator's right hand grasps the proximal metatarsal shafts from the lateral aspect, with the thumb contacting dorsally and the fingers plantarly. His forearm is supinated (see Fig. 6-46*A*). For *supination*, the operator's right hand grasps the proximal metatarsal shafts from the medial aspect, with the thumb contacting dorsally and the fingers plantarly. His forearm is pronated (see Fig. 6-46*B*).

M—The right hand rotates the metatarsals, as a unit, into pronation or supination.

These techniques are used to restore pronation and supination to the forefoot.

The remaining joints of the foot—the intermetatarsals, the metatarsophalangeals, and the interphalangeals may be mobilized in the same manner as that described for the corresponding joints of the hands. Specific intertarsal movements (*e.g.*, between cuboid and calcaneus, cuboid and navicular) may be produced in a manner similar to the specific intercarpal movements used for the hand.[7,18]

Fig. 6-45. Dorsal-plantar glide of naviculocuneiform joint.

Fig. 6-46. Rotation of cuneiform-metatarsal and cuboid-metatarsal joints: (A) pronation and (B) supination.

REFERENCES

1. Burke GL: Backache from Occiput to Coccyx. Vancouver, MacDonald, 1964
2. Cookson JC, Kent BE: Orthopedic manual therapy— An overview. Phys Ther 59:136–146, 1979
3. Cyriax J: Textbook of Orthopaedic Medicine, Vol 1, Diagnosis of Soft Tissue Lesions, 8th ed. London, Balliere Tindall, 1983
4. Cyriax J: Textbook of Orthopaedic Medicine, Vol 2, Treatment by Manipulation, Massage and Injection, 11th ed. London, Balliere Tindall, 1984
5. Fisher AGT: Treatment by Manipulation, 5th ed. New York, Paul B. Hoeber, 1948
6. Hood W: On so-called bone-setting: Its nature and results. Lancet 7:344–349, 1871
7. Kaltenborn FM: Manual Therapy for the Extremity Joints, 3rd ed. Oslo, Olaf Norlis Bokhandel, 1980
8. Maigne R: Orthopedic Medicine. Springfield, IL, Charles C Thomas, 1972
9. Maitland GD: Vertebral Manipulations, 5th ed. Stoneham, MA, Butterworth & Co, 1986
10. Marlin T: Manipulative Treatment for the General Practitioner. London, Edward Arnold & Co, 1934
11. Mennell JB: The Science and Art of Joint Manipulation. London, J & A Churchill, 1949
12. Mennell JMcM: Joint Pain. Boston, Little, Brown & Co, 1964
13. Mixter WJ, Barr JS: Rupture of the intervertebral disc with involvement of the spinal canal. N Engl J Med 211:210–215, 1934
14. Nwuga VC: Manipulation of the Spine. Baltimore, Williams & Wilkins, 1976
15. Paris, SV: The Spinal Lesion. Christ Church, New Zealand, Pegasus Press, 1965
16. Smith RL: At Your Own Risk: The Case Against Chiropractice. New York, Trident Press, 1969
17. Stoddard A: Manual of Osteopathic Technique. London, Hutchinson, 1978
18. Svendsen B, Moe K, Merritt R: Joint Mobilization Laboratory Manual. Loma Linda, CA, Loma Linda University, 1981
19. Webster GV: Concerning Osteopathy. Norwood, MA, Plimpton Press, 1921

RECOMMENDED READINGS

Cyriax J, Coldham M: Textbook of Orthopaedic Medicine, Vol 2, Treatment by Manipulation, Massage, and Injection, 11th ed. Baltimore, Williams & Wilkins, 1984

Cyriax JH, Cyriax PJ: Illustrated Manual of Orthopaedic Medicine. Stoneham, MA, Butterworth & Co, 1983

Evjenth O, Hamberg J: Muscle Stretching in Manual Therapy—A Clinical Manual, Vol 1, the Extremities. Alfta, Alfta Rehab Forlag, 1985

Kaltenborn FM: Manual Therapy for the Extremity Joints, 3rd ed. Oslo, Olaf Norlis Bokhandel, 1980

Kaltenborn FM: Manual Mobilization of the Extremity Joints, Vol 2, Advanced Treatment Techniques. Oslo, Olaf Norlis Bokhandel, 1986

Lewit K: Manipulative Therapy of the Locomotor System. Boston, Butterworths, 1985

Maitland GD: Peripheral Manipulation, 2nd ed. Stoneham, MA, Butterworth & Co, 1977

Svendsen B, Moe K, Merritt R: Joint Mobilization Laboratory Manual: Extremity Joint Testing and Selected Treatment Techniques. Loma Linda, CA, Loma Linda University, 1981

7 Automobilization Techniques for the Extremities

Darlene Hertling

Automobilization (self-mobilization) techniques are specific joint-mobilization procedures that the patient performs. These passive exercises to maintain or increase joint mobility must be carefully taught to the patient.

Automobilization techniques of the spine were well known prior to 1975 through the work of Kaltenborn and his school. Then in 1975 the first of a series of articles by Rohde on automobilization techniques of the extremities appeared in East Germany. Automobilization techniques were first investigated and developed at the Fochkrankenhaus und Forschungsinstitut für Physiotherapie, Mahlow.[11–14] The extremity techniques described place emphasis on increasing capsular extensibility in order to restore painless range of motion to a joint. The primary indication for these techniques is painful limitation of joint movement due to loss of capsular extensibility.

Traditional home programs have, for the most part, stressed active or passive motions (performed at times with a wand or pulley) that are often poorly controlled by the patient, thus leading to further pain and stiffness.[3,10] According to Rohde, these techniques often compress the joint surfaces while having little or no effect on the joint capsule.[11,13] The logical and most effective approach in the management of capsular restriction is increasing capsular extensibility through techniques applied directly to the joint. Among the advantages cited by Rohde are the following:

— Major emphasis is placed on a pain-free position at the end of a range, in which mobilization can be most effective with regard to capsular stretch.
— Often the patient can control pain more easily than the therapist can.
— The patient can perform automobilizations several times a day independently. This reduces the time and expense of formal treatment sessions in a physical therapy department.
— Increased range of motion is possible without excessive force.
— Little or no equipment is required; anything that is needed usually is available in the home.
— The techniques are simple, easy to apply, and are not time consuming.

Furthermore, it is probable that the oscillatory nature of the techniques reduces pain by increasing proprioceptive input to "the gate"[1,8,9] (see Chapter 3, Pain).

Some of the disadvantages of automobilization techniques would appear to include the following:

— Some of the positions that the patient must assume in order to employ automobilizations are awkward and often difficult if there is limitation or pain elsewhere (e.g., spine or other joints).
— The variety of techniques is somewhat limited for some joints, such as the hip, because of poor accessibility. Some techniques may not be possible or are poorly managed at certain joints.
— Automobilization techniques of the finger joints require that the patient be able to stabilize one part and mobilize another with the same hand. This is somewhat difficult, though not impossible.
— The movements cannot be observed once the patient is independent, and the techniques may not be carried out correctly.

ROHDE'S PRINCIPLES FOR AUTOMOBILIZATION OF THE EXTREMITIES

For most automobilization techniques, the patient either holds one part of the extremity from movement or provides a fulcrum over which movement can take place. Mobilization is carried out by the patient's hand, or in some cases, by use of his body weight. Rohde's approach is a form of oscillatory treatment, similar to Maitland's approach.[8] It employs movements that are smooth and regular. These gentle, rhythmic oscillations are performed at the end of motion 10 to 20 times (one or two oscillations per second, or up to three to four per second in chronic conditions) without using excessive force. The basic rules for automobilization are essentially the same as those for other mobilization techniques (see Chapter 6, Peripheral Joint Mobilization Techniques).

—The part must be completely relaxed if treatment is to be effective.
—The handgrip (or stabilizing belt) should be firm but should not produce pain.
—The patient's position must be comfortable, easy to maintain, and must allow complete control of the movements.

According to Rohde, it is also important that

—The patient know the goals and principles of automobilization thoroughly.
—The patient be well motivated.
—The techniques be precise, easy to understand, and simple in nature.[11,13]
—The patient be seen periodically to determine whether the techniques are being carried out correctly and are effective. They should be discontinued once normal range is achieved.

In general, automobilization is indicated in subacute or chronic painful conditions of the joints that have resulted in a capsular pattern of restriction, and for which restoration of range of motion appears possible. Rohde lists the following indications and contraindications:[11]

Indications
Arthrosis (*e.g.,* degenerative joint disease)
Chronic inflammatory diseases of the joints (*e.g.,* chronic polyarthritis or monarticular rheumatoid arthritis)
Sudeck-Leriche syndrome (reflex sympathetic dystrophy)
Postimmobilization stiffness (*e.g.,* following casting)
Capsular atrophy (*e.g.,* hemiplegia)

Contraindications
Hypermobility
Acute inflammatory conditions or very painful conditions in which the end point cannot be reached without pain (gentle traction may be useful in such instances)

Patients with limited intelligence or who are very awkward
Advanced cerebrosclerosis

GENERAL CONSIDERATIONS

It is important that both the history and the physical examination be carried out (see Chapter 4, Assessment of Musculoskeletal Disorders). The examination might include the neighboring joints as well as relevant spinal levels. From this examination you should determine where to place emphasis in treatment and the general treatment approach (*e.g.,* mobilizations, manipulations, and/or soft-tissue techniques).

Automobilizations are usually started after the acute phase, but this will vary somewhat with the nature of the pathology. Usually a 2-week training period is required, after which the patient can become independent. Frequent re-evaluations are necessary. The frequency and intensity of automobilizations should correspond to the patient's condition and clinical picture. In chronic conditions, it is recommended that these techniques be carried out one to two times initially. They may be increased gradually to three or more times daily. In subacute conditions, three times weekly is suggested.[11]

Prior to automobilization, some form of heat or cold therapy may be used, such as mild moist heat for subacute conditions, and more intense heat for chronic conditions (*e.g.,* hot packs if given at home). For certain joints, such as those of the hand, foot, elbow, or knee, some of the techniques may be carried out in a warm bath. This is not practical for the shoulder or hip joint. Frequently, additional treatment of the soft tissue may be indicated. Rohde suggests the following:[11]

Self-massage (*e.g.,* the upper trapezius in shoulder joint problems)
Proprioceptive neuromuscular facilitation techniques (*e.g.,* hold–relax techniques to reduce muscle tightness and encourage relaxation)[16]
Isometric exercises (*e.g.,* for muscle weakness)[16]
Pendulum or free swinging exercises with a weight, as advocated by Rössler and Kohlrausch, to increase range of motion and permit relaxation.[6,15] Although these exercises are somewhat similar to Codman's pendulum exercises for the shoulder, exercises for the trunk and lower extremity are also described.[2] In addition, they incorporate relaxation techniques similar to those of Jacobson.[5]

In general, automobilization techniques should begin with distraction or inferior glide techniques. These are particularly useful in the early stages for managing pain (gentle traction may even be started in the acute phase) and prior to other automobilization techniques. A particularly effective variation is the use of hold–relax techniques applied directly before a specific automobilization.[16] These techniques, in which the patient performs an isometric contraction of the antagonists in order to reflexively inhibit a particular muscle group, are particularly useful just before shoulder automobilizations into internal and external rotation. Automobilization techniques are gradually added to the patient's program based on the ongoing clinical evaluation. For example, following distraction or inferior glide techniques at the shoulder, the patient would incorporate flexion, extension, and internal rotation techniques. Finally abduction and external rotation techniques, which are more likely to produce pain and spasm, would be added.

Once the basic principles of mobilization and automobilization techniques are understood, the therapist can create any number of automobilization techniques and exercises.[4] Examples of shoulder joint techniques follow. In general, you should begin with inferior glide or distraction, emphasizing caudal shift of the humeral head in the glenoid cavity. Although automobilization techniques of the foot and hand have been described by Rohde, we will limit our discussion to those of the major large joints.[12] Only a few of the more important techniques of the elbow, knee, and hip will be described.

Note: For the sake of simplicity, all of the techniques to be described in this chapter are applied to the patient's *right* extremity, except where indicated. In the automobilization techniques, the left hand usually will be performing the mobilizations. (E—equipment; P—patient; MH—mobilizing hand; M—movement)

AUTOMOBILIZATION TECHNIQUES FOR THE SHOULDER

1. *Inferior Glide* — Long-axis extension (Fig. 7 – 1)
    E — A high-back chair that is well padded with a blanket or towel on the back of the chair
    P — Sitting, with the right arm over the back of the chair, the axilla firmly fixed over the back of chair
    MH — Grasps the arm just proximal to the humeral epicondyles so as to gain a purchase on them. An alternate handhold would be to grasp the forearm just above the styloid processes.
    M — An inferior glide is produced by pulling directly downward toward the floor while

Fig. 7 – 1. Inferior glide (long-axis extension) of glenohumeral joint may be performed (*A*) manually or (*B*) by using a weight.

employing rhythmic oscillations (Fig. 7 – 1*A*).

Note: A variation of this technique, which Rohde tested, is to use a weight in the hand (*e.g.*, a bucket of sand) and to perform gentle, pivotlike motions at the end (Fig. 7 – 1*B*).

2. *Inferior Glide* — Shoulder adduction with distraction ventrally (Fig. 7 – 2)
    E — A firm pillow or towel roll placed in the axilla
    P — Standing, with the arm positioned across the chest
    MH — Grasps the forearm just above the styloid processes. MH pulls the arm rhythmically across the chest (into adduction) and downward, resulting in a slight separation

Fig. 7 – 2. Inferior glide of glenohumeral joint: (*A*) shoulder adduction with distraction ventrally; (*B*) shoulder adduction with distraction dorsally.

of the head of the humerus in the glenoid cavity (Fig. 7–2*A*).

Note: Distraction dorsally may be carried out in a similar fashion if the patient has sufficient internal rotation to place her forearm behind her back. In this case, the elbow is flexed and the MH employs rhythmic oscillations behind the patient's back in a downward direction dorsally (Fig. 7–2*B*).

3. *Inferior Glide*—Shoulder abduction when the patient has less than 90° abduction (Fig. 7–3)

   P—Sitting sideways to a table, the right arm is positioned comfortably at the end of painless abduction with the muscles relaxed. The elbow is extended with the hand, and the forearm is fixed on the table.

  MH—Contacts the anterior, superior aspect of the proximal humerus below the acromion

   M—An inferior glide is produced by pushing directly downward toward the floor, with rhythmic oscillations.

4. *Inferior Glide*—Shoulder abduction (when the patient has more than 90° abduction) (Fig. 7–4)

   P—Standing with the right side facing a wall. The arm is positioned comfortably in abduction so that the forearm rests on the wall, with the elbow in 90° flexion.

  MH—Contacts the anterior-superior aspect of the proximal end of the humerus below the acromion

   M—An inferior glide is produced by pushing directly downward toward the floor with rhythmic oscillations. A stronger capsular stretch can be employed by bending the knees and using body weight to assist in the movement.

5. *Inferior Glide*—Shoulder flexion (when the patient has less than 90° flexion) (Fig. 7–5)

Fig. 7–4. Inferior glide (shoulder abduction for 90° or more abduction) of glenohumeral joint (left arm).

   P—Sitting facing a table. The right forearm is positioned comfortably at the end of painless flexion with the muscles relaxed. A pillow wedge is used under the forearm to provide fixation of the hand and forearm.

  MH—Contacts the anterosuperior aspect of the proximal humerus below the acromion

   M—An inferior glide is produced by pushing directly downward toward the floor, with rhythmic oscillations.

6. *Inferior Glide*—Shoulder flexion (when the patient has more than 90° flexion) (Fig. 7–6)

   P—Standing facing a wall. The right forearm, with the elbow bent to 90° flexion, is positioned at the end of range on the wall for fixation.

  MH—Contacts the anterosuperior aspect of the

Fig. 7–3. Inferior glide (shoulder abduction for 90° or less abduction) of glenohumeral joint.

Fig. 7–5. Inferior glide (shoulder flexion for 90° or less flexion) of glenohumeral joint.

Fig. 7–6. Inferior glide (shoulder flexion for 90° or more flexion) of glenohumeral joint.

proximal end of the humerus below the acromion

M—An anterior glide is produced by pushing directly downward toward the floor, with rhythmic oscillations. A stronger capsular stretch may be employed by lowering the body weight.

7. *Anterior Glide*—Shoulder extension (Fig. 7–7)

P—Sitting, with the back to a table. The right arm is positioned comfortably at the limits of painless extension with the muscles relaxed. The elbow is extended with the right hand fixed on the table. The trunk is in a flexed position.

MH—Contacts the posterosuperior aspect of the proximal humerus just below the acromion

M—An anterior glide is produced by moving the arm in a ventral, caudal direction, with rhythmic oscillations.

8. *Shoulder Internal Rotation* (Fig. 7–8)

P—Sitting sideways to a table. The right upper arm is positioned so that its entire extent is

Fig. 7–8. Internal rotation of glenohumeral joint.

braced against the table. To do this the patient bends his trunk to the side toward the upper arm. The elbow is flexed to 90°.

MH—Grasps the dorsal aspect of the wrist with the thumb, and with the fingers wrapped around the ventral aspect

M—The arm is internally rotated as far as possible with rhythmic oscillations carried out at the end of range.

9. *Shoulder External Rotation* (Fig. 7–9)

P—Sitting sideways to a table. The right upper arm is positioned so that its entire extent is braced against the table. To do this the patient bends his trunk to the side toward the upper arm. The elbow is flexed to 90°.

MH—Grasps the ventral aspect of the wrist

M—The forearm is externally rotated, and rhythmic oscillations are carried out at the end of range.

Note: Hold–relax techniques are particularly useful with rotation techniques of the shoulder.

AUTOMOBILIZATION TECHNIQUES FOR THE ELBOW

1. *Humeroulnar Joint*—Medial-lateral tilt (side-bending oscillations) (Fig. 7–10)

Fig. 7–7. Anterior glide (shoulder extension) of glenohumeral joint.

Fig. 7–9. External rotation of glenohumeral joint.

Fig. 7–10. Medial-lateral tilt (side-bending oscillations) of humeroulnar joint.

P — Standing in a doorway with the right forearm and hand fixed against the wall. The elbow is in slight flexion or close to the limit of extension.

MH — Grasps the upper arm near the humeral epicondyles

M — Keeping the forearm stationary, the MH moves the humerus medially or laterally, effecting a medial or lateral tilt of the humeroulnar joint.

2. *Humeroulnar Joint* — Distraction in flexion (Fig. 7–11)

P — Sitting, with the shoulder abducted 90°. The upper arm is supported on a table. (A kitchen counter is usually a good height.) The elbow is flexed over a firm pillow or towel roll.

MH — Is placed over the lower arm and dorsum of hand

M — Slow, gentle, oscillating movements are performed downward in the direction of flexion.

Fig. 7–11. Distraction in flexion of humeroulnar joint.

Fig. 7–12. Valgus tilt of femorotibial joint.

AUTOMOBILIZATION TECHNIQUES FOR THE KNEE

1. *Femorotibial Joint* — Valgus tilt (Fig. 7–12)

E — A couch or chair moved slightly away from a wall

P — Stands on the right side of the chair with his back to the wall. The right foot is placed on the seat of the chair with support on the medial aspect of the foot to provide fixation. The posterior aspect of the thigh should be in contact with the back of chair, and the buttocks in contact with the wall for additional support. The hip should be in slight flexion so that it is not locked in extension.

MH — The patient leans his trunk well forward so that his left forearm will be in line with the direction of movement. The forearm is supinated, with the heel of the left hand contacting the lateral aspect of the femoral and tibial condyles. The fingers wrap around the knee posteriorly for additional support.

M — The left hand gently moves the knee into valgus tilt, taking care to avoid any flexion or extension of the knee.

Note: Varus tilt may be carried out in the reverse fashion.

2. *Femorotibial Joint* — Forced (gentle) flexion (Fig. 7–13)

P — Supine, lying with the hip flexed slightly above 90°. The knee is flexed over a firm pillow or towel roll which acts as a fulcrum.

MH — Both hands contact the lower leg over the anterior aspect with the fingers interlaced.

Fig. 7–13. Posterior glide (gentle forced flexion) of femorotibial joint (left leg).

M—Gentle flexion, with oscillations, is performed.

Note: Forced flexion may also be done in a sitting position. The right hip is completely flexed so that the thigh is supported on the chest. The knee is flexed over the right forearm, which now acts as a fulcrum and gives additional support. The left MH contacts the lower leg over the anterior aspect and carries out gentle flexion of the knee.

3. *The Patellofemoral Joint*—Medial-lateral glide (not illustrated)

P—Long-sitting on a firm cot or the floor, with the knee slightly flexed over a firm pillow or towel roll. (A sitting position in a chair may be used, with the leg extended, the knee slightly flexed, and the foot fixed to the floor.)

MH—Both thumb pads contact the lateral or medial patellar border. The remaining fingers rest over the anterior aspect of the patient's leg. The elbows are extended as much as possible.

M—A medial or lateral glide of the patella can be produced by leaning the trunk forward and to one side. The glide is effected by movement of the trunk rather than any part of the hand (see Chapter 6, Peripheral Joint Mobilization Techniques).

Note: Superior-inferior glide may also be performed by contact of the thumb pads on the superior or inferior borders of the patella, with the rest of the hand resting over the medial and lateral aspects of the knee.

AUTOMOBILIZATION TECHNIQUES FOR THE HIP

1. *Inferior Glide or Long-Axis Extension* (Fig. 7–14)

E—A comfortable, snug-fitting ankle strap and a stationary wall- or table-hook for attachment to the ankle strap

P—Supine, the right leg extended, and the ankle strap attached to the end of table- or wall-

Fig. 7–14. Inferior glide (long-axis extension) of hip joint.

hook. The left lower extremity is flexed, with the foot on the table or floor.

M—The left leg pushes downward and upward to push the body away from the fixed point, thus transmitting a traction force on the right lower extremity.

2. *Distraction in Sidelying* (Fig. 7–15)

This particular technique, described by Rohde, represents a combination of distraction and a muscle-strengthening exercise.[11] In this case, the gluteus medius, which is commonly weak in most hip conditions, is exercised.

P—Lying on the right side, close to one side of a table. A firm pillow or blanket roll is placed between the legs in the groin area. The left hip is extended at the hip with the lower leg off the edge of the table. A sandbag or ankle cuff with a weight is applied to the left ankle.

M—The left leg is actively raised against the pull of the weight and held for a few seconds; the patient then relaxes, allowing the leg to fall into adduction, with the hip in slight extension, over the edge of the table. Slight oscillatory motion will occur naturally at the end of range.

Fig. 7–15. Distraction (sidelying) of hip joint (left leg).

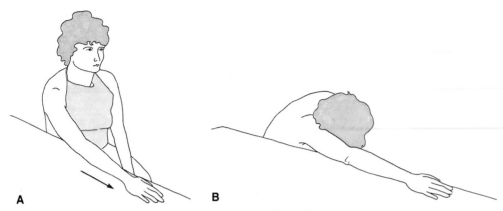

Fig. 7–16. Passive shoulder flexion (sitting): (*A*) starting position; (*B*) end position.

PASSIVE EXERCISE

Additional exercises that are particularly useful in a home program for painful extremity joints have been advocated by Dontigny and Grimsby.[3,4] They allow the patient to passively stretch his own joints by moving the body in relationship to the stabilized extremity. This type of movement affords an excellent stretch, minimizes incorrect movements by the patient, and allows for a greater degree of pain-free movement. Grimsby maintains that when passive exercise is used for the hip, shoulder, or ankle, the patient uses the concave surface of the joint to mobilize. By so doing, the patient avoids considerable pain and achieves a greater range of motion, because rolling and gliding occur in the same direction.[4] It would also appear—if we compare these exercises to the traditional approach of movement of the extremity in relationship to the body—that using a closed kinetic chain (through the stabilized extremity) provides greater joint stability as well as a more normal pattern of movement. Examples of these types of exercises are described for the shoulder.

PASSIVE SHOULDER EXERCISES

1. *Shoulder Flexion*
   a. *Sitting* (Fig. 7–16)
      P—Sits at side of table with the forearm resting on table
      M—Patient flexes trunk and head while sliding the arm forward along the edge of table so that the shoulder is moved passively into flexion.
   b. *Standing* (Fig. 7–17)
      P—Stands facing a high counter top (or high window ledge or bookshelf). He rests his hand, palm down, on the edge of the counter with the elbow extended.
      M—The patient lowers his body weight to move the shoulder passively into flexion.

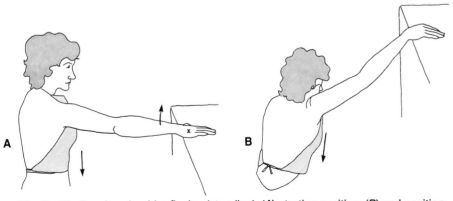

Fig. 7–17. Passive shoulder flexion (standing): (*A*) starting position; (*B*) end position.

Fig. 7–18. Passive shoulder extension: (*A*) starting position; (*B*) end position.

2. *Shoulder Extension* (Fig. 7–18)

   P—Stands with his right side to the table and positions the right hand on the table, with the arm at the side and the elbow extended

   M—Maintaining the right hand in a fixed position on the table, he walks forward to produce shoulder extension through the painless range of motion available.

3. *Shoulder Extension—Alternate Technique* (Fig. 7–19)

   P—Stands with his back to table and grasps the edge of table with both hands

Fig. 7–19. Alternate technique for passive shoulder extension: (*A*) starting position; (*B*) end position.

Fig. 7–20. Passive shoulder abduction (sitting): (*A*) starting position; (*B*) end position (left arm).

   M—The patient then lowers his body weight as he allows the elbows to flex and the shoulders to extend.

4. *Shoulder Abduction*

   a. *Sitting* (Fig. 7–20)

   P—Sits at side of a table and rests his forearm on the table, with the forearm supinated and the shoulder slightly abducted

   M—The patient sidebends the upper trunk to the left from the waist while sliding the arm across the table so that the shoulder is moved into abduction as the lower trunk moves away from the table.

   b. *Standing* (Fig. 7–21)

   P—Stands with his right side facing a high counter top (or high window ledge or bookshelf). He rests his hand on the surface with the forearm slightly supinated, elbow extended, and shoulder abducted through partial range.

   M—The patient lowers his body weight, allowing his shoulder to move passively into abduction and external rotation.

5. *Shoulder Internal Rotation* (Fig. 7–22)

   P—Stands with his left side toward a door frame. He places the back of his hand against the frame so that it will remain fixed with his

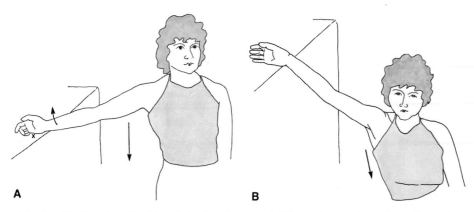

Fig. 7-21. Passive shoulder abduction (standing): (A) starting position; (B) end position.

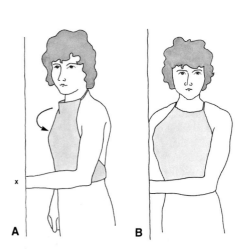

Fig. 7-22. Passive internal rotation of shoulder: (A) starting position; (B) end position (left arm).

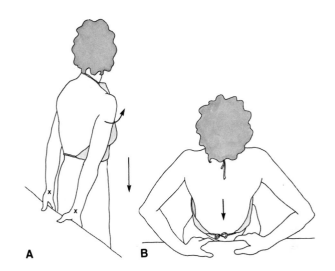

Fig. 7-23. Alternate technique for passive internal rotation of shoulder: (A) starting position; (B) end position.

Fig. 7-24. Passive external rotation of shoulder (sitting): (A) starting position; (B) end position.

Fig. 7–25. Passive external rotation of shoulder (standing): (*A*) starting position; (*B*) end position (left arm).

elbow flexed 90°. The upper arm remains at the side with the elbow held close to the trunk.

M—The patient walks forward as he rotates toward his left forearm to produce passive internal rotation of the shoulder.

6. *Shoulder Internal Rotation — Alternate Technique* (Fig. 7–23)

P—Stands with his back to the table and grasps the edge of the table with both hands

M—The patient lowers his body weight slowly, allowing the elbows to bend and the shoulders to abduct and internally rotate.

7. *Shoulder External Rotation*

a. *Sitting* (Fig. 7–24)

P—Sits at the side of the table with the forearm resting on the table, the shoulder abducted, and the elbow flexed

M—The patient flexes his trunk and head forward toward the table allowing the shoulder to be moved passively into external rotation.

b. *Standing* (Fig. 7–25)

P—Stands facing a door frame. He places the palmar surface of his hand against the frame so that it will remain fixed. The elbow is flexed 90°. The upper arm remains at the side with the elbow held close to the trunk.

M—The patient walks backward, rotating his

body away from his left arm to produce passive external rotation of the shoulder.

Similar exercises can be designed for the hip (such as the "all-fours" or crawling position) and for other extremity joints.

REFERENCES

1. Casey KL, Melzack R: Neural mechanism of pain: A conceptual model. *In* Way EL (ed): New Concepts in Pain and Its Clinical Management: Philadelphia, F A Davis, 1967
2. Codman EA: The Shoulder. Boston, Thomas Todd Co, 1934
3. Dontigny RL: Passive shoulder exercises. J Phys Ther 50:1707–1709, 1970
4. Grimsby O: Personal communication, 1977
5. Jacobson E: Progressive Relaxation. Chicago, University of Chicago Press, 1938
6. Kohlrausch W, Kohlrausch A: Bewegungstherapie und Rehabilitation bei Erkrankungen der Extremitätengelenke. *In* Grober J, Stieve FE (eds): Handbuch der Physiokalischen Therapie, BD II/1. Stuttgart, Gustav Fischer Verlag, 1971
7. Lewit K: Manuelle Therapie (im Rahmen der ärtlichen Rehabilitation). Leipzig, J A Barth, 1973
8. Maitland G: Peripheral Manipulation. Ontario, Butterworth & Scarborough, 1976
9. Melzack R, Wall PD: Pain mechanisms: A new theory. Science 150:971, 1965
10. Robins V: Should patients with hemiplegia wear a sling? J Phys Ther 49:1029, 1970
11. Rohde J: Die Automobilisation der Extremitätengelenke (I). Zeitschrift für Physiotherapie 27:57, 1975
12. Rohde J: Die Automobilisation der Extremitätengelenke (II). Zeitschrift für Physiotherapie 28:51, 1976
13. Rohde J: Die Automobilisation der Extremitätengelenke (III). Zeitschrift für Physiotherapie 28:121, 1976
14. Rohde J: Die Automobilisation der Extremitätengelenke (IV). Zeitschrift für Physiotherapie 28:427, 1976
15. Rössler H: Die Physikalische Therapie. Stuttgart, Gustav Fischer Verlag, 1968
16. Voss D, Ionta MK, Myers BJ: Proprioceptive Neuromuscular Facilitation, 3rd ed. Philadelphia, Harper and Row, 1985

RECOMMENDED READING

Lewit K: Manipulative Therapy of the Locomotor System. Boston, Butterworth, 1985, pp 243–255.

8 *Friction Massage*

Randolph M. Kessler

Massage, as is true of most forms of manual therapy, is a method of treatment that has been viewed with considerable controversy by the medical community. The "laying on of hands" of any sort tends to be associated with charlatanism. Its value, if any, is frequently felt to be of a psychological nature or the result of the placebo phenomenon. This attitude is not necessarily unfounded, for several reasons. First, those who have advocated the use of massage have often done so on the basis of nonscientific or non-physiological mechanisms that the medically oriented professional cannot always accept. Reflex zones, trigger points, fibrositic nodules, and meridians have all been identified as areas to which massage may be directed, but have never been identified as true anatomical or physiological entities. Secondly, there is little empiric or direct scientific evidence for the efficacy of massage. It tends to be used on the basis that it "seems to work;" it makes the patient feel better. So, while there is little question among clinicians who employ massage as a therapeutic measure that it has some value, its value is not well documented. This is primarily because massage is often used for the relief of painful conditions in which there are few associated pathologic signs. This makes reliable measurement of the possible effects of treatment a difficult problem in research design and technology. Finally, the use of massage by lay practitioners, especially in situations of questionable moral standards, has contributed to the adverse connotations often associated with its use.

The result of the prevailing attitudes toward massage is that it is often not used in the treatment of some conditions for which it might have a significant therapeutic effect. Furthermore, massage is time-consuming, occasionally strenuous, often boring, and relatively costly. Therefore, the clinician as well as the patient may at times avoid it. On the other hand, massage is often employed in circumstances in which it is unnecessary or its therapeutic effect is questionable.

In order to avoid the inappropriate use of any treatment, the clinician should consider not only the objectives but how these objectives fit into the overall plan of management. Although for many conditions seen clinically our primary goal is long-term relief of pain, we cannot necessarily justify the use of massage solely on the basis that it helps relieve pain. While massage may certainly provide *temporary* pain relief in many conditions, it does not necessarily contribute to the *long-term* relief of pain, which requires resolution of the pathologic state. Massage should not be used unless the clinician can rationalize that its use contributes to resolving the physical pathologic process. Such a rationale should have a well-accepted physiologic basis. Otherwise, not only will massage not help the patient to feel better, but because of its often pleasurable effects, it may actually reinforce the disease state. The therapist can better expect that treatment of the pathologic process will relieve pain, rather than that relief of pain will improve the patient's condition.

There are several types of conditions for which a particular form of massage, when appropriately administered, may have a direct or indirect effect upon the pathologic state. Deep stroking in the presence of certain edematous conditions may assist in the resolution of fluid accumulations. A variety of massage techniques can be used to reflexively promote muscle relaxation for more effective mobilization of a part. This may certainly be useful when abnormal muscle tension is an important factor in the perpetuation of the pathologic process (see Chapter 9, Relaxation). Deep frictions and kneading types of massage may assist in restoring mobility between tissue interfaces or may increase extensibility of individual structures. Deep massage also tends to increase circulation to the area treated, which may be desirable in certain cases. These effects are generally well described in traditional massage textbooks, along with descriptions of related massage techniques.[2-4]

PRINCIPLES OF DEEP TRANSVERSE FRICTION MASSAGE

A particularly important massage technique in the management of many common musculoskeletal disorders is deep transverse friction massage. Its importance and the rationale and technique of application have not been well described in the traditional literature.

As discussed under pathologic considerations in Chapter 2, Arthrology, many of the chronic musculoskeletal disorders seen clinically are manifestations of the body's response to fatigue stresses. Tissues tend to respond to fatigue stresses by increasing the rate of tissue production. Thus, prolonged abnormal stresses to a tissue will lead to tissue hypertrophy, provided that the nutritional status of the tissue is not compromised and that the stress rate (the rate of tissue breakdown) does not exceed the rate at which the tissue can repair the microdamage. Under continuing stress, if nutrition to the tissue is affected or if the rate of tissue breakdown is excessive, the tissue will gradually atrophy and weaken to the point of eventual failure. Tissues that normally have a low metabolic rate (usually those that are relatively poorly vascularized) are most susceptible to such degeneration. Such tissues include articular cartilage, intra-articular fibrocartilage, tendons, and some ligaments. On the other hand, those tissues with good vascularity and a normally high rate of turnover, such as cancellous bone, muscle, capsular tissue, and some ligaments, are more likely to respond by undergoing hypertrophy. This results in increased density of the structural elements. Of course, even these structures may not be able to keep up with the rate of tissue breakdown if the stress rate is too high or under conditions of reduced nutrition (*e.g.*, hypovascularity).

Under conditions of mildly increased stress rates, the body has the ability to adapt adequately, and no pathologic state (*i.e.*, pain, inflammation, or dysfunction) results. Such conditions might even include situations of high-magnitude stresses if the high stress levels are induced gradually and the stresses are intermittent enough to allow an interval for adequate repair to take place. A typical example is the individual engaging in vigorous athletic activities who goes through a period of gradual training. The training period allows for adequate maturation of new tissue so that structural elements become oriented in ways that best attenuate energy without yielding. Such energy attenuation requires that there be a sufficient mass of tissue to provide some resistance to deformation, but it also requires that the structure be adequately extensible to minimize the strain on individual structural elements. To increase the ability of a structure to attenuate the energy of work done on it (a force tending to deform the structure), new collagen is produced to increase the tissues' total ability to resist the force. However, this new collagen must be sufficiently mobile to permit some deformation. The less it deforms, the greater the resistance the tissue must offer. The greater the resistance it must offer, the greater will be the internal strain on individual collagen fibers or bony trabeculae. The greater the strain on individual structural elements, the greater the rate of microdamage. As the rate of microdamage increases, so does the likelihood of pain and inflammation. As you can see, a more massive tissue is not necessarily one that will permit normal functioning under increased stress. It must also be deformable, and deformability requires time for the new structural elements (collagen fibers and bony trabeculae) to assume the proper "weave."

The effect of the weave, or orientation, of structural elements in contributing to the extensibility of a structure as a whole can be appreciated by examining a Chinese "finger trap" (Fig. 8–1). You can lengthen and shorten the finger trap without changing the length of any of the individual fibers composing it. Its extensibility is due entirely to the weave of the fibers and interfiber mobility. Thus, you can apply an extending force to the structure without inducing internal strain on any of the individual fibers. If the fibers were not in the proper weave or if they were to stick to one another, the deforming force would be met with greater resistance by the structure and greater internal strain to individual fibers. The body adapts to mildly increased stress rates by laying down collagen precursors which, in response to imposed stresses, polymerize into collagen fibers. The fibers become oriented in the proper weave to allow deformability of the tissue.

Under abnormally high stress levels or altered nutritional conditions, the body's attempt to adapt may be inadequate. The particular structure may not be able to produce new tissue fast enough, or the new tissue that is produced may not have sufficient time or proper inducement to mature. In the former situation, the tissue will degenerate, whereas in the latter, pain and inflammation are likely to result if stresses continue. Tissue degeneration must be treated by reducing stress levels and/or increasing nutrition to the tissue, depending on the underlying cause. Typical examples of such tissue degeneration would include the degradation of articular cartilage in degenerative joint disease, and the lesions that commonly affect the soft tissues of the diabetic foot. Articular

Fig. 8–1. A Chinese finger trap before and after being extended illustrates the extensibility of structural elements.

cartilage, being avascular and having a normally low metabolic turnover, does not adapt well to increased stress levels and is thus susceptible to fatigue degradation. The diabetic foot may have a nutritional deficit because of vascular changes and possibly increased stresses secondary to reduced sensory feedback, leaving it abnormally susceptible to tissue breakdown.

Situations in which the new tissue does not mature adequately are typically those in which the stress levels are not sufficient to cause degeneration but are too excessive to allow time for normal tissue modeling. In bone, the condition is referred to as *sclerosis;* in capsules, ligaments, and tendons, it may be referred to as *fibrosis.* In both situations there is often a normal or increased amount of tissue, but the tissue is not sufficiently deformable to attenuate the energy of loading from use of the part. This can cause pain, inflammation, and/or increased stresses to adjacent tissues. Correction of such conditions requires that stress levels be reduced while stresses sufficient to stimulate normal tissue modeling are maintained. In addition, normal extensibility of the structure must be restored. This requires that interfiber mobility be increased. The nutritional status of the tissue must also be considered.

There are many common musculoskeletal disorders that may be related to abnormal or inadequate tissue modeling. Bony sclerosis typically occurs in degenerative joint disease when there are abnormal compressive stresses to a joint. Most tendinitis can be attributed to continued abnormal stresses to a tendon, which preclude adequate tissue modeling and create a structure that is not suffi-

ciently deformable. This is especially true of the condition often referred to as *tennis elbow*, in which the origin of the extensor carpi radialis brevis becomes fibrosed, and a chronic inflammatory process arises. Rotator cuff tendinitis, usually involving the supraspinatus or infraspinatus regions of the tendinous cuff, is a very common disorder in which normal modeling is compromised by hypovascularity to the area of involvement. Often these lesions at the shoulder progress to a stage at which gradual degeneration and eventual failure ensue. It is likely that the capsular fibrosis associated with "frozen shoulder" is a similar disorder of tissue modeling; the joint capsule hypertrophies in response to increased stress levels, but in doing so loses its extensibility. Abnormal tissue modeling will also result when a tissue is immobilized during the repair phase of an inflammatory process. Thus, a fracture may "heal," but normal modeling of bony trabeculae requires resumption of normal stress levels. Similarly, a joint capsule will become fibrosed when the joint is immobilized following arthrotomy; collagen is laid down in response to the traumatic inflammatory process affecting the synovium, but the lack of movement permits an unorganized network of fibers that forms abnormal interfiber bonds (adhesions) that do not extend normally when the part is moved.

The approach to treatment of conditions in which continued stresses have not allowed the structure to mature adequately must include measures to reduce stresses to the part. We must consider means of reducing loading of the part as well as means of preventing excessive internal strain. Reduced loading might be accomplished through control of activities, the use of orthotic devices to control alignment or movement, or the use of assistive devices such as crutches. Also, to reduce loading of a particular tissue, the capacity of other tissues to attenuate more of the energy of loading might be increased. This is often done by increasing the strength and activities of related muscles. Thus, if we wish to reduce the likelihood of excessive loading of the anterior talofibular ligament, the peroneal muscles should be strengthened. However, we can also strap the ankle to provide additional afferent input to reflexively enhance the ability of the peroneals to contract.

Reduction of stress levels alone, however, will not assure that adequate maturation will take place. As mentioned earlier, stress to the part is a necessary stimulus for the restoration of normal alignment of structural elements. This apparent paradox is understood when we consider that reducing stress is necessary in order to allow new tissue to be laid down and reconstituted, while at the same time some stress is necessary to optimize the nutritional status of the part and to effect proper orientation and mobility of the new tissue. Consequently, in the case of most chronic musculoskeletal disorders, resolution is not likely to take place with either complete rest of the part or unrestricted use. A judgment must be made, then, as to the appropriate activity level for a particular disorder and the rate at which normal activities can be resumed. This judgment must be based on data gained from an examination that reflects the nature and extent of the pathologic process as well as etiologic considerations. Knowledge of the healing responses of musculoskeletal tissues and of their responses to various stress conditions must also be applied.

In situations in which significant reduction of activities is necessary in order to allow healing to occur, there are measures that the therapist can, and should, take. The therapist must help prevent undue dysfunction that may result from a mass of tissue being laid down as an unorganized, adherent cicatrix, and from the atrophy of related muscle groups that is likely to take place. There are few conditions, even of an acute inflammatory nature, in which some gentle range of motion and isometric muscle exercises cannot be performed during the healing process without detrimental effects.

Some of the chronic disorders that tend to be the most persistent are minor lesions of tendons and ligaments. These are often refractory to treatments such as rest and anti-inflammation therapy because they are not chronic inflammatory lesions *per se*, but pathologic processes resulting from abnormal modeling of tissue in response to fatigue stresses. Therefore, while rest allows new tissue to be produced,

that which is produced is not of normal extensibility because of the lack of a proper orientation of structural elements, abnormal adherence of structural elements to one another, and adherence to adjacent tissues. In some situations, most notably rotator cuff tendinitis, inadequate tissue nutrition is also a factor. Because the lack of extensibility that accompanies "healing" of these lesions, the structure becomes more susceptible to internal strain when stresses are resumed and less able to attentuate the energy of loads applied to it. The result is recurrence of a low-grade inflammatory process each time use of the part is resumed. The most common of these disorders are supraspinatus tendinitis at the shoulder, tendinitis of the origin of the extensor carpi radialis brevis (tennis elbow), tendinitis of the abductor pollicis longus or extensor pollicis brevis tendons at the wrist (de Quervain's disease), coronary ligament sprain at the knee, and anterior talofibular ligament sprain.

In such chronic, persistent lesions of tendons and ligaments — and occasionally muscle — procedures to promote normal mobility and extensibility of the involved structure are important components of the treatment program. Passive or active exercises that impose a longitudinal strain on the involved structure may be incorporated. However, this creates the risk of maintaining the weakened or unresolved state of healing by contributing to the rate of tissue microdamage. That is probably why these disorders tend not to resolve spontaneously with varying degrees of activity. Too little activity results in loss of extensibility; too much activity does not allow for adequate healing. The appropriate compromise is difficult to judge.

Another method of promoting increased extensibility and mobility of the structure, while reducing stress levels and allowing healing to take place, is the use of deep transverse friction massage. This is a form of treatment advocated primarily by Cyriax, but unfortunately not widely adopted to date.[1] It involves applying a deep massage directly to the site of the lesion in a direction perpendicular to the normal orientation of fibrous elements. This maintains mobility of the structure with respect to adjacent tissues and probably helps to promote increased interfiber mobility of the structure itself without longitudinally stressing it. It may also promote normal orientation of fibers as they are produced. This effect might be likened to the effect of rolling your hand over an unorganized pile of toothpicks; eventually the toothpicks will all become oriented perpendicular to the direction in which the hand moves. In some pathologic processes, such as rotator cuff tendinitis, in which the etiology may be related to a nutritional deficit arising from hypovascularity, the hyperemia induced by the deep friction massage may also contribute to the healing response.

Although these effects of friction massage are highly conjectural, they are based on sound physiological and pathologic concepts. Further support is provided by the often dramatically favorable results obtained clinically when friction massage is appropriately incorporated in a treatment program. Studies are needed, however, to substantiate the physiological effects and the clinical efficacy of friction massage in these chronic disorders. Designing a legitimate clinical study would be difficult because most of the disorders for which friction massage seems to be effective do not present with measurable objective signs, and documentation of subjective improvement is usually unreliable. Basic studies of the effects of friction massage, however, may be fashioned after previous investigations into the effects of exercise, immobility, and other variables on the healing and maturation of collagen tissue. Until we have more concrete evidence of the value of friction massage, its use must be justified on the above considerations combined with "educated empiricism."

CLINICAL APPLICATIONS

INDICATIONS

Friction massage is indicated for chronic conditions of soft tissues—usually tendons, ligaments, or muscles—arising from abnormal modeling of fibrous elements in response to fatigue stresses or accompanying resolution of an acute inflammatory disorder. The intent is to restore or maintain the mobility of the structure with respect to adjacent tissues and to increase the extensibility of the structure under normal loading conditions. The approach is to allow for increased energy-attenuating capacity of the part with reduced strain to individual structural elements. Typical conditions in which friction massage is often indicated include

Tendinitis
Supraspinatus or infraspinatus (shoulder)
Tennis elbow
de Quervain's (wrist)
Peroneal tendinitis (ankle or foot)

Subacute or chronic ligamentous sprains
Intercarpal ligament sprains (wrist)
Coronary ligament sprains (knee)
Minor medial collateral ligament sprains (knee)
Minor anterior talofibular or calcaneocuboid ligament sprains (ankle)

Acute signs and symptoms should be resolved at the time at which friction massage is used (see criteria for acute *versus* chronic conditions in Chapter 5, Concepts of Management).

TECHNIQUES

The part should be well exposed and supported so as to reduce postural muscle tone. The structure to be treated is usually put in a position of neutral tension. It should be positioned so that the site of the lesion is easily accessible to the fingertips. If adherence between a tendon and its sheath is suspected, then the tendon should be kept taut to stabilize it while the sheath is mobilized during the massage.

The therapist should be seated, if possible, with the elbow supported to reduce muscle tension of more proximal parts. The pad of the index finger, middle finger, or thumb is placed directly over the involved site (Figs. 8-2, 8-3). The remaining fingers should be used to provide further stabilization of the therapist's hand and arm. *No lubricant is used;* the patient's skin must move along with the therapist's fingers.

Fig. 8-2. Transverse friction massage to the supraspinatous tendon.

Fig. 8-3. Transverse friction massage to the common extensor tendon at the lateral humeral epicondyle.

Beginning with light pressure, the therapist moves the skin over the site of the lesion back and forth, in a direction perpendicular to the normal orientation of the fibers of the involved part. The amplitude of movement is such that tension against the skin at the extremes of each stroke is minimal. This is necessary to avoid friction between the massaging fingers and the skin, which might well produce a blister. Friction may be further avoided by using the thumb and finger of the opposite hand to gather the skin in somewhat toward the area being massaged. The rate of movement should be about two or three cycles per second and should be rhythmical.

At the beginning of the massage, the patient may feel mild to moderate tenderness. This should not be a deterrent. However, after 1 or 2 minutes of treatment with light pressure, the tenderness should have subsided considerably. If it has not, or if tenderness has increased, treatment is stopped. At that point the therapist should consider whether pressure used at the initiation of the massage was excessive. Continuing or increasing tenderness is very rare, however; more often the massage has an anesthetic effect. As the tenderness subsides after 1 or 2 minutes, the pressure should be increased somewhat. The patient may feel some tenderness again. After about two more minutes, the therapist should again determine if the tenderness has subsided. If it has not, he should discontinue for that session; if it has subsided, he again increases the pressure and massages for about two more minutes. During the final 2 minutes of massage, the therapist should feel that the depth of massage is sufficient to affect the involved structure.

During the first treatment, the massage should be stopped after 5 or 6 minutes and the key signs reassessed. If it is a muscular or tendinous lesion, the painful resisted movement is checked; if it is a ligamentous lesion, the painful joint-play movement is retested. The patient should feel some immediate improvement. If he has not, the therapist should consider whether the technique of treatment was appropriate, assuming that the disorder is one for which friction massage is indicated.

With successive treatments, the depth of massage is always gradually increased, as described above, and the length of treatment is gradually increased by about 3 minutes in each session, working up to 12 or 15 minutes each session. However, treatment should not be continued during a particular session nor should the depth of massage be increased if the tenderness to massage increases or does not subside during treatment. Responses will vary, of course, with the patient and with the nature of the disorder. In some cases the duration of treatment must be increased more slowly than in others. There are few conditions that do not resolve after six to ten sessions over 2 or 3 weeks, provided that other components of the treatment program are appropriately carried out and provided that friction massage is indicated.

It is not unusual for a patient to feel some increased "soreness" following the first or second sessions, but this must be distinguished from exacerbation of symptoms. Some skin or soft-tissue tenderness and soreness are to be expected. This would occur whether the patient did or did not have an underlying problem and should not be misconstrued by the therapist or patient as worsening of the condition, so long as key symptoms and signs related to the patient's condition are no worse.

A common mistake during treatment by friction massage is the development of skin blisters or abrasions. These result either from fingernails that are too long or from poor technique that causes friction between the massaging finger and skin. Another common mistake is for the therapist to apply the massage to the area of pain rather than to the site of the lesion. The two areas do not necessarily coincide.

In addition, the therapist must avoid overstressing the more distal joints of his thumb and fingers when performing the massage. This is especially important if friction massage is being used frequently. Such stresses can be reduced by stabilizing the distal interphalangeal joint of the massaging finger with a free finger, as shown in Figure 8–3, and by alternating fingers during a particular treatment session.

Friction massage should be avoided when the nutritional status of the skin is compromised and in cases of impaired vascular response. These would typically include patients on long-term, high-dose, steroid drug therapy and patients with known peripheral vascular disease.

Specific techniques for friction massage of the supraspinatus tendon and extensor carpi radialis brevis are described below.

Supraspinatus Tendon

Light to deep transverse frictions are given over the tendon. The patient sits comfortably on a chair, and the arm is put in a neutral or somewhat extended position with the lower arm supported. The therapist sits at the patient's side. A position of neutral or slight humeral extension brings the tendon forward into a position in which the site of the lesion is easily accessible to the fingertip. (see Fig. 8–2). The therapist identifies the site of the supraspinatus tendon lying between the greater tubercle of the humerus and the acromion process. It is essential that the tendon be accurately located by knowledge of anatomy; it cannot be distinguished by palpation. The pad of the therapist's middle finger, reinforced by the index finger (or *vice versa*), is placed directly over the site of the lesion, which is always just proximal to the tendon insertion on the greater tubercle. The thumb is used to stabilize the arm. The therapist applies friction in a direction perpendicular to the normal orientation of the tendon, using the thumb both as fulcrum and to maintain pressure. The thumb and fingers of the opposite hand support and gather the skin over the shoulder to avoid friction between the massaging finger and skin.

This is the most valuable treatment in the management of supraspinatus tendinitis and is a key compo-nent of the treatment program (see Chapter 10, The Shoulder and Shoulder Girdle). A similar technique is used for the other tendons of the rotator cuff.

"Tennis Elbow"

Light to deep frictions are given to the affected fibers of the extensor carpi radialis brevis at the anterior aspect of the lateral humeral epicondyle. The patient sits with the lower arm supported; the elbow is flexed and the forearm is supinated to allow easy access of the massaging finger or thumb. The therapist sits at the side, facing the patient. One hand supports at the elbow. The massaging hand is placed so that the thumb is over the affected fibers (see Fig. 8–3). Counterpressure is applied by the fingers lying against the medial proximal aspect of the forearm. The thumb is drawn across the site of the lesion in a direction perpendicular to the fibers by alternate supination and pronation of the forearm, using the fingers as a fulcrum. The therapist may also use the index or long fingers for massage, as described for friction massage to the supraspinatus tendon.

REFERENCES

1. Cyriax J, Coldham M: Textbook of Orthopaedic Medicine, Vol 2, Treatment by Massage, Manipulation and Injection, 11th ed, pp 8–12. London, Baillière Tindall, 1984
2. Rogoff JB (ed): Manipulation, Traction and Massage, 2nd ed. Baltimore, Williams & Wilkins, 1980
3. Tappin FM: Healing Massage Techniques: A Study of Eastern and Western Methods. Reston, VA, Reston Publishing, 1978
4. Wood EC: Beard's Massage: Principles and Techniques, 3rd ed. Philadelphia, WB Saunders, 1981

RECOMMENDED READINGS

Chamberlain GJ: Cyriax's friction massage: A review. J Orthop Sports Phys Ther 4:16–22, 1982
Cyriax J: Deep friction. Physiotherapy 63:60–61, 1977
Cyriax J, Coldham M: Textbook of Orthopaedic Medicine, Vol 2, Treatment by Manipulation, Massage, and Injection, 11th ed. London, Baillière Tindall, 1984
Palastanga N: Connective tissue massage. *In* Greive GP (ed): Modern Manual Therapy of the Vertebral Column. New York, Churchill Livingstone, 1986
Walker JM: Deep transverse frictions in ligament healing. J Orthop Sports Phys Ther 6:89–94, 1984

9 *Relaxation*

Darlene Hertling and Daniel Jones

THE REVIVAL OF RELAXATION TECHNIQUES AND THE DEVELOPMENT OF RELATED TECHNIQUES

Relaxation techniques are being used by physical therapists and other health professionals more than ever before. The concept of relaxation has had a long and varied history. In the early part of this century, Jacobson introduced a form of therapy based on muscular quiescence known as *progressive relaxation*.[19] American interest in the topic of relaxation waned during the 1940s and 1950s. It was not until the introduction of systematic desensitization by Wolpe in 1958, in which progressive relaxation played an important role, that American interest in this topic was once again renewed.[54]

Systematic desensitization is one of the most widely used behavioral therapy techniques to employ relaxation. It is a method used for breaking down neurotic anxiety-response habits in a step-by-step fashion.[55] Relaxation is used as a physiological anxiety-inhibiting state. The subject is first exposed to a weak anxiety-arousing stimulus, which is repeated until the stimulus progressively loses its ability to evoke anxiety. Successively stronger stimuli are applied and similarly treated until the habit is overcome, or the trainee gains some control over it. Relaxation training has since become an integral part of many behavioral procedures; the principles of behavioristic psychology, behavior modification, stress management, and related techniques often employ relaxation training.

Relaxation techniques and related techniques have also found their way into the newly established pain clinics. The prototype, and now probably the largest and best-organized clinic, was begun in 1961 by Bonica and White, of the University of Washington Medical School.[37] Other pain clinics have been formed at other hospitals and clinics both here and abroad. There is evidence that many psychological approaches are able to produce some measure of pain relief. According to Sternbach, these include desensitization techniques (in which exposure to pain and the opportunity to gain some kind of control over it helps to relieve it or to make it bearable), hypnotic suggestion techniques, and progressive relaxation.[46]

Interest in relaxation and related techniques has been further augmented by increased self-awareness and by what has been called the "body boom" of the 1960s and 1970s.[29] It has led to increased concern with relaxation, posture, getting in touch with one's body, and thereby one's emotions. Ultimately, it has to do with healing the body and, hopefully, the mind as well. According to Kruger, "The body boom has begot a widely assorted, though in many ways a cohesive family of both medical and nonmedical therapists who do body work—the father of the breed, Reich, the mother, Yoga, and the family estate Esalen, California, which is considered the mecca of the American Human Potential Movement."[29]

Recent research demonstrates that we are more capable of controlling our bodily and psychological processes than was previously believed.[4,20,33,41–43,55] The defining mark of the "new body therapies" is their attention to exercise, relaxation, massage, and body and human potential.

Theoretical principles include an understanding of the relationship between the body and character structure (first developed by psychoanalyst Wilhelm Reich) and existentialist, physiological, behavioral, and sociologic theories.

Therapeutic practices include a variety of psychophysiological methods for making use of bodily processes to reduce tension and anxiety. Among them are the following methods:

—The revival of ancient Asian disciplines such as yoga, T'ai chi, and Zen awareness training, and their western modifications
—Principles of behavioristic psychology and behavior modification

—Sophisticated instrumentation of Western technology, such as biofeedback

—The neo-Reichian approach of bioenergetics, best known through the work of Lowen and of Kelemann.[31,32] Body movements and verbalization are used to release blocked or repressed energy and to reintegrate body and mind.

—The Alexander technique, which changes body alignment by increasing awareness of posture and by the use of suggestion and gentle repositioning of the limbs[1,2]

—The rediscovery of dance therapy. An example is the Feher School of Dance and Relaxation, which works extensively with back problems. It is considered a form of dynamic or active distraction used for relaxation purposes.[29]

—A variety of massage techniques, including massages for different parts of the body to promote relaxation and well-being, and more recently, acupressure massage and acupuncture.[3,13,14,48,53] Chapman of the University of Washington Pain Clinic has experimented with acupuncture. He believes that one of its effects is to bring about relaxation very quickly, and that it may tend to reduce physiological stress reactions.[37]

—The revival of the Jacobson relaxation technique, including newer techniques such as the Lamaze technique (associated with natural childbirth), autogenic training (a medical therapy based on sensory awareness devised by J. H. Schultz, a German neurologist), and the relaxation response or Benson's technique (meditation on a single word or color)[4,33,41,47]

—Differential relaxation techniques of body parts and systems through respiration exercises, such as Fuchs' functional relaxation and Jencks' respiration exercises for use in daily-life activities and coping with stress.[25,26]

COMPONENTS OF THE STRESS RESPONSE

Research during the past decade in the management of stress and the application of relaxation and related techniques has received an increasing amount of attention. The existing literature on relaxation and related states is extremely diverse. The foundations on which this body of research rests range from age-old meditative disciplines of Asia to contemporary research on behavior modification, and the newest approach, biofeedback, is often combined with relaxation techniques.

Components of the stress response identified by theorists include physiological, psychosomatic, psychological, and sociologic aspects. Selye has spent almost four decades of laboratory research on the physiological mechanism of adaptation to the stress of life.[42,43] From his studies on overstressed animals, he observed nonspecific changes, which he called the *general adaptation syndrome*, and specific responses that depend on the kind of stressor and on the part of the organism involved. He established a stress index that comprises some major pathologic results of overstress, including enlargement of the adrenal cortex, atrophy of lymphatic tissues, and bleeding ulcers. He has further defined certain pathologic consequences of long-term stress as *diseases of adaptation*. Among these he classified stomach ulcers, cardiovascular disease, high blood pressure, connective tissue disease, and headaches.

Mason, one of the most distinguished investigators of the psychological and psychiatric aspects of biologic stress, suggests that emotional stimuli are the most common stressors.[36] They are reflected in the endocrine, autonomic, and musculoskeletal systems (Fig. 9–1). We know that every individual will not elicit the same syndrome even with the same degree of stress. Likewise, it is known that the same stressor can cause different lesions in different individuals, which can selectively enhance or inhibit one of the stress effects. Conditioning may be internal (*i.e.*, genetic predisposition, past experience, age, sex) or external (*i.e.*, treatment with certain hormones, drugs, dietary factors). Under the influence of such conditioning factors a normally well-tolerated degree of stress may be pathogenic and may cause diseases of adaptation that selectively affect predisposed areas of the body. Any kind of activity sets our stress mechanism in motion. However, whether the heart, gastrointestinal tract, or musculoskeletal system will suffer most depends largely on accidental conditioning factors. Although all parts of the system are exposed equally to stress, it is the weakest link that breaks down first.

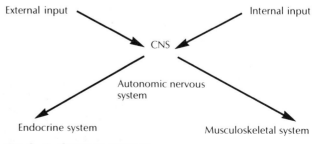

Fig. 9–1. Common stresses.

Stimulus

(Dependent on psychological interpretation)

Frequent stressor ——————————— Specific effect

(Prevents body returning
to baseline levels of function)

(response stereotype,
particular individual)

Failure in homeostatic mechanism

Fig. 9–2. Scheme illustrating onset of stress-related disorders.

Sternbach has described a scheme for the onset of stress-related disorders and the resultant failure in the homeostatic mechanism to prevent the body from returning to a baseline level of function in many cases.[45] For example, frequent stressors cause an increase in blood pressure. Often, as the result of failure in the homeostatic mechanism, the system readjusts to a new level of increased blood pressure (Fig. 9–2). Similarly, Brown has pointed out that muscle behavior under stress is translated into muscle holding or tension.[5] If stressors are frequent, the following two muscle events occur: (1) muscle tension becomes sustained at higher levels, and (2) the tightness of the muscles causes them to be hyperactive. Under normal conditions, an appropriate adjustment is made by the central muscle control system. Special nerve cells in the muscle tissue sense when a fiber is contracting, how fast it is tensing, and other complex aspects of muscle contraction. The system seems to become inefficient, however, with continued stress or rumination about the stress, since the length of time muscle fibers have been tense does not seem to be relayed to the central mus-

cle control system. As a result, the muscles have little chance to recover from increased tension. Tension becomes sustained at higher levels and may continue to increase. If muscles are not given relief from tension by relaxation or a change of activity, the muscle fibers physiologically "adapt" to states of increased tension.

Hess produced the changes associated with the fight-or-flight response by stimulating a part of the cat's brain within the hypothalamus.[15,18] By stimulating another area within the hypothalamus, he demonstrated a response whose physiologic changes were similar to those measured during the practice of relaxation, that is, a response opposite the fight-or-flight response (ergotropic response). He described this as a protective mechanism against overstress that belongs to the trophotropic system and promotes a restorative process (Fig. 9–3).

Benson believes the trophotropic response described by Hess in cats is the relaxation response in humans.[4] Both of these opposing responses are associated with physiologic changes, and each appears to be controlled by the hypothalamus. Because the

Ergotropic response	Trophotropic response
Primarily sympathetic	Primarily parasympathetic
Excitement, arousal	Relaxation
Mobilization of body	Energy conservation
↑ HR, BP, R	↓ HR, BP, R
↑ Blood sugar	↑ GI function
↑ Muscle tension	↓ Muscle tension
Pupil dilatation	Pupil constriction
↑ O_2 consumption	↓ O_2 consumption
↑ CO_2 elimination	↓ CO_2 elimination

Fig. 9–3. Effects of the ergotropic and trophotropic responses (BP, blood pressure; HR, heart rate; R, respiration; GI, gastrointestinal).

fight-or-flight response and the relaxation response are in opposition, one counteracts the effects of the other. This is why Benson and Wallace feel the relaxation response is so important; through its use the harmful effects of inappropriate elicitation of the fight-or-flight response are counteracted. They indicate that most of the relaxation therapies evoke the same physiologic changes as the relaxation response.

ROLE OF PHYSICAL THERAPY

One of the common symptoms physical therapists see in many of their patients today is tension pain related to neuromuscular hypertension. Many feel that muscle tension or stress is actually a partial or complete cause of heart attack, cerebrovascular accident, peripheral and neurovascular syndromes, chronic musculoskeletal problems, and the common headache. Most physical therapists would agree that a chronic pain patient who is tense will invariably take much longer to treat and need more time to recover. Experience seems to indicate that many musculoskeletal disorders have more severe and/or more prolonged symptoms when muscular tension is a factor. Since this appears to be true, then certainly we should be aware of tension symptoms in the evaluation process and should develop skills to treat the tension factor in these patients.

Tension may not only prolong a condition but may be the primary factor in the causation of dysfunction. Tension tends not only to aggravate the condition, thus compounding the pathology, but it may actually bring to light what would otherwise have been a subclinical pathologic process. Holmes and Wolff believe that in many instances the primary local cause of backache is minimal, but the muscle tension produced by anxiety and emotional stress causes secondary pain in the back that may outlast and exceed the primary pain.[40] In any event, both the cause of the habitual holding—the tension itself—and the subclinical pathologic process will require treatment.

NEUROMUSCULAR HYPERTENSION

What is neuromuscular hypertension? Certainly we contract muscle isotonically or isometrically all day long, be it small muscle movement of the eyes, or the action of the quadricep, hamstring, and gastrocnemius muscles when running, or some normal activity that requires muscle contraction between the two extremes. This involves normal muscular effort, or normal energy expenditure. We also seem to have a remarkable ability to recruit muscular effort when faced with an emergency situation. Humans, however, are creatures of habit and can become accustomed to contracting these muscles subconsciously. This is when problems occur. One gets used to bracing or holding or continuous movement and then carries that muscular effort over into activities that should require a small amount of effort. This is

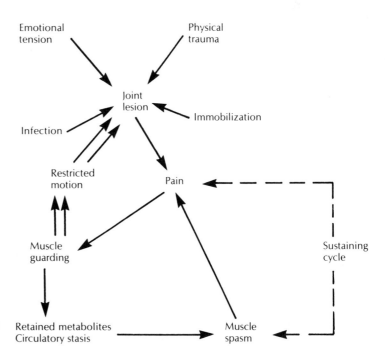

Fig. 9-4. Mechanism by which irritation leads to joint dysfunction.

learned behavior. Excess tension may even carry over into periods in which there should be minimal effort, such as lying down or sleeping.

Should some medical condition develop, this tension factor immediately prohibits the natural healing process. Jacobson says, "Acute conditions may occur after intense or prolonged pain or distress from whatever source, whether physical, as a trauma, angina or colic, or mental, as a fright, bereavement, quarrel or loss."[20] Our society probably perpetuates this holding or contracting habit. The pressures of occupation, family, church, and friends contribute to the overuse of muscle tissue and increased neuromuscular excitability. Whatmore and Kohli describe this as a pathophysiological state made up of errors in energy expenditure.[52]

The chronic musculoskeletal problems that therapists are confronted with are seldom found to be associated with only one factor, but with a number of factors. Emotional tension, physical trauma, infection, immobilization, or various combinations may lead to joint dysfunction resulting in a sustaining cycle of pain, muscle guarding, retained metabolites, and restricted motion (Fig. 9–4).

Physical therapy plays an important role in the local relief of tension pain associated with neuromuscular hypertension. Often localized tension may be relieved by heat and massage. Joint mobilization of the involved part is often the most effective treatment for breaking up this sustaining cycle. But physical therapy can also act at a deeper level to relieve underlying muscle holding or tension by teaching the tense individual to relax the body and mind through conscious relaxation during normal daily activities.

TYPES OF RELAXATION AND RELATED TECHNIQUES

For habitual holding itself, Jacobson's approach has been used in physical therapy almost since its beginning. Jacobson's approach to instructing relaxation has been found to be very suitable in our work and certainly is the most well known in the United States. However, a large number and variety of techniques and combinations of techniques are now being used by physical therapists, as well as other medical practitioners. These include Benson's relaxation response, transcendental meditation, Schultz and Luthe's autogenic training, among others. It is generally felt that individual differences and the diversity of needs require a wide choice of techniques. A review of clinical reports suggests that a judicious mix

of techniques may obtain the best results.[5] Of the many techniques now available to us, most carry similar requirements, most notably the need for practice, a quiet atmosphere, a comfortable position, and a passive and receptive attitude.

Indications are numerous. Jacobson cites some of the following:[20]

— Acute neuromuscular hypertension
— Chronic neuromuscular hypertension
— States of fatigue and exhaustion
— States of debility
— Various preoperative and postoperative conditions
— Sleep disturbances
— Alimentary spasm and peptic ulcers

Some of the most common stress-related conditions treated by physical therapists include

— Tension headaches
— Migraine headaches
— High blood pressure
— Pulmonary disease (asthma and emphysema)[44]
— Muscle guarding
— Spasticity
— Arthritis and related disorders
— Bell's palsy
— Cerebral palsy
— Burns (before treatment with debridement and range of motion exercises)
— Various chronic pain conditions associated with muscle tension (*e.g.*, cervical strain, adhesive capsulitis)

Types of relaxation and related techniques are difficult to pinpoint, but basically there are two types — the somatic or physical approach, and the cognitive or mental approach. Many techniques employ a combination of both approaches. Such a great variety of psychophysiological methods are available to us that only a general survey will be made here, with detail given to some of the more familiar ones. Physical approaches may primarily emphasize passive distraction (*e.g.*, Jacobson's technique, Praskauer massage, and respiratory techniques) or active or dynamic distraction (*e.g.*, Feldenkrais's awareness through movement, T'ai chi, or the Alexander technique). Those that stress the mental or cognitive approach include meditation, sensory awareness techniques, autogenic training, and sentic cycles. The outline of Psychophysiological Methods of Relaxation and Related Techniques lists only a few of the more commonly used methods of relaxation and related techniques that are practiced in the United States and Europe today. Many excellent techniques have been omitted.

Psychophysiological Methods of Relaxation and Related Techniques

Active Tonus Regulation (Stokvis, Netherlands)

Ideomotor movements are used to prove the influence of mind over body. Suggestions for relaxation of muscles, respiration, and mind are used to induce an altered state of consciousness.[26]

Alexander Technique (Alexander, England)

Kinesthetics is the key word in the Alexander lexicon. The core of this technique is helping people to become aware of when and where their bodies are tense. Proper alignment of head on spine is used to correct physical misalignments, attitudes, and behavior.[1,2]

Autoanalysis (Bezzola, Switzerland)

A simple technique in which the body serves as its own excellent biofeedback instrument through attention to and verbalization of successive internal sensations to induce deep mental and physical relaxation.[26]

Autogenic Training (Schultz, Germany)

One of the four major relaxation techniques now being used that developed directly from the therapeutic practice of hypnosis for relaxation. The complete program is divided into three categories of exercises: autosuggestion about relaxation; single-focus meditation (as in yoga); and meditation on abstract qualities. The first series of exercises is primarily used by physical therapists, and occasionally the second.[33,41]

Awareness through Movement (Feldenkrais, Israel)

Sensory awareness involving movements of limbs, breathing, facial expressions, and self-massage for balance of tension and postural alignment. Feldenkrais, an expert body therapist from Israel, is now living in California and offers courses to health professionals.[13,14]

Functional Relaxation (Fuchs, Germany)

Slow, relaxed exhalations and breathing rhythms are used for differential relaxation of the body parts and systems. Gentle hand contact by the therapist and later by the patient is used to detect inhibiting tension. It is considered a medical therapy requiring a therapist's guidance.[26]

Hatha Yoga (India)

Hatha yoga exercises require both physical manipulation and concentration on awareness of body activities. Assumption of certain postures and controlled breathing are used to induce altered states of consciousness.[11,49]

Meditation Techniques

Whether of Hindu, Zen, Buddhist, or other origin, meditation behavior usually entails concentration of attention and awareness of a single idea, object, or point inside or outside the body. Many Western modifications have been developed for their usefulness as antidotes to the stress of ordinary living. Although meditative practices were not originally designed to be relaxation techniques, the experience of relaxation is a by-product of most such techniques.[10,51,53]

Muscular Therapy (Benjamin, U.S.)

An approach to tension relief that combines deep massage, tension-release exercises, body-care techniques, and postural re-education. The tension-release exercises make use of the neo-Reichian approach of bioenergetics.[3]

Nyingma System (India)

A system of physical exercises, posture, breathing, and massage is used as a basis for sensory awareness and relief of emotional tension. The Nyingma Institute is located in Berkeley, California, and workshops are offered for psychotherapists, physical therapists, and other health professionals.[53]

Passive Movements (Michaux, France)

Passive movement of relaxed body parts, without the active participation of the subject, to induce both physical and mental relaxation.[26]

Progressive Relaxation (Jacobson, U.S.)

Most widely known of the four major relaxation techniques. Alternate tensing and relaxing of skeletal, respiratory, and facial muscles are used to induce physical and mental relaxation.[19–24]

Proskauer Massage (Proskauer, U.S.)

Also called *breath therapy*. Exhalation and inhalation are coupled with an extremely light and delicate massage to different muscle groups so that the massage is timed with the rhythm of the breathing exercise. Meditation and imagery are used to enhance physical and mental relaxation.[29,53]

Relaxation Response (Benson, U.S.)

From the collected writings of the East (meditation) and the West (autogenic training), Benson has devised a simplified method of eliciting the relaxation response. It consists of two basic categories of exercises: autosuggestion about relaxation, and single-focus meditation usually on the mantra "one."[4]

Respiration of Special Accomplishment (Jencks, U.S.)

Self-suggesting technique coupled with breathing rhythm to enhance relaxation or invigoration, warmth or coolness, for use in daily-life activities and coping with stress. Jencks' exercises can easily be adapted for use in physical therapy as well as in psychotherapy.[25,26]

Self-Hypnotism (Pierce, U.S.)

Attention, with closed eyes, to tensing the skeletal muscles of the body part to a point of fatigue. Attention is then shifted to another body part to bring about automatic complete relaxation. This is followed by a series of eye exercises. Finally, imagery is used as a method of distracting attention to further enhance relaxation.[39,53]

Sensory Awareness Training (Grindler, Germany)

Sensory awareness training originated about 100 years ago in Europe as a training method for performing artists. Several of the teachers later emigrated to the United States. The earliest and perhaps most significant work with sensory awareness training was done by Elsa Grindler (1885–1961).[26] A large number and variety of exercises have evolved, including autogenic training. Most of the therapeutic techniques are used for inducing physical relaxation through sensory awareness of muscle tension and inhibited breathing.

Sentic Cycles (Clynes, U.S.)

A behavioral therapy technique composed of eight sentic states or self-induced emotional states. Clynes, a psychophysiological researcher, has demonstrated the close relationship between emotional states and predictable physiological change.[8]

Systematic Desensitization (Wolpe, U.S.)

A behavioral therapy technique in which progressive relaxation is used (following Jacobson) in conjunction with behavioral management techniques. The client develops a series of "scenes" or "visualizations" that are called forth in a hierarchial order based on their fear-evoking ability while attempting to remain relaxed.[54,55]

Transcendental Meditation (T.M.) (Maharishi Mahesh Yogi, United States)

A form of meditation adapted to Western concepts and philosophic background most often used as an adjunct to therapeutic relaxation techniques, including EMG biofeedback.[34,50] Graduates are required to meditate for twenty minutes per day using a mantra that has been assigned to them.

Credited courses in T.M. have been given in dozens of colleges and universities in the United States and abroad.

The two major techniques used by physical therapists in the United States are progressive relaxation and autogenic training. Various types of meditation, massage, breathing, and sensory awareness techniques are also employed and are often combined with other techniques. With the exception of self-hypnosis, hypnosis is used primarily by other health professionals in the management of painful conditions of the musculoskeletal system as well as cancer, alcohol and drug abuse, natural childbirth, and others.

RELAXATION AND MASSAGE

An invaluable tool in the management of common musculoskeletal disorders is massage. However, since World War II, there seems to have been a general decrease in the use of massage for these conditions, perhaps because massage is time consuming, sometimes strenuous, and demands skill on the part of the person giving the treatment. It is also possible that increased knowledge and sophistication of equipment has made basic massage too simple to use. Another reason is, unfortunately, that the basis for its use has been empiric rather than scientific. However, many therapists, including these authors, believe that experience has shown massage to be an extremely important and beneficial tool. Surely it is not the total answer, but as with heat or cold, exercise, relaxation, mobilization, and electrical stimulation, massage as part of our repertoire helps us treat our patients more effectively.

When discussing massage we could talk about stroking and effleurage, pétrissage and kneading, friction, percussion, ice, mechanical vibration, or connective tissue massage. We could cover direction (centrifugal *versus* centripetal or proximal *versus* distal), pressure, rate and rhythm, media, positions of patient and clinician, duration, and frequency. However, we have chosen to let you review this basic material and its history in the literature, what little there seems to be. One of the better sources is *Massage: Principles and Techniques*, by Beard and Wood.[56]

As mentioned earlier, much has been written about massage, although little scientific study has been done to tell us what physiological effects massage has on various body tissues. In one study of injured muscle, animal muscle tissue was subjected to a crushing injury and later examined microscopically. One group of animals was left untreated, while another group received massage. The untreated group showed the following results:

1. Dissociation into fibrillae of muscular fibers as shown by well-marked longitudinal striation
2. Hyperplasia (sometimes simple thickening of the connective tissue)
3. Increase, in places, of the number of nuclei in the connective tissue
4. Interstitial hemorrhages
5. Enlargement of blood vessels, with hyperplasia of their adventitious coats
6. Sarcolemma was usually intact, but in one section, a multiplication of nuclei was seen, resembling somewhat an interstitial myositis.

The treated group, on the other hand, showed the following results:

1. Normal appearance of muscle
2. No secondary fibrous bands separating the muscle fibers
3. No fibrous thickening around the vessels
4. Greater general bulk of the muscle
5. No signs of hemorrhages

It has been concluded from this study and others that massage may lessen the amount of fibrosis that inevitably develops in immobilized, injured, or denervated muscle. Even when there has not been injury, there are innumerable situations that will cause a metabolic imbalance within the soft tissue. Observation, and particularly palpation, will reveal abnormal muscle tissue that is often hard, well defined, stringy, and painful. Massage will benefit this uninjured but abnormal tissue, too.

Clinical Application

Massage should usually follow application of heat or cold, and should be done in a relaxing rhythm, with media of the therapist's choice. One should have good hand contact, but most importantly, the massage should be deep. That means the therapist must feel for abnormal tissue (hard and tender) during the palpation portion of massage and gradually restore that tissue to its normal soft, elongated, nontender state. This appears to increase circulation, decrease pain sensitivity, and promote relaxation; it certainly reduces tension or stress to the tissues with which the muscle comes in contact.

Because muscle is the only tissue in the body that contracts, it follows that excessive or continuous contraction, especially for prolonged periods of time, can only lead to abnormality. It is interesting to note that over the years many patients, after a few treatments of vigorous deep massage, experience considerable relief from arthritis, adhesive capsulitis, tension headaches, and so forth. Patients also tend to become unhappy if there is a change in personnel to someone who gives a gentler massage. From a practical standpoint, we must realize that acute conditions cannot tolerate deep massage immediately. Occasionally, there will be patients who never tolerate deep massage. Usually the extremely tense individual who is unwilling to change his daily habits is in this category. However, it is important to realize that some muscles become so tense that the patient has a very difficult time relaxing the tissue without some massage. If mobilization is used, it is common sense that the least amount of force used will add to the safety of patient treatment. Therefore, massage prior to mobilization can be extremely useful. On the other hand, a joint restriction can sometimes cause localized protective spasm, which will be relieved by restoring the normal mobility to the joint by mobilization.

In 1963 Kopell and Thompson discussed various surgical procedures for the relief of certain peripheral entrapment neuropathies.[27] It has been found that massage, stretching, mobilization, and exercise can provide relief from symptoms in these same conditions. This seems to indicate the tense, spasmodic, or contracted muscle is at least partly the cause of the symptoms in some of these entrapment conditions.

MUSCLE RE-EDUCATION

Although massage is a valuable tool in relieving tension in muscle, it is imperative that the patient be taught how to relax his muscles in order to achieve prolonged good results. This requires a learning process like that for any other skill we have learned — riding a bike, tying our shoes, reading, playing a sport, or driving a car. It is essentially muscle re-education, a skill physical therapists have used in their practice for years. To teach relaxation, we must develop a muscle awareness in the student. This means practice on the part of the patient.

One way for the patient to develop muscle awareness is to lie down in a comfortable position in a quiet place and practice, in an easy way, three things — the "basic three." The first is belly or abdominal breathing. Explain to the patient that chest breathing requires contraction of various muscles from neck to chest. Since relaxation of muscle tissue is the desired result, and not contraction, abdominal breathing is the method of choice. As the lungs expand with inspiration, their normal space is taken up in the chest cavity. More space can be given to the expanding lungs by allowing the diaphragm, which separates the chest from the abdominal cavity, to be pushed down into the abdominal cavity. Consequently, the external appearance and feel is that the abdomen rises. With exhalation the pressure is reversed; the air is expelled easily, and the diaphragm returns to its normal position. The normal habit of tension is rapid, shallow, chest breathing or sighing types of patterns. Abdominal breathing with a slow, rhythmical, average amount of air is extremely important for relaxation.

Secondly, the patient should "let all the muscles go." Explain that this means no movement and no holding or bracing. Instruct the patient that it is best to have a couple of pillows under the knees to protect the low back. The legs must roll outward, that is, be externally rotated, in order to relax the various hip muscles. One or two pillows may be placed under the head to support the mid-cervical area. The arms may be flexed with the hands resting on the abdomen but not touching or interlocked, or the muscle will tend to contract. Or they may be extended and externally rotated if the bed or plinth allows complete support of the arms.

Several key areas should be pointed out for the patient to "let go." For example, the eyes should not be closed quickly, since this is a contraction, but gradually after a few minutes have passed. Muscle relaxation can never be forced or done with determined effort because relaxation is a negative effort rather than a positive effort of contraction. Point out the various forms of muscle that contract or relax for facial expression and the contraction of the tongue with speech. The neck, upper back, arms, legs, and low back can all be pointed out again as areas where the patient "lets go" or "turns the power off."

The third aspect of the "basic three" is thinking about letting go without hard concentration. Learning, of course, requires some mental energy, and relaxation as a means of combating tension is definitely a learning process. So, by having the patient think—not concentrate hard—about letting go of that residual tension in the various areas of the body mentioned above, he can learn to relax. As Jacobson states, "The mind and body are one operating unit, not two, and this operating unit is based on muscle contractions."[22] Thus, letting the muscle go in itself will help to put the mind at ease.

PROGRESSIVE RELAXATION

One of the most widely accepted tools used in learning relaxation is the contract–relax method commonly known as *Jacobson's progressive relaxation*. By teaching the patient to contract a muscle and develop recognition of the tension signals, or effort,

he can begin to recognize tension as it occurs in daily life. This is followed by a period of "letting go," "turning the power off," "going negative," or whatever term is most meaningful to a particular patient. In other words, effort is discontinued, and the fibers of that muscle lengthen as relaxation takes place.

The patient is asked to practice 60 minutes each day in a quiet room free from intruders and phone calls. The following eight instructions for steps to be followed consecutively during the first period are adapted in part from Jacobson's *Self-Operations Control Manual.*[22]

Arm Practice
1. Lying on your back with arms at sides, leave eyes open 3 to 4 minutes.
2. Gradually close eyes and keep them closed during the entire hour.
3. After 3 to 4 minutes with eyes closed, bend left hand back. Observe the control sensation 1 to 2 minutes, and how it differs from the strains in the wrist and in the lower portion of the forearm.
4. Go negative for 3 to 4 minutes.
5. Again bend left hand back and observe as described in 3.
6. Go negative once more for 3 to 4 minutes.
7. Bend left hand back a third and last time, observing the control sensation 1 to 2 minutes.
8. Finally, go negative for the remainder of the hour.

Eight similar steps are taken in the second period, except that the left wrist is flexed instead of extended. The same eight instructions apply during every period of the entire course except that the motion performed will vary with the number of the period. The motion indicated for a period is usually performed three times at intervals of several minutes.

It should be noted that this does not apply to every third period of practice. During these sessions all motion is omitted, and the patient simply relaxes for the entire hour ("zero period"). In this way, the person avoids forming the bad habit of tensing a part before relaxing it.

The sequence of the movements performed each day and the periods for relaxation of the left arm are as follows:

Period	Left Arm
1	Bend hand back (wrist extension)
2	Bend hand forward (wrist flexion)
3	Relax only (no contraction)
4	Bend at elbow (elbow flexion)
5	Straighten arm (elbow extension)
6	Relax only
7	Progressive tension and relaxation of whole arm

Day seven, and each subsequent period of progressive tension and relaxation of the entire part, involves slowly tightening the entire part—a gradual and continuous increase in the amount of muscle contraction. When the part has become moderately tense, the patient gradually and slowly relaxes, contracting less and less for the remainder of the 60 minutes.

Periods eight through 14 follow exactly the same procedures as periods one through seven, except with the right arm. The periods then continue to other areas of the body as follows:

Period	Left Leg
15	Bend foot up (dorsiflexion)
16	Bend foot down (plantar flexion)
17	Relax only
18	Raise foot (knee extension)
19	Bend at knee (knee flexion)
20	Relax only
21	Raise knee (hip flexion)
22	Press lower thigh down (hip extension)
23	Relax entire leg
24	Progressive tension and relaxation of entire leg

Following the pattern described above, Periods 15 through 24 are focused on the left leg, and Periods 25 through 34 are focused on the right leg.

Period	Trunk
35	Pull in abdomen (contraction of abdominals)
36	Arch back slightly (spinal extension)
37	Relax abdomen, back, and legs
38	Observe a deeper breathing pattern
39	Bend shoulders back (contraction of interscapular muscles)
40	Relax only
41	Lift left arm forward and inward (pectorals)
42	Lift right arm forward and inward
43	Relax only
44	Elevate shoulder (upper trapezius and levator scapulae)

Periods 45 through 50 are focused on neck practice.

Period	Neck
45	Bend head back
46	Bend chin toward chest (neck flexion)
47	Relax only
48	Bend head left (left side flexion)
49	Bend head right
50	Relax only

Finally, Periods 51 through 62 are eye-region practice.

Period	Eye Region Practice
51	Wrinkle forehead
52	Frown
53	Relax only
54	Close eyelids tightly
55	Look left with lids closed
56	Relax only
57	Look right with lids closed
58	Look up
59	Relax only
60	Look down with lids closed
61	Look forward with lids closed
62	Relax only

This progressive relaxation can continue into visualization practice, speech-region practice, and practice in other positions, such as sitting, and in activities of daily living as explained in Jacobson's *Self-Operations Control Manual.*[22]

Another variation of Jacobson's progressive relaxation is a tool that has been used for years called the "relaxation lesson." The instructions given to the patient are as follows:

> Begin with diaphragmatic breathing; then do some combination breathing with the chest and diaphragm. Settle into a nice rhythmic breathing pattern, with the abdominal muscles relaxed, and the diaphragm doing all the work. Do this lying on your back with the proper supports so that you relax best. Coordinate the following exercises with the breathing rhythm. All exercises should be done with minimal effort; the relaxation period is most important. Concentrate so that you may establish new habits for your muscles.

—Bend fingers, wrist, and elbow (flexion pattern). Relax.

—Straighten fingers, pull back wrist, and stiffen elbow (extension). Let go.

—Roll arm inward (inward rotation). Let go.

—Roll arm outward (outward rotation). Relax

—Bend hip, knee, push foot down, curl toes (flexion). Let go.

—Pull toes and foot up, stiffen knee, push straight leg into bed (extension). Relax.

—Roll leg inward (rotation). Relax.

—Roll leg outward (outward rotation). Let go.

—Check breathing pattern and rhythm, thinking back to each arm and each leg. They should feel heavy and relaxed. As a muscle relaxes, it softens and lengthens. Concentrate; the exercise is not more important than the rest period.

—Squeeze buttocks together (attempt to use gluteals and sphincters). Relax.

—Arch back (erector spinae group). Let go.

—Pinch shoulder blades back toward spine (rhomboids). Let go.
—Pull shoulders forward (pectorals). Relax.
—Pull shoulder to ears (upper trapezius). Let go.
—Push shoulders toward knees (depressors). Relax.
—Pull abdominals in and relax. This alters breathing rhythm, so once again check your breathing. It should be belly breathing.
—Turn chin to right, left, and straight ahead. Release all the neck muscles.
—Push back of head into bed (neck extensors). Let go.
—Lift head (neck flexors). Relax.
—Pull corners of mouth downward. Let go (platysma fish breathing).
—Raise eyebrows and wiggle scalp. Let go.
—Frown. Relax.
—Squeeze eyelids tightly together. Let go.
—With eyes lightly closed and without moving head, turn eyes right, left, up, down and straight ahead. Relax.
—Squeeze jaws together. Relax jaw muscles so mouth drops almost open.
—Push tongue against roof of mouth. Relax tongue.
—Swallow. Relax.
—Review mentally. Concentrate on feeling relaxed.

> Minimum practice on this lesson is 1 hour per day—two 30-minute periods, six 10-minute periods, four 15-minute periods, or three 20-minute periods. Check your breathing hourly and practice diaphragmatic breathing 5 minutes out of every hour. You must establish new habits to break the pain–tension cycle.

The two contract–relax tools explained above are slight variations of methods of teaching relaxation. The important point is to determine, after evaluating the patient, which method of practice will best suit the patient so that he may learn to relax his muscles. As the patient progresses in his ability to relax, the method will also certainly change and progress. Sometimes isolation of contract–relax is effective. With adhesive capsulitis, learning to relax the rotator cuff muscles can be effective. Learning to extend the neck can relieve tension headaches. Relaxation of the fingers and wrist extensors is valuable in treating tennis elbow.

The patient must develop some understanding of what relaxation is, which means that those of us doing the teaching must have a greater understanding of the muscle relaxation process. However, the key to success is practice and repetition on the part of the patient. Because muscle relaxation is learned, the patient must practice. As mentioned before, 60 minutes is the recommended time period for daily practice. Frequently, the patient is so tense that he finds it extremely difficult to practice 60 continuous minutes, and shorter periods must be used. In very difficult cases, 5 minutes of practice out of each waking hour can be done. With contract–relax methods the emphasis must always be on the "letting go" phase. Patients will tend to emphasize the contraction phase of the exercises. You must carefully explain and repeat and reemphasize that the "going negative" or "power off" phase is what is important. It is often helpful to tell the patient that even if he does every movement correctly but does not spend time "letting go" after the movement, the program will not be worth the paper it is printed on. On the other hand, even if half the movements are incorrect, but the patient really relaxes those muscles following the contraction, then muscle relaxation will be achieved.

Biofeedback

A comment about biofeedback or electromyography (EMG) equipment is appropriate at this time. As noted in Jacobson's *Progressive Relaxation*, these methods have been used for years.[20] EMG equipment can reveal baseline data regarding the amount of muscle tension initially present and can indicate progress at a later date. Biofeedback equipment used a few times can help the patient to understand through sight and sound what muscle relaxation is. However, like muscle relaxant medications that do not seem to have solved tension conditions, biofeedback appears to be just another crutch for the patient if used as the relaxation method. The key to relaxation appears to be learning and practice on the part of the patient. The patient must accept the major responsibility in combating neuromuscular hypertension problems. The therapist is present to help, to teach, to clarify, to encourage, and to explain.

Practical Application

Learning to sense muscle relaxation is only the first step in the progressive relaxation process, just as in reading, learning the alphabet and the phonetic sounds are the basic steps. The learning is valuable when the letters and sounds are put into words— words with meaning. The same applies to relaxation. Until we begin to adapt our ability to relax to our daily lives, we have nothing more than a tool of no practical value. Practicality comes with continuing periods of awareness of what our muscles are doing throughout the waking hours. By checking ourselves for muscle tension during various activities (*e.g.,* working, driving, walking, eating, participating in recreational activities) we begin to realize how much we contract muscles excessively. Thus, we can begin to let go. Over time, the relaxation of muscle rather than the contraction becomes the habit pattern; relaxation acquires practical value in our lives. Reminders to help us become aware of muscle habits can be helpful. For example, we might use time to develop a mental connotation with relaxation. Every time we look at our watch, or the radio mentions the time, or someone says it is time for lunch or asks what time it is, we can check ourselves. However, reminders must be changed every few days, or the mental connotation will itself become a habit, and the needed awareness of muscle activity will not develop.

AUTOGENIC TRAINING

Autogenic training was developed by Schultz, a German neurologist, from investigations of hypnosis begun around 1900.[33,41] Two basic mental exercises are used: (1) the standard exercises, and (2) the meditative exercises. The six standard exercises are physiologically oriented. The verbal content of the standard formula is focused on the neuromuscular system (heaviness of the limbs), the vasomotor system (warmth of the limbs and coolness of the forehead), the cardiovascular system, and respiratory mechanism. These exercises are practiced several times a day until the patient is able to shift to a less stressful state or the trophotropic state described by Hess.

A reduction of afferent stimuli requires observation of the following points:

—The exercises should take place in a quiet room with moderate temperature and reduced illumination.
—Restrictive clothing should be loosened or removed.
—The body should be as relaxed as possible, and the eyes closed. Three distinctive postures have been found adequate—a horizontal posture; a reclining arm-chair posture; and a simple, relaxed, sitting position.
—The subject's attitude toward the exercises should not be tense or compulsive but of a "let it happen" nature, referred to as *passive concentration*.

The first exercise of the autogenic standard series aims at muscular relaxation. Right-handed individuals should start out with passive concentration on the right arm and heaviness, for example, "My right arm is comfortably heavy." Once the patient achieves the feeling of heaviness in the right arm, and the feeling spreads to the other extremities regularly, the formula is extended to include the other limbs (left arm, both arms, right leg, left leg, both legs, arms and legs). Concentration on heaviness continues until heaviness can be experienced more or less regularly in all four extremities. This may be achieved in 2 to 8 weeks.

Subsequently, passive concentration on warmth is added, starting with the right arm and warmth—"My right arm is comfortably warm." The warmth formula follows the same progressive procedures used for heaviness until all the extremities become regularly heavy and warm. This training on peripheral vasodilation may require another period of 2 to 8 weeks.

After having learned to establish the feeling of heaviness and warmth, the trainee continues with passive concentration on cardiac activity by using the formula, "Heartbeat calm and regular," or just passively observing the heart beat. This is followed by the respiration formula "Respiration regular—it breathes me," or passively observing the breathing rhythm.

The last two, or final, exercises of the physiologically oriented standard exercises concern the abdominal region ("Solar plexus comfortably warm") and the cranial region, which should be cooler than the rest of the body ("My forehead is cool" or "Forehead pleasantly cool").

After the standard formulas have been repeated four to seven times in the sequence described, the altered state of consciousness is ended in a manner similar to awakening from a deep sleep by stretching, inhaling, or yawning, and gradually opening the eyes. Activation phrases are used, such as "I feel life and energy flowing through my legs, hips, solar plexus, chest, and arms. The energy makes me feel light and alive."

As training progresses, and after all six formulas have been added successively and mastered, they may be shortened. The time needed to establish these exercises effectively may require several months (4 to 6 months according to Schultz). In modern practice, however, Schultz or Luthe's autogenic training techniques have been modified to reduce training to a minimum of 6 weeks, so that a whole "round" can be practiced in 1 hour.[5] After several months of practice, the subject should be able to achieve the induced altered state of consciousness by simply thinking "heaviness—warmth—heartbeat and respiration—solar plexus—forehead."

The meditative exercises are reserved for the trainee who has mastered the standard exercises.

They focus primarily on certain mental functions, single-focus mental concentration (as in yogic meditation), and finally meditation on abstract qualities of universal consciousness, much as in yogic or Zen meditation. The standard series of exercises and the single-focus meditation are primarily used in medical or psychological treatment.

Certainly, the autogenic standard exercises concentrate on somatic attention and have a similar effect as progressive relaxation. According to Benson the first five standard exercises have been found to be the most effective in producing the relaxation response.[4] The meditative exercises that give an important role to single-focus concentration or to imagery are more cognitive in nature. They elicit subjective and physiological changes that are different from those that follow the practice of somatic procedures.

Clinical Application

The clinical usefulness of autogenic training in the treatment of muscular disorders, according to Luthe and Schultz, is largely based on the following factors:[33]

— Muscular relaxation
— Improved local circulation
— Decreased stimulation of pain
— Reduction of unfavorable reactivity to emotional stress
— Possible favorable effects on deviation of certain metabolic and endocrine functions
— Reduction or elimination of relevant medications
— Promotion of the patient's active participation in treatment

Regular practice of autogenic training has been found particularly helpful in relieving complaints associated with arthritis and related disorders (rheumatoid arthritis, osteoarthritis), nonarticular rheumatism (fibromyositis, myalgia), and cervical-root and low-back syndromes (particularly when associated with nerve-root pressure, such as lumbago–sciatic syndrome).

When musculoskeletal disorders involve the spine in conditions such as ankylosing spondylitis, degenerative joint disease, or herniation of a vertebral disk, autogenic training may prove to be very helpful when used in combination with other forms of treatment. In such cases, the patient should be encouraged to learn all the standard exercises, with particular emphasis on the heavy and warm formulas. In addition, topographically adapted special formulas are used. Topographically specific heaviness and warmth formulas may cover the entire length of the spine or may be used with passive concentration on a particular area (e.g., "The lower part of my spine is heavy" or "My pelvis is warm"). When used to cover the entire length of the spine, dynamic mental contact has a better effect. This implies that the mental contact does not remain fixed on a given topographic area but shifts progressively over different sections of the spine starting with the cervical section and moving to the coccygeal area, while the mental process of passive concentration (e.g., "My spine is very warm") continues. The mental control travels repeatedly down the spine and is followed by concentration on the arms and legs.

Similarly, in musculoskeletal disorders affecting the joints of the extremities the emphasis is on frequent practice of the first two standard exercises (heavy and warm formulas) with relatively prolonged passive concentration on the affected area (e.g., "My right knee is warm" or "My right shoulder is warm").

Variations

Benson and Wallace have devised a simplified method incorporating a modification of the standard autogenic exercises and single-focus attention.[4] Deep relaxation of the muscles, concentrating on heaviness and warmth, begins with the feet and progresses proximally to the calves, thighs, back, neck, arms, and shoulders. This method uses *one* as a mantra, while the patient breathes in and out for 10 to 20 minutes during the program. Benson and Wallace suggest that there is not a single method that is unique in eliciting the relaxation response, and that any one of the age-old or newly developed techniques may produce the same physiological results, regardless of the mental device used.

Jencks has designed an interesting variation of autogenic training for children. Her variation includes all aspects of Schultz's standard formula but works through imagery instead of Schultz's precise meditative exercises.[25] Sensory awareness is aroused through images, for which suggestions are made in the form of Erickson's therapeutic double binds.[12] Jencks refers to this approach as the "autogenic rag doll."

Autogenic training has been found to be a useful adjunct to massage. Frances M. Tappin, a physical therapist and foremost authority on massage, states, "Since one purpose of massage is relaxation and relief of stress, it will be doubly effective if the one doing the massage can provide autogenic phrases to increase the effectiveness of massage."[48] She feels this is particularly true in situations where tension is a major part of the patient's problem. She suggests a series of autogenic phrases developed by Alyce and Elmer Green of the Menninger Clinic that tend to bring the patient closer to the alpha brain rhythm, which is associated with feelings of calm.[16]

Alpha waves (slow brain waves) increase during the practice of relaxation but are not commonly found in sleep. Although we still do not know the significance of alpha waves, we do know that they are present when people feel relaxed.[4,5]

AN INTEGRATED RELAXATION APPROACH

Many physical therapists now use a combination of techniques or an integrated system using a sequential approach. Such an approach is best exemplified in a training program developed by Budzynski, Director of the Biofeedback Institute in Denver.[6,7] A gross awareness of muscle tension is acquired by moving from one form of relaxation to another in order of difficulty. The trainee progresses only after he has mastered a less difficult technique. His training program consists of three major components: progressive relaxation, autogenic training, and finally, a form of stress management combining autogenic training with systematic desensitization. There are six exercise elements that build upon each other to produce simultaneous mind–body relaxation. The approach may be used independently or as an adjunct to biofeedback or related clinical procedures.

The first set of exercises is used to develop a gross awareness of muscle tension using a modification of progressive relaxation. Once the trainee can perform the exercises to the therapist's satisfaction, he moves on to differential relaxation (also developed by Jacobson). This allows the trainee to integrate his ability to relax into everyday living situations.[24] Along with practice twice a day, the patient is encouraged to become aware of specific tension areas in his body throughout the day.

The third set of exercises uses the autogenic formulas designed to develop further "muscle sense" with useful cognitive responses. The emphasis is on limb heaviness.

The fourth set moves on to limb heaviness and warmth, and the fifth to the forehead and the face. The fifth set is intended to bring together all of the components learned in the first five.

The final set employs systematic desensitization, a behavioral therapy approach combined with the relaxation techniques. The therapist typically assists the client in developing a series of scenes or visualizations. These are then listed in a hierarchical order, based on their fear-evoking quality. The client begins by visualizing the scene that has the fewest anxiety- or fear-provoking properties. This scene is repeated until the trainee can visualize it while remaining relaxed. He then moves to the next scene.

GUIDELINES FOR ADMINISTERING RELAXATION TECHNIQUES IN MUSCULOSKELETAL DISORDERS

EVALUATION

The most obvious candidates for relaxation techniques that physical therapists see are patients with chronic back and neck problems. These conditions are often the result of many varying factors. The role of our urbanized, overstressed, under-exercised life in the etiology of premorbid states — of which neck and back pain are often the first symptoms — needs special consideration. Today, the initial attack of back pain is frequently precipitated by emotional problems, tension, or unaccustomed work or athletic activities. These causes are often masked by or combined with true mechanical factors, but rarely are they entirely missing. Therefore, when taking the case history, do not overlook physical signs of emotional stress and muscle tension. We need to emphasize the overall picture of the patient rather than concentrate on the local mechanical problems only.

Subjective Examination for Tension

An examination should always be conducted (see Chapter 4, Assessment of Musculoskeletal Disorders) for the extremities and for mechanical problems of the spine, which have been discussed and described by authors such as Cyriax, Grieve, and Maitland, among others.[9,17,35] In addition, it may be necessary to further develop the history as it relates to tension and stress factors. The results of stress are often expressed as secondary manifestations, such as irregular sleeping habits, gastrointestinal problems, headaches, and so forth. People under stress experience a wide variety of physical responses, anxiety or restlessness, and emotional symptoms.

The nature of the patient's work and the manner in which the predominant activities of daily life are performed are important clues to whether the patient is under tension. The following are some areas that may need to be explored:

Nature of work—Does the patient like his or her work, superiors, and co-workers? Is the job competitive and stressful?

Way the work is performed—Do the daily activities require repetitive movements of the body? Does the activity allow free movement, or does the patient maintain a fixed position for prolonged periods?

Driving—Commuting for long periods of time is often a source of tension not only from the standpoint of maintaining a fixed position, but also as a source of constant daily irritation from heavy traffic.

Physical activities—Does the type of work provide much exercise? If not, what if anything, does the patient do to compensate for lack of exercise? What is the nature of such activity, and how often is it performed?

Home and family—Is there illness in the family? If married, is the marriage relationship satisfactory? Are there children? The home situation is often an important source of tension.

People under stress may experience a wide variety of physical symptoms. These may include:

Cardiovascular and respiratory symptoms—Does the patient experience chest pain, a rapid or racing heart beat, difficult breathing, or shortness of breath? Does he have a problem with high blood pressure?

Eye, ear, nose, and throat symptoms, headaches or head pain—A special cause or starting point of neck pain may be related to grinding and clenching of the teeth. Does the patient frequently experience nasal stuffiness, hoarseness, or difficulty swallowing? Are there frequent migraine or tension headaches? Does the patient experience transient somatic effects such as dizziness or fainting?

Digestive disorders—Does the patient experience frequent stomach problems, a peptic ulcer syndrome, or a "nervous" stomach? Is he or she frequently bothered by indigestion, constipation, or nausea?

Endocrine imbalances—The most frequent endocrine disorders causing muscle pain are hypothyroidism and estrogen deficiency.[28] Does the patient tire easily, require a lot of sleep, or have a weight problem? Is there increased or decreased perspiration? Are there problems with dysmenorrhea or an irregular menstrual cycle?

Muscle-tension pain—Patients often describe only the leading, most severe symptoms and forget a multitude of others that momentarily seem unimportant. Has there been excessive muscle tension or pain in other parts of the body (jaw, forehead, legs, shoulders)? Has the patient been bothered by stiff, sore, or cramping muscles? If so, where?

There must be close observation of whether the pain is primary or secondary. For example, did pain cause the stress or *vice versa?*

Stress is often accompanied by symptoms of anxiety or restlessness. Inquiry or observation during the interview may be useful in determining if some of the following manifestations are present:

—Chewing the lips, grinding and clenching the teeth, and biting fingernails
—Pacing
—Increased eating, smoking, or drinking
—Difficulty falling asleep, waking up feeling exhausted, and being keyed up and jittery during the day.

Stress is also accompanied by a variety of emotions. Possibly the most important question concerns the emotional stability of the patient. This aspect is often hard to obtain by direct questioning, but is frequently revealed in the course of the interview and treatment program. The patient's medical chart is also a useful source of information.

And finally, we will want to know

—In what type of situation does the patient become aware of unwanted tension? What is the environment, what is he or she doing at the time, and how?
—Is there any warning signal that tension may be coming on? Any thoughts or behaviors that are an indication of tension?
—When does the patient experience the most tension during a day?
—How does the patient experience tension? If the patient states that he or she feels "nervous," what does this actually mean?
—How does the patient deal with anxiety or unwanted tension?
—What does the patient feel is the source of the tension?

Closer inquiry in these areas and others may pinpoint the source of tension and thereby make it possible to influence it.

Many times the history will indicate that tension is a factor, especially under the following circumstances:

—Symptoms have an insidious onset, with a number of general symptoms of a vague and aching quality
—Symptoms are related to a specific injury or particular activity and have taken a long time to improve or have actually become worse

— The patient tires easily and has general symptoms of fatigue
— There is morning pain and stiffness, aggravated by activity—at times only a minor amount of activity—and relieved by rest. (These patients many times have difficulty sleeping. They may tell you, "I never have been able to relax.")
— Particular problems have become recurrent. For example, the patient may have experienced a third or fourth episode of shoulder pain, or problems in the other shoulder as well. When muscle tension is involved, problems tend to recur.
— When questioned about medications, the patient indicates he has taken muscle relaxants in the past.
— The patient has gone from doctor to doctor without a specific diagnosis, or has been told he has a "functional illness."
— A specific condition has been identified which is known to be related to muscle tension (e.g., adhesive capsulitis of the shoulder or various types of tendinitis)
— There are general health problems related to tension and fatigue.

A useful term for measuring the client's stress profile is the "Symptoms of Stress Checklist," a questionnaire that measures the ways people respond to stressful situations.[30] Sets of questions dealing with physical, psychological, or behavioral responses are included. The questionnaire is filled out by the patient during the first week, or it may be filled out prior to the examination. Many other such evaluation forms are now available. They are not only a useful source of information, but many can also be used to assess the patient's progress during the training session and at its end.

Physical Examination for Tension

The physical part of evaluation may reveal many signs that point to tension. The first time you see the patient you will see that he is not resting or is constantly moving. For instance, the patient may prefer to stand rather than sit in the waiting room. Once you begin the examination you may observe constant shifting of position in the chair, shifting and movement of arms or legs, use of arms in talking, constant movement of eyes, actual tremors, restlessness, rapid and short breathing patterns or constant sighing, diminished concentration, irritability, and other signs of apparent overactivity of the skeletal muscles.

Inspection can be a relevant part of the examination for tension problems. Bony structure and alignment may be unremarkable, although subcutaneous soft tissues and the skin are affected (i.e., hard, stringy muscle fiber, and adherent skin). You may determine this during palpation. Atrophy from tension fatigue, muscles that are well defined because of contraction in the muscle tissue, or poor general posture may be observed on inspection.

Selective tissue tension tests may elicit some positive signs as well. The patient may hesitate to move actively. There may be hypersensitivity to pain or general anxiety. Or he may move quickly rather than in the requested slow and deliberate pattern.

Passive testing is a key test for tension-related conditions, since it may be impossible to do a pure passive motion—the patient will actually assist you in moving the part. Even after you carefully explain to the patient that you would like him to completely let go, he will continue to assist. Patients often state that they are not aware of using their muscles. It thus becomes important in the remaining examination and treatment to stop frequently to point out that you want the patient to let go, and to explain relaxation. The patient quickly learns that by stopping movement or touching a particular muscle you can feel assistance or resistance, and therefore, he must "let go."

Be aware that although assistance is the most prevalent sign with passive movements, tense patients may actually resist movements. A hypersensitivity to pain and a muscle spasm or muscle tension end feel will occur. Apparent involvement of joint-play movements are more apt to be encountered because of resistance on the part of the patient. There will be involuntary, hyperactive muscle contractions that tend to prohibit testing of various joint-play movements. Many joint-play movements will appear painful, again because of the hyperactive muscle activity. Resistive testing will demonstrate a quick contraction on the part of the patient, and there will usually be several areas that have a pain response, rather than one or two specific movements. A general weakness may be prevalent. Neuromuscular tests may demonstrate hypersensitive responses to various stimuli, and will usually produce hyperactive responses when deep-tendon reflexes are tested.

Palpation will elicit distinct signs when tension is present. The skin is often tender and dry, has an elevated temperature, and is adherent to underlying tissue. Palpation of subcutaneous tissue, in particular muscle, is a key test. The muscle will feel hard and stringy and will be tender to palpation. It is difficult to distinguish between muscle tissue that is tense and that which is in spasm. Both are hard, but it is safe to assume that if several muscle groups are hard and tender, as well as numerous anatomic areas, there is a tension factor involved rather than pure protective spasm. Muscle tissue in a relaxed state is soft, pliable, not tender to palpation, and the various fibers are elongated. With tension (muscle is the only tissue in the body that contracts) there is just the opposite effect of the relaxed state, and this can be readily palpated.

Clearly, before initiating a program of relaxation training, the therapist must decide if it is realistic to expect that increasing relaxation skills will be a significant factor in alleviating the patient's problems. If the tension occurs in response to a serious problem in the patient's life, it must be dealt with differently (even though relaxation can be beneficial here as well). However, relaxation training can be helpful as a means of eliminating or reducing physical complaints, such as a headache or low-back pain, when there are no strictly organic bases for the complaint that can be treated more directly by other means.

MANAGEMENT

A thorough knowledge of and experience with relaxation procedures, as well as the use of other clinical skills, are essential to effective relaxation training. Relaxation techniques are seldom used alone, because in most cases the patient's problem is combined with true mechanical factors, muscle imbalances and pain, emotional or behavioral problems, and so on. Relaxation training is an integral part of many behavioral procedures. Principles of behavioristic psychology, behavior modification, and biofeedback are often employed in conjunction with relaxation training but are beyond the scope of this chapter. These methods are discussed and described in many excellent books and articles in the literature.

The first session of relaxation training is perhaps the most important. The therapist should

1. Explain and justify the procedures so that the patient can understand and accept the rationale underlying relaxation training.
2. Instill a feeling of confidence in the technique as well as enthusiasm for carrying out necessary "homework." Success at learning relaxation skills requires regular practice once they have been learned in the training session.
3. Explain and set up long-term and short-term goals. An intermediate goal is for the patient to be able to relax at any time using any or all of the techniques that work best for him or her. The ultimate goal is to produce relaxation independent of conditioned responses.

The Physical Setting

A suitable setting for training should be provided. Eliminate all sources of extraneous stimulation. Relaxation should take place in a quiet, dimly lit, attractive room. An important consideration is the chair or couch that the patient uses during relaxation training. Recliner chairs are considered ideal. A treatment table may be used as long as the basic requirement of complete support and comfort are met.

The client should wear loose-fitting, comfortable clothing. Glasses, contact lenses, watches, and shoes should be removed to reduce extraneous stimulation and to allow free movement.

The therapist must be aware of self, touch, and tone of voice. The voice should be used as an instrument to facilitate the relaxation process. How the therapist speaks is just as important as what is actually said. You should speak softly, and the pace of speech should gradually be reduced as the session progresses.

Directing the Procedure

The therapist directs the sequence of events, which will vary with the training technique employed. The clinical training should generally be continued until the therapist is convinced that the patient is performing a set of exercises correctly and that deep relaxation has in fact been achieved. This can usually be determined through questioning after the session and by nonverbal clues that are observed during the treatment session (*e.g.*, fidgeting in the chair).

Postrelaxation questioning should follow each session in order to determine if problems exist, and whether an alternative strategy should be employed. The patient's report usually is a sufficiently reliable guide to his or her ability to relax and is most helpful as an aid in modifying the approach to that patient. Ask the patient to describe what relaxation feels like, as well as more specific questions regarding any problems that occurred during the session. It is important to ask if anything that was said or done during the session made it more difficult to relax, and what statements or techniques seem to facilitate relaxation so that they can either be eliminated or emphasized in subsequent sessions.

Assigned Home Programs

A home program of relaxation may be started from the very beginning or as soon as the therapist is convinced that the patient is performing a set of exercises correctly. Self-administered relaxation is ideally suited for problems in which tension is a major component and easily lends itself for use in "homework" assignments between therapy sessions. In general, self-administered relaxation can provide benefits as a treatment in itself, or it can be used in conjunction with additional therapeutic techniques.

The importance of practicing cannot be overemphasized to the patient. Relaxation is a skill that improves with practice. The trainee is usually required to practice once or twice a day (varying with the training technique employed, *e.g.*, anywhere from two 10-minute sessions to a single 1-hour session). In many cases, you will find that frequent, shorter sessions will be more effective for some patients. Advise the patient to practice at times when he or she is under minimal or no pressure. For example, just before bedtime is often recommended, although the best times will vary from patient to patient. It is not advisable to practice on a full stomach.

As the patient becomes more and more proficient in relaxation skills, the number of daily practice sessions as well as the time spent can gradually be reduced. Gradually the patient should be weaned away from both therapist and any instrumentation used. The patient must learn to rely on the learned awareness and control, along with other self-generating aids, so that tension can be reduced at any time in day-to-day stressful situations.

Devices may be used to foster home practice and to incorporate these habits into routine activities of daily living. Some clinicians have used small parking-meter timers that can be set to buzz at hourly intervals to remind the patient to practice for anywhere from 30 seconds to 3 minutes. Patel uses an interesting reminder system, instructing patients to use everyday sounds such as ringing telephones or church bells.[38] Others use visual reminders such as stop lights, so that each time the patient comes to a lengthy stop in traffic, he practices his techniques. Others have patients replace their coffee breaks at work with relaxation breaks. Obviously, it is best if the patient will also allot long periods every day for serious practice in a conducive environment.

Standard relaxation tapes made from Jacobson's and Schultz and Luthe's relaxation techniques, which have been modified to reduce training time, are readily available commercially and are often used in home practice. Budzynski's relaxation approach described earlier is also available on tape. Tape practice, according to Brown, should be used with a bit of caution, however, and should be considered on an individual patient basis. Recent research indicates that recorded relaxation instruction may actually result in increased EMG tension levels in some patients.[5] Tape recorders offer far more flexibility than prerecorded tapes. Each relaxation session can be recorded during the clinical session on a tape recorder provided by the patient, which he can then take home for practice between sessions. This has several advantages. The relaxation technique can be modified to meet the patient's own needs and can become progressively shorter as the patient becomes more skilled in his learning techniques.

Tapes used for home practice have also been found to be useful for patients who have difficulty relaxing in the presence of a therapist. Patients may be started on relaxation learning in this way, and then at a later date start clinical practice with the therapist.

It is usually advisable for patients to do other homework as well. Patients may be requested to chart their painful activities during the day or to record situations that make them tense. This type of record keeping is useful in documenting the patient's progress as well as in helping to pinpoint sources of tension. Encourage the patient to make frequent body checks for muscle tension during the day in order to become more aware of the environment and of tension-causing factors.

Invariably, the patient will need activities of daily living (ADL) training to improve gait, posture, body mechanics, and ways of conserving energy and reducing tension. The most difficult step of all is transferring this learning to the patient's day to day living.

ASSESSING THE PATIENT'S PROGRESS

To assess the success of relaxation training, the therapist can employ several kinds of information — clinical observation, the subjective report of the patient with the help of a subjective stress profile or anxiety-scale evaluation, and objective indicators of relaxation. Important indicators of progress that may be gained by observing the patient during the clinical session include physical signs, such as less observable movement, a reduction in the breathing pattern during the course of the session, and a peaceful, relaxed appearance (a relaxed open jaw or a sleepy-eyed appearance following successful relaxation). The patient's ability to gain deep relaxation in shorter and shorter periods of time is also an indicator.

There should be signs of symptomatic improvement. Furthermore, stimuli that once called forth muscle-tension or "fibrositis" pain (backache) no longer do so under the same condition. By deconditioning the muscle-tension habit or anxiety response that has been partly responsible for his problem, he brings about a proportionate reduction of the symptoms.

Secondary manifestations should decline. Stress-dependent reactions, whether migraines, intestinal cramps, grinding and clenching the teeth, or difficulty falling asleep, can also be used as measures of improvement. A reduction or termination of drugs to reduce pain or encourage muscle relaxation is also a useful indicator of improvement.

It is often an advantage to have objective indicators of relaxation. Jacobson has used EMG.[21] Recently, more convenient equipment, such as EMG biofeedback, have become available. They can be used as methods of evaluation, and as treatment to facilitate relaxation by translating muscle potential into auditory or visual feedback to the patient. Other physiological measurements might include cardiovascular measurements (heart rate, blood pressure, skin temperature) and the use of brain wave biofeedback (electroencephalogram). Fortunately, the patient's report usually serve as a sufficiently reliable guide that relaxation skills have been a significant factor in alleviating his problems.

RESEARCH

To date, quantitative research in this area of relaxation and related techniques has been relatively scant. However, caution should be used in applying these techniques, because there may be side-effects. Symptoms ranging from insomnia to hallucinatory behavior and withdrawal have been reported when relaxation techniques have been practiced for long periods or to excess.[53] Clearly, additional research is needed to test and clarify the numerous hypotheses presented in the current literature. Therapists can help by documenting the claims made for relaxation and for specific treatment strategies that seem to be most effective. And, finally, therapists should review the current studies involving relaxation for possible areas of clinical research as they apply to physical therapy and musculoskeletal disorders.

Relaxation has been found to be a successful alternative for drugs and numerous types of back surgery. Major advantages include cost effectiveness and the fact that the patient may make a contribution to treatment. Relaxation is not a "magic bullet" and will not cure joint dysfunction or other musculoskeletal disorders. It is, however, a key to reducing the muscle tension, anxiety, nervousness, and stress, that may lead to a variety of physical and psychological disabilities.

REFERENCES

1. Alexander FM: The Use of Self. London, Re-Education Publications, 1910
2. Barlow W: The Alexander Technique. New York, Alfred A Knopf, 1973
3. Benjamin BE: Are You Tense? The Benjamin System of Muscular Therapy: Tension Relief Through Deep Massage and Body Care. New York, Pantheon Books, 1978
4. Benson H: The Relaxation Response. New York, Avon Books, 1976
5. Brown BB: Stress and the Art of Biofeedback. New York, Harper & Row, 1977
6. Budzynski TH: Relaxation Training Program. New York, Bio Monitoring Audio Cassette Publications, 1977
7. Budzynski TH, Stoya J, Adler C: Feedback-induced muscle re-education: Application to tension headaches. Behav Ther Exp Psychiatry 1:205–211, 1970
8. Clynes M: Toward a view of man. *In* Clynes M, Milsum J (eds): Biomedical Engineering Systems. New York, McGraw–Hill, 1970
9. Cyriax J, Coldham M: Textbook of Orthopaedic Medicine, Vol 1, 11th ed. London, Baillière Tindall, 1984
10. Davis M, Eshelman ER, McKay M: The Relaxation and Stress Reduction Workbook, 2nd ed. Oakland CA, New Harbinger, 1982
11. Devi I: Yoga for Americans. Englewood Cliffs, NJ, Prentice–Hall, 1959
12. Erickson MH, Ross EL: Varieties of double bind. Am J Clin Hypn 17:143–157, 1975
13. Feldenkrais M: Body and Mature Behavior. New York, International University Press, 1949
14. Feldenkrais M: Awareness Through Movement. New York, Harper & Row, 1972
15. Gellhorn E: Principles of Autonomic–Somatic Interactions. Minneapolis, University of Minnesota Press, 1967
16. Green E, Green A: The ins and outs of mind body energy. *In* Science Year 1974: World Book Science Annual. Chicago, Field Enterprises Corporation, 1973
17. Grieves CP: Mobilisation of the Spine, 3rd ed. New York, Churchill Livingstone, 1979
18. Hess WR: Functional Organization of Diencephalon. New York, Grune & Stratton, 1957
19. Jacobson E: Progressive Relaxation. Chicago, University of Chicago Press, 1929
20. Jacobson E: Progressive Relaxation, 4th ed. Chicago, University of Chicago Press, 1962
21. Jacobson E: Anxiety and Tension Control. Philadelphia, JB Lippincott, 1964
22. Jacobson E: Self-Operations Control Manual. Chicago, National Foundation for Progressive Relaxation, 1964
23. Jacobson E: Tension in Medicine. Springfield, IL, Charles C Thomas, 1967
24. Jacobson E: You Must Relax. New York, McGraw–Hill, 1970

25. Jencks B: Respiration for Relaxation, Invigoration, and Special Accomplishment. Salt Lake City, Jencks, 1974
26. Jencks B: Your Body: Biofeedback at Its Best. Chicago, Nelson Hall, 1977
27. Kopell HR, Thompson AL: Peripheral Entrapment Neuropathies. Baltimore, Williams & Wilkins, 1963
28. Kraus H: Clinical Treatment of Back and Neck Pain. New York, McGraw–Hill, 1970
29. Kruger H: Other Healers, Other Cures. New York, Bobbs–Merrill, 1974
30. Leckie M, Thompson E: Symptoms of Stress Checklist. Seattle, University of Washington, 1977
31. Lowen A: Physical Dynamics of Character Structure. New York, Grune & Stratton, 1958
32. Lowen A: Breathing, Movement and Feeling. New York, Institute for Bioenergetics Analysis, 1965
33. Luthe W (ed): Autogenic Therapy, Vols. 1–6. New York, Grune & Stratton, 1969–1972
34. Maharishi MY: The Science of Being and Art of Living. London, International SRM Publications, 1966
35. Maitland GD: Vertebral Manipulations, 3rd ed. London, Butterworth, 1972
36. Mason JW: A re-evaluation of the concept of nonspecificity in stress theory. Psychol Res 8:323–333, 1971
37. Mines S: The Conquest of Pain. New York, Grosset & Dunlap, 1974
38. Patel C: Randomized controlled trial of yoga and biofeedback in management of hypertension. Lancet 2:93–95, 1975
39. Pierce F: Mobilizing the Midbrain. New York, GP Putnam's Sons, 1924
40. Ruch, TC: The nervous system: Sensory function. *In* Fulton JF (ed): Textbook of Physiology. Philadelphia, WB Saunders, 1955
41. Schultz JH, Luthe W: Autogenic Training: A Psychophysiologic Approach in Psychotherapy. New York, Grune & Stratton, 1959
42. Selye H: The Stress of Life. New York, McGraw–Hill, 1956
43. Selye H: Stress Without Distress. Philadelphia, JB Lippincott, 1974
44. Sinclair JD: Exercise in pulmonary disease. *In* Basmajian JV (ed): Therapeutic Exercise, 3rd ed. Baltimore, Williams & Wilkins, 1976
45. Sternbach RA: Psychophysiological bases of psychosomatic phenomena. Psychosomatics 7:81–84, 1966
46. Sternbach RA: Strategies and tactics in the treatment of patients with pain. *In* Crue BL (ed): Pain and Suffering: Selected Aspects. Springfield, IL, Charles C Thomas, 1970
47. Stewart E: To lessen pain: Relaxation and rhythmic breathing. Am J Nurs 76:958–959, 1976
48. Tappin FM: Healing Massage Techniques: A Study of Eastern and Western Methods. Reston, VA, Reston Publishing, 1978
49. Vishnudevahada S: The Complete Illustrated Book of Yoga. New York, Julian Press, 1960
50. Wallace RK: Physiological effects of transcendental meditation. Science 167:1751–1754, 1970
51. Wallace RK, Benson H: The physiology of meditation. Sci Am 226:84–90, 1972
52. Whatmore GB, Kohli DR: Dysponesis: A neurophysiologic factor in functional disorders. Behav Sci 13:102–124, 1968
53. White J, Fadiman J (eds): Relax: How You Can Feel Better, Reduce Stress and Overcome Tension. The Confucian Press, 1976
54. Wolpe J: Psychotherapy by Reciprocal Inhibition. Stanford, Stanford University Press, 1958
55. Wolpe J: The Practice of Behavior Therapy, 2nd ed. New York, Pergamon Press, 1973
56. Wood EC, Becker PD: Beard's Massage, 3rd ed. Philadelphia, WB Saunders, 1981

RECOMMENDED READINGS

Achterberg J: Imagery in Healing: Shamanism and Modern Medicine. Boston, New Science Library, 1985

Bakal DA: Headache: A biophysical perspective. Psych Bull 32:369–382, 1975

Benson H, Beary JF, Carol MP: The relaxation response. Psychiatry 37:37–46, 1974

Benson H, Kotch JB, Crassweler KD: The relaxation response: A bridge between psychiatry and medicine. Med Clin North Am 61:929–938, 1977

Bohachick P: Progressive relaxation training in cardiac rehabilitation: Effect on psychologic variables. Nurs Res 22:283, 1984

DiCara L: Learning in the autonomic nervous system. Sci Am 222:30–39, 1970

Dixon HH, O'Hara M, Peterson RD: Fatigue contractor of skeletal muscle. Northwest Medicine 66:812–816, 1967

Gellhorn E: Autonomic Imbalances and the Hypothalamus. Minneapolis, University of Minnesota Press, 1957

Green K, Webster J, Beiman I, Rosmarin D, Holliday P: Progress and self-induced relaxation training: Their relative effects on subjective and autonomic arousal of fearful stimuli. J Clin Psychol 37:309–315, 1981

Kahn RL: Some propositions toward a researchable conceptualization of stress. *In* McGrath JE (ed): Social and Psychological Factors in Stress. New York, Holt, Rhinehart & Winston, 1970

Kiely WF: From the symbolic stimulus to the pathophysiological response: Neurophysiological mechanism. Int J Psychiatry Med 5(4):515–529, 1974

Lazarus RS: Psychological Stress and Coping Process. New York, McGraw–Hill, 1966

Lazarus RS: Psychological stress and coping in adaptation and illness. Int J Psychiatry Med 5(4):321–333, 1974

Levi L (ed): Emotions: Their Parameters and Measurement. New York, Raven Press, 1975

Lipoloski ZJ, Lipsitt D, Whybrow PC (eds): Psychosomatic Medicine. New York, Oxford University Press, 1977

Lynn SJ, Rhue JW: Hypnosis, imagination and fantasy. Journal of Mental Imagery 11:101–113, 1987

Marks DF: Theories of Image Formation. New York, Brandon House, 1986

McGrath J (ed): Social and Psychological Factors in Stress. New York, Holt, Rinehart & Winston, 1970

McKay M, Davis M, Fanning P: Thoughts and Feelings: The Art of Cognitive Stress Intervention. Richmond, CA, New Harbinger Publications, 1981

Moss GE: Illness, Immunity and Social Interaction. New York, John Wiley & Sons, 1973

Rinehart RE: Modern concepts in rheumatology. Northwest Medicine 56:578–581, 1957

Rinehart RE: Evaluation of behavior. Chicago, Chicago Physical Biological Sciences LTD, 1975

Rinehart RE, Dixon HH: Muscular dysfunction. Northwest Medicine 60:707, 1961

Rubin R: Mind–brain–body interaction: Elucidation of psychosomatic intervening variables. *In* Pasnau RO (ed): Consultation–Liaison Psychiatry, pp 73–85. New York, Grune & Stratton, 1975

Selye H: Forty years of stress research: Principal remaining problems and misconceptions. Can Med Assoc J 115:53–56, 1976

Selye H: History and present status of the stress concept. *In* Goldberger L, Breznits S (eds): Handbook of Stress: Theoretical and Clinical Aspects. New York, The Free Press, 1982

Sheikh A: Imagery: Current Theory, Research, and Application. New York: John Wiley & Sons, 1983

Squires S: The power of positive imagery: Visions to boost immunity. American Health 6:56–61, 1987

Stein M, Schiavi RE, Canerino M: Influence of brain and behavior on the immune system. Science 191:435–440, 1976

Stoyva J, Budzynski TH: Cultivated low arousal—An antistress response? *In* Dicra LV (ed): Recent Advances in Limbic and Autonomic System Research. New York, Plenum Press, 1978

Wadden T: Relaxation therapy for essential hypertension: specific or nonspecific effects? J Psych Res 28:53–61, 1984

RELAXATION AND RELATED TECHNIQUES

Benson H: Beyond the Relaxation Response. New York, Berkeley Books, 1984

Benson H, Beary JF, Carol MP: The relaxation response. Psychiatry 37:37–45, 1974

Bernstein D, Borkovic T: Progressive relaxation training: A manual for the helping profession. Champaign, IL, Research Press, 1973

Brena S: Yoga and Medicine. New York, Penguin Books, 1972

Bry A: Visualization: Directing the Movies of Our Mind. New York, Barnes & Noble, 1979

Carasso, RL: Treatment of cervical headache with hypnosis, suggestive therapy and relaxation techniques. Am J Clin Hypn 27(4):216–218, 1985

Dimotto JW: Relaxation. Am J Nurs 84:754–758, 1984

French AP, Tupin JP: Therapeutic application of a simple relaxation method. Am J Psychother 28:282–287, 1974

Frownfelter DL: Relaxation principles and techniques. *In* Frownfelter DL (ed): Chest Physical Therapy and Pulmonary Rehabilitation. Chicago, Year Book Medical Publishers, 1978

Goleman DJ, Schwartz GE: Meditation as an intervention in stress reactivity. J Consult Clin Psychol 44(3):456–466, 1976

Grzesiak RC: Relaxation techniques in treatment of chronic pain. Arch Phys Med Rehabil 58:270–272, 1977

Hillenberg JB, Collins FL: The importance of home practice for progressive relaxation training. Behav Res Ther 21:633–642, 1983

Kabot–Zinn J, Lipworth L, Burney R: The clinical use of mindfulness meditation for the self-regulation of chronic pain. J Behav Med 8:163–190, 1985

Kutz I, Borysenko J, Benson H: Meditation and psychotherapy: A rationale for the integration of dynamic psychotherapy, the relaxation response, and mindfulness meditation. Am J Psychol 142:1–8, 1985

Lehrer PM, Woolfolk RL, Rooney AJ, McCann B, Carrington P: Progressive relaxation and meditation: A study of psychophysiological and therapeutic differences between two techniques. Behav Res Ther 21:651–662, 1983

Leshan L: How to Meditate. New York, Bantam, 1974

Lysebeth AV: Yoga Self-Taught. New York, Barnes & Noble, 1973

Mitchell L: The Mitchell Method of Physiological Relaxation. *In* McGuigan FJ, Sime WE, Macdonald Wallace J: Stress and Tension Control, 2nd ed. New York, Plenum Press, 1984

Morse DR, Martin JS, Furst ML, Dublin LL: A physiological and subjective evaluation of meditation, hypnosis and relaxation. Psychosom Med 39(5):304–324, 1977

Rathbone JL: Relaxation. Philadelphia, Lea & Febiger, 1969

Roccia L, Rogora GA: Agopuntura e rilassamento. Minerva Med 67:1918–1920, 1976

Schilling D, Poppen R: Behavioral relaxation training and assessment. J Behav Ther Exp Psychiatry 14:99–107, 1983

Showers M: Physical therapy and muscle reeducation. *In* Tension Control. Chicago, Chicago Physical Biological Sciences, LTD, 1975

Wallace RK, Benson H: The physiology of meditation. Sci Am 226:84–90, 1972

White J: What is Meditation? New York, Doubleday, 1974

Yorkston JF, Sergeant JD: Simple method of relaxation. Lancet 2:1319–1321, 1960

MANAGEMENT OF STRESS

Bandler R, Grinder J: Frogs into Princes. Moab, UT, Real People Press, 1979

Beach CW, Marshall MG: Tension Control at Michigan

State University. East Lansing, MI, American Association of Tension Control, 1974

Bonica J, Fordyce WE: Operant Conditioning for Chronic Pain. Springfield, IL, Charles C Thomas, 1974

Coburn J, Manderino MA: Stress inoculation: An illustration of coping skills training. Rehabilitation Nursing 11:14–17, 1986

Dettmar DM: The effect of stress release in indices of mandibular dysfunction. Aust Dent J 32(1):39–41, 1987

Fletcher DJ, Bezanson D: Coping with stress. How to help patients deal with life's pressure. Postgrad Med 77(4):93–96,99–100, 1985

Fordyce W: Behavioral Methods for Chronic Pain and Illness. St. Louis, CV Mosby, 1976

Goldfried MR, Merbaum M: Behavior Change Through Self-Control. New York, Holt, Rinehart & Winston, 1973

Holzman PS: On learning and seeing oneself. J Nerv Ment Dis 148:198–209, 1969

Hutchings D, Reinbing R: Tension headaches: What form of therapy is most effective? Biofeedback Self Regul 1:183–190, 1976

Kanter FH: Self management methods. *In* Kanter FH, Goldstein AP (eds): Helping People Change. New York, Pergamon Press, 1975

Mandel AR, Keller SM: Stress management in rehabilitation. Arch Phys Med Rehabil 67(6):375–379, 1986

McGuighan FJ, Sime WE, Mcdonald WJ (eds): Stress and Tension Control, 2nd ed. New York, Plenum Press, 1983

Meichenbaum D: Toward a cognitive theory of self-control. *In* Schwartz GE, Shapiro D (eds): Consciousness and Self-Regulation. New York, Plenum Press, 1976

Miller NE: Visceral learning and other additional factors potentially applicable to psychotherapy. International Psychiatry Clinic 6:294–312, 1968

Muse M: Stress-related post-traumatic chronic pain syndrome: Behavioral treatment approach. Pain 25(3):389–394, 1986

Ost LG: Applied relaxation: Description of a coping technique and review of controlled studies. Behav Res Ther 25:397–409, 1987

Schwartz GE: Self-regulation of response patterning: Implications for psychophysiological research and therapy. Biofeedback Self Regul 1:7–30, 1976

Schwartz GE, Shapiro D (eds): Consciousness and Self-Regulation. New York, Plenum Press, 1976

Steinmetz J, Blankenship J, Brown L, Hall D, Miller G: Managing Stress Before It Manages You. Palo Alto, CA, Bull Publishing, 1982

Stoyva J, Anderson C: A coping rest model of relaxation and stress management. *In* Goldberger L, Breznitz S (eds): Handbook of Stress: Theoretical and Clinical Aspects. New York, The Free Press, 1982

Whatmore G, Kohli K: The Physiopathology and Treatment of Functional Disorders, Including Anxiety States and Depression and the Role of Biofeedback Training. New York, Grune & Stratton, 1974

BIOFEEDBACK TECHNIQUES

Blanchard E, Young L: Clinical applications of biofeedback training: A review of evidence. Arch Gen Psychiatry 30:573–588, 1974

Budzynski T: Biofeedback procedures in the clinic. Seminars in Psychiatry 5(4):537–547, 1973

Budzynski T, Stoyva J, Adler CS, Mullaney DJ: EMG biofeedback and tension headache: A controlled outcome study. Psychosom Med 35:484–496, 1973

Davis M, Eshelman ER, McKay M: The Relaxation and Stress Reduction Workbook, 2nd ed. Oakland, CA, New Harbinger Publications, 1982

Funch DP, Gale EN: Biofeedback and relaxation therapy for chronic temporomandibular joint pain. Consult Clin Psychol 52:928–935, 1984

Gaarder K, Montgomery P: Clinical Biofeedback: A Procedural Manual. Baltimore, Williams & Wilkins, 1977

Lynch JJ: Biofeedback: Some reflection on modern behavioral science. Seminars in Psychiatry 5(4):551–562, 1972

Miller N: Biofeed: Evaluation of new technique. N Engl J Med 290:685, 1974

Peck C, Kraft G: Electromyographic biofeedback for pain related to muscle tension: A study of tension headache, back and jaw pain. Arch Surg 112:889–895, 1977

Schwartz GE, Shapiro D: Biofeedback and essential hypertension: Current findings and theoretical concerns. Seminars in Psychiatry 5:591–603, 1973

Sterman L: Clinical biofeedback. Am J Nurs 75:2006–2009, 1975

Stoyva J: Self-regulation: A context for biofeedback. Biofeedback Self Regul 1:1–6, 1976

Stoyva JM: Guidelines in cultivating general relaxation: Biofeedback and autogenic training combined. *In* Basmajian JV (ed): Biofeedback: Principles and Practice for Clinicians. Baltimore, Williams & Wilkins, 1983

Turin A, Johnson W: Biofeedback therapy for migraine headaches. Arch Gen Psychiatry 33:517–519, 1976

Venables PH, Martin I (eds): Manual of Psychophysiological Methods. Amsterdam, North Holland Pub., 1966

Wells N: The effect of relaxation on postoperative muscle tension and pain. Nursing Research 31:236–238, 1982

Part Two
CLINICAL APPLICATIONS —
PERIPHERAL JOINTS

10 The Shoulder and Shoulder Girdle

Randolph M. Kessler and Darlene Hertling

REVIEW OF FUNCTIONAL ANATOMY

OSSEOUS STRUCTURES

The osseous components of the functional shoulder girdle include the upper thoracic vertebrae, the first and second ribs, the manubrium, the scapula, the clavicle, and the humerus (Fig. 10–1).[70] For this complex to function adequately, the spine must be stable. To achieve full arm elevation, the upper thoracic vertebrae must be able to extend, rotate, and sidebend to the ipsilateral side and the bodies of the first and second ribs must be able to descend and move posteriorly (with vertebral rotation). The manubriosternal, costomanubrial, and sternoclavicular joints must permit the manubrium to sidebend and rotate to the ipsilateral side.

The acromioclavicular and sternoclavicular joints provide the mobility of the scapulothoracic mechanism. Movement of the glenohumeral joint provides between 90° (active) and 120° (passive) elevation. For full elevation of the arm, scapular rotation, clavicular elevation, and thoracic extension must accompany humeral elevation. During ipsilateral elevation the upper thoracic vertebrae must be able to extend, rotate, and sidebend to the ipsilateral side while the lower thoracic vertebrae must sidebend away from the side of motion. For full vertical elevation to be obtained, exaggeration of lumbar lordosis becomes necessary and is achieved by action of the spinal muscles.[38] Although the joints act interdependently and in concert, it is necessary to discuss structure and movement of these joints individually in order to understand their functions and significance.

Glenohumeral Joint

The *humeral head,* in the anatomic position, faces medially, slightly posteriorly, and superiorly. The head forms almost half a sphere, with an angular value of about 150°. It forms an angle of about 45° with the humeral shaft (Fig. 10–2).

The glenoid cavity faces laterally, forward, and superiorly. It has an angular value of only 75°. This incongruity between the humeral head and the glenoid cavity is partially compensated for by the fibrous or fibrocartilaginous glenoid labrum, which serves to deepen the glenoid cavity. The glenoid is pear-shaped—narrow superiorly and wider inferiorly.

Acromioclavicular Joint

The clavicle is S-shaped, the lateral third being concave anteriorly (Fig. 10–3). This provides for extra motion during elevation of the arm (see under Biomechanics). The articular surface of the clavicle is convex. The concave articular surface of the acromion process faces medially and somewhat anterosuperiorly. This joint is oriented in such a way that a strong compression force tends to cause the clavicle to override the acromion. This is what occurs in an acromioclavicular separation, usually caused by a fall on the tip of the acromion.

Sternoclavicular Joint

The sternal end of the clavicle is somewhat bulbous, and is convex in the frontal plane while having a slight concavity anteroposteriorly. It articulates with the upper lateral edge of the manubrium, as well as with the superior surface of the medial aspect of the cartilage of the first rib. It tends to extend above the superior surface of the manubrium by as much as one half its width.

Scapulothoracic Mechanism

The scapulothoracic joint complex or mechanism (see Fig. 10–4) is not a true anatomic joint, because it has none of the usual joint characteristics. Movements are inescapably associated with the sternocla-

169

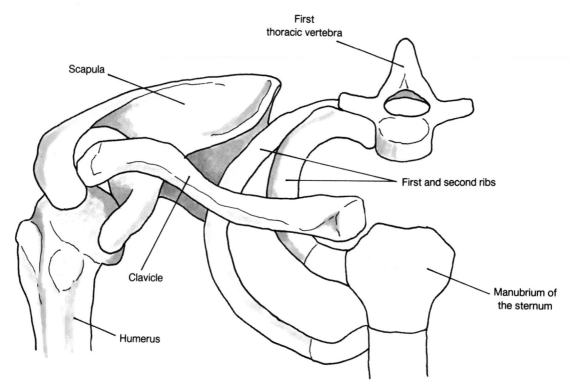

Fig. 10-1. Osseous components of the functional shoulder girdle.

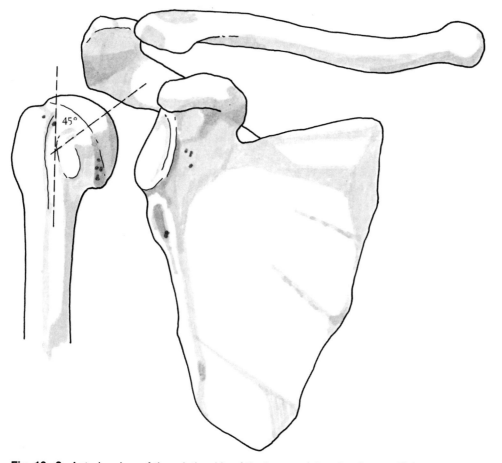

Fig. 10-2. Anterior view of the relationship of the bones of the glenohumeral joint.

vicular and acromioclavicular joints. These two anatomic joints and the functional thoracic joint form a closed kinetic chain in which movement in one joint invariably causes motion in the other.

The scapula, viewed from above at rest, makes an angle of about 30° with the frontal plane (Fig. 10-3A). It makes an angle of about 60° with the clavicle, viewed from above.

The medial portion of the scapular spine usually lies level with the T3 spinous process, wheras the inferior angle lies level with the T7 or T8 spinous process. The medial border lies about 6 cm lateral to the thoracic spinous processes.

LIGAMENTS

Glenohumeral Joint

The articular capsule of the glenohumeral joint (Fig. 10-4) is quite thin and lax with redundant folds situated anteroinferiorly when the arm is at rest. This allows a full range of elevation. Because of the laxity of the joint capsule, the head of the humerus can be distracted laterally about 2 cm in the cadaver, with the arm in a position of slight abduction. With the arm at the side, the superior joint capsule remains taut, whereas the remainder of the capsule assumes a forward and medial twist. The tendons of the supraspinatus, infraspinatus, teres minor, and subscapularis blend with the fibers of the joint capsule.

The glenohumeral ligaments provide some reinforcement to the capsule anteriorly, helping to check external rotation.

The middle glenohumeral ligament limits lateral rotation up to 90° abduction and is an important anterior stabilizer of the shoulder joint.[77] The inferior glenohumeral ligament is the thickest of the glenohumeral structures and attaches to the anterior, inferior, and posterior margins of the glenoid labrum.[74,80] It strengthens the capsule anteriorly and inferiorly, helping to prevent anterior subluxation and dislocation.[77]

The coracohumeral ligament strengthens the superior capsule and is important in maintaining the glenohumeral relationship. The downward pull of gravity on the arm is counteracted largely by the superior capsule and the coracohumeral ligament. From the root of the coracoid process, it extends to the greater and lesser tubercles of the humerus beneath the supraspinatus tendon. The ligament blends with the rotator cuff and fills in the space between the subscapularis and the supraspinatus muscles.[68] Tension develops mainly in the anterior band during extension and in the posterior band during flexion.

The anterior band, running somewhat anteriorly to the vertical axis about which rotation occurs, checks external rotation and perhaps extension. The tension in the posterior band is felt to be a factor in assisting the glenohumeral ligament in medial rotation of the shoulder during flexion.[10,66]

The transverse humeral ligament traverses the intertubercular (bicipital) groove, acting as a retinaculum for the tendon of the long head of the biceps.

Acromioclavicular Joint

The major ligaments of the acromioclavicular joint (see Fig. 10-4) are the superior and inferior acromioclavicular ligaments and the coracoclavicular ligaments. The superior and inferior ligaments offer some protection to the joint and help prevent overriding of the clavicle on the acromion.

Although situated away from the joint, the coracoclavicular ligaments are of the most importance in providing acromioclavicular joint stability.

The trapezoid ligament lies almost horizontally in the frontal plane and is positioned in such a way that it can check overriding, or lateral, movement of the clavicle on the acromion. It also helps prevent excessive narrowing of the angle between the acromion and clavicle (viewed from above), as occurs with protraction.

The conoid ligament is oriented vertically, medial to the trapezoid ligament, and is twisted upon itself. It primarily checks superior movement of the clavicle on the acromion; it also prevents excessive widening of the scapuloclavicular angle. As the arm is abducted, the scapula rotates in such a way that the inferior angle swings laterally and superiorly. This movement increases the distance between the clavicle and the coracoid process, pulling the conoid ligament taut. This tightening causes posterior or external (backward axial) rotation of the clavicle, bringing the acromioclavicular joint back into apposition (because of the "s" shape of the clavicle). It is necessary for full elevation of the arm (see under Biomechanics).

These ligaments suspend the scapula from the clavicle and transmit the force of the superior fibers of the trapezius to the scapula.[19] Anteriorly, the space between the ligaments is filled with fat and frequently a bursa. In up to 30% of subjects the bony components may be opposed closely and may form a coracoclavicular joint.[19,55]

The coracoacromial ligament, together with the acromion and the coracoid process, form an important protective arch over the glenohumeral arch (see Fig. 10-4).[56] The arch forms a secondary restraining

Fig. 10-3. Acromioclavicular, sternoclavicular, and scapulothoracic articulations shown *(A)* at rest, *(B)* in retraction, and *(C)* in protraction.

socket for the humeral head, preventing dislocation of the humeral head superiorly. This arch can be the site of impingement on the greater tubercle, supraspinatus tendon, or subdeltoid bursa in cases of abnormal joint mechanics.

Sternoclavicular Joint

The relatively lax sternoclavicular joint capsule is reinforced anteriorly by the anterior sternoclavicular ligament, posteriorly by the posterior sternoclavicular ligaments, and superiorly by the interclavicular ligament (Fig. 10-5). The costoclavicular ligament lies just lateral to the joint. Its anterior fibers run superiorly and laterally, and check elevation and lateral movement of the clavicle. The posterior fibers run superiorly and medially from the first rib, and check elevation and medial movement of the clavicle.

An intra-articular disk is attached above to the clavicle and below to the first costal cartilage and the sternum. It is especially important in helping to prevent medial dislocation of the clavicle, which can occur with a fall on the outstretched arm or on the point of the shoulder. Invariably the clavicle will break or the acromioclavicular joint will dislocate before the sternoclavicular joint dislocates medially.

This is true in spite of the fact that the medial sloping of the joint surfaces and the superior overlap of the clavicle on the sternum would seem to make the joint susceptible to medial dislocation.

BURSAE

There are usually considered to be eight or nine bursae about the shoulder joint. Practically speaking, only two are worth considering here, because of their clinical significance.

Subacromial or Subdeltoid Bursa

The subacromial or subdeltoid bursa extends over the supraspinatus tendon and distal muscle belly beneath the acromion and deltoid muscle. At times it extends beneath the coracoid process (Fig. 10-6A). It is attached above to the acromial arch and below to the rotator cuff tendons and greater tubercle. It does not normally communicate with the joint capsule but may in the case of a rotator cuff tear. This is seen on arthrogram as dye leaking over the top of the supraspinatus tendon. The bursa is susceptible to impingement beneath the acromial arch, especially if it is inflamed and swollen (Fig. 10-6B). Inflammation of the bursa is often attributed to rupture of a supra-

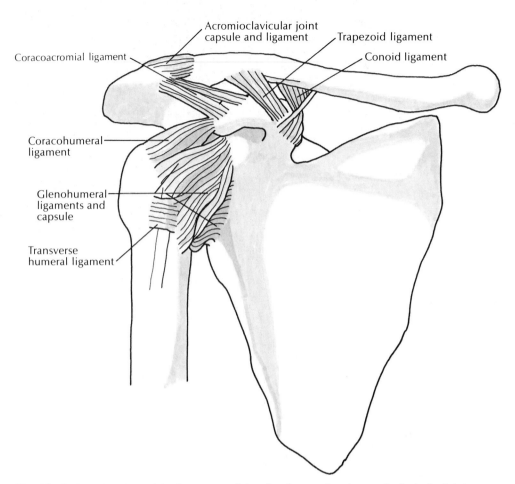

Fig. 10-4. Anterior view of the ligaments of the glenohumeral and acromioclavicular joints.

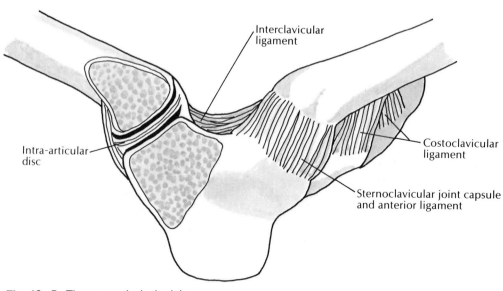

Fig. 10-5. The sternoclavicular joint.

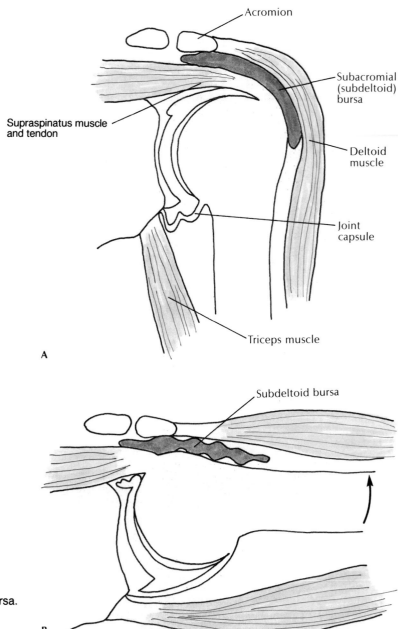

Fig. 10-6. (A) The subacromial (subdeltoid) bursa. (B) As the humerus elevates, the bursal tissue gathers beneath the acromion.

spinatus calcium deposit superiorly into the underside of the bursa.

Subscapular Bursa

The subscapular bursa overlies the anterior joint capsule and lies beneath the subscapularis muscle. It communicates with the joint capsule and fills with dye on arthrography. Articular effusion may be manifested clinically by an anterior swelling, owing to distension of the bursa (Fig. 10-7).

VASCULAR ANATOMY OF THE ROTATOR CUFF TENDONS

The tendons of the rotator cuff include the supraspinatus, infraspinatus, teres minor, and subscapularis. As implied by the term *rotator cuff*, they do not exist as discrete tendons but blend to form a continuous cuff surrounding the posterior, superior, and anterior aspects of the humeral head. The fibers of the tendinous cuff attach to the articular capsule of the glenohumeral joint by blending with it. This allows the cuff to provide dynamic stabilization of the joint.

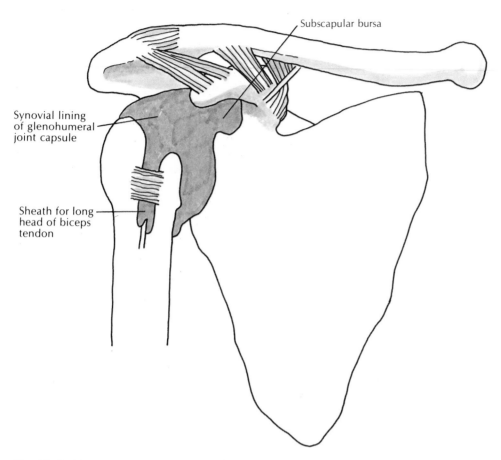

Subscapular bursa

Synovial lining
of glenohumeral
joint capsule

Sheath for long
head of biceps
tendon

Fig. 10–7. The subscapular bursa.

The rotator cuff is a frequent site of lesions—usually of a degenerative nature—in response to fatigue stresses. Lesions usually affect the supraspinatus, and to a lesser extent, the infraspinatus portions of the cuff. Since such degeneration often occurs with normal activity levels, the nutritional status of this frequently involved area of the cuff is of particular interest. Most fatigue or degenerative lesions occur either from increased stress levels or from a nutritional deficit.

The primary blood supply to the rotator cuff tendons is derived from six arteries, three of which contribute in virtually all individuals, and three of which are sometimes absent (Fig. 10–8).[63] The posterior humeral circumflex and the suprascapular arteries are usually present; they supply primarily the infraspinatus and teres minor areas of the cuff. The subscapularis is supplied by the anterior humeral circumflex artery, which is usually present; the thoracoacromial artery, which is occasionally absent; and the suprahumeral and subscapular arteries, which are often absent. The supraspinatus region receives its supply primarily from the thoracoacromial artery which, as mentioned, is not always present. This artery anastomoses with the two circumflex arteries, which also contribute some to the supraspinatus region.

The most significant feature of the blood supply to the rotator cuff is that the supraspinatus and, to a lesser extent, the infraspinatus regions of the cuff are areas that are often considerably hypovascular with respect to the rest of the tendinous cuff. This has been confirmed by injection studies as well as by histologic sections. In Rothman and Parke's investigation, it was found that, regardless of age, the supraspinatus region was hypovascular in 63% of 72 specimens, and that the infraspinatus region was hypovascular in 37%.[73] It was further noted that when the infraspinatus was undervascularized, so was the supraspinatus. Hypovascularity was demonstrated in the subscapularis region in only 7% of the specimens.

Clinically, the relative incidence of tendinitis in these tendons correlates well with the above relative incidences of hypovascularity. Also, the incidence of shoulder tendinitis tends to increase with advancing age, which is consistent with the findings that tendon hypovascularity, in general, progresses with age.[63]

It is proposed that the hypovascularity in the supraspinatus region is at least partly the result of pressure applied to the underside of the tendon by the superior aspect of the humeral head as the tendon passes around and over its insertion on the greater tubercle of the humerus.[50]

BIOMECHANICS

JOINT STABILIZATION

As indicated in the discussion of functional anatomy, the glenohumeral joint capsule is relatively lax. This is somewhat unique, because most joints rely primarily on their capsules and ligaments to maintain proper orientation of joint surfaces during movement and in response to external forces. The shoulder joint capsule does provide some stabilization of the joint when the arm is at the side, and it does help to guide movement of the joint. At the shoulder, however, the muscles also play an essential role in these functions. The shoulder, then, relies on active and passive stabilizing components to maintain joint integrity. This is necessary at the glenohumeral joint because the incongruent bony constituents confer little intrinsic stability, such as is present at the hip joint.

When the arm hangs freely to the side, the superior joint capsule and coracohumeral ligament are normally taut, and the plane of the glenoid cavity faces somewhat upward. A vertical force produced by the weight of the hanging arm is met by a reactive tensile force to the superior joint capsule. The result of these two forces is a force that tends to pull the head of the humerus in against the upward-facing glenoid cavity (Fig. 10–9). In this way the tightness of the superior joint capsule and the orientation of the glenoid stabilize the humerus when the arm hangs freely at the side. Little or no muscle contraction by the deltoid or the rotator cuff muscles is necessary to prevent inferior subluxation of the humerus, even when some weight is held in the hanging hand.[3,4]

Once the arm is elevated from the side in any plane, tension is lost in the superior joint capsule so that it can no longer contribute to the maintenance of joint integrity (Fig. 10–10). Now the rotator cuff muscles, supraspinatus, subscapularis, and teres minor must contract to hold the humerus in a proper orientation with respect to the glenoid cavity during movement of the arm (Fig. 10–11). In this way, the rotator cuff tendons, which blend with the joint capsule, provide for stabilization of the glenohumeral joint when the arm is held away from the side.[3,4,5,35]

Clinically there are some common conditions in which these normal stabilizing mechanisms are compromised. The two common causes are alterations in the normal structural alignment of the bony constituents of the shoulder girdle, and rotator cuff muscle weakness. In a person with a thoracic kyphosis, the scapula follows the contour of the thorax and assumes a downward rotated position; the glenoid cavity no longer faces upward. Also, in this position the freely hanging humerus assumes a position of relative abduction with respect to the scapula, and tension is lost in the superior joint capsule (Fig. 10–12). In this situation, the rotator cuff muscles must contract to maintain joint integrity with the arm at the side, thus preventing inferior subluxation of the humerus. Therefore, the person with a thoracic kyphotic deformity must maintain increased tone in the rotator cuff muscles to compensate for the loss of capsular stabilization. It is possible that thoracic kyphosis is an etiologic factor in some cases of frozen shoulder. The increased tone of the rotator cuff muscles results in increased tensile stresses to the joint capsule, with which the rotator cuff tendons blend (Fig. 10–13). The increased stress to the capsule stimulates an increase in collagen production, which leads to a gradual loss of extensibility of the capsule — in other words, capsular fibrosis.

In the patient with shoulder girdle muscle paresis, a similar situation may exist; the weakness of the scapular muscles allows the scapula to assume a downward rotated position on the chest wall (Fig. 10–14A). The common condition in which this occurs is hemiplegia following a stroke. In these individuals, rotator cuff muscle activity may also be reduced, and the arm is predisposed to inferior subluxation because of the loss of active and passive stabilizing components (Fig. 10–14B)

INFLUENCE OF THE GLENOHUMERAL JOINT CAPSULE ON MOVEMENT

The orientation and configuration of the shoulder joint capsule play a major role in determining the degree and type of movement that occur at the joint. When the arm hangs freely to the side the fibers of the joint capsule are oriented in a forward and medial twist (Fig. 10–15).[37] Because the plane of the scapula is oriented midway between the frontal and sagittal planes, this capsular twist is increased with abduction (elevation in the frontal plane) and decreased with flexion (elevation in the sagittal plane) (Fig. 10–16). Thus, as the arm swings into abduction, the increasing twist in the joint capsule begins to pull the head of the humerus in tightly against the glenoid

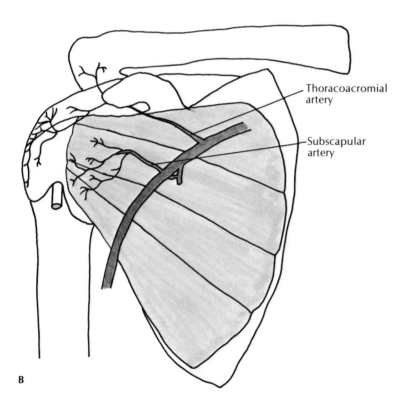

Fig. 10–8. Vascular supply of the rotator cuff muscles: *(A)* posterior view; *(B)* anterior view, showing the thoracoacromial and subscapular arteries; and *(C)* anterior view, showing the suprahumeral and anterior humeral circumflex arteries.

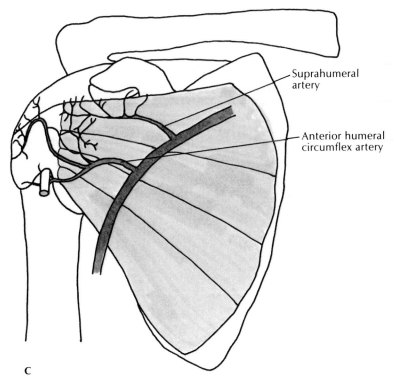

Suprahumeral
artery

Anterior humeral
circumflex artery

Fig. 10–8. *Continued.*   C

Fig. 10–9. Vertical and reactive tensile forces to the superior joint capsule when the arm is hanging freely at the side.

Fig. 10–10. During elevation of the arm, tension is lost in the superior joint capsule.

Fig. 10–11. Rotator cuff muscles contract to hold the humerus in proper orientation with respect to the glenoid during movement of the arm.

Fig. 10–12. In a person with thoracic kyphosis, (A) the scapula assumes a downward, rotated position so that the glenoid fossa no longer faces upward, and (B) the freely hanging humerus assumes a position of relative abduction with loss of tension in the superior joint capsule.

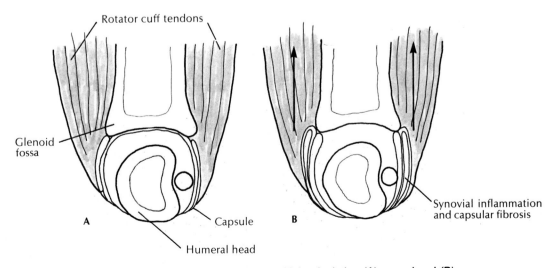

Fig. 10–13. Transverse section of the glenohumeral joint depicting (A) normal and (B) increased cuff tension.

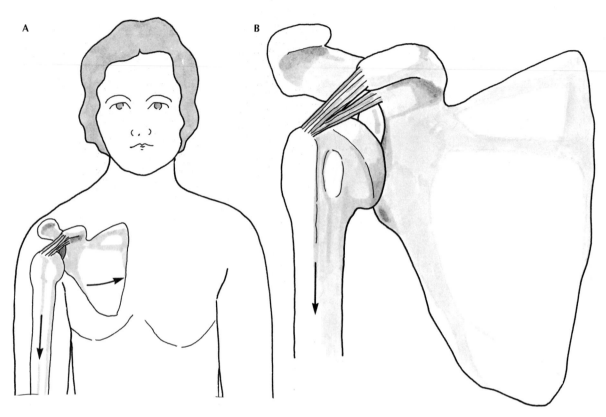

Fig. 10–14. In the person with shoulder-girdle muscle paresis, *(A)* the scapula assumes a downward, rotated position on the chest wall, and *(B)* reduced rotator-cuff tension predisposes to inferior subluxation.

cavity, and the tension in the capsular fibers gradually increases as the twisting continues. The tension eventually causes the capsule to pull the humerus around into external rotation (Fig. 10–17). This external rotation untwists the joint capsule and allows further movement to occur. If the humerus were not to rotate externally, the joint would lock at the midrange of abduction from the combined effects of abnormal compression of joint surfaces and excessive tension on the capsular fibers. The external rotation that occurs also causes the greater tubercle to clear the coracoacromial arch during abduction.[16,35,47] In this way, the external rotation of the humerus that takes place during abduction is a passive phenomenon occurring as a result of the twisted configuration of the glenohumeral joint capsule, combined with the fact that abduction involves movement out of the plane of the scapula in a direction that tends to increase the twist. If lateral rotation does not occur, full movement is restricted because the joint locks and the greater tubercle impinges on the acromial arch (Fig. 10–18).

A common condition in which external rotation of the humerus becomes restricted is frozen shoulder.

With capsular fibrosis at the shoulder, the anterior joint capsule becomes especially tight. The capsule adheres to the anterior aspect of the humeral head while the redundant folds of the capsule situated anteroinferiorly adhere to one another.[60] It is important for the clinician to realize that in the presence of capsular tightness at the shoulder, abduction is restricted by locking and impingement. This movement should not be forced until external rotation is gained.

MUSCULAR FORCE COUPLE

The rotator cuff muscles act with the deltoid muscle in a force-couple mechanism during elevation to guide the humerus in its movement on the glenoid cavity.[21,35,47,72] The force of elevation, together with active downward pull of the short rotator muscles, establishes the muscle force couple necessary for elevation of the limb. When the arm is by the side, the direction of the deltoid muscle force is upward and outward with respect to the humerus, whereas the force of the infraspinatus, teres minor, and subscapularis is downward and inward. The force of the del-

Fig. 10–15. Anterior view of the orientation of the fibers of the joint capsule when the arm hangs freely at the side.

toid muscle, acting below the center of rotation, is opposite that of the force of the three rotator muscles applied above the center of rotation and produces a powerful force couple.[8]

Some anatomists have considered the primary function of the supraspinatus muscle to be only the initiation of abduction, thus necessitating contraction of the rotator cuff muscle in order for the arm to be swung from the side. However, Howell and associates have observed that in the shoulder with a paralyzed supraspinatus muscle, the deltoid can initiate and generate a significant torque from 0° to 30° elevation in the plane of the scapula.[34]

For the glenohumeral joint to be stable and functional within its range, the muscles must generate sufficient force throughout the entire range. The deltoid is well suited in two ways to fulfill this need. First, the muscle fibers are in a multipennate arrangement.[30,70] Functionally, this means that there is less change in length of each fiber while providing maximal force during contraction. For a muscle to be powerful, it must develop maximal tension over the range as quickly as possible. This is accomplished better in a multipennate arrangement. Therefore,

multipennate muscles are more powerful than muscles with parallel fibers.

The second reason that the deltoid is well designed to provide stability to the glenohumeral joint is related to its attachments. Arising from the scapular spine, acromial arch, and clavicle, the deltoid has a broad base and a large muscle mass. More importantly, the origins can be raised during humeral elevation. This scapular rotation decreases the range over which the deltoid needs to contract during humeral elevation, which in turn increases muscle power throughout the entire range. The combination of the multipennate design and movable origin is of considerable functional advantage for the deltoid and glenohumeral joints.[18]

Absence of the supraspinatus muscle alone, provided the shoulder is pain free, produces a marked loss of force in higher ranges of abduction. The force of abduction is lost rapidly and by 90° of combined humeral and scapular motions, the weight of the arm can barely be lifted against gravity.[8] However, in complete loss of deltoid muscle function, the rotator cuff (including the supraspinatus muscle) can produce abduction of the arm with 50% of the normal

A

B

Fig. 10–16. Capsular twist is *(A)* decreased with flexion and *(B)* increased with abduction.

Fig. 10–17. Capsular pull results in external rotation of the humerus and "untwisting" of the capsule during abduction.

Fig. 10–18. Locking of the joint and impingement of the greater tubercle results if lateral humeral rotation does not occur during abduction.

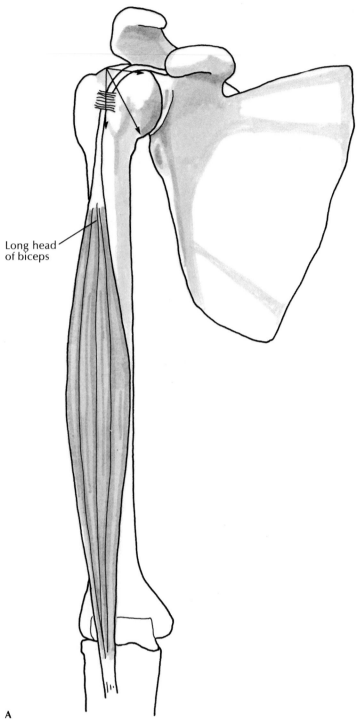

Long head
of biceps

A

Fig. 10–19. Long head of biceps acts in the muscular-force couple to create *(A)* vertical and reactive tensile forces and *(B)* moment arm during humeral elevation.

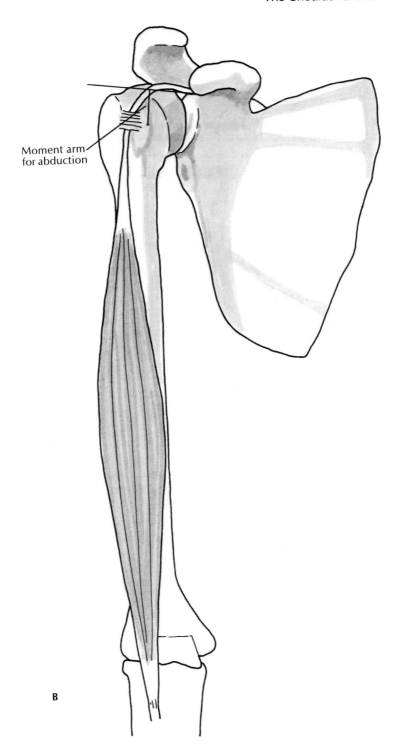

Moment arm
for abduction

B

force.[8] It can be concluded that the supraspinatus and deltoid muscles are equally responsible for producing torque about the shoulder joint in the functional planes of motion.

Another example of a force couple is the combined action of the three parts of the trapezius muscle and the serratus anterior.[49] The serratus acts as a force couple with the trapezius during upward rotation of the glenoid fossa by tracking the scapula anteriorly, laterally, and superiorly.[16]

The long head of the biceps also aids in humeral head depression because of the way the tendon acts as a pulley around the superior aspect of the humerus.[35,47] If the arm is externally rotated so that the bicipital groove faces laterally, the long head of the biceps works as a pulley to assist in abduction of the arm (Fig. 10–19).

The clinician who deals with stroke patients, or any patient with diffuse paralysis of the shoulder musculature, must be aware of the importance of the rotator cuff muscles in guiding glenohumeral movement. If passive range of motion of the shoulder is performed in such cases, the head of the humerus must be guided into inferior glide (depression) passively during flexion and abduction. If it is not, the subacromial tissues may be subjected to repeated trauma. This may explain the onset of shoulder pain in many of these patients as sensation to the shoulder returns. It also emphasizes that "routine" range of motion be performed by a skilled professional.[58]

ANALYSIS OF SHOULDER ABDUCTION

When we consider function at the shoulder, we must be concerned with the contribution of several joints in addition to the glenohumeral articulation. These include the acromioclavicular joint, the sternoclavicular joint, the articulation between the scapula and the thorax, the joints of the lower cervical and upper thoracic spine, and the articulation between the coracoacromial arch and the subacromial tissues. An analysis of the functioning of each of these structures during abduction of the arm emphasizes the importance of a normal interplay between the components of the shoulder complex.

During the first 15° to 30° abduction, much of the movement occurs at the glenohumeral joint, although this varies among individuals.[26,35,45] During this early phase, the muscles controlling the scapula contract to stabilize the scapula against the chest wall, preparing it for subsequent movement. Because the glenohumeral joint capsule is twisted forward and medially at the starting position, and because abduction is a movement of the humerus out of the plane of the scapula, the medial twist of the capsule begins to increase as abduction proceeds.*[37]

Beginning at 15° to 30° abduction, the scapula begins to move to contribute to elevation of the arm. In doing so, it moves forward, elevates, and rotates upward on the chest wall. Much of this movement of the scapula can occur because of movement at the sternoclavicular joint; the clavicle protracts about 30°, elevates about 30°, and rotates backward around its long axis about 50°.[20,35,47] The acromioclavicular joint contributes much less to scapular movement because its planar joint surfaces do not allow much angular movement. The scapula does rotate some at the acromioclavicular joint at the beginning of scapular movement. Viewed from above, the angle between the scapula and clavicle narrows as the scapula slides around and forward on the chest wall (see Fig. 10–3C). The rotation which the scapula undergoes in the frontal plane, with respect to the clavicle, causes the conoid ligament to tighten. Since this ligament attaches to the backside of the clavicle, as it pulls tight, it pulls the clavicle into a backward axial rotation. As the angle between the scapula and clavicle narrows (as viewed from above), the joint close-packs quite early. However, because the clavicle rotates axially and because it is S-shaped, the joint surfaces maintain a more constant relationship than they would otherwise. Furthermore, less movement is required of the acromioclavicular joint because of this axial rotation and the shape of the clavicle (Fig. 10–20). Thus, out of the approximate total 60° that scapular movement contributes to elevation of the arm, about 30° occurs at the sternoclavicular joint, and the remaining 30° occurs from the combined effects of clavicular rotation, which cause the clavicular joint surface to face upward, and the movement that occurs at the acromioclavicular joint.

From 15° or 30° of abduction the humerus continues to elevate with respect to the scapula through a total of 90° to 110°.[7,26,35,45,47] The humerus contributes about 10° of movement for every 5° contributed by scapular motion. As the humerus elevates, the greater tubercle begins to approximate the coracoacromial arch, and the capsular fibers continue to twist medially. Once a certain amount of tension develops in the joint capsule, the capsule pulls the humerus around into a lateral axial rotation, causing the greater tubercle to be directed behind and be-

---

* The increasing medial twist is a result of medial conjunct rotation from movement of the humerus around the medial axis as defined at the beginning of movement. This occurs because abduction is an impure swing in which the humerus moves out of the plane of the scapula.

The Shoulder and Shoulder Girdle **189**

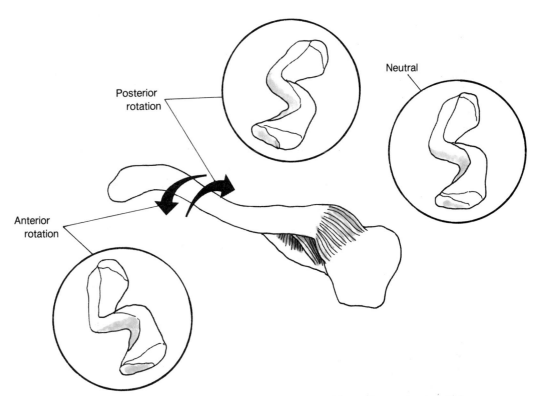

Posterior
rotation

Neutral

Anterior
rotation

Fig. 10–20. Clavicular rotation in the sagittal plane, as viewed from the proximal end of the clavicle and the frontal plane.

neath the acromion. As this occurs the subdeltoid bursal tissue is gathered proximally beneath the acromion (see Fig. 10–6). If the bursa is distended, or if the tubercle rides too high or does not rotate laterally, subacromial impingement will occur with either loss of movement or chronic trauma to the subacromial tissues, or both.

The combined glenohumeral and scapular movements contribute about 160° to the full range of abduction. The remaining movement occurs as a result of movement at the lower cervical and upper thoracic spines. If both arms are raised simultaneously, extension occurs at these regions. If unilateral abduction is performed, the spine bends away from the side of arm movement. The contribution of spinal movement to the full 180° elevation of the arm is often overlooked. The person with a fixed spinal deformity, such as a thoracic kyphosis, cannot be expected to demonstrate full elvation of the arm.

EVALUATION OF THE SHOULDER

A general approach to evaluation of soft-tissue lesions is discussed in Chapter 4, Assessment of Musculoskeletal Disorders. However, there are additional concepts and techniques specific to evaluation of the shoulder region.

The shoulder and the arm are common sites of referred pain from other areas, such as the myocardium, cervical region, and diaphragm. Usually the history will suggest the origin of pain. If not, a scan examination consisting of active motion of the neck and all major upper-extremity joints, with passive over-pressure at the extremes of each motion, may be useful in reproducing the pain and suggesting the site of the lesion. In discussing examination of the shoulder itself, we assume that the physician's examination, the history, or the scan examination has localized the lesion to the shoulder region. The clinician's in-depth examination clarifies the nature and extent of the lesion so that prescribed treatment modalities may be safely and effectively applied and establishes a baseline for judging progress.

I. History
  A. *Specific questions* for shoulder lesions include the following:
    1. Does the pain ever spread to below the elbow?
    2. Can the patient lie on the shoulder at night?

3. Is the patient able to use the arm to comb his or her hair?

4. Can the patient reach into a hip pocket or fasten a bra behind her?

5. Can the patient eat comfortably with the arm?

6. Does it hurt to put on or remove a shirt or jacket?

7. Is it difficult to perform activities that require reaching above shoulder level?

B. *Site of pain*—Except in acromioclavicular joint sprains, pain is seldom felt at the shoulder itself but rather over the lateral brachial region. It may spread to all or any part of the limb that is innervated by that spinal segment, from which the glenohumeral joint structures are primarily derived, usually the C5 segment or, in the case of acromioclavicular problems, the C4 sclerotome (see Figs. 3–1, 3–3, and 4–2).

C. *Nature of pain*—Common lesions at the shoulder tend to be aggravated by use and relieved by rest. Patients with capsular lesions give a history of painful limitation, especially with movements into external rotation and abduction. Patients with noncapsular lesions often present with painful "twinges" during various functions, such as donning a jacket or reaching above shoulder level.

In the case of acute bursitis, which is relatively rare, the pain may become quite intense and is often felt even at rest.

D. *Onset of pain*—Except in athletic settings, a history of trauma does not accompany most common shoulder lesions. More often, the onset is insidious, as is the case in tendinitis or capsular tightening. In these, the onset is very gradual, whereas in acute bursitis, the patient notes a rapid buildup of pain over 12 to 72 hours.

E. *General health*—The final set of subjective questions should consider the patient's general health, in particular disorders of the cardiac and visceral organs that may cause pain to be referred to the shoulder region (*e.g.*, diaphragmatic irritation, cardiac ischemia, gallbladder problems, pancreatic disease).[11]

II. Physical Examination

A. *Observation*

1. Posture of the arm and shoulder girdle

a. Does the patient hold arm close to side or across chest?

b. Does the patient tend to support arm?

2. Function, particularly dressing, and general willingness to use arm

B. *Inspection*

1. Structure. Observe the patient in relaxed standing position for

a. Upper spinal curvatures

b. Shoulder heights

c. Bony relationships—acromioclavicular joint; acromion-to-greater tubercle distance; sternoclavicular joint

d. Position of scapulae

e. Rotary position of humerus hanging freely at the side, as judged by the orientation of the epicondyles and antecubital space

f. Step deformities over the shoulder. Such a deformity may be caused by an acromioclavicular deformity, with the distal end of the clavicle lying superior to the acromion process. Flattening of the normally round deltoid may indicate an anterior dislocation of the glenohumeral joint or atrophy of the deltoid muscle. If deformity appears when traction is applied to the arm, it may be secondary to multidirectional instability, leading to inferior subluxation. This deformity is referred to as a *sulcus sign*.[52,65]

2. Soft tissues. With patient in sitting position, observe for

a. Atrophy—especially over the shoulder girdles

b. Swelling

   i. Anteriorly for joint effusion

   ii. Laterally for bursal swelling

   iii. Entire extremity for edema, as from reflex sympathetic dystrophy

c. General contours—note asymmetries

3. Skin (entire extremity and shoulder girdle)

a. Color

b. Moisture

c. Texture

d. Scars and blemishes

C. *Selective tissue tension tests*

1. Active movements (sitting). Prior to observing ipsilateral movements of the shoulder girdle, observe synchrony of motion or identical movements of the shoulder girdle bilaterally.[67] Have the patient simultaneously and sequentially abduct the arms to 90° with the elbows in 90° flexion and neutral glenohumeral rotation; horizontally extend and externally rotate the shoulders. By observing from the rear, one can notice asynchrony in such areas as shoulder elevation, indicating use of the upper trapezius to assist in abducting the arm; oscillating movements of the scapula, indicating the inability to fixate the scapula; muscle fasciculations, indicating local muscle weakness or fatigue; and excessive lateral rotation of the scapula during external rotation, indicating a tight anterior capsule which limits external rotation.

    a. Observation

        i. Routine active movements of the shoulder girdle—protraction, retraction, elevation, circumduction, and depression

        ii. Detailed examination with applied passive overpressure at the limits of each active shoulder movement

          — Flexion and extension (observe the scapulohumeral rhythm posteriorly)

          — Abduction — determine whether a painful arc exists

          — Horizontal adduction

          — External rotation — arm at side with forearm at 90° flexion

          — Internal rotation with back of hand moving up between scapulae

        iii. Note these factors:

          — Willingness to move

          — Limited range and what appears to limit it

          — Quality of movement

          — Nature of end feel

          — Presence of crepitus

          — Presence and nature of pain

          — Presence of a painful arc

2. Passive movements (supine)

    a. Perform

        i. Flexion and extension

        ii. Internal/external rotation (with elbow bent and arm at 45° abduction)

        iii. Abduction—note painful arc

        iv. Horizontal adduction

    b. Record

        i. Range of motion

        ii. Pain

        iii. End feel

        iv. Crepitus

3. Resisted isometric movements (supine)

    a. Strong isometric contractions with the arm close to the side (parentheses indicate tendons most commonly involved if test is positive)

        i. Internal rotation (subscapularis)

        ii. External rotation with arm close to side (infraspinatus)

        iii. External rotation with arm at 75° abduction (teres minor)

        iv. Abduction with arm close to side (supraspinatus)

        v. Elbow flexion (long head of biceps)

        vi. Forearm supination (biceps)

        vii. Others as necessary for differentiation of the status of the musculotendinous tissue (see Chapter 6, Peripheral Joint Mobilization Techniques).

    b. Record whether strong or weak, painful or painless

4. Joint-play movements (supine) (see Chapter 6, Peripheral Joint Mobilization Techniques)

    a. Tests

        i. Inferior glide

        ii. Lateral glide

        iii. Anterior glide

        iv. Posterior glide

        v. Backward glide

        vi. Backward and downward glide

        vii. Backward and outward glide

        viii. Scapular rotations

    b. Compare to other arm and record

        i. Amplitude of joint play (normal, restricted, hypermobile)

        ii. Presence of pain or muscle guarding

    c. Passive joint-play movements may need to include tests for the cervical and upper thoracic spine and the following related joints:

        i. Sternoclavicular joint

        ii. Acromioclavicular joint

        iii. Scapulothoracic mechanism

        iv. Costovertebral joints

D. *Neuromuscular tests.* These tests may be performed if neurologic involvement is suspected, such as that following anterior humeral dislocation, or that accompanying a cervical nerve root impingement (see Chapter 4, Assessment of Musculoskeletal Disorders).

1. Included might be upper extremity muscle testing, sensory testing, and reflex testing (see Chapter 4, Table 4–1).

2. Cervical root tension test.[24,25,27,39,54] Methods for testing for movements of the cervical nerve roots or their sleeves by applying tension are not yet clear cut.[54] However, when shoulder pain is cervical in origin, symptoms can frequently be reproduced by tension tests which have been described by Elvey.[24,25] One sequence for carrying out a cervical root tension test is outlined below.[27]

  a. The patient lies supine with the arm at the side, the elbow straight, and the arm slightly extended. Passively abduct the arm to the point of pain provocation.

  b. Release the abduction tension to a position just short of provoking the symptoms, then externally rotate the limb gently until pain is again elicited.

  c. Release the external rotation to a position just short of provoking the symptoms, then supinate the forearm while holding the arm steady.

  d. Carefully flex the elbow, without other movements added, and assess the pain response.

Note: When abnormal tension signs are present, treatment should be aimed at the neural tissue rather than capsular or muscle tissue.[26]

E. *Palpation*

  1. Skin

    a. Temperature over joint regions and entire extremity

    b. Moisture, especially distally

    c. Mobility of skin over subcutaneous tissues

    d. Tenderness, especially if neurologic involvement is suspected

    e. Texture

  2. Soft tissues

    a. Consistency, tone, and mobility of shoulder girdles and brachial region

    b. Swelling. Joint effusion may be palpable anteriorly; bursal effusion may be noted laterally

    c. Pulse. Radial pulse tests (*e.g.,* Adson's maneuver) may be carried out if thoracic outlet syndrome is suspected. Be sure to compare to the opposite side.

    d. Tenderness. Referred tenderness over the lateral brachial region accompanies most common shoulder lesions. Don't be misled.

  3. Bones and soft-tissue attachments

    a. Bony relationships

      i. Acromioclavicular joint

      ii. Sternoclavicular joint

      iii. Acromion-to-greater-tubercle distance

    b. Tenderness

      i. Tenoperiosteal junctions of the supraspinatus, infraspinatus, subscapularis, teres minor, and biceps

      ii. Acromioclavicular joint

      iii. Sternoclavicular joint

    c. Bony contours

F. *Special Tests*—Only those special tests that the examiner feels have relevance should be performed. If the patient's signs, symptoms, or dysfunction have not been reproduced, additional tests that can be performed include:

  1. Locking test.[17,53] The patient lies supine with the arm initially at the side of the body. The examiner's forearm is used to stabilize the lateral border of the scapula, and the clavicle is stabilized by placing the supinated hand under the shoulder and over the trapezius to prevent shoulder-girdle elevation (Fig. 10–21). With the other hand, the operator flexes the patient's elbow and extends the humerus on the glenohumeral joint with slight internal rotation. The humerus is abducted until it reaches a position where it becomes locked and further movement is impossible, resulting in compression against the inferior surface of the acromion. Normally this maneuver is painless. In some shoulder abnormalities the locking position may not be obtainable and may be painful.

  2. Quadrant test.[17,53] The locking position is obtained as described above. The arm is carried forward by first relaxing the pressure on the abducted arm so that it can be moved anteriorly from the coronal plane. The small arc of movement that can be felt during this anterior and rotation movement is known as the *quadrant position.* The humeral head is now unlocked; the arm and forearm are rotated externally and then brought up toward full flexion to a vertical position over the subject's head (Fig. 10–22), producing stress on the anteroinferior joint capsule. The degree and site of pain should be observed.

    Overpressure is applied to the arm, moving it backward, which increases the stress on the joint capsule and compresses

Fig. 10–21. Locking position of the shoulder causing compression to the subacromial physiological joint.

the acromioclavicular joint. The range of this movement in the sagittal plane should be noted. Patients with joint laxity will demonstrate a pronounced forward movement of the humeral head into the antero-superior portion of the axilla.

3. Anterior stability test. To test for anterior stability of the shoulder, either an apprehension test or a modification of the quadrant test may be used. When using the quadrant test, the shoulder is placed in the quadrant position and the examiner moves the head anteriorly. This maneuver may be repeated at varying degrees of abduction, feeling for anterior subluxation.[2]

Fig. 10–22. Quadrant position of the shoulder.

To perform the apprehension test (with the patient sitting), the examiner holds the patient's arm with the shoulder in 90° abduction and the elbow in 90° flexion (Fig. 10–23). Externally rotate the forearm with some arm extension. Any apprehension or pain felt by the patient suggests subluxation or prior dislocation. This test can also indicate a rotator cuff lesion or labrum tear.[2]

4. Impingement syndrome test. An impingement test is positive when pain is elicited by internal rotation of the humerus in the forward-flexed position (horizontal adduction). The examiner flexes the arm (elbow flexed, forearm pronated) passively (Fig. 10–24). This maneuver tends to drive the greater tubercle under the acromial arch. The significant structures involved are the supraspinatus and the biceps tendon.[14]

5. Test for bicipital tendinitis. The patient's pain may be reproduced by stretching or contracting (isometrically) the biceps tendon. While resisting elbow flexion with one hand, the examiner simultaneously palpates over the bicipital groove with the other hand. A number of special tests have been devised to reveal involvement of the biceps muscle or tendon and the integrity of the transverse humeral ligament; these include the Yergason test, Lippman test, Ludington test, and Booth and Marve transverse humeral ligament test.[7,44,48,84]

G. *Miscellaneous.* Because the shoulder and

Fig. 10-23. Apprehension test for anterior stability consists of abduction and lateral rotation of the humerus *(A)*, combined with forward and downward pressure on the humeral head *(B)*. When performed at 90° or more abduction, the test stresses the inferior glenohumeral ligament; when performed at 45° abduction, it stresses the subscapularis and middle glenohumeral ligament.

upper extremity articulate with the thorax and spine, they function as a kinetic chain. Involvement of costosternal and costovertebral joints and the upper thoracic and cervical spine can all refer symptoms to the shoulder and may need to be checked. Because thoracic outlet syndrome includes pain in the shoulder, specific tests should be used to rule it out; these include the Adson maneuver, hyperabduction test, and the costoclavicular syndrome test (see Chapter 19, The Cervical Spine).[1,33,46,76] Other conditions that can cause or contribute to thoracic outlet syndrome include fascial fusions of muscles, malunion of old clavicular fractures, the presence of a cervical rib, pseudarthrosis of the clavicle, and exostosis of the first rib.

H. *Ancillary Tests.* After completion of the comprehensive physical examination, there are additional tests that may be indicated to provide supplemental information for confirmation of a diagnosis. When possible, evaluation of power and endurance and objective recordings of strength can be valuable. Isokinetic testing is effective in following the progress of a rehabilitation program.[82]

Nerve conduction studies have proven beneficial in diagnosing specific neurologic lesions. If it is necessary to further evaluate the intra-articular aspects of the shoulder joint for exact diagnosis, arthrography, arthrotomography, computed tomography, and arthroscopy are available. The use of arthrography for the shoulder has been of

Fig. 10-24. Shoulder impingement syndrome test for possible involvement of the supraspinatus and biceps tendons.

principle value for evaluation of rotator cuff pathology.[16]

COMMON LESIONS

IMPINGEMENT SYNDROME

The impingement symptom complex primarily involves the coracoacromial arch intruding on the rotator cuff, subacromial bursa, or biceps tendon.[14] There are three theories regarding the factors involved in the development of impingement syndrome: the mechanical–anatomic theory; the vascular compromise theory; and the theory proposed by Perry,[69] which implicates kinesiologic factors that limit scapular rotation or promote uncoordinated muscular activity.

Neer, a strong advocate of the mechanical–anatomic theory, recognizes three stages of the syndrome (1) a benign, self-limiting, over-use syndrome, (2) the development of thickening and fibrosis followed by repeated episodes of the first stage, and (3) development of bony changes including spurs and eburnation of the humeral tuberosity leading to possible complications such as rotator cuff tears.[62]

Tendinitis at the shoulder is a very common disorder. It occurs in young active individuals as well as in older persons, and about equally in males and females. In the case of a younger person it may be caused by activities such as tennis, racquetball, or baseball, which increase the stress levels to the rotator cuff tendons. In the older person it is more likely to be a degenerative lesion. Because of the relatively poor blood supply near the insertion of the supraspinatus, nutrition to the area may not meet the metabolic demands of the tendon tissue. The resultant focal cell death sets up an inflammatory response, probably due to the release of irritating enzymes and dead tissue acting as a foreign body.[21,50] The body may react by laying down scar tissue or calcific deposits. Such calcific deposits may be visible on radiographs; however, they are often seen in the absence of symptoms and, conversely, they are not always present in known cases of tendinitis. Superficial migration of these deposits with rupture into the underside of the subdeltoid bursa is thought to be a major cause of acute bursitis at the shoulder.[51] Because of the poor blood supply to the region, adequate repair may not take place, and the lesion may develop into an actual tear in the tendon.

The degenerative lesions tend to be persistent, with little likelihood of spontaneous resolution. The combined effects of poor blood flow and continued stress to the tendon do not allow for adequate maturation of the healing tissue. It is not unusual for a patient to describe a history of several years of constant or intermittent problems with the shoulder. This by no means should suggest that such patients cannot be helped, since they do respond well, and often dramatically, to the program outlined below. Transverse friction massage is an essential component of the treatment program in chronic cases. The beneficial effects of friction massage in such cases are not well understood. However, it is proposed that an increase in the mobility of the developing, or developed, scar tissue takes place without stressing the tendon longitudinally (see Chapter 8, Friction Massage). This prevents the healing tissue from being continually retorn during daily activities.

A factor that may contribute to chronicity and recurrence is weakening of the rotator cuff muscles from reflex inhibition or from actual disuse. Such weakening would predispose to subacromial impingement during elevation of the arm and further mechanical irritation to the site of the lesion. Rotator cuff strengthening is, therefore, an important part of the treatment program. However, if recent or repeated steroid injections to the tendon have been performed, it is necessary to proceed gradually with the strengthening program. Although local steroids do relieve the pain through inhibiting the inflammatory response, they have an antianabolic effect on connective tissue, which may result in structural weakening of the injected tendon.[79]

The differential diagnosis of shoulder pain has been well documented in other publications, and specific conditions afflicting athletes have also been reported.[2,9,29,31,67,75]

According to Cahill, the four types of pathologic processes most often neglected are glenohumeral instability, primary acromioclavicular lesions, groove syndrome, and quadrilateral space syndrome. Of these conditions, glenohumeral instability is the one most frequently confused with impingement syndromes.[14] It should be apparent that treatment for impingement syndrome will not benefit the patient with instability.

I. History
   A. *Site of pain*—Lateral brachial region, possibly referred below to the elbow in the C5 or C6 sclerotome
   B. *Nature of pain*—Sharp twinges felt on various movements, such as abduction, putting on jacket, or reaching above shoulder level

C. *Onset of pain*—Usually gradual with no known trauma. May be related to occupational or recreational overuse. May have been present for many months, or even years.

II. Physical Examination

A. *Active movements*—Relatively full range of motion. Often a painful arc is present at midrange of abduction. There is usually slight limitation and pain at full elevation due to pinching of the lesion between the greater tubercle and the posterior rim of the glenoid cavity.

B. *Passive movements*
1. Essentially full range of motion
2. Pain at full elevation, but full range of motion is usually present
3. May be a painful arc on rotation and abduction
4. May be pain on stretch of the involved tendon (*e.g.*, on full internal rotation in the case of supraspinatus or infraspinatus tendinitis)

C. *Resisted movements*—The key test
1. Maximal isometric contraction of the relevant muscle will reproduce the pain.
2. In the case of simple tendinitis, the contraction will be fairly strong; if an actual tear exists, it will be weak.
3. The supraspinatus is the most commonly involved tendon.
4. Others (biceps, subscapularis, teres minor) are rarely involved.

D. *Palpation*
1. Tenderness usually over the involved tendon, near its insertion
2. Usually referred tenderness over the lateral brachial region. *Don't be misled.*

E. *Inspection*
1. Usually negative
2. Some atrophy may be noted if a chronic tear exists.

III. Management.
The presence or absence of a calcific deposit, as demonstrated by radiographs, should not affect the treatment plan.

A. *Ultrasound*
1. Resolution of inflammatory exudates
2. Increased blood flow to assist the healing process
3. May provide some pain relief although persistent pain is usually not a problem

B. *Friction massage*—A key component of the treatment program
1. To form mobile scar

2. The hyperemia induced by the massage may enhance blood flow to the area to assist the healing response.

C. *Instruction in appropriate use of the arm*
1. Strict avoidance of activities that may cause impingement or tension stress at the site of involvement while formation of painless scar takes place
2. Gradual return to normal use as healing progresses

D. *Restrengthening* of involved muscles and other measures to restore normal joint mechanics

General Guidelines

In most of cases of tendinitis at the shoulder, perhaps the only dispensable component of the above program is the use of ultrasound. In the authors' experience, failure to appropriately institute any of the remaining measures will increase the likelihood that treatment will be unsuccessful or that the patient will suffer a recurrence. The younger person whose primary complaint is pain during recreational activities such as baseball or racquetball must be advised that temporary abstinence from certain activities is an essential remedial measure. However, restricting activities to "resting" the part is usually not sufficient in itself to effect a resolution of the pathology, although the reduction in pain experienced may often suggest this. Usually, resumption of activities will be accompanied by a recurrence of the previous symptoms because simply resting the part does not ensure the development of a mature, mobile cicatrix. This is also true for the older person, who may experience pain during normal daily activities. Although appropriate control of activities is usually necessary for resolution of the problem, it alone is usually not adequate. The use of friction massage and, perhaps more importantly, restrengthening exercises, should not be excluded.

The therapist must, through a complete history, become aware of the patient's habitual daily activities. This is important because the patient often engages in activities that may contribute to the problem without actually realizing it. Such "fatigue" pathologies typically result from the cumulation of otherwise asymptomatic stresses. Activities that particularly need to be avoided are those involving repetitive elevation of the arm to shoulder level or above.

The importance of strengthening exercises can be appreciated by understanding the key role the muscles play in the normal functioning of the shoulder joint. As mentioned earlier, the supraspinatus is largely responsible for maintaining adequate depression of the humeral head during abduction. In the presence of a weak supraspinatus, the head of the humerus will tend to ride high in the glenoid during elevation of the arm because of the disproportionate contraction of the deltoid. This would predispose to impingement of the greater tubercle, along with its tendinous attachments, against the coracoacromial arch. Thus, in cases of tendinitis there is a tendency toward muscle atrophy from reflex inhibition or disuse that may often be a factor in prolonging the pathologic process.

Remedial strengthening exercises are best performed with the arm close to the side to prevent the possibility of impingement and reflex inhibition during performance of the exercises.

During the early stages of rehabilitation, isometric exercises are performed with the shoulder in a neutral position following warm-up. *Warm-up* may be defined as an increase in body heat by active muscular use for the purposes of lowering soft-tissue viscosity and enhancing body chemical and metabolic functions in order to protect and prepare the body for more aggressive physical activity.[7,43] General central muscular body activity may be used (*e.g.,* calisthenics or riding a stationary bicycle) or local exercises (*e.g.,* saw or pendulum exercises).[12,28] Active muscular activity is likely to be more productive than passive means of heating, because passive heating does not enhance the metabolic and cardiac factors that are also important.[64] The position of the shoulder can be altered in several ways to enhance isometric strengthening of appropriate muscle groups at different angles and lengths in the pain-free range.[28] If pain from joint compression occurs, the use of manual resistance and slight traction to the joint as resistance is given is helpful. Ice is frequently used to reduce postexercise soreness. However, the value of ice alone has been recently questioned, based on experimental data.[83]

As range of motion improves and healing progresses, the patient is graduated to isotonic exercises for the rotator cuff muscles with manual resistance, free weights, or elastic tension cord resistance (isoflex exercises). Isoflex exercises are convenient (particularly for home programs) and effective, and they allow unlimited arcs of motion with both concentric and eccentric muscle training.[23,28,64]

To strengthen the supraspinatus, the patient should stand with the arm at the side and rotate the shoulder internally to pronate the forearm. Then, moving the arm in a diagonal direction of abduction, the patient should aim to achieve 90° abduction at 30° to 40° in front of the coronal position. This position aligns the muscle parallel to arm movement (in the plane of the scapula), and in this position the electromyographic output of the supraspinatus is greatest.[36]

A strong rotator cuff is necessary to depress the humeral head in the glenoid during overhead activities.[40] It is therefore important to first attain a strong rotator cuff before initiating shoulder elevation above 90°. Range of motion can be increased gradually as long as impingement is avoided.

Two exercises that are also important in the prevention of impingement are shoulder shrugs and push-ups with the arm abducted to 90°.[12] These exercises strengthen the upper trapezius and serratus anterior, providing normal scapular rotation and thus allowing the acromion to elevate without contracting the rotator cuff.

Shoulder elevation above 90° should be initiated with a D1F (flexion–adduction–external rotation) proprioceptive neuromuscular (PNF) pattern before advancing to D2F (flexion–abduction–external rotation) pattern.[78] Rotator cuff dysfunction may result in both reduced humeral depression and external rotation.[6,13,15] Neer has reported that the functional arc of shoulder elevation is not lateral, as previously thought, but forward. This results in the suprahumeral structures being impinged against the anterior part of the acromion in cases where the humerus is internally rather than externally rotated.[61]

The advanced phase of rehabilitation concentrates on the progressive return to normal function. In general the patient continues self-stretching of the rotator cuff and inferior capsule as normal strength and endurance return (see Chapter 7, Automobilization Techniques for the Extremities). During this phase, exercises may be performed on an exercise machine (*e.g.,* Nautilus®, Universal®). Free weights should be used until the patient can safely transfer to the exercise machines for resistive exercise.[12] Pool therapy can be a very effective functional modality for power and endurance training using PNF patterns with hand paddles facilitated by the isokinetic resistance of water.[26]

Total body fitness should be initiated no later than the early part of the advanced stage of rehabilitation. This program should consist of exercises to develop cardiovascular fitness, leg strength, and endurance.[59] This is especially important for athletes who engage in sports that predominantly use the muscles of the upper extremity, but also require strong lower extremities. It is important to maintain the central cardiovascular system by general aerobic conditioning. A specific aerobic exercise to enhance the endurance of the upper extremity muscle group consists of sitting behind a stationary bike and pedalling with the hands.

Rehabilitation following surgical repair of the rotator cuff is lengthy and characterized by slow progress. The surgical techniques are beyond the scope of this text, but are well documented in the literature.[7,20,42,58,75,81] Rehabilitation requires an average of 12 to 14 months for an athlete to return to a level of activity that was maintained prior to the injury.[27] General mobilization to restore accessory motion should be initiated following immobilization. Caudal glides of the humeral head should be emphasized to increase the available space between the acromion and humerus (see Chapter 6, Peripheral Joint Mobilization Techniques). A program of general shoulder strengthening, capsular stretching, and specific rotator cuff strengthening exercises should be continued as long as the patient uses the shoulder to any great degree in activities of daily living and sports.[12]

Many injuries of the shoulder can be classified as overuse problems resulting from repetitive stresses with minimal abnormalities.[77] Abnormalities that represent deficits in strength, flexibility, or technique are often easily remedied through appropriate intervention by a skilled therapist.

The successful use of friction massage requires precision with respect to the site of application and the intensity or depth of application (see Chapter 8, Friction Massage). If for some reason it is not practical for the patient to be followed regularly for treatment, instruction of a family member in the technique of application or instruction to the patient in self-administration should be considered. However, application by a skilled and experienced practitioner is preferred, when feasible, to ensure that the appropriate technique is used and to accurately monitor and document results. As athletic activities or activities involving repetitive elevation of the arm are resumed, instructing the patient in self-administered friction massage prior to engaging in the particular function may be an important preventive measure.

ADHESIVE CAPSULITIS—FROZEN SHOULDER

Capsular tightening at the shoulder is also a common disorder, usually referred to as *frozen shoulder* or *adhesive capsulitis*. The majority of cases seen by physical therapists are those in which no specific cause can be determined for the stiffening. It affects women more often than men, and middle-aged and older persons more often than younger persons. It is probable that some of the so-called idiopathic cases of frozen shoulder come about from an alteration in

scapulohumeral alignment, as occurs with thoracic kyphosis. This is consistent with the fact that women are more frequently affected, since women are also more predisposed to developing thoracic kyphosis than men. Some believe this problem to be a progression of rotator cuff lesions, in which the inflammatory/degenerative process spreads to include the entire joint capsule, resulting in capsular fibrosis.[21,51,57] While this may be so in some cases, there are two major contradictions to this proposal: rotator cuff tendinitis affects men and women fairly equally, whereas frozen shoulder is much more common in women; and persons with a frozen shoulder rarely present with coexistent tendinitis, as evidenced by the absence of pain on resisted movement.

It is commonly said that these people stop using the arm because for some reason it is painful, and motion is therefore lost from disuse. In our experience, this is rarely the case. Instead, the loss of motion is responsible for the pain. The patient continues to use the arm until the restriction of motion progresses to the extent that it interferes with daily activities. It is not until this point that the patient feels much pain or is aware of a problem with the arm. The woman first notices that it is difficult to comb her hair and fasten a bra. She may also be awakened at night when rolling onto the affected side. The man notes difficulty reaching into the hip pocket and combing his hair, and may be similarly awakened at night. Because much shoulder motion can be lost before interfering with daily activities of persons in this age group, these patients invariably do not seek medical help until the shoulder has lost about 90° abduction, 60° flexion, 60° external rotation, and 45° internal rotation. In fact, it is somewhat rare to see a patient present with significantly more, or significantly less, than this amount of movement. Of course, there are some cases of capsular tightening at the shoulder that are associated with particular disease states or conditions. Conditions that might result in capsular tightness at the glenohumeral joint include:

—*Degenerative joint disease*—This is rare at the shoulder and, if present, is relatively asymptomatic.
—*Rheumatoid arthritis*—The smaller joints of the hand and feet are usually affected first.
—*Immobilization*—For example, following fracture of the arm, forearm, or wrist, or dislocation of the shoulder.[32]
—*Reflex sympathetic dystrophy* (see Chapter 12, The Wrist and Hand Complex). This condition may follow certain visceral disorders such as a myo-

cardial infarction, or it may follow some trauma, such as a Colles' fracture. Capsular stiffening of the joints of the hand, wrist, and shoulder is a common component of this syndrome. A frozen shoulder occurring in conjunction with a reflex sympathetic dystrophy is usually more refractory to treatment, probably because of the abnormal pain state that tends to accompany the disorder.

I. **History**
   A. *Site of pain* — Lateral brachial region, possibly referred distally into the C5 or C6 segment
   B. *Nature of pain* — Varying from a constant dull ache to pain felt only on activities involving the movement into the restricted ranges. The patient is often awakened at night when rolling onto the painful shoulder.
   C. *Onset of pain* — Very gradual. May be related to minor trauma, immobilization, chest surgery, or myocardial infarction. More commonly, no cause can be cited.

II. **Physical Examination**
   A. *Active movements* — Limitation of motion in a capsular pattern: little glenohumeral movement on abduction, much difficulty and substitution getting the hand behind the neck. Usually there is some limitation when flexing the arm or trying to put the hand behind the back.
   B. *Passive movements* — Limitation in a capsular pattern: external rotation is markedly restricted, abduction moderately restricted, flexion and internal rotation are somewhat limited.
      1. May be limited to pain with a muscle-guarding end feel (acute)
      2. May be limited by stiffness with a capsular end feel (chronic)
   C. *Joint play* — Restriction of most joint-play movements, especially inferior glide
   D. *Resisted isometric movments* — Strong and painless, unless a tendinitis also is present
   E. *Palpation* — Often referred tenderness over the lateral brachial region. There is often a feeling of increased muscle tone, with induration over the lateral brachial region.
   F. *Inspection* — Often negative. Observe for a surgical scar.

III. **Acute vs. Chronic**
   A. *Acute*
      1. Pain radiates to below the elbow.
      2. The patient is awakened by pain at night.
      3. On passive movement, limitation is due to pain and muscle guarding, rather than stiffness *per se*.
   B. *Chronic*
      1. Pain is localized to the lateral brachial region.
      2. The patient is not awakened by pain at night.
      3. On passive movement, limitation is due to capsular stiffness, and pain is felt only when the capsule is stretched.
   C. *Subacute* — Some combination of the above findings

IV. **Management**
   A. *Acute stage*
      1. Relief of pain and muscle guarding to allow early, gentle mobilization
         a. Ice or superficial heat
         b. Grade I or II joint-play oscillations
      2. Maintenance of existing range of motion and efforts to gently begin increasing range of motion
         a. Grade I or II joint-play mobilization. At this stage it is often best to perform these with the patient lying prone and the arm hanging freely at the side of the plinth. Inferior glide is particularly comfortable for most patients and is usually most helpful in relieving muscle spasm. This is an important movement to perform because the spasm, which is usually present in the acute stage, causes the humerus to assume a superior position in the glenoid cavity, further interfering with normal joint mechanics.
         b. Initiation of active assisted range of motion exercises at home, such as automobilization techniques, wand and pendulum exercises.
      3. Instruction in isometric strengthening exercises, especially for the rotator cuff muscles. The movement associated with isotonic exercises will usually cause pain and reflex inhibition, thus reducing their effectiveness.
      4. Prevention of excessive kyphosis and shoulder-girdle protraction. When appropriate, provide instruction in postural awareness for the upper trunk and shoulder girdles such that the patient learns to differentiate proprioceptively between a kyphotic, protracted posture and a relatively upright, retracted position. A sys-

tem of regular "postural checks" should be incorporated into the patient's daily activities.

5. Gradual progression of the above program as the condition becomes more chronic (see below)

B. *Chronic stage* — Increase the extensibility of the joint capsule, with special attention to the anteroinferior aspect of the capsule.

1. Ultrasound preceding or accompanying stretching procedures.
2. Specific joint mobilizations with emphasis on the anteroinferior capsular stretch (see Chapter 6 Peripheral Joint Mobilization Techniques and Chapter 7, Automobilization Techniques for the Extremities)

General Guidelines

When using specific joint mobilization techniques in the presence of a chronically tight joint, the primary objective is to stretch the joint capsule. In order to do so the more vigorous, grade IV, techniques must be used. It is usually best, however, to commence with grade I or II oscillations in preparation for more intensive stretching. The lower grades of oscillations promote reduced muscle spasm and pain, probably by increasing large-fiber, sensory input. Perhaps the best technique to use at the initiation of glenohumeral mobilization is *inferior glide* with the arm to the side, because this technique, especially, seems to induce relaxation. For this reason, this is also a good technique for relieving the "cramping" sensation a patient may experience during more vigorous movements.

Prior to or during capsular stretching procedures, you may use ultrasound to help increase the extensibility of the tissue. For example, perform the anteroinferior capsular stretch while an assistant directs ultrasound to the anteroinferior aspect of the joint. Specific joint mobilization techniques are most effective when used in conjunction with the motions they are intended to restore, such as inferior glide simultaneous with abduction or flexion, posterior capsular stretch with internal rotation, and anterior capsular stretch with external rotation. It is also possible to combine passive stretching with appropriate accessory movements (*e.g.*, flexion with inferior glide or abduction with inferior glide).

Instruct the patient in home range of motion exercises. These are necessary to maintain gains made in treatment and to use as a measure to help increase movement. A major goal of the treatment program is to promote independence in mobilization procedures. Once approximately 120° abduction, 140° flexion, and 60° external rotation are achieved, many patients will continue to make satisfactory improvement in range of motion by continuing on a supervised home exercise program. From the outset, though, it is difficult for most patients to make substantial gains in range of motion with home exercises alone; skillfully applied passive movement will significantly accelerate improvement in the early phases of treatment. The probable reason for this is that in the relatively acute stage, the reflex muscle spasm that accompanies active movement of the joint prevents the patient from exerting an effective stretch to the joint capsule — he simply fights against his own muscles. The therapist skilled in the use of passive joint mobilization procedures is able to localize the stretch to specific portions of the joint capsule and carefully graduate the intensity of the stretch to avoid eliciting protective muscle contraction. Also, the therapist can combine joint-play movements with certain movements of the arm to reduce cartilaginous or body impingement at the extremes of movement. For example, while moving the arm into abduction, the therapist can passively move the head of the humerus inferiorly to prevent impingement of the greater tubercle against the acromial arch, which would tend to occur from the loss of external rotation and from a loss of inferior glide of the joint. By doing so, muscle spasm is reduced and a more effective stretch to the inferior capsule is effected. In fact, until significant gains in external rotation are made, the patient should not be instructed to stretch into abduction on his own, because attempts to do so may traumatize the subacromial tissues more than stretching the inferior aspect of the joint capsule.

It must be emphasized that the primary goal of treatment is restoration of painless functional range of movement and that regaining full movement of the arm is not always realistic. This is especially true for individuals with some degree of increased thoracic kyphosis, because full elevation of the arm involves extension of the upper thoracic spine. For these patients "normal" elevation is usually about 150° to 160°. Range of motion of the uninvolved shoulder should serve as a guide for setting treatment goals.

In the more acute cases of frozen shoulder, the patient's major complaint is often the inability to get a good night's sleep. Each time the patient rolls onto the involved side, he is awakened by pain. The resultant fatigue adds to the patient's general debilitation. Fortunately, with appropriate management this is usually the first aspect of the problem to resolve. In fact, subjective improvement, in the form of significant reduction in night pain, will usually precede any evidence of objective improvement, such as increased range of motion. It has been our experience that one or two sessions of gentle joint play oscillations, especially into inferior glide, preceded by superficial heat or ice, will frequently be sufficient to alleviate nocturnal symptoms. This leads us to speculate whether the night pain may be more related to the fact that the joint is compressed in a position in which the humerus is held into a cephalad malalignment by muscle spasm, rather than being the result of compression of an inflamed joint capsule. At any rate, it seems that relaxation of the associated muscle spasm is one of the more important measures in reducing pain in the acute phase.

In the chronic stage, pain is primarily the result of repeated tensile stresses to the tight joint capsule during daily activities. Treatment should be directed primarily toward increasing range of motion, although some restriction of activities may be warranted. For the most part, however, in the chronic stage, encourage the patient to use the arm as much as tolerable to minimize habitual disuse, which can be a factor in perpetuating the disorder.

Some authors claim that adhesive capsulitis is a self-limiting disorder, and that spontaneous resolution can be expected in about 12 months' time.[58,63,79] This has not been consistent with our clinical experience. Even if it were the case, this should not be used as a reason for not instituting active treatment because, with appropriate therapy, satisfactory results can be expected within no longer than 3 to 4 months. The only frequent exception is when a frozen shoulder results as part of a sympathetic reflex dystrophy. These cases are often quite refractory to conservative management and may require supplementary measures such as sympathetic blocks or manipulation under anesthesia.

Although in most cases of frozen shoulder the prognosis for functional recovery is good, the time frame of recovery is rarely linear. Improvement tends to be characterized by spurts and plateaus. Both the therapist and the patient should be cognizant of this to avoid undue frustration during periods of limited progress.

ACUTE BURSITIS

Acute bursitis is relatively rare and is thought by many to occur secondary to calcific tendinitis, in which the deposit migrates superficially into the floor of the subdeltoid bursa.[57]

I. **History**
   A. *Site of pain*—Lateral brachial region, possibly referred distally
   B. *Nature of pain*—Intense, constant, dull, sometimes throbbing pain. The patient may present with the arm in a sling, or supporting the arm at the elbow with the uninvolved hand. During this acute period, very little relief is found in any position. All movements are reported to be painful.
   C. *Onset of pain*—May be a history suggestive of a chronic tendinitis. The acute pain, however, usually arises over a period of 12 to 72 hours, with a gradual buildup of pain over this period.

II. **Physical Examination**
   A. *Active movements*—Marked restriction in all planes with evidence of rather severe pain on attempts to elevate the arm
   B. *Passive movements*—Restricted by pain in a noncapsular pattern with an "empty" end feel; no resistance is felt to movement, but the patient insists that movement be ceased because of intense pain. Rotation with the arm at the side may be fairly free, but abduction past 60° or flexion past 90° is usually not permitted because of complaints of severe pain.
   C. *Resisted movements*—There may be some hesitation to perform a maximal contraction, with perhaps some pain on resisted abduction, owing to squeezing of the inflamed bursa. When carefully tested, however, most contractions are strong and painless.
   D. *Palpation*—Possibly some warmth and swelling noted over the region overlying the subdeltoid bursa. There is usually considerable tenderness in this area.
   E. *Inspection*—Often unremarkable. Possibly some visable swelling laterally at the side of the bursa

III. **Management**
   A. *Early stages*
      1. Resolution of the acute inflammatory process
         a. Ice or superficial heat
         b. Support of the arm with a sling to reduce postural tone in the muscles adjacent to the bursa, thereby relieving pressure to the inflamed area
      2. Maintaining range of motion—Gentle active-assisted exercises such as wand and pendulum exercises
   B. *Chronic stage*

With the above measures, it is rare for the condition to remain "acute" for longer than a few days. Resolution of the acute stage is characterized by the absence of pain at rest and localization of pain to the lateral brachial region. The patient is able to actively elevate the arm to at least 90° flexion or abduction.

1. Resolution of chronic inflammatory process. Bursitis at the shoulder and of the trochanteric bursa are, in our experience, the two conditions in which the use of ultrasound to provide relief of symptoms, in the presence of a subacute or chronic inflammation, will often have an unequivocally beneficial effect. The increased blood flow induced by the local heat apparently aids in a more rapid resolution of inflammatory irritants and debris.

   Unlike tendinitis or frozen shoulder, acute bursitis at the shoulder tends to be self-limiting over a period of several weeks. With appropriate therapy few patients have significant pain or disability 2 weeks after the onset of acute symptoms. However, because calcific rotator cuff tendinitis is often a preexisting condition, it is important as the acute phase of the bursitis resolves to test for the presence of tendinitis, the clinical signs of which may be obscured by the acute symptoms of bursitis. If tendinitis does exist, appropriate treatment measures should be instituted (see previous discussion on tendinitis).

2. Restoration of full range of motion, joint play, and strength
   a. Instruction in home range of motion procedures
   b. Specific joint mobilization (automobilization or passive movements) if warranted
   c. Instruction in home strengthening exercises.

OTHER LESIONS

There are, of course, other more serious lesions that commonly affect the shoulder, such as anterior dislocation and acromioclavicular joint separation. These are usually not seen by a physical therapist until they have been treated by the physician with prolonged immobilization, or perhaps surgery followed by immobilization. At this point, the therapist no longer deals with the original injury so much as with the effects of immobilization. As a result, the goals and techniques of management in such cases are often essentially the same as those for a patient with capsular tightness. There are, however, some special considerations with which one should be familiar, depending on the original problem. For example, surgery for recurrent anterior dislocation may be performed with the specific intent of limiting external rotation to help provide some anterior stabilization.[15,21] Or, following an anterior dislocation, it may be desirable for the sake of preventing recurrence to allow the anterior capsule to heal in a tightened state. In both cases emphasis on regaining external rotation will be less than what it might be in other cases of capsular tightness. Certain surgical fixations for acromioclavicular separation, such as those involving insertion of a screw from the clavicle to the coracoid, may permanently restrict normal clavicular axial rotation. As long as such a screw is still in place, full elevation of the arm should not be expected; it can only occur if the screw should break.

Although it is not within the scope of this book to discuss them at length, the therapist must be familiar with these other types of injuries, the current surgical procedures, and such special considerations as those mentioned above.

REFERENCES

1. Adson, AW, Coffey JR: Cervical Rib. Ann Surg 85:839, 1961
2. Andrews JR, Gillogly S: Physical examination of the shoulder in throwing athletes. *In* Zarins B, Andrews JR, Carson WG (eds): Injuries to the Throwing Arm. Philadelphia, WB Saunders, 1985
3. Basmajian JV: Factors preventing downward dislocation of the abducted shoulder joint. J Bone Joint Surg 41(A):1182–1186, 1959
4. Basmajian JV: Weight-bearing by ligaments and muscles. Can J Surg 4:166–170, 1961
5. Basmajian JV: Surgical anatomy and function of the arm–trunk mechanism. Surg Clin North Am 43:1471–1482, 1963
6. Basmajian JV: Muscles Alive: Their Functions Revealed by Electromyography, 4th ed. Baltimore, Williams & Wilkins, 1977
7. Bateman JE, Welsh RP: Surgery of the Shoulder. Saint Louis, CV Mosby, 1984
8. Bechtol CO: Biomechanics of the shoulder. Clin Orthop 146:37–41, 1980
9. Blackwell TA: Throwing injuries to the shoulder. *In* Donatelli R (ed): Physical Therapy of the Shoulder. New York, Churchill Livingstone, 1987
10. Blakely RL, Palmer ML: Analysis of rotation accompanying shoulder flexion. Phys Ther 64:1214–1216, 1984

11. Booth RE, Marvel JP: Differential diagnosis of shoulder pain. Orthop Clin North Am 6(2):353–379, 1975

12. Brewster CE, Shields CL, Seto JL, Morrissey MC: Rehabilitation of the upper extremity. *In* Shields CL (ed): Manual of Sports Surgery, pp 62–90. New York, Springer–Verlag, 1987

13. Brunnstrom S: Clinical Kinesiology. Philadelphia, FA Davis, 1962

14. Cahill BR: Understanding shoulder pain. Inst Course Lect 34:332–336, 1985

15. Calliet R: Shoulder Pain. Philadelphia, FA Davis, 1981

16. Codman EA: The Shoulder. Boston, Thomas Todd, 1934

17. Corrigan B, Maitland GD: Practical Orthopaedic Medicine. Boston, Butterworth, 1985

18. DeLuca CJ, Forrest WJ: Force analysis of individual muscles acting simultaneously on the shoulder joint during isometric abduction. J Biomech 6:385–395, 1973

19. Dempster WT: Mechanisms of shoulder movement. Arch Phys Med Rehabil 46:49–67, 1965

20. DePalma AF: Surgical anatomy and function of the acromioclavicular and sternoclavicular joints. Surg Clin North Am 43:1541–1550, 1963

21. DePalma AF: Surgical anatomy of the rotator cuff and natural history of degenerative periarthritis. Surg Clin North Am 43:1507–1521, 1963

22. DePalma AF: Surgery of the Shoulder, 2nd ed. Philadelphia, JB Lippincott, 1973

23. Dominguez RH, Gajda R: Total Body Training. New York, Warner Books, 1982

24. Elvey RL: Brachial plexus tension test and the pathoanatomical origin of arm pain. *In* Idczack RM (ed): Aspects of Manipulative Therapy. Carlton, Australia, Lincoln Institute of Health Sciences, 1981

25. Elvey RL: The investigation of arm pain. *In* Grieves GP (ed): Modern Manual Therapy of the Vertebral Column. New York, Churchill Livingstone, 1986

26. Fish GH: Some observations of motion at the shoulder joint. Can Med Assoc J 50:213–216, 1944

27. Grieves GP: Mobilisation of the Spine: Notes on Examination, Assessment and Clinical Methods, 4th ed. New York, Churchill Livingstone, 1984

28. Freedman L, Munro R: Abduction of the arm in the scapular plane: Scapular and glenohumeral movements. J Bone Joint Surg 48(A):1503–1510, 1966

29. Halbach JW, Tank RT: The shoulder. *In* Gould JA, Davies GJ (ed): Orthopaedic and Sports Physical Therapy. St Louis, CV Mosby, 1985

30. Hart DL, Carmichael SW: Biomechancis of the shoulder. J Orthop Sports Phys Ther 6:229–234, 1985

31. Hawkins RJ, Kennedy JC: Impingement Syndrome in Athletes. Am J Sports Med 8:151–157, 1980

32. Heppenstall RB: Fractures of the proximal humerus. Orthop Clin North Am 6(2):467–475, 1975

33. Howell JW: Evaluation and management of thoracic outlet syndrome. *In* Donatelli R (ed): Physical Therapy of the Shoulder. New York, Churchill Livingstone, 1987

34. Howell SM, Imobersteg M, Seger DH, Marone PJ: Clarification of the role of the supraspinatus muscle in shoulder function. J Bone Joint Surg 68(A):398–404, 1986

35. Inman VT, Saunders JB, Abbott LC: Observations of the function of the shoulder joint. J Bone Joint Surg 26(A):1–30, 1944

36. Jobe FW, Moynes DR: Delineation of diagnostic criteria and a rehabilitation program for rotator cuff injuries. Am J Sports Med 10:336–339, 1982

37. Johnston TB: The movements of the shoulder joint: Plea for the use of the 'plane of the scapula' as plane of reference for movements occuring at the humeroscapular joint. J Bone Joint Surg 25(B):252–260, 1937

38. Kapandji IA: The Physiology of the Joints, Vol 1: Upper Limb. New York, Churchill Livingstone, 1970

39. Kenneally M, Rubenach H, Elvey RL: The upper limb tension test: The SLR test of the arm. *In* Grant R (ed): Physical Therapy of the Cervical and Thoracic Spine. New York, Churchill Livingstone, 1988

40. Kent BE: Functional anatomy of the shoulder complex: A review. Phys Ther 51:867–888, 1971

41. Kessell L, Walson M: The painful arc syndrome. J Bone Joint Surg 59(B):166–172, 1977

42. Kisner C, Colby LA: Therapeutic Exercises: Foundations and Techniques. Philadelphia, FA Davis, 1985

43. Lehmann F, Warren CG, Scham SM: Therapeutic Heat and Cold. Clin Orthop 99:207–245, 1974

44. Lippman RK: Frozen shoulder: perarthritis: bicipital tenosynovitis. Arch Surg 47:283–296, 1943

45. Lockhart RD: Movements of the normal shoulder joint. J Anat 64:288–302, 1936

46. Lord JW, Rosati LM: Neurovascular compression syndromes of the upper extremity. Clinical Symposia 23:3–23, 1971

47. Lucas DB: Biomechanics of the shoulder joint. Arch Surg 107:425–432, 1973

48. Ludington NA: Rupture of the long head of biceps flexor cubiti muscle. Ann Surg 27:358–363, 1923

49. MacConaill MH, Basmajian JV: Muscles and Movements: A Basis for Human Kinesiology. Baltimore, Williams & Wilkins, 1969

50. MacNab I: Local steroids in orthopaedic conditions. Scott Med J 17:176–186, 1972

51. MacNab I: Rotator cuff tendinitis. Ann R Coll Surg Engl 53:271–287, 1973

52. Magee DJ: The shoulder. *In* Magee DJ: Orthopedic Physical Assessment. Philadelphia, WB Saunders, 1987

53. Maitland GD: Peripheral Manipulations. Boston, Butterworths, 1977

54. Maitland GD: Vertebral Manipulations, 5th ed. Boston, Butterworths, 1986

55. Matsen FA: Biomechanics of the shoulder. *In* Frankel VH, Nordin M (ed): Basic Biomechanics of the Skeletal System. Philadelphia, Lea & Febiger, 1970

56. Moore KL: Clinically Oriented Anatomy. Baltimore, Williams & Wilkins, 1980

57. Moseley HF: The natural history and clinical syn-

dromes produced by calcific deposits in the rotator cuff. Surg Clin North Am 43:1489–1492, 1963

58. Moseley HF: Shoulder Lesions, 3rd ed. New York, Churchill Livingstone, 1969

59. Morehouse L, Gross L: Maximum Performance. New York, Simon & Shuster, 1977

60. Najenson T, Yacibovich E, Pikelni S: Rotator cuff injury in shoulder joints of hemiplegic patients. Scan J Rehabil Med 3:131–137, 1971

61. Neer OS II: Anterior acromioplasty for chronic impingement syndrome in the shoulder. J Bone Joint Surg 54(A):41–50, 1972

62. Neer OS II: Impingement lesions. Clin Orthop 173:70–77, 1983

63. Neviaser JS: Adhesive capsulitis of the shoulder: A study of pathological findings in periarthritis of the shoulder. J Bone Joint Surg 27:211–222, 1945

64. Nirschl R: Rehabilitation of the athlete's elbow. *In* Morrey BR (ed): The Elbow and Its Disorders, pp 524–525. Philadelphia, WB Saunders, 1985

65. Norris TR: Diagnostic technique for shoulder instability. Instr Course Lect 34:239–257, 1985

66. Palmer L, Blakely R: Documentation of medial rotation accompanying shoulder flexion: A case report. Phys Ther 68:55–58, 1986

67. Pappas AM, Zaacki RM, McCarthy CF: Rehabilitation of the pitching shoulder. Am J Sports Med 13(4):223–235, 1985

68. Peat M: Functional anatomy of the shoulder complex. Phys Ther 66:1855–1865, 1986

69. Perry J: Anatomy and biomechanics of the shoulder in throwing, swimming, gymnastics and tennis. Clin Sports Med 2:247–270, 1983

70. Pettman E: The "functional" shoulder girdle. International Federation of Orthopaedic Manipulative Therapists, Vancouver, BC, 1984

71. Radin E: Relevant biomechanics in the treatment of musculoskeletal injuries and disorders. Clin Orthop 146:2–3, 1980

72. Rothman RH, Marvel JP, Heppenstall RB: Anatomical considerations in the glenohumeral joint. Orthop Clin North Am 6(2):341–352, 1975

73. Rothman RH, Parke BB: The vascular anatomy of the rotator cuff. Clin Orthop 41:176–186, 1965

74. Sarrafian SK: Gross and functional anatomy of the shoulder. Clin Orthop 173:11–18, 1983

75. Shields CL: Manual of Sports Surgery. New York, Springer–Verlag, 1987

76. Smith KF: The thoracic outlet syndrome: A protocol of treatment. J Orthop Sports Phys Ther 1(2):89–97, 1979

77. Spencer J, Turkel MA, Ithaca MC, Panio MW, Marshall JL: Stabilizing mechanism preventing anterior dislocation of the glenohumeral joint. J Bone Joint Surg 63(A):1208–1217, 1981

78. Sullivan PE, Markos PD, Minor MA: An Integrated Approach to Therapeutic Exercise: Theory and Clinical Application. Reston, Virginia, Reston Publication, 1982

79. Turek SL: Orthopaedics: Principles and Their Applications, 4th ed. Philadelphia, JB Lippincott, 1984

80. Warwick R, Williams P (eds): Gray's Anatomy, 35th British ed. Philadelphia, WB Saunders, 1973

81. Watson–Jones RR: Fractures and Joint Injuries. Vol 2, 4th ed. Baltimore, Williams & Wilkins, 1960

82. Wooden MJ: Isokinetic evaluation and treatment of the shoulder. *In* Donatelli R (ed): Physical Therapy of the Shoulder. New York, Churchill Livingstone, 1987

83. Yackzan L, Adams C, Francis KT: The effects of ice massage on delayed muscle soreness. Am J Sports Med 12:159–165, 1984

84. Yergason RM: Supination sign. J Bone Joint Surg 13(A):160, 1931

RECOMMENDED READINGS

Aronen JG, Regan K: Decreasing the incidence of recurrence of first time anterior dislocations with rehabilitation. Am J Sports Med 12:283–291, 1984

Atwater AE: Biomechanics of overarm throwing movements and injuries. Exerc Sport Sci Rev 7:43–85, 1979

Moynes DR: Prevention of injury to the shoulder through exercise and therapy. Clin Sports Med 2:413–422, 1983

Pappas AM, Zawacki RM, Sullivan TJ: Biomechanics of baseball pitching: A preliminary report. Am J Sports Med 13:216–222, 1985

Zarins B, Rowe CR: Current concepts in the diagnosis and treatment of shoulder instability in athletes. Med Sci Sports Exerc 15:444–448, 1984

11 *The Elbow*

Randolph M. Kessler and Darlene Hertling

REVIEW OF FUNCTIONAL ANATOMY

OSTEOLOGY

At the distal anterior end of the humerus there are two articular surfaces: the trochlea, which is pulley shaped, somewhat like an hourglass or spool lying on its side, and the capitellum, which forms most of a sphere mediolaterally and half of a sphere anteroposteriorly. The lateral epicondyle extends laterally above the capitellum for attachment of the extensor muscles. The medial epicondyle is the site of attachment of the flexor–pronator group. The coronoid fossa lies immediately above the trochlea, and the radial fossa is immediately above the capitellum. These fossae receive the coronoid process and the anterior rim of the radial head, respectively, on full elbow flexion (Fig. 11–1).

If one looks laterally, or medially, the distal humerus angulates anteriorly such that the longitudinal axis of the trochlea is directed anteriorly, 45° to the shaft of the humerus. As implied above, the hemisphere of the capitellum faces anteriorly, with the articular surface having an angular value of about 180° (Fig. 11–2).

Posteriorly (Fig. 11–3), the large, deep olecranon fossa accepts the olecranon process on full elbow extension. At times it communicates with the coronoid fossa. The trochlear articular surface, with its median groove, extends posteriorly. The groove usually runs obliquely, distally, and laterally; the medial half of the trochlea extends farther distally than the lateral half does. The asymmetry of the trochlea causes the ulna to angulate laterally on the humerus when the elbow extends. This abduction of the forearm on full extension is referred to as the *carrying angle* of the elbow.

The radial head is concave on its superior surface for articulation with the convex capitellum. Viewed from above, the radial head is slightly oval, being longer anteroposteriorly, so that with pronation it is displaced slightly laterally (Fig. 11–4).

The proximal ulna consists of the olecranon and the coronoid process, between which is the trochlear notch. With the elbow extended, the trochlear notch faces anteriorly and superiorly, corresponding to the 45° angulation of the distal humerus (see Fig. 11–2A). Lying inferiorly and medially to the trochlear notch is the radial notch, which faces laterally for articulation with the radial head (see 11–1).

The angulation of the distal humerus and trochlear notch of the proximal ulna allows about 160° elbow flexion and 180° extension. The angulation is necessary in order to provide room for the anterior muscle groups of the arm and forearm, which approximate on elbow flexion (Fig. 11–5). Any bony malalignment that interferes with these critical angles (*e.g.,* following a supracondylar fracture) will make normal movement impossible.

LIGAMENTS

The capsule of the elbow is reinforced by medial and lateral collateral ligaments. These ligaments serve to restrict medial or lateral angulation of the ulna on the humerus. They also help prevent dislocation of the ulna from the trochlea. Each collateral ligament consists of anterior, intermediate, and posterior fibers. The anterior fibers of both help reinforce the annular ligament of the radioulnar articulation (Fig. 11–6). The capsule is strengthened anteriorly by an anterior oblique ligament (Fig. 11–7).

The annular ligament runs from the anterior margin of the radial notch of the ulna around the radial head to the posterior margin of the radial notch. It is lined with articular cartilage so that with pronation and supination the radial head articulates with the capitellum of the humerus and the radial notch of the ulna, as well as with the annular ligament (see Figs. 11–6 and 11–7).

The joint capsule of the elbow encloses the humeroulnar joint, the radiohumeral joint, and the proxi-

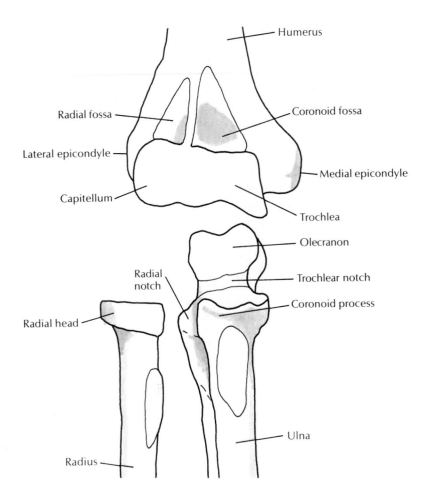

Fig. 11-1. Bones of the right elbow.

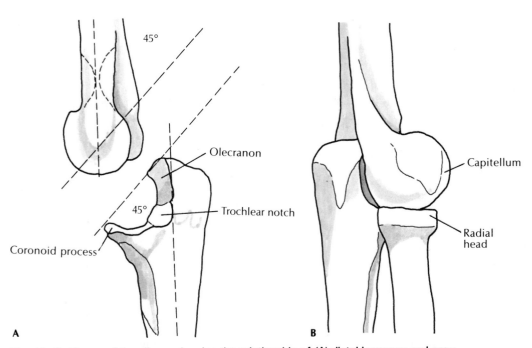

Fig. 11-2. Bones of the elbow, showing the relationship of *(A)* distal humerus and proximal ulna and *(B)* proximal radius (lateral view).

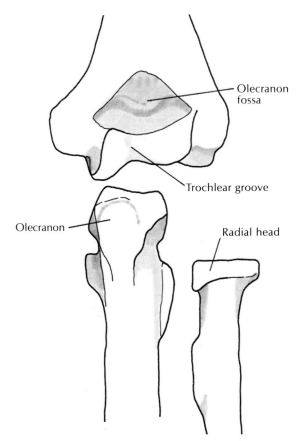

Fig. 11–3. Posterior view of bones of the elbow.

Olecranon
fossa

Trochlear groove

Olecranon

Radial head

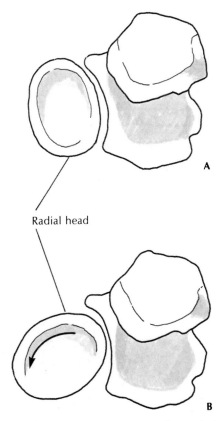

Radial head

A

B

Fig. 11–4. Relationship of proximal radius and ulna in *(A)* pronation and *(B)* supination, as viewed from above.

Fig. 11–5. Elbow in flexion.

Fig. 11–6. Ligaments of the elbow viewed (A) laterally and (B) medially.

mal radioulnar joint (Figs. 11–6 through 11–8). Some anatomists describe the existence of a quadrate ligament (ligament of Denucé) at the distal border of the annular ligament whose anterior fibers become taut on forearm supination and whose posterior fibers become taut on pronation (Fig. 11–8).[11,40,62]

BURSAE

The olecranon bursa overlies the olecranon posteriorly, lying between the superior olecranon and the skin. It may become inflamed from trauma, prolonged pressure ("student's elbow"), or other inflammatory afflictions such as infection and gout (Fig. 11–9).

TENDINOUS ORIGINS

The flexor–pronator muscles of the wrist have their tendinous origins at a common aponeurosis that originates at the medial epicondyle of the humerus. The wrist extensor group has its common aponeurotic origin at the lateral epicondyle. From superior to inferior on the humerus, the brachioradialis inserts first, followed by the extensor carpi radialis longus, the extensor carpi radialis brevis, and the remaining extensor muscles (Fig. 11–10). The extensor carpi radialis brevis is the uppermost muscle to attach to the common extensor tendon. The extensor carpi radialis longus and the brachioradialis do not contribute to the common tendon but rather attach above the epicondyle.

The extensor carpi radialis brevis is important

Fig. 11–7. Anterior view of the ligaments of the elbow.

Fig. 11–8. The quadrate ligament.

clinically since its tendon is most frequently involved in cases of lateral tennis elbow.

Although it originates in part from the common extensor tendon, the extensor brevis also has proximal attachments to the lateral collateral ligament of the elbow, and often to the annular ligament (see Fig. 11–10).

Deep to the tendon of the extensor brevis, and just distal to its insertion at the lateral epicondyle, there is a small space normally filled with loose, areolar connective tissue. This is termed the *subaponeurotic space*[19] and is bordered on the ulnar side by the extensor digitorum tendon and distally by the attachment of the brevis to the annular ligament (see Fig. 11–10). Surgical findings commonly reveal granulation tissue in this space in cases of lateral tennis elbow. Histologic studies show hypervascularization and the ingrowth of numerous free nerve endings into this space with granulation.[8,19] The granulation probably represents the reactions of adjacent tissues to chronic irritation of the extensor brevis origin resulting from tension stresses.[19,47]

On full forearm pronation, with the elbow extended, the orientation of the extensor carpi radialis brevis becomes such that proximally it is stretched over the prominence of the radial head (see Fig. 11–4). This fulcrum effect from the radial head adds to the normal tensile forces transmitted to the origin of this muscle when stretched during combined wrist flexion, forearm pronation, and elbow extension.[47] This may in part explain the susceptibility of this tendon to chronic inflammation at or near its attachment.

NERVES AND ARTERIES

Blood Supply

Blood supply to the elbow joint is usually abundant. The medial portion of the elbow is supplied from superior and inferior ulnar collateral arteries and two ulnar recurrent arteries. The lateral portion is

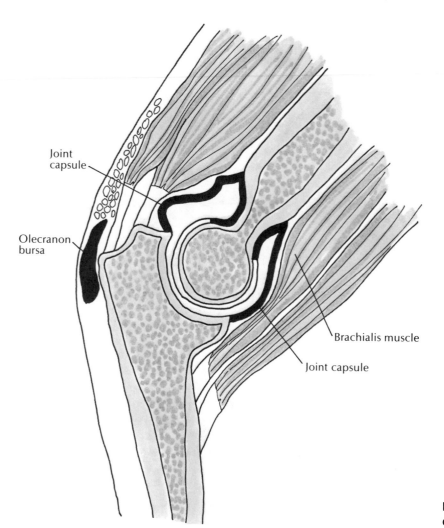

Joint
capsule

Olecranon
bursa

Brachialis muscle

Joint capsule

Fig. 11–9. Sagittal section through the elbow.

supplied by radial and middle collateral branches of the profunda artery and radial and interosseous recurrent arteries.[36,42]

Innervation

Joint branches are believed to be derived from all the major nerves crossing over this joint (i.e., radial, median, ulnar), including contributions from the musculoskeletal nerves. The variations and relative contributions have been documented by Gardner.[16] A detailed description of the nerves near the level of or close to the elbow joint can be found in other sources.[2,11,16,21,27,36,51,61,63] The reader will benefit from studying sagittal and anteroposterior diagrams that depict some of the anatomical relationships (Figs. 11–11 through 11–13).

Clinically the examiner must be aware of potential injury or pinching of various nerves near the level of the elbow. For example, for the most part, resistant

lateral tennis elbow may be caused by lateral epicondylitis and its associated fascial tears or calcification.[64] On occasion, persistent complaints may be due either to compression of the posterior interosseous nerve or to a combination of persistent localized epicondylitis and nerve compression.[7, 53,58]

Of the several entrapment syndromes near the level of the elbow, the ulnar tunnel syndrome is the most common.[10,25,34,61,63–66,69,71–73] The ulnar nerve at the elbow passes behind the medial epicondyle in a groove that is converted into a osseofibrous canal, the cubital tunnel, by the arcuate ligament that runs from the medial epicondyle to the olecranon process (see Fig. 11–11).[10,73] The arcuate ligament is taut at 90° flexion and lax in extension. An entrapment neuropathy of the ulnar nerve is common especially after prolonged sitting, overuse of the elbow, or repeated microtrauma from occupations that involve leaning on the elbow.[10]

Next in frequency of occurrence is the posterior

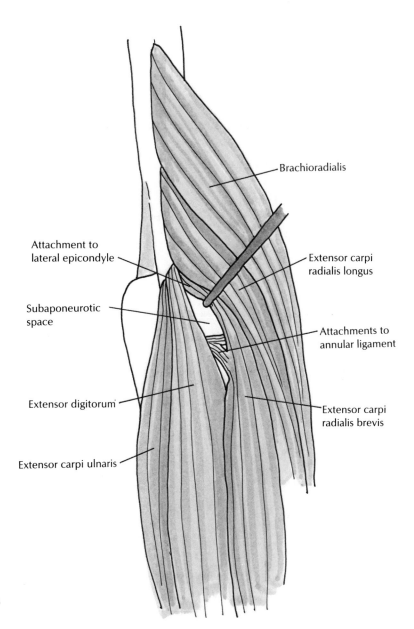

Brachioradialis

Extensor carpi
radialis longus

Attachment to
lateral epicondyle

Subaponeurotic
space

Attachments to
annular ligament

Extensor digitorum

Extensor carpi
radialis brevis

Extensor carpi ulnaris

Fig. 11–10. Lateral view of the tendinous
origin of the forearm muscles.

interosseous nerve syndrome or radial tunnel syndrome.[7,14,20,26,37,41,44,46,51,52,56,60,64–66,69,70] The most common compression site of the posterior interosseous nerve is as it passes under the fibrous origin of the extensor carpi radialis and then pierces the supinator muscles (in the region of the arcade of Frohse) to pass along the interosseus membrane, where it supplies the extensor muscles of the forearm, to reach the wrist (see Fig. 11–12).[4,41,46,52,56,60]

The anterior interosseous nerve syndrome and pronator syndrome, which involves the median nerve, are somewhat less common. The median nerve may be compressed just prior to the anterior interosseous branch on entering the forearm beneath the edge of the lacertus fibrosis of the biceps,

resulting in the pronator syndrome (see Fig. 11–13),[34,43,55] while the anterior interosseous nerve is occasionally pinched or entrapped as it passes between the two heads of the pronator teres.[15,32,35,38,54,57,61,64,74]

There are still other types of entrapment neuropathies, although much rarer, that one should be aware of. One is median nerve entrapment, which is occasionally combined with that of the brachial artery caused by a supracondylar spur and/or Struther's ligament (see Fig. 11–13C).[17,27,63,66] Another is ulnar nerve entrapment caused by Struther's arcade, which is said to be fibers arising from the medial head of triceps that interweave to the intermuscular septum (see Fig. 11–11A).[30,63,64]

Arcade of Struthers

Ulnar nerve

Median Nerve

Medial intermuscular septum

A

Fig. 11–11. The ulnar nerve: Anatomical distribution of the ulnar nerve crossing the intermuscular septum, passing under the arcade of Struthers (A) and the cubital tunnel at the elbow (B).

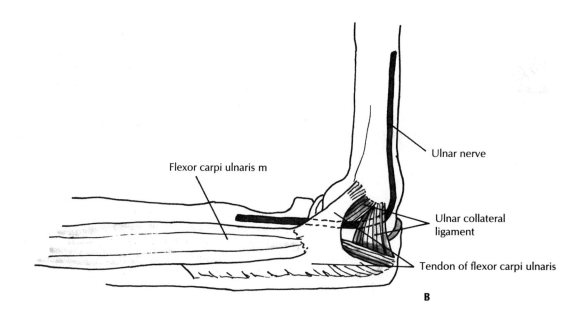

Flexor carpi ulnaris m

Ulnar nerve

Ulnar collateral ligament

Tendon of flexor carpi ulnaris

B

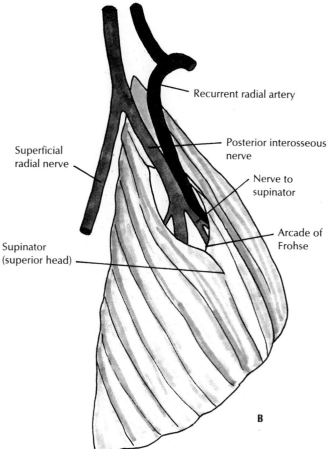

Fig. 11–12. *(A)* The radial nerve and its major forearm branches, the posterior interosseous nerve and the superficial radial nerve. *(B)* Enlarged view of the posterior interosseous nerve and its relationship to the supinator muscle and the arcade of Frohse.

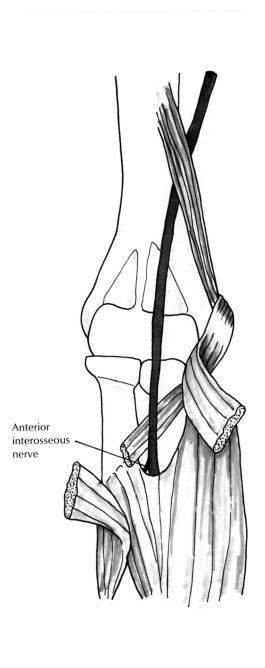

Fig. 11-13. The median nerve, proximal to the lacertus fibrosus *(A)*, the lacertus fibrosus released exposing the anterior interosseous nerve *(B)*, and the ligament of Struthers, an anomalous structure *(C)*.

EVALUATION OF THE ELBOW

HISTORY

Routine questions to be pursued during evaluation of patients with common musculoskeletal disorders are discussed in Chapter 4. However, the following questions are of particular concern when evaluating patients with elbow disorders:

1. What activities (*e.g.*, athletic or occupational) do you engage in that involve vigorous or repetitive use of the arm? (Except for the arthritides, the majority of elbow conditions noted are traumatic conditions or degenerative conditions, such as tennis elbow, that become active with certain activities.)
2. Are any other joints involved? (Except for the degenerative or traumatic lesions, rheumatoid arthritis is one of the few remaining causes of elbow pain of local origin.)

The elbow is largely derived from C6 and C7 and may, therefore, be the site of referred pain from other structures of the same segmental derivation; it may also refer pain to other structures in these segments.

PHYSICAL EXAMINATION

I. **Observation**
   A. *Posture and attitude in which the arm is held*
   B. *Functional use of the arm during gait, dressing, and other activities*
II. **Inspection** (include the entire extremity)
   A. *Structure.* Observe the extremities with patient in a relaxed, standing position
      1. Shoulder height
      2. Elbow carrying angle (valgus – varus angle)
      3. Elbow flexion – extension angle
      4. Positions of medial and lateral epicondyles, radial head, and olecranon
   B. *Soft tissue*
      1. Atrophy. Observe and measure the girth of arm or forearm.
      2. Swelling
         a. Marked posterior swelling is usually bursal swelling.
         b. Articular effusion is often visible anteriorly as well as posteriorly.
      3. General contours
   C. *Skin*
      1. Color changes
      2. Scars or blemishes
      3. Moisture
      4. Texture
III. **Selective tissue tension tests**
   A. *Active movements* (sitting)
      1. Observe
         a. Elbow flexion – extension
         b. Forearm pronation – supination (with elbow at 90°)
         c. Wrist flexion – extension
      2. Apply slight overpressure. Assess effect on pain; assess end feel; feel for crepitus.
      3. Record significant findings relating to range of motion, pain, end feel, and crepitus.
   B. *Passive movements* (supine for optimal stabilization)
      1. Tests
         a. Elbow flexion – extension with the shoulder flexed, extended, and in neutral positions for constant-length phenomenon in case of muscular pain and tightness
         b. Elbow pronation – supination
         c. Wrist flexion with ulnar deviation (the elbow is held extended and the forearm pronated, stretching the common extensor tendon)
         d. Wrist extension with the forearm supinated and elbow extended (common flexor – pronator tendon stretched)
      2. Record range of motion, pain, crepitus, and type of end feel.
   C. *Joint-play movements*
      1. Tests (see Chapter 6 Peripheral Joint Mobilization Techniques)
         a. Inferior glide of the ulna on the humerus
         b. Medial-lateral (valgus – varus) movement of ulna on humerus
         c. Superior-inferior glide of the radius
         d. Anterior-posterior movement of radial head
         e. Rotation of the radial head
         f. Anterior-posterior glide of distal radioulnar joint
      2. Record significant findings related to the degree of mobility and the presence of pain and muscle guarding.
   D. *Resisted isometric movements (supine)*
      1. Resisted wrist movements. The patient is asked to grip the examiner's hand and squeeze strongly. If elbow pain is reproduced, additional isometric contractions of the wrist are examined (*i.e.*, wrist flexion and extension).

2. Resisted elbow movements. The four elbow movements of flexion, extension, supination, and pronation are tested next using isometric contractions.
3. If referred pain from more proximal regions is suspected, include resisted isometric contraction tests of shoulder and cervical spine movements.
4. Record whether the resisted isometric contraction is strong or weak and whether it is painful or painless.

IV. **Palpation**
   A. *Skin*
      1. Temperature—Especially over brachialis and joint
      2. Moisture—Especially over the hand and forearm
      3. Texture
      4. Mobility of skin over subcutaneous tissues, especially after immobilization
      5. Tenderness—Primarily if neurologic involvement is suspected (*e.g.*, ulnar nerve lesion)
   B. *Subcutaneous soft tissues*
      1. Consistency, tone, and mobility
      2. Swelling. Joint effusion is often palpable anteriorly by ballottement.
      3. Tenderness
         a. Common tendon insertions
         b. Soft-tissue attachments
   C. *Bones*
      1. Bony relationships—Especially the position of the radial head
      2. Tenderness—Tenoperiosteal junctions of common flexor and common extensor groups
      3. Bony contours
   V. **Other**—Results of roentgenograms, laboratory tests, and electromyograms, if available

COMMON LESIONS

ELBOW TENDINITIS

Elbow tendinitis is a very common disorder affecting the elbow. The tendon most commonly involved is the extensor carpi radialis brevis, at or near its insertion at the lateral epicondyle.[6,8,13,19,47] At times, other common extensor tendons will also be involved concurrently or, rarely, by themselves. Much less frequently, the common flexor tendon is involved at the tenoperiosteal junction. Even more uncommon is tendinitis of the triceps at its attachment to the olecranon. Confusion about the pathology and treatment

of tennis elbow has plagued the medical community since the 19th century. Surgical studies have clearly identified classic tennis elbow as tendinitis, which Nirschl and Pettrone have divided into lateral, medial, and posterior areas and have classified on an anatomical basis.[48,50]

Lateral tennis elbow. Lateral tendinitis (lateral epicondylitis) primarily involves the extensor carpi radialis brevis and occasionally involves the extensor digitorum, extensor carpi radialis longus, and, more rarely, the extensor carpi ulnaris.[48,50]

Medial tennis elbow. Medial tendinitis (also known as golfer's elbow or medial epicondylitis) primarily involves the pronator teres and flexor carpi radialis and occasionally the palmaris longus, flexor carpi ulnaris, and flexor digitorum superficialis. An additional factor is compression neurapraxia of the ulnar groove.[49]

Posterior tennis elbow. Tendinitis of the triceps at its attachment to the olecranon is rare. It typically follows sudden severe strain to the triceps tendon (*e.g.*, in javelin throwers), as the arm is fully extended.[10]

Tendinitis affecting the elbow is rarely of acute traumatic origin. Except in sports medicine clinics, most patients presenting with tennis elbow do not relate the onset or aggravation of the problem to athletic endeavors such as tennis. Even when the chief complaint is the development of pain during some activity, the onset is usually gradual and pain is felt most *after* the activity. This is because lateral tennis elbow is usually a "degenerative" disorder; it represents tissue response to fatigue stresses. The inflammatory response, which characterizes the disorder, is an attempt to speed up the rate of tissue production to compensate for an increased rate of tissue microdamage (*e.g.*, collagen fiber fracturing). The increased microdamage rate occurs because of greater internal strain to the tendon fibers over time. This might come about from some increase in use of the tendon, for example, with carpentry, pruning shrubs, or tennis. It may also occur with normal activity levels if the capacity of the tendon to attenuate tensile loads is reduced. This typically occurs with aging, in which a loss of the mucopolysaccharide chondroitin sulfate makes the tendon less extensible; more of the energy of tensile loading must be absorbed as internal strain to collagen fibers rather than by deformation of the tissue. The explanation for the susceptibility of the extensor carpi radialis brevis to excessive strain is probably related to the added tensile load imposed on the tendon by the radial head when the tendon is stretched (*e.g.*, wrist flexion, elbow extension, and forearm pronation). In this position the tendon is further stretched over the prominence of the radial head.[47] Because the development of tennis elbow may be due to age-related tissue changes, most patients presenting with this problem are 35 years old or older.[6,8,13]

Lateral tennis elbow is classically a very persistent disorder that does not tend toward spontaneous resolution. If the patient with tennis elbow continues to perform activities that stress the tendon, the immature collagen that is produced in an attempt at repair continues to break down before it has the chance to adequately mature and the chronic inflammatory process continues. If the part is completely immobilized, there may not be adequate stress to the new collagen to stimulate maturation, in which case the scar will again break down on resumption of activities. In order for treatment to be successful, this dilemma must be resolved.

Medial tennis elbow characteristically occurs with wrist flexor activity and active pronation, as in pitching a baseball and pull-through strokes of swimming.[49] Typically it occurs in middle-aged patients, often those involved in sports or occupational activities that require a strong hand grip and an adduction movement of the elbow.

Posterior tennis elbow consists of intrinsic overload of the triceps attachment in activities that cause a sudden snapping of elbow extension. Pain is reproduced on fully resisting extension of the elbow while the patient stands with the elbow flexed and forearm fully supinated.

According to Nirschl, it should be appreciated that the primary overload abuse in tendinitis is caused by intrinsic concentric muscular contraction.[47] Curwin and Standish maintain that decreased flexibility causes the muscles to be overstretched during eccentric contraction and overloading of the extensors.[12] They advocate that maximum strengthening of the muscles must necessarily include eccentric work since this is the nature of the force producing the injury and since eccentric exercise produces greater tensile force on the tendon.

Examination and Management

I. **History**
   A. *Site of pain*
      1. Lateral tennis elbow—Over the lateral humeral epicondyle, often referred into the C7 segment, down the posterior forearm into the dorsum of the hand, and perhaps into the ring and long fingers
      2. Medial tennis elbow—Over the medial epicondyle, rarely referred into the ulnar aspect of the forearm

3. Posterior tennis elbow—Over the posterior compartment of the elbow
   B. *Onset of pain*—Usually gradual. May be related to wrist extension activities in lateral tennis elbow, such as grasping, hitting a backhand at tennis, or pruning shrubs, or to wrist flexion and pronation activities in medial tennis elbow. The patient rarely recalls a sudden onset of pain during these activities, however. At times a direct blow to the epicondyle will initiate the problem.
   C. *Nature of pain*—Varies from a dull ache or no pain at rest to sharp twinges or straining sensation with activities as mentioned above. Lateral tennis elbow is particularly aggravated by grasping activities because the wrist extensors must contract to stabilize the wrist during use of the finger flexors. Medial tennis elbow is made worse by repeated wrist flexion movements and gripping.

II. **Physical examination**
   A. *Active movements*—Usually fairly painless. In more severe cases of lateral tennis elbow, there may be some pain with active wrist flexion with the elbow in extension from the stretch placed on the tendon. Active wrist extension does not usually produce enough tension to reproduce the pain. Similarly, there may be some pain with active wrist extension with the elbow extended in medial tennis elbow, but usually not on active wrist flexion.
   B. *Passive movements*
      1. One of the key tests that should reproduce the pain in lateral tennis elbow is full passive wrist flexion with ulnar deviation, forearm pronation, and elbow extension. Passive elbow movements alone are painless.
      2. Full wrist extension with supination and elbow extension reproduces the pain in medial tennis elbow.
   C. *Resisted isometric movements*—The other key test is resisted wrist extension (with the elbow extended) reproducing the pain in lateral tennis elbow; resisted wrist flexion reproduces pain in medial tennis elbow. At times, resisted pronation is painful in medial tennis elbow. Resisted elbow extension with the elbow in flexion and forearm fully supinated is a key test for posterior tennis elbow.
   D. *Joint-play movements*—Should be full and painless.
   E. *Palpation*
      1. Rather exquisite tenderness occurs usually over the epicondyles in medial and lat-

eral tennis elbow. An area of tenderness may be palpated over the insertion of the triceps tendon into the olecranon in posterior tennis elbow.

2. In lateral tennis elbow, the tenderness may often extend down into the muscle belly. Less often, the tenderness is felt superior to the epicondyle at the insertion of the extensor carpi radialis longus.

3. There may be some warmth noted over the respective epicondyle and olecranon.

F. *Inspection* — Usually no significant findings

G. *Differential diagnoses.* Other entities include de Quervain's tenovaginitis (See Chapter 12, The Wrist and Hand Complex) and extensor carpi ulnaris tendinitis at the wrist; pronator syndrome in the forearm, and radial nerve entrapment accompanying lateral epicondylitis at the elbow.[9,33] Associated problems can appear either independently or in combination with the various forms of tennis elbow tendinitis.[49] These may include ulnar nerve neurapraxia,[49] carpal tunnel syndrome,[47,50] intra-articular abnormalities, joint laxity,[29,45,75] and associated soft-tissue or myofascial trigger point syndromes.[3,5,20,24,31,67,68] The multiplicity of conditions and treatments found in the literature is typified by Cyriax's coverage of tennis elbow.[13]

Gunn attributes the tennis elbow symptoms in one group of patients to reflex localization of pain from radiculopathy of the cervical spine.[22,23] Maigne has observed that about 60% of cases with clinical epicondylitis have minor intervertebral derangement at C5–C7 or C6–C7 levels on the side of the tennis elbow.[39] About one half of these cases are associated with some degree of periarthritis of the elbow and thus are considered mixed forms.

III. Management

A. *Goals*

1. Restoration of normal, painless use of the involved extremity
2. Prevention of recurrence

B. *Objectives*

1. Resolution of the chronic inflammatory process
2. Maturation of the scar (healed area of the tendon). The new collagen must be sufficiently "strong" and extensible to withstand the tensile stresses imposed by the patient's particular activity level; there must be an appropriate amount of tissue that is oriented to attenuate tensile stresses with a minimum of internal strain.
3. Restoration of strength and extensibility to the muscle–tendon complex

C. *Techniques*

1. Acute cases. Lateral tennis elbow is, by nature, a chronic disorder, but as indicated in the criteria suggested in Chapter 4, some patients may present with acute symptoms and signs associated with lateral tennis elbow; pain is referred into the entire forearm and perhaps the hand, and occasionally up the back of the arm. There may be some pain at rest, and some degree of muscle spasm is elicited when the tendon is stressed passively or by resisted movements.

In such cases, the immediate goal is to promote progression to a more chronic state assisting in the resolution of the acute inflammation.

a. Instruct the patient to apply ice to the site of the lesion several times a day. The physical therapy modality of high-voltage galvanic stimulation has been helpful in relieving pain and inflammation.[49]

b. Continued stress to the tendon must be prevented. If the patient presents with acute symptoms and signs as outlined above, this is best achieved by immobilization of the wrist, hand, and fingers (not the elbow) in a resting splint. In some cases a simple wrist cock-up splint will suffice, since this will obviate the need for the wrist extensors to contract when the finger flexors are used. Activities involving grasping, pinching, and fine finger movements must be restricted. This is often the most difficult component of the program to institute but at the same time the most important at this stage. The effectiveness of any other treatment measures will be compromised if the patient continues to engage in activities that stress the lesion site. This requires, for example, that a carpenter take some time off from work or temporarily change duties, that a tennis player abstain from playing for a while, and that persons who enjoy knitting, sewing, or gardening temporarily alter their activities.

c. A few times a day, the patient should remove the splint and actively move the wrist into flexion, the forearm into pronation, and the elbow into extension, simultaneously, to minimize loss of extensibility of the muscle and tendon. This should be done *gently*, avoiding significant discomfort, and very slowly to prevent high strain-rate loading of the tissue.

   If appropriate instructions are given and the patient faithfully follows the outlined program, progression to a more chronic status should occur over a period of a few (*i.e.*, 3 to 5) days.

2. Chronic cases (lateral tennis elbow). If pain is fairly localized over the lateral elbow region and there is little or no pain at rest, the disorder should be treated as chronic tendinitis.

   a. Advise the patient explicitly as to the appropriate level and type of activity that may be performed. Strong, repetitive, grasping activities, such as hammering, and activities that particularly stress the tendon, such as tennis, must be restricted until there is very little pain on resisted isometric wrist extension and little or no pain when the tendon is passively stretched (wrist flexion, forearm pronation, and elbow extension). Such activities must be resumed very gradually, with some protection of the part. Protection may be provided by counterforce bracing with an inelastic cuff worn firmly around the proximal forearm (the forearm extensors for lateral tennis elbow and the forearm flexors for medial tennis elbow). The concept of elbow bracing for tennis elbow was initially introduced by Ilfeld in 1965.[28] Nirschl later introduced a wider device curved for better fit and support of the conical shape of the forearm.[47] In theory, constraining full muscle expansion when muscles contract should diminish the potential force generated in the muscle. Cybex testing and biomechanical studies, which have demonstrated both angular velocity and the sequence of the electromyographic re-

cording of muscular activity, have confirmed the clinical validity of this concept.[48,49] If the use of such a device is instituted, the therapist should gradually wean the patient from it as strength, mobility, and painless function increase.

   Also, as normal activities are resumed, certain adaptations may be implemented to minimize the stresses that may be imposed on the wrist extensors. For example, the tennis player typically receives high strain-rate loading to the wrist extensor group when using a backhand stroke if the ball strikes the racquet above the center point of the strings. This produces a moment arm about which the force of the ball hitting the racquet can create a high pronatory torque. If the wrist extensors are somewhat weak, the wrist might also be forced into flexion. The combined effects of the active and passive tension created in the wrist extensor group result in high loading of the extensor tendons. The passive component can be minimized by hitting the ball on center and by having adequate wrist extensor strength to keep the wrist from flexing. The passive pronatory torque can also be reduced by increasing the diameter of the racquet handle. Other considerations would include the tension of the strings on the racquet head and the flexibility of the racquet shaft. High string tension and low racquet flexibility will result in reduced attenuation of forces by the racquet and, therefore, greater transmission of high strain rate forces to the arm. Also, the larger the head on the racquet, the greater the potential moment arm about which pronatory forces can act. Thus, a tennis player might benefit from taking lessons to improve the likelihood of hitting the ball on center, from reducing string tension, and from using a relatively flexible racquet with a handle of maximum tolerable diameter and a head of standard size. Each patient's activities should be similarly assessed for ways to reduce the loads imposed on the wrist extensor group.

b. Ultrasound and friction massage should be used to assist in the resolution of the chronic inflammatory process and to promote maturation at the site of healing.

Resolution of inflammatory exudates, such as lysosomal enzymes and other cellular "debris," may be enhanced by the increased blood flow stimulated by the heating effects of the ultrasound. Ultrasound must often be applied under water because of the irregular surface contour of the lateral elbow region.

Friction massage is an essential component of the treatment program. Its beneficial effects in cases of tendinitis are not well understood but are probably related to the induced hyperemia and the mechanical influence it may have on tissue maturation (see Chapter 8, Friction Massage). The hyperemic effects are of greatest importance in cases of tendinitis that may be related to hypovascularity, for instance, at the shoulder. Hyperemia does not seem to be a significant factor in the etiology of tennis elbow, however, and this may in part explain why friction massage is effective over a shorter period of time in cases of rotator cuff tendinitis than it is on cases of tennis elbow. The mechanical effects of the deep massage may promote orientation of immature collagen along the lines of stress. This would be an important factor in pathologic disorders, such as tennis elbow, in which some type of mechanical stimulus is necessary for adequate tissue maturation. Use of deep transverse massage may assist in tissue maturation without imposing a longitudinal stress to the healing tendon tissue and, therefore, without continued rupturing of fibers at the site of the lesion. Thus, the defect heals with a maximum degree of tissue extensibility and is less likely to be overstressed as use of the part is resumed. This seems to be a solution to the dilemma mentioned above. If the patient continues to use the part, he or she perpetuates the problem by producing continued damage at the lesion site; if the patient completely immobilizes the part, there is no stimulus for tissue maturation, and as soon as activity is resumed, the healed tissue begins to break down.

c. Strength and mobility must be restored. As symptoms and signs indicate improvement, the patient must resume activities gradually. Excessive internal strain to the tendon can be minimized during stressful activities by optimizing tissue extensibility. No vigorous activities should be allowed until it is determined if the muscle–tendon complex has sufficient extensibility. Following the ultrasound and friction massage, the therapist should gently and slowly stretch the tissue by holding the elbow extended, the forearm pronated, and the wrist ulnarly deviated, while flexing the wrist and fingers. The patient is instructed to perform this stretch at home, emphasizing that it must be performed slowly and gently. The patient should notice a stretching sensation but no pain. As vigorous activities such as tennis, carpentry, and gardening are resumed, the patient can be taught to administer friction massage for a few minutes prior to engaging in the activity.

Also, before a normal activity level is resumed, it is important to be sure that good forearm strength has been restored. In lateral tennis elbow, wrist extensor strengthening exercises are always necessary, since the muscles will invariably undergo atrophy from disuse and reflex inhibition. Good extensor strength is necessary to protect the tendon from high strain-rate passive loading, which may occur with many types of activities. A convenient method of wrist extensor strengthening is to have the patient tie a rope that is 3 feet long to the center of a 1-inch dowel and a weight to the end of the rope; the patient grasps both ends of the dowel and rotates it toward him until the entire rope becomes wrapped around the dowel. This can be repeated as appropriate; the weight may be varied as necessary.

Forearm rehabilitative exercises to increase muscle power, flexibility, and endurance are important concepts.

Continued strengthening of uninjured areas as well as protective exercise sequences for the injured area are necessary. Isometric, isotonic, isokinetic, and isoflex exercises are all used. Isoflex exercises consist of muscular strengthening, employing both concentric and eccentric training, using the resistance of an elasticized tension cord.[49] Maximum strengthening of the muscles must necessarily include eccentric exercise.[12]

d. Local anti-inflammatory therapy, such as infiltration with a corticosteroid, is commonly used in cases of tendinitis. It must be emphasized that although symptomatic improvement is often dramatic, such treatment has only temporary value. It has no lasting beneficial effect on the pathologic process and certainly does not influence etiologic factors. At best, it should be considered as an adjunct to management in the acute state. Too often other important components of the treatment program are ignored when an apparent "cure" is heralded by dramatic symptomatic improvement.

POSTIMMOBILIZATION CAPSULAR TIGHTNESS

Patients with restricted movement at the elbow from capsular tightness are often referred to physical therapists. Since capsular restriction from degenerative joint disease at the elbow is rare, the patients with capsular restriction who are seen by physical therapists are usually those whose elbows have been immobilized. The only other frequent cause of capsular restriction at this joint is inflammatory arthritis (usually rheumatoid arthritis but occasionally traumatic arthritis).

The common injuries for which management may involve elbow immobilization include fractures of the arm or forearm (humeral shaft fractures, supracondylar fractures, and Colles' fractures are the most common) and elbow dislocations (usually posterior dislocation of the ulna on the humerus).

I. History. Determine a time frame of events that indicates the date of injury, dates of subsequent surgeries (if any), duration of immobilization, and date of removal of supports or splints. Any suggestion of complications following the injury or immobilization, such as vascular dysfunction, should be noted. Determine whether there have been previous attempts at remobilization,

and if so, what these entailed. Assess the patient's functional disability in terms of limitations on dressing or grooming and on occupational and recreational activities. These should be documented and used as a means by which to judge progress.

II. Physical examination. The key sign is limitation of motion in a capsular pattern. However, take note of any complication that may have ensued.

A. *Reflex sympathetic dystrophy* (see Chapter 12, The Wrist and Hand Complex)

1. Key signs include capsular restriction of all or most upper extremity joints, to varying degrees; generalized edema of the forearm and hand; trophic changes in skin and nails (glossy smooth skin, hyperhidrosis, hypohidrosis, cyanosis, brittle or ridged nails); and dysesthesias, with pain hypersensitivity even to light touch. Roentgenograms often reveal marked osteopenia, especially of the bones of the hand and wrist.

2. The exact cause of this disorder is not known. It is especially prevalent in patients who have sustained a Colles'-type fracture. It is believed to be related in some way to nerve trauma (such as trauma to the median nerve in Colles' fracture), the degree of edema, immobilization, and psychological factors. Preventive measures to be taken during the period of immobilization should include frequent active exercise of the free joints (usually shoulder and fingers) and regular periods of elevation of the involved extremity.

   Development of a true reflex sympathetic dystrophy, often referred to as a shoulder–hand syndrome, can be a significant complicating factor in the rehabilitation program following immobilization. The marked articular restrictions and pain hypersensitivity make efforts at remobilization especially difficult.

B. *Malalignment of bony fragments.* This is occasionally seen following a supracondylar fracture at the elbow and invariably follows a Colles' fracture (see Chapter 12, The Wrist and Hand Complex).

Elbow malalignment is easily detected by observing the carrying angle of the arm and by assessing structural alignment. With a supracondylar fracture, the distal fragment tends to displace posteriorly and medially

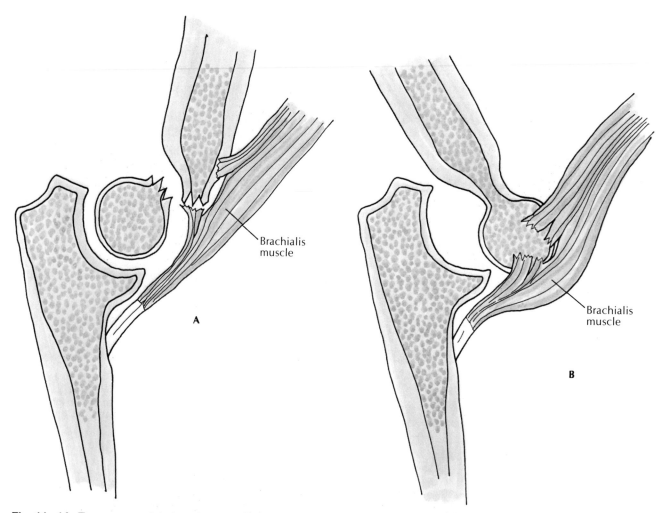

Fig. 11–14. Two common injuries of the elbow that result in displacement of bony parts are *(A)* supracondylar fracture and *(B)* posterior dislocation of ulna on humerus.

with an angulation medially. Rotational displacement, medial or lateral displacements, and posterior or anterior displacements are not significant in the young person, since these usually resolve with remodeling of the bone. Angular displacements, however, tend to persist. Typically, the malalignment following a supracondylar fracture presents as a decrease or reversal of the normal carrying angle. The medial epicondyle is positioned higher than the lateral epicondyle, and the olecranon becomes directed medially. Such malalignment usually does not result in a functional deficit but may be cosmetically unacceptable.

C. *Brachialis contusion.* The displacement of bony parts that accompanies supracondylar elbow fractures and elbow dislocations may result in a contusion to the distal brachialis muscle belly, which overlies and is in close contact with the distal end of the humerus (Fig. 11–14). The consequence of such a contusion may be eventual metaplasia of the contused portion of this muscle into osseus tissue, a condition referred to as myositis ossificans.[1,18] Myositis ossificans usually results in permanent restriction of motion at the elbow; extension is restricted more than flexion.

It is questionable whether mobilization of the part (active, passive, prolonged, or otherwise) actually affects the eventual outcome. It is believed by some that the condition is often the result of overzealous attempts to remobilize the part. This may indeed be the case if the brachialis muscle is stretched. In cases of capsular restriction, however, in which the stretch is applied to the anterior capsule rather than the brachialis muscle, it is doubtful that any form of mobilization would predispose to development of myositis ossificans of the brachialis muscle. It is probable that the development of myositis ossificans, following injuries in which the brachialis muscle is traumatized, occurs as an inevitable event resulting from the original injury.

The therapist must be protected medicolegally in the event that myositis ossificans should occur. This can be done by *(1)* recognizing the two common conditions (supracondylar fracture and posterior dislocation) that especially predispose to development of myositis ossificans and *(2)* distinguishing between capsular and muscular restriction of motion at the elbow. Fortunately, fractures and dislocations at the elbow occur primarily in children. Because of this, remobilization is not a major problem and passive mobilization is seldom required. However, if mobilization procedures are requested for a patient whose extremity has been immobilized following a supracondylar fracture or elbow dislocation, the therapist must take certain precautions. First, the cause of the restriction is determined. Limitation of extension more than flexion with an elastic end feel is very suggestive of a muscular restriction. The constant length phenomenon is used to determine whether it is biceps or brachialis. Limitation of motion in a capsular pattern with a capsular end feel suggests a capsular restriction. Stretching a tight elbow flexor muscle in such a case must not be done vigorously, except in cases of persistent restriction of elbow extension, and then only with agreement of the referring physician and with the patient's understanding.

Second, whether the restriction appears to be capsular or muscular, the therapist must attempt to detect any signs of inflammation of the brachialis muscle. This is done by palpating for a hematoma or excessive tenderness over the distal brachialis muscle belly. Any suggestion of inflammation or hematoma of the distal brachialis muscle belly should preclude vigorous mobilization, barring the stipulations indicated above. Regardless of the intensity of the mobilization program, the therapist would do well to record thermistor readings over the distal brachialis region before and after each treatment session. A rise in temperature that persists over, for example, a 24-hour period might indicate that the intensity of the pro-

gram should be reduced, especially if a muscular restriction is at fault.

III. Management of capsular tightness
  A. *Acute* (see criteria for acute vs. chronic in Chapter 5). Since most capsular elbow restrictions are those that follow immobilization after injury, they will rarely be found in an acute stage, since the acute inflammatory process subsides during the period of immobilization.
   1. Provide relief of pain and muscle guarding using ice, superficial heat, and grade I and II joint-play movements.
   2. Maintain existing range of motion and increase movement as pain and guarding abate.
    a. Use gentle joint-play movements, grades I and II.
    b. Initiate an active-assisted home range of motion exercise program.
   3. Strengthen progressively muscles controlling the shoulder, elbow, forearm, and wrist as necessary. Use isometrics in acute stage, since joint movement might cause reflex inhibition of the muscles to be strengthened.
  B. *Chronic*
   1. Ultrasound to tight capsular tissues along with or followed by capsular stretching, with joint-play mobilization techniques (see Chapter 6). If the therapist is treating a stiff elbow following a radial head resection, special attention should be given to preventing the development of a valgus contracture at the elbow by use of the "varus tilt" mobilization technique. The radius tends to migrate superiorly since the radial head no longer abuts the capitellum of the humerus. This may also result in problems at the distal radioulnar joint.
   2. Progression of home program to include prolonged stretch as tolerated and as indicated.
   3. Progression of home strengthening program, including exercises to increase flexibility, endurance, and eccentric control.

REFERENCES

1. Ackerman LV: Extra-osseous localized non-neoplastic bone and cartilage formation (so-called myositis ossificans). J Bone Joint Surg 40(A):279–298, 1958

2. Anson BJ, McVay CB: Surgical Anatomy, 5th ed, vol 2. Philadelphia, WB Saunders, 1971

3. Bernhang AM: The many causes of tennis elbow. NY State J Med 79:1363–1366, 1979

4. Blom S, Hele P, Parkman L: The supinator channel syndrome. Scand J Plast Reconstr Surg 5:71–73, 1971

5. Bowden BW: Tennis elbow. J Am Osteopath Assoc 78:97–98, 101–102, 1978

6. Boyd HB: Tennis elbow. J Bone Joint Surg 55(A):1183–1187, 1973

7. Capener N: The vulnerability of the posterior interosseous nerve of the forearm. J Bone Joint Surg 48(B):7:770–773, 1966

8. Coonard RW: Tennis elbow: Its course, natural history, conservative and surgical management. J Bone Joint Surg 55(A):1177–1182, 1973

9. Cooney WP III: Bursitis and tendinitis in the hand, wrist and elbow. Minn Med 8:491–494, 1983

10. Corrigan B, Maitland GD: Practical Orthopaedic Medicine. Boston, Butterworths, 1985

11. Cunningham DJ: Myology. In Romanes GJ (ed): Textbook of Anatomy, 12th ed. New York, Oxford University Press, 1981

12. Curwin S, Standish WD: Tendinitis: Its Etiology and Treatment, pp 115–132, Lexington, MA, Collamore Press, 1984

13. Cyriax J: Textbook of Orthopaedic Medicine, Vol I, The Diagnosis of Soft Tissue Lesions, 8th ed, pp 168–181. London, Ballière Tindall, 1982

14. Dharapak C, Nimberg GA: Posterior interosseous nerve compression: Report of a case caused by traumatic aneurysm. Clin Orthop 101:225–228, 1974

15. Farber JS, Bryan RS: The anterior interosseous nerve syndrome. J Bone Joint Surg 50(A):521–523, 1968

16. Gardner E: The innervation of the elbow joint. Anat Rec 102:161–174, 1948

17. Gessini L, Jandolo B, Pietrangeli A: Entrapment neuropathies of the median nerve at and above the elbow. Surg Neurol 19:112–116, 1983

18. Gilmer WS, Anderson LD: Reaction of soft somatic tissue which may progress to bone formation: Circumscribed myositis ossificans. South Med J 52:1432–1448, 1959

19. Goldie I: Epicondylitis lateralis humeri. Acta Chir Scand [Suppl] 339:3–119, 1964

20. Goldman S, Honet JC, Sobel R, Goldstein AS: Posterior interosseous nerve palsy in the absence of trauma. Arch Neurol 21:435–441, 1969

21. Grant JCB: Upper Limb In Basmajian JV (ed): Grant's Methods of Anatomy, 10th ed. Baltimore, Williams & Wilkins, 1980

22. Gunn CC, Milbrant WE: Tennis elbow and the cervical spine. Can Med Assoc J 114:803–809, 1976

23. Gunn CC, Milbrandt WE: Tennis elbow and acupuncture. Am J Acupuncture 5:61–66, 1977

24. Hagert GC, Lunborg G, Hansen T: Entrapment of the posterior interosseous nerve. Scand J Plast Reconstr Surg 11:205–212, 1977

25. Hayashi Y, Kohimc, Kohno TH: A case of cubital syn-drome caused by the snapping of the medial head of the triceps brachii muscle. Hand Surg 9A:96–99, 1984

26. Hayerl GG, Lundborg G, Hanson T: Entrapment of the posterior interosseous nerve. Scand J Plast Reconstr Surg 11:205–212, 1977

27. Hollinshead WH: Anatomy for Surgeons, Vol 3, The Back and Limbs, 3rd ed, pp 341–435. New York, Harper & Row, 1982

28. Ilfeld FW, Field SM: Treatment of tennis elbow: Use of special brace. JAMA 195:67–70, 1966

29. Indelicato PA, Jobe FW, Kerlan RK, Carter VS, Shields CL, Lomardo Sl: Correctable elbow lesions in professional baseball players: A review of 25 cases. Am J Sports Med 7:72–75, 1979

30. Kane E, Daplan EB, Spinner M: Observation of the course of the ulnar nerve in the arm. Ann Chir 27:487–496, 1973

31. Kelly M: Pain in the forearm and hand due to muscular lesions. Med J Aust 2:185–188, 1947

32. Kiloh LG, Nevin S: Isolated neuritis of the anterior interosseous nerve. Br Med J 1:850–851, 1952

33. Kopell HP, Thompsen WAL: Pronator syndrome. N Engl J Med 259:713–715, 1958

34. Kopell HP, Thompsen WAL: Peripheral Entrapment Neuropathies. Baltimore, Williams & Wilkins, 1963

35. Lake PA: Anterior interosseous nerve syndrome. J Neurosurg 41:306–309, 1974

36. Langman J, Woerdeman MW: Atlas of Medical Anatomy. Philadelphia, WB Saunders, 1976

37. Lister GD, Belsole RB, Kleinert HE: The radial tunnel syndrome. J Hand Surg 4:52–60, 1979

38. Maeda K, Miura T, Komada T, Chiba A: Anterior interosseous nerve paralysis: Report of 13 cases and review of Japanese literature. Hand 9:165–171, 1977

39. Maigne R: Tennis elbow (epicondylitis). In Liberson WT (ed): Orthopedic Medicine, A New Approach to Vertebral Manipulations, pp 244–254. Springfield, IL, Charles C Thomas, 1972

40. Martin BF: The annular ligament of the superior radioulnar joint. J Anat 92:473–482, 1958

41. Mayer JH, Mayfield PH: Surgery of the posterior interosseous branch of the radial nerve. Surg Gynecol Obstet 84:979–982, 1947

42. Morrey BF: The Elbow and Its Disorders. Philadelphia, WB Saunders, 1985

43. Morris HH, Defers BH: Pronator syndrome: Clinical and electrophysiological features in seven cases. J Neurol Neurosurg Psychiatry 39:461–464, 1976

44. Mulholland RC: Non-traumatic progressive paralysis of the posterior interosseous nerve. J Bone Joint Surg 48(B):781–785, 1966

45. Newman JH, Goodfellow JW: Fibrillation of the head of the radius: One cause of tennis elbow. J Bone Joint Surg 57(B):115, 1975

46. Nielson HO: Posterior interosseous nerve paralysis caused by a fibrous band compression of the supinator muscle: A report of four cases. Acta Orthop Scand 47:304–307, 1976

47. Nirschl RD: Tennis elbow. Orthop Clin North Am 4:787–800, 1973

48. Nirschl RD: Medial tennis elbow: The surgical treatment. Presented at the annual meeting of the American Academy of Orthopedic Surgeons. Atlanta, March 1, 1980

49. Nirschl RD: Muscle and tendon trauma: Tennis elbow. In Morrey BF (ed): The Elbow and Its Disorders. Philadelphia, WB Saunders, 1985

50. Nirschl RD, Pettrone F: Tennis elbow: The surgical treatment of lateral epicondylitis. J Bone Joint Surg 61(A):832–839, 1979

51. Omer G, Spinner M: Peripheral Nerve Problems. Philadelphia, WB Saunders, 1980

52. Riordan DC: Radial nerve paralysis. Orthop Clin North Am 5:283–287, 1974

53. Roles NC, Maudsley RH: Radial tunnel syndrome: Resistant tennis elbow as a nerve entrapment. J Bone Joint Surg 54(B):499–508, 1972

54. Rosk MR: Anterior interosseous nerve entrapment: Report of seven cases. Clin Orthop 142:176–181, 1979

55. Seyffarth H: Primary myoses in the m. pronator teres as a cause of lesions of the n. medianus (the pronator syndrome). Acta Psychiatr Scand [Suppl] 74:251–256, 1951

56. Sharrard WJW: Posterior interosseous neuritis. J Bone Joint Surg 48(B):777–780, 1966

57. Sharrard WJW: Anterior interosseous neuritis: Report of a case. J Bone Joint Surg 50(B):804–805, 1968

58. Somerville EW: Pain in the upper limb. Proceedings of the British Orthopaedic Association. J Bone Joint Surg 45(B):620–621, 1963

59. Spinner M: The anterior interosseous nerve syndrome with special attention to its variations. J Bone Joint Surg 52(A):84–94, 1970

60. Spinner M: The arcade of Frohse and its relationship to posterior interosseous nerve paralysis. J Bone Joint Surg 50(B):809–812, 1968

61. Spinner M: Injuries to the Major Branches of Peripheral Nerves of the Forearm, 2nd ed. Philadelphia, WB Saunders, 1978

62. Spinner M, Kaplan EB: The quadrate ligament of the elbow: Its relationship to the stability of the proximal radioulnar joint. Acta Orthop Scand 41:632–647, 1970

63. Spinner M, Kaplan EB: The relationship of the ulnar nerve to the medial intermuscular septum in the arm and its clinical significance. Hand 8:239–242, 1976

64. Spinner M, Linschied RL: Nerve entrapment syndromes. In Morrey BF (ed): The Elbow and Its Disorders, pp 691–712. Philadelphia, WB Saunders, 1985

65. Spinner M, Spencer PS: Nerve compression lesions of the upper extremity: A clinical and experimental review. Clin Orthop 104:46–67, 1974

66. Tajima T: Functional anatomy of the elbow joint. In Kashiwagi d (ed): Elbow Joint. Amsterdam, Elsevier Science Publishers, 1985

67. Travel JG, Simons DG: Myofascial Dysfunction—The Trigger Point Manual. Baltimore, Williams & Wilkins, 1983

68. Van Rossum J, Buruma OJS, Kamphuisen HAC, Onvlee GJ: Tennis elbow—a radial tunnel syndrome. J Bone Joint Surg 60(B):197–198, 1978

69. Wadsworth TG: The external compression syndrome of the ulnar nerve at the cubital tunnel. Clin Orthop 124:189–204, 1977

70. Wadsworth TG: The Elbow. New York, Churchill Livingstone, 1982

71. Wadsworth TG: Entrapment neuropathy in the upper limb. In Birch R, Brook D (eds): Operative Surgery, The Hand. pp 469–486. London, Buttersworths, 1984

72. Wadsworth TG: The cubital tunnel syndrome. In Kashiwagi D (ed): Elbow Joint. Amsterdam, Elsevier Science Publishers, 1985

73. Wadsworth TG, Williams JR: Cubital tunnel external compression syndrome. Br Med J 1:662–666, 1973

74. Wiens E, Lau SCK: The anterior interosseous nerve syndrome. Can J Surg 21:354–357, 1978

75. Woods GW, Tullos HS, King JW: The throwing arm: Elbow joint injuries. J Sports Med [Suppl] 1(4):43–47, 1973

RECOMMENDED READINGS

An KW, Morrey BF: Biomechanics of the elbow. In Morrey BF (ed): The Elbow and Its Disorders, pp 43–61. Philadelphia, WB Saunders, 1985

Bowling RW, Rockar PA: The elbow complex. In Gould JA, Davies GJ (eds): Orthopedic and Sports Physical Therapy. St. Louis, CV Mosby, 1983

Brewster CI, Shields CL, Seto TL, Morrissey MC: Rehabilitation of the upper extremity. In Shields CL (ed): Manual of Sports Surgery. New York, Spinger-Verlag, 1987

Corrigan B, Maitland GD: Practical Orthopedic Medicine. Boston, Butterworths, 1983

Heppenstall RB: Injuries of the elbow. In Heppenstal RB (ed): Fracture Treatment and Healing. Philadelphia, WB Saunders, 1980

Kisner C, Lynn AC: Therapeutic exercises: Foundations and Techniques, pp 281–296. Philadelphia, FA Davis, 1986

La Freniere JG: "Tennis elbow": Evaluation, treatment and prevention. Phys Ther 59:742–746, 1979

London JT: Kinematics of the elbow. J Bone Joint Surg 63(A):529–535, 1981

Murtagn JE: Tennis elbow, description and treatment. Aust Fam Physician 7:1307–1310, 1978

Nirshl RP: Rehabilitation of the athlete's elbow. In Morrey BF (ed): The Elbow and Its Disorders, pp 523–529. Philadelphia, WB Saunders, 1985

Nirshl RP, Pettrone FA: Tennis elbow: The surgical treatment of lateral epicondylitis. J Bone Joint Surg 61(A):832–839, 1979

Nirshl RP, Sobel J: Conservative treatment of tennis elbow. Phys Sports Med 9:43–54, 1981

Priest JD, Braden V, Gerberich SG: The elbow and tennis. I and II. Phys Sports Med 8:80–91, 77–85, 1980

Tucker K: Some aspects of post-traumatic elbow stiffness. Injury 9:216–220, 1978

12 *The Wrist and Hand Complex*

Darlene Hertling and Randolph M. Kessler

REVIEW OF FUNCTIONAL ANATOMY

THE WRIST COMPLEX

Osteology

Distal End of Radius. The radius flares distally, and this end is much larger than the distal end of the ulna. It extends farther laterally than medially. The distal lateral extension of the radius is the radial styloid process. The radial styloid normally extends about 1 cm farther distally than the ulnar styloid (Fig. 12–1).

The medial aspect of the distal radius is a concave surface anteroposteriorly. The medial concavity is the ulnar notch, which articulates with the head of the ulna, allowing pronation and supination to occur. The distal end of the radius is triangular in its transverse cross section. The distal articular surface of the radius is composed of two concave facets, one for articulation with the scaphoid and one for articulation with the lunate (Fig. 12–2). The distal articular surface of the radius faces slightly palmarly (average of 10°) and somewhat ulnarly (average of 20°) (Fig. 12–3).

Distal End of Ulna. The distal end of the ulna flares only mildly compared with the distal end of the radius. The ulnar styloid process is a small conical projection from the dorsomedial aspect of the distal end of the ulna. The radial aspect of the ulnar head is convex anteroposteriorly. It is cartilage-covered for articulation with the ulnar notch of the radius during pronation and supination (see Figs. 12–1 and 12–2).

The distal end of the ulna is somewhat circular on transverse cross section, except for the irregularity formed by the styloid process dorsomedially. The distal surface of the ulna is covered with articular cartilage for articulation with the articular disk (not with the carpals). There is movement between the ulna and disk primarily on pronation and supination, during which the disk must sweep across the distal end of the ulna.

Carpals. The proximal row of carpals consists of the triquetrum, pisiform, lunate, and scaphoid bones. The scaphoid has a biconvex articular surface proximally for articulation with the lateral facet of the distal end of the radius. The lunate is also convex proximally and articulates with the medial facet of the distal radius and with the articular disk in positions of radial deviation. The triquetrum has a small convex articular surface proximally. This surface is in contact with the ulnar collateral ligament when the wrist is in neutral position and articulates with the articular disk primarily in positions of ulnar deviation. The flexor carpi ulnaris tendon inserts onto the pisiform bone, which lies palmarly over the triquetrum.

The distal end of the scaphoid consists of two distal articular surfaces. The radial surface of the distal scaphoid is convex for articulation with the concave surface formed by the combined proximal ends of the trapezoid and trapezium. The ulnar articulating surface of the distal scaphoid is concave and faces somewhat palmarly and ulnarly. It articulates with the proximal end of the capitate. The distal surface of the lunate is quite concave anteroposteriorly but less so mediolaterally. It grasps the convex proximal end of the capitate and also articulates, to a lesser extent, with the hamate. The distal surface of the triquetrum is concave for articulation with the hamate (see Figs. 12–1 and 12–2).

There is some movement between the bones of the proximal row of carpals. For this reason each of the proximal carpals is lined with articular cartilage on its radial or ulnar surfaces, or both, to allow for such movement.

Ulnarly to radially, the distal carpals comprise the hamate, capitate, trapezoid, and trapezium (see Fig. 12–1). As indicated previously, the combined proximal surfaces of the hamate and capitate form a convex surface that articulates with the concave surface formed by the combined distal surfaces of the trique-

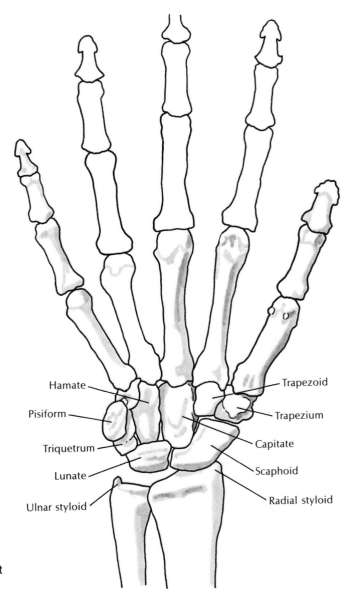

Fig. 12–1. Palmar aspect of the bones of the right wrist and hand.

trum, lunate, and scaphoid (see Fig. 12–2). The combined proximal surfaces of the trapezoid and trapezium form a concave surface for articulation with the convex distal articular surface of the scaphoid. The distal end of the trapezium is a sellar surface that articulates with the correspondingly sellar surface of the proximal aspect of the first metacarpal. The trapezoid articulates distally with the second metacarpal, the capitate with the third metacarpal, and the hamate with the fourth and fifth metacarpals (see Fig. 12–1).

Because there is a small amount of movement between adjacent bones of the distal row, these are also lined with articular cartilage radially and ulnarly to allow for such intercarpal movement.

The carpals, taken together, form an arch in the transverse plane that is concave palmarly. This arch deepens with wrist flexion and flattens on wrist extension. The "hook" of the hamate, a rather large prominence on the palmar aspect of the hamate, and the pisiform bone, situated on the palmar aspect of the triquetrum, form the ulnar side of this arch. The trapezium, which tends to be oriented about 45° from the plane of the palm, and the radial aspect of the scaphoid, which curves palmarly, form the radial side of the arch. The flexor retinaculum, or transverse carpal ligament, traverses this arch (Fig. 12–4). The flexor ulnaris tendon inserts onto the pisiform. When this muscle contracts it pulls on the pisiform, causing tightening of the flexor retinacu-

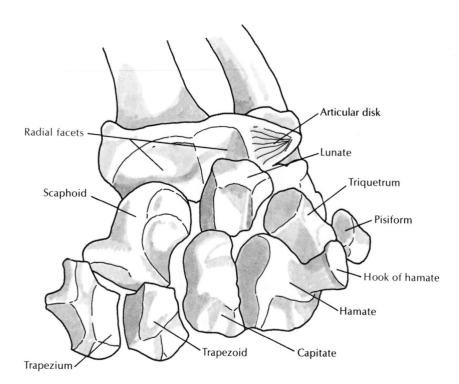

Radial facets

Scaphoid

Trapezium

Trapezoid

Capitate

Articular disk

Lunate

Triquetrum

Pisiform

Hook of hamate

Hamate

Fig. 12-2. Inferior aspect of the lower end of the radius and ulna and the carpal bones of the hand.

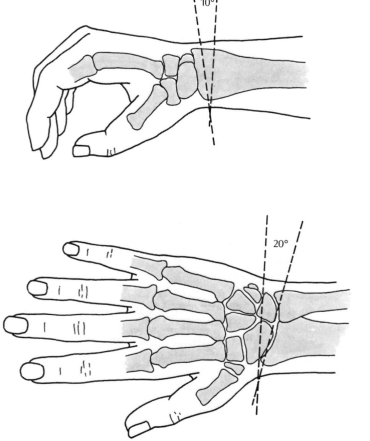

10°

20°

Fig. 12-3. Normal wrist alignment.

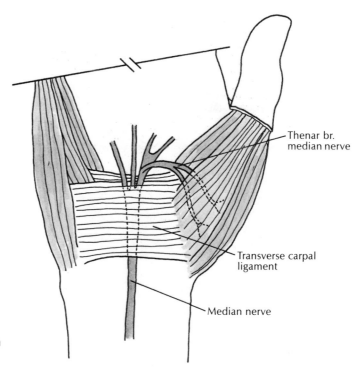

Fig. 12-4. Transverse carpal ligament and median nerve.

lum. This tightening deepens the transverse carpal arch.

Ligaments, Capsules, Synovia, and Disk

The articular cavity of the distal radioulnar joint is usually distinct from the articular cavity of the radiocarpal joint, which is also separate from that of the midcarpal joint. The carpometacarpal joints often share a common joint cavity which, in some cases, communicates with the midcarpal joint (Fig. 12-5).

The distal radioulnar joint is bordered proximally by the lax "sacciform recess" in the capsule, which loops proximally between the radius and ulna. Distally this joint is bordered by the triangular articular disk. This fibrocartiligenous disk attaches ulnarly to the ulnar styloid process and radially to the ulnar margin of the distal radial articular surface. It is what separates the distal radioulnar joint from the radiocarpal joint. Anteriorly and posteriorly the margins of the disk attach to the joint capsule. The superior aspect of the disk is a cartilage-lined concave surface for articulation with the distal end of the ulna. As implied above, the disk moves with the radius on pronation and supination and must therefore sweep across the distal end of the ulna on these movements. During flexion and extension of the wrist the disk remains stationary relative to the ulna. With this movement the lunate or triquetrum, or both, articu-

lates with the distal surface of the disk, which is also concave and cartilage-covered. The disk, then, provides two articular surfaces for the ulna and carpals, respectively, separates the adjacent joint cavities, and binds together the distal ends of the ulna and radius (see Fig. 12-5).

The radiocarpal joint is bordered proximally by the radius and the articular disk. Distally it is bordered by the three proximal carpals and their respective interosseous ligaments, which are flush with the continuous convex articular surface formed by the proximal carpals. Medially and laterally the joint is bordered by the strong ulnar and radial collateral ligaments. Both collateral ligaments attach proximally to the styloid processes. Distally, the ulnar ligament attaches to the triquetrum and pisiform; the radial ligament attaches to the scaphoid and trapezium. Palmarly and dorsally, the capsule of this joint is reinforced by the palmar radiocarpal ligament and the dorsal radiocarpal ligament (Fig. 12-6). Palmarly, there is also an ulnocarpal ligament. These ligaments ensure that the carpals follow the radius during pronation and supination. Synovium lines the capsuloligamentous structures mentioned, as well as the interosseous ligaments between triquetrum and lunate and between scaphoid and lunate.

The articulations between the proximal and distal carpal bones are enclosed in a common joint cavity.

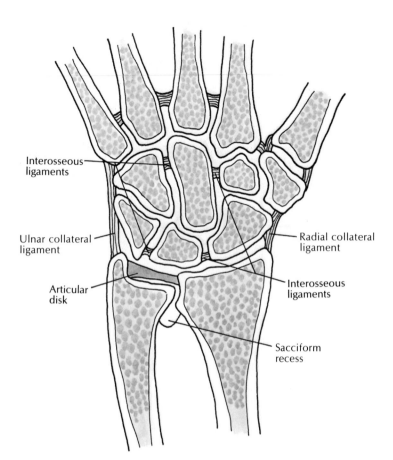

Interosseous ligaments

Ulnar collateral ligament

Articular disk

Radial collateral ligament

Interosseous ligaments

Sacciform recess

Fig. 12–5. Cross section through the articulations of the wrist, showing the synovial cavities.

Anatomically, the midcarpal joint is considered the compound joint between the two rows of carpals. However, functionally, as explained in the section on biomechanics, the distinction is not so simple. Proximally, the midcarpal joint is bordered by the scaphoid, lunate, and triquetrum and their interosseous ligaments, which as mentioned intervene between the proximal ends of these bones. In this way the intercarpal articulations between the proximal carpals are enclosed within the midcarpal joint cavity. Distally, the midcarpal joint is bordered by the distal carpals and their interosseous ligaments, which intervene about midway, or further distally, between the distal carpals. Occasionally an interosseous ligament intervenes between capitate and scaphoid, dividing the midcarpal joint into medial and lateral cavities. Since an interosseous ligament is often missing between trapezoid and trapezium, the midcarpal joint often communicates with the common joint cavity of the carpometacarpal joints (see Fig. 12–5). Medially and laterally, extensions of the ulnar and radial collateral ligaments connect the triquetrum to the hamate and the scaphoid to the trapezium. There are also dorsal and palmar intercarpal

ligaments between the bones of the two rows. Palmarly these intercarpal ligaments are often referred to as the radiate ligament since they tend to radiate outward from the capitate (Fig. 12–6).

Palmar and dorsal intercarpal ligaments also connect the carpals within a row. The pisohamate ligament (from the pisiform to the hook of the hamate) and the pisometacarpal ligament (to the base of the fifth metacarpal) are believed to be continuations of the flexor carpi ulnaris tendon that attaches to the pisiform (see Fig. 12–6). The joint between the pisiform and triquetrum is usually distinct from the other joints mentioned, having its own joint capsule and synovial-lined cavity.

THE HAND COMPLEX

The hand consists of five digits, or four fingers and a thumb. There are 19 long bones distal to the carpals and 19 joints that make up the hand complex. These are divided in five rays, with each ray making up a polyarticulated chain comprising the metacarpals and phalanges. The base of each metacarpal articulates with the distal row of carpals.

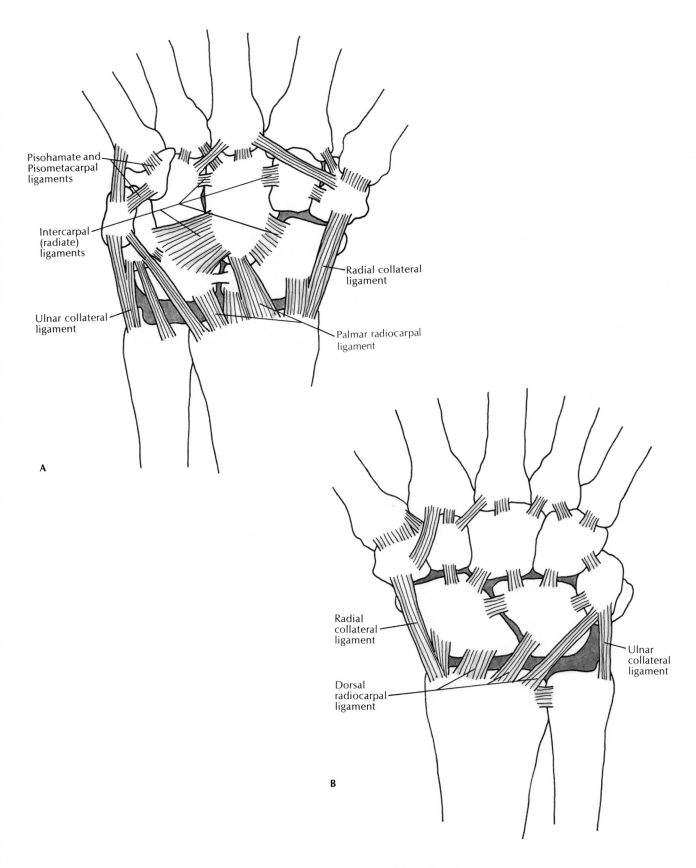

Fig. 12-6. Palmar aspect *(A)* and dorsal aspect *(B)* of the ligaments of the right wrist and metacarpus.

Carpometacarpal Joints of the Fingers

In the carpometacarpal joint area there are two stable joints that permit little or no motion: the carpometacarpal joints of the index and middle fingers. There are also two very mobile joints: the carpometacarpal joints of the thumb and the little finger.[91] Since thumb function differs significantly from that of the other digits, it will be examined separately. The second metacarpal articulates primarily with the trapezoid and secondarily with the trapezium, capitate, and third metacarpal (see Fig. 12–1). The trapezoid is mortised in the base of the index metacarpal base, affording a very secure fixation.

The middle or third metacarpal articulates primarily with the capitate and is also bound to the adjacent second and fourth metacarpal (see Fig. 12–1). Therefore all the carpals in the distal carpal row and the index and middle metacarpal bases are firmly joined and function together as a single osseoligamentous unit, the fixed stable portion of the hand.[70]

The little finger metacarpal articulates with the hamate and fourth metacarpal (see Fig. 12–1). The hamate is a saddle-like joint, and its articulation with the little metacarpal resembles that of the thumb carpometacarpal joint but is not as mobile.[91] The articular surface of the base of the fifth metacarpal is convex in the volardorsal direction and concave in the radioulnar axis.[96]

The ring finger metacarpal base articulates with the hamate primarily in a joint similar to that of the little finger but with even less motion permitted. It also articulates with the capitate as well as the middle and little finger metacarpals (see Fig. 12–1).

While the little finger carpometacarpal joint is considered a saddle joint with two degrees of freedom, the other finger carpometacarpal joints are plane synovial joints with one degree of freedom: flexion–extension.[54,82] Their proximal surface may be considered concave and the distal end, convex.

The capsular pattern of restriction is limitation of motion equally in all directions. All are supported by strong transverse and weaker longitudinal ligaments volarly and dorsally (see Fig. 12–6). It is this ligamentous structure that controls the total range of motion available at each carpometacarpal joint. The function of the carpometacarpal joints of the fingers is primarily to contribute to the hollowing of the palm to allow the hand and digits to conform optimally to the shape of the object being held.[82]

Carpometacarpal Joint of the Thumb

The carpometacarpal joint of the trapezium–thumb metacarpal joint is a very mobile articulation. Although described as a saddle-type joint, it is actually a reciprocally biconcave joint resembling two saddles whose concave surfaces are opposed to each other at right angles or 90° rotation (Fig. 12–7). All motions are possible, including circumduction.[16,91] The carpometacarpal articulation is specialized to produce automatic axial rotation of the first metacarpal during angular movements. Zancolli[119] offers the concept that the trapezium is formed by two different types of joints. One part, the saddle area, occupies the center of the articular surfaces and takes part in simple angular movements. The other part is located on the palmar side and is an ovoid area that represents a ball-and-socket joint for complex rotatory movements. The saddle part of the joint favors the circumduction motion to the motion of opposition. The trapezium is firmly bound to the trapezoid and indeed to the entire distal carpal row and has virtually no independent motion.

According to Zancolli,[119,120] the greatest stability of the first metacarpal is achieved after complete pronation in the position of full opposition when ligamentory tension, muscular contraction, and joint congruence produce the maximal effect in achieving stabilization of pinch. Opposition with simultaneous pronation (or axial rotation) is sequentially abduction, flexion, and adduction of the first metacarpal. Axial rotation occurring in the carpometacarpal joint is made possible because of the laxity of the joint capsule and the joint configuration.[18,82,119,120] The tension in the ligaments combined with muscle activity of opposition and reposition form couples (paired parallel forces) that produce this axial rota-

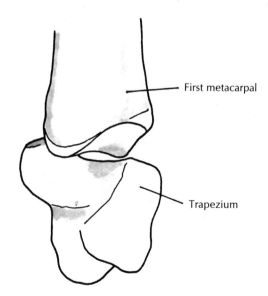

Fig. 12–7. Schematic representation of the saddle-shaped carpometacarpal articulation of the thumb.

First metacarpal

Trapezium

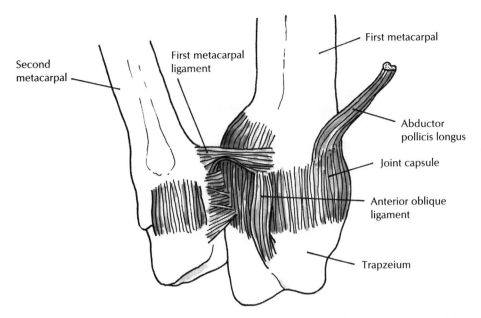

Fig. 12–8. Volar view of the right first carpometacarpal joint and the arrangement of the ligaments.

tion. The function of muscles crossing the joint is essential. According to Kauer,[56] the close structural relationship between the tendon of the abductor pollicis longus and the first carpometacarpal joint influence the restraining and directing function of the ligamentous system. The functional significance of the movement of opposition can be appreciated when one realizes that use of the thumb against a finger occurs in almost all forms of prehension.[82]

The strongest carpometacarpal joint ligament is the deep ulnar or anterior oblique carpometacarpal ligament that unites the tubercle of the trapezium and the volar beak of the metacarpal base (Fig. 12–8).[96] Extrinsic support is provided by the extensor pollicis longus and the origin of the thenar muscles.

Metacarpophalangeal Joints of the Fingers

The distal metacarpophalangeal joints of the fingers are made of an irregular spheroidal (convex) metacarpal head proximally and the concave base of the first phalanx distally (Fig. 12–9A). They are multiaxial condyloid joints and primarily allow flexion and extension but also abduction, adduction, and some axial rotation. The most extensive movements are flexion and extension. The average flexion range is 90° to 95°, but hyperextension of 20° to 30° and even as much as 45° is common. The articular surface of the metacarpal head is rounded dorsally and is flat volarly (see Fig. 12–9A). It has 180° of articular surface in the sagittal plane with the predominant portion lying volarly. This is apposed to approximately

20° of articular surface on the phalanx, resulting in poorly mated surfaces.[82]

The joint is surrounded by a capsule that is lax in extension and in conjunction with the poorly mated surfaces allows some passive axial rotation of the proximal phalanx in this position (Fig. 12–10).[82] The primary ligament support of the metacarpophalangeal joint includes two lateral collateral ligaments, two accessory collateral ligaments, and the volar plate (Figs. 12–10 and 12–11). The volar plate or ligament is a thick, tough fibrocartilaginous structure that firmly inserts into the volar base of the proximal phalanx. Proximally it thins out to become nearly membranous at its metacarpal attachment. The volar plate with the two accessory ligaments on the sides enlarges the cavity of the metacarpophalangeal joint, permitting the head of the metacarpal to remain in the articular cavity as the metacarpophalangeal joint flexes (see Fig. 12–10). During flexion, this thin proximal portion folds in like the billows of an accordion or a telephone booth door.[91] The plate also helps to restrict the hyperextension that is permitted by the loose capsule. Distally and laterally the volar plate on both sides is attached to a lateral collateral ligament and in its midposition laterally, to an accessory ligament (see Fig. 12–11). The four volar plates of the metacarpophalangeal joints also blend with and are interconnected by the transverse metacarpal ligament, which connects the adjacent lateral borders of the index, middle, ring, and little fingers. While the dorsal surface of the volar plate is in contact with the head of the metacarpal, the volar sur-

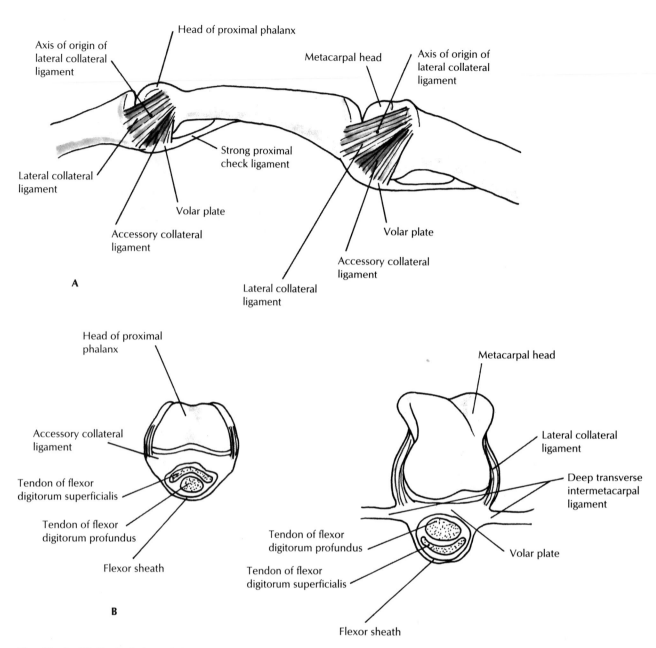

Fig. 12-9. *(A)* Sagittal view of the metacarpophalangeal and interphalangeal joints of the fingers. *(B)* Anterior view of metacarpal and proximal phalanx head.

face of this ligament is in contact with the flexor tendon. The volar plate and transverse metacarpal ligament form the dorsal wall of the vaginal ligament, which forms a tunnel and completely surrounds the flexor tendons (see Fig. 12-9). The flexible attachment of the volar plate to the phalanx permits the plate to glide distally along the volar surface of the metacarpal head without restricting motion during flexion and also prevents impingement by the joint of the long flexor tendons (Fig. 12-12).

The metacarpophalangeal joint is the most stable in maximal flexion since the lateral collateral ligaments are stretched tautly in this position and the accessory collateral ligaments offer additional stability by firmly holding the volar plate against the volar surface of the metacarpal head (see Fig. 12-12). The capsule also becomes taut in this close-packed position (see Fig. 12-10). In extension the capsule and lateral collateral ligaments are lax and the metacarpophalangeal joint is relatively mobile,

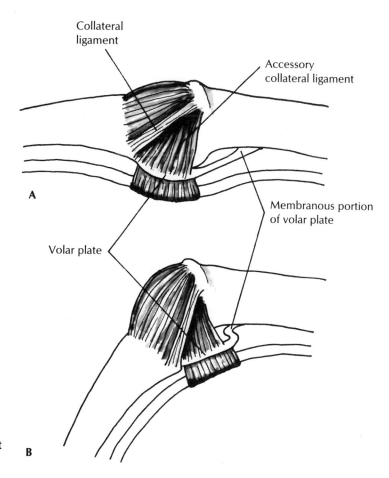

Collateral ligament

Accessory collateral ligament

Membranous portion of volar plate

Volar plate

A

B

Fig. 12–10. The metacarpophalangeal joint during flexion *(A)* and extension *(B)*.

permitting abduction and adduction as well as some axial rotation by the intrinsic muscles. Disparity of the articular surfaces and laxity of the ligaments at these joints allows for considerable passive range of movement in all positions of these joints except the close-packed position. Together with the transverse metacarpal arch, the passive movements at the metacarpophalangeal joints enhance the plasticity of the hand and facilitate its adaptability to the size and shape of the object being grasped.[89]

The asymmetry of the metacarpal heads as well as the difference in length and direction of the collateral ligaments explains why the ulnar inclination of the digits normally is greater than radial inclination.[104] The normal ulnar inclination of the fingers occurs at the metacarpophalangeal joints, being most marked in the index finger. Inclination is less in the middle and little finger and almost nonexistent in the ring finger. Normal ulnar inclination is due to a number of anatomical factors, which have been the subject of numerous studies in recent years.[33,40,42,95,119]

Metacarpophalangeal Joint of the Thumb

The metacarpophalangeal joint of the thumb is a semicondyloid-type articulation between the head of the first metacarpal and base of its proximal phalanx. Two sesamoid bones are constantly present extra-capsularly on its volar surface: a somewhat larger lateral sesamoid and a medial sesamoid (Fig. 12–13).[96] The joint has two degrees of freedom: flexion, extension, abduction, adduction, and limited axial rotation.[55] The capsule is inserted in the ridge separating the articulation of the proximal phalanx and the metacarpal. The capsule is reinforced on each side by the collateral ligaments similar to those of the other metacarpophalangeal joints. Each collateral ligament is inserted into a tubercle on the base of the phalanx and into the corresponding sesamoid (Fig. 12–14). The two sesamoids are incorporated into the fibrocartilage of the volar plate.[96] The tunnel of the flexor pollicis longus is intimately connected to the volar plate so the tunnel is an integral part of the apparatus, connecting the lateral liga-

Metacarpal head

Accessory collateral ligament

Volar plate

Lateral collateral ligament

Base of proximal phalanx

Fig. 12–11. Metacarpophalangeal joint with collateral ligaments divided.

ments and the volar plate with the sesamoids. The volar plate is attached firmly to the proximal phalanx but loosely to the metacarpal, and it is the proximal attachment that has given way, with irreducible dislocation.[16]

There is considerable individual variation in joint ranges depending on the anatomical configuration of the single broad condyle of the metacarpal.[11] Flexion ranges from 5° to 100°, with an average of about 75°.[91] If the head is round, 90° to 100° flexion is achieved. If it is flat (only 10% to 15% of cases), little flexion is possible. The main functional contribution of the first metacarpophalangeal joint is to provide additional range to the thumb pad in opposition and to allow the thumb to grasp and contour to objects.[82] The literature contains little information on the function of the sesamoids. The most common belief is that they increase the leverage of certain muscles connected with the tendons running to these joints.[96]

Interphalangeal Articulations of the Fingers

The interphalangeal joints of the digits are each composed of the head of a phalanx and the base of the phalanx distal to it (see Fig. 12–9). Each is a true synovial hinge joint that functions uniquely in flexion and extension with one degree of freedom. From a clinical standpoint, each phalanx has a head (caput) or a distal end with a convex surface and a body (corpus) and a base or proximal end with a concave surface.[51] The head of each phalanx, divided into two condyles separated by a cleft, fits the contiguous articular surface of the phalangeal base and articulates in a tongue-in-groove configuration (see Fig. 12–9).[91] Their trochlear-shaped articulations are closely congruent through excursion of the joint.[104]

The proximal interphalangeal joint has its greatest range of flexion and extension of any digital joint

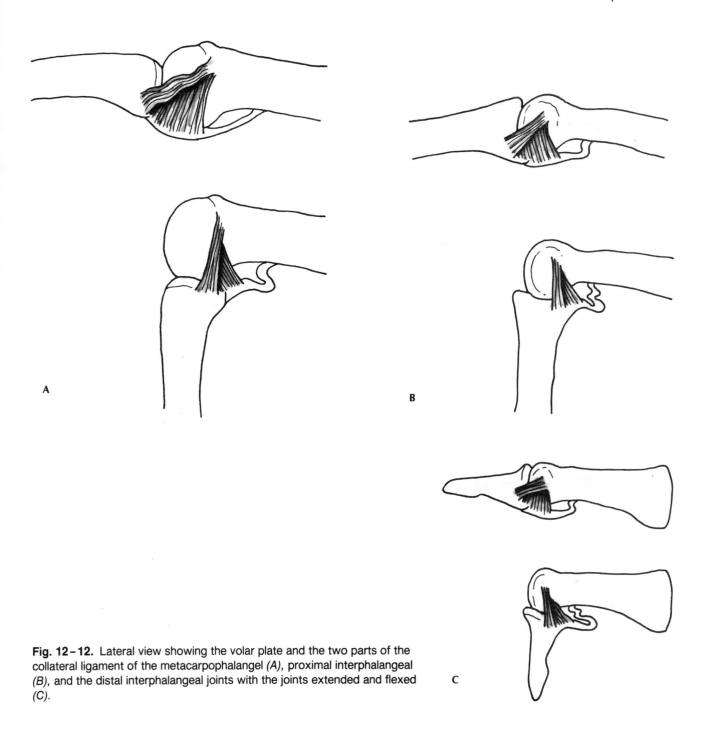

Fig. 12–12. Lateral view showing the volar plate and the two parts of the collateral ligament of the metacarpophalangel *(A)*, proximal interphalangeal *(B)*, and the distal interphalangeal joints with the joints extended and flexed *(C)*.

with an average of 105°. The intrinsic ligamentous support of the proximal interphalangeal joint resembles that of the metacarpophalangeal joint and includes two lateral collateral ligaments, two accessory collateral ligaments, and a volar plate (see Fig. 12–12B). The volar plate, which prevents hyperextension, has a thick distal insertion and two check ligaments proximally inserted on the middle phalanx (Fig. 12–15). It is interesting that traumatic ruptures

of the volar plate occur in the thicker distal insertion rather than the proximal insertion.[104] The fibrous flexor sheath is inserted on the volar plate on the base of the phalanx proximally and distally. This differs from the insertion at the metacarpophalangeal joint, where the flexor sheath inserts on the volar plate and base of the proximal phalanx but not on the metacarpal. This arrangement involving the collateral ligaments, volar plate, and flexor sheath is the key to

Fig. 12-13. Inner view of the metacarpophalangeal joint of the right thumb. The capsule and lateral ligaments are excised with the parts attached shown. The volar plate with the sesamoids is shown at the bottom of the joint.

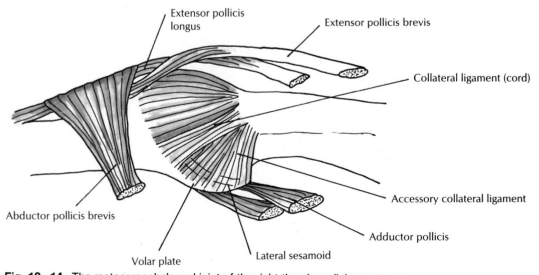

Fig. 12-14. The metacarpophalangel joint of the right thumb, radial aspect.

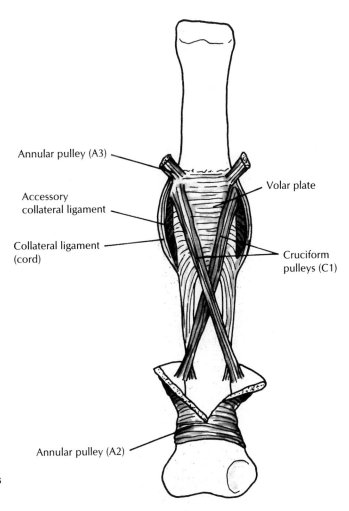

Annular pulley (A3)

Accessory
collateral ligament

Collateral ligament
(cord)

Volar plate

Cruciform
pulleys (C1)

Annular pulley (A2)

Fig. 12–15. Schematic representation of the proximal interphalangel joint and the arrangement of the components of the flexor sheath and volar plate.

interphalangeal stability.[26] Little hyperextension of this joint is possible in contrast to the metacarpophalangeal joint.

The distal interphalangeal joint resembles the proximal interphalangeal joint in function and ligamentous structure but has less stability and allows some hyperextension, giving a larger pulp contact (see Fig. 12–12C). Distal interphalangeal flexion rarely exceeds 80°, but hyperextension is greater than at the proximal interphalangeal joint because the distal interphalangeal joint's volar plate does not possess the check ligaments proximally.[91]

The total range of flexion–extension available to the index finger is 100° to 110° at the proximal interphalangeal joints and 80° at the distal interphalangeal joint. The range at each joint increases ulnarly, with the proximal and distal joints achieving 135° and 90°, respectively, in the little finger.[82]

Interphalangeal Joint of the Thumb

The interphalangeal joint of the thumb is structurally and functionally similar to the distal interphalangeal joints of the fingers. It is a trochlear type of articulation, allowing mainly flexion and extension with a slight degree of axial rotation toward pronation. Axial rotation, in fact, occurs at all three joints of the thumb: (1) trapeziometacarpal—automatic longitudinal rotation at a saddle joint; (2) metacarpophalangeal—active longitudinal rotation at a condylar joint through the action of the lateral thenar muscles; and (3) interphalangeal joint.[52,53]

At the end of the extension range, motion is restricted by the volar plate. There is considerable variation in the amount of extension permitted, with many normal subjects having the ability to hyperextend the joint.[16] Lack of extension of this joint, if

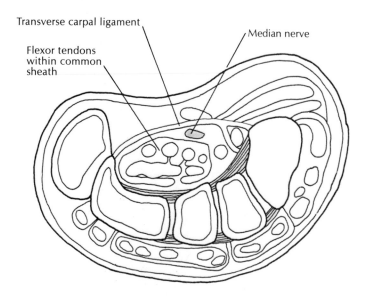

Transverse carpal ligament

Median nerve

Flexor tendons within common sheath

Fig. 12–16. Cross-section of the wrist through the carpus, demonstrating the relationship of the median nerve to the flexor tendons and transverse carpal ligaments (flexor retinaculum).

greater than 15°, is functionally more disabling then lack of flexion.[104]

TENDONS, NERVES, AND ARTERIES

These structures are not discussed in detail here. The reader will benefit from studying cross-sectional diagrams that depict anatomical relationships of these structures (Fig. 12–16). The relationships described below are of most importance clinically.

As mentioned, the transverse carpal ligament (flexor retinaculum) forms a roof over the palmar arch of the carpal bones (see Figs. 12–4 and 12–16). Through the resulting tunnel pass the tendons of the flexor digitorum profundus and flexor digitorum superficialis. These tendons are all enclosed in a common synovial sheath. The flexor carpi radialis tendon and the flexor pollicis longus tendon also pass through the "carpal tunnel," each enclosed in a separate sheath. Superficial to the common flexor tendon sheath and deep to the flexor retinaculum passes the median nerve. At the distal end of the tunnel the nerve divides into several digital branches, one of which turns rather sharply around the distal border of the flexor retinaculum to innervate the thenar muscle (see Fig. 12–4). "Carpal tunnel syndrome" is the result of compression of the median nerve within the tunnel or, occasionally, of just the thenar branch of the nerve as it turns around the distal border of the retinaculum. The palmaris longus tendon and the ulnar nerve and artery pass superficially to the flexor retinaculum. The nerve and artery travel beneath the flexor carpi ulnaris tendon, then radially to the pisiform bone before dividing to enter the hand.

The tendons of the extensor pollicis brevis and the abductor pollicis longus are enclosed in a common sheath as they pass across the lateral aspect of the distal radius. Inflammation of this sheath, or of the tendons within the sheath, is a fairly common disorder, referred to as *de Quervain's disease,* or tenosynovitis. These tendons form the radial side of the "anatomical snuff box." The extensor pollicis longus tendon passes around Lister's tubercle on the dorsal aspect of the distal radius in a pulley-like fashion. It turns obliquely toward the thumb to form the ulnar side of the "snuff box." The radial artery travels laterally to the flexor carpi radialis tendon before turning deep beneath the abductor pollicis longus and extensor pollicis brevis tendons. It becomes superficial dorsally and can be palpated in the anatomical snuff box.

At the level of the fingers the long flexor tendons are attached to the volar aspect by three fibrous sheaths: the first lies just proximal to the metacarpal head, the second on the palmar surface of the proximal phalanx, the third on the same surface of the second phalanx (Fig. 12–17). These form fibrous tunnels or digital pulleys along with the slightly concave osseous palmar surface of the phalanges. Between these three sheaths the tendons are held down by annular oblique and cruciate fibers that cover the metacarpophalangeal and proximal interphalangeal joints in a crosswise position (see Fig. 12–15). The two digital pulleys constitute the most important elements of the flexor tendon sheaths; the cruciate pulleys play an accessory role.[94] Synovial sheaths allow gliding of the tendons within their tunnels.

Anatomically, it is worth noting that the synovial

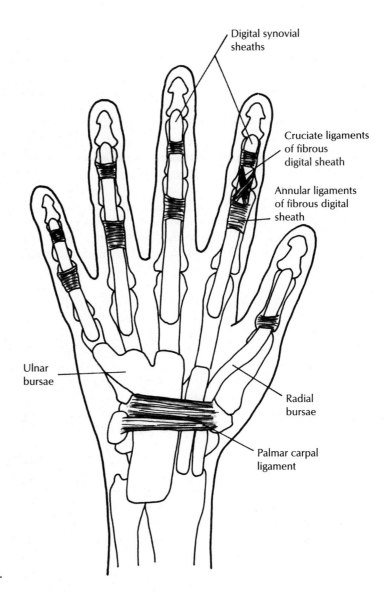

Digital synovial
sheaths

Cruciate ligaments
of fibrous
digital sheath

Annular ligaments
of fibrous digital
sheath

Ulnar
bursae

Radial
bursae

Palmar carpal
ligament

Fig. 12-17. Bursae and lumbrical sheaths of hand.

sheaths of the flexor tendons start in the forearm proximal to the flexor retinaculum (see Fig. 12-16). The skin creases on the flexor aspect of the fingers, except for the proximal crease, lie immediately proximal to the corresponding joints and at this level the skin is directly in contact with the synovial sheath, which can be readily infected.[54]

The long extensor muscles of the hand also run along fibro-osseous tunnels, but since their course on the whole is convex these tunnels are less numerous. They are only seen at the wrist, where the tendons become concave outward during extension.[54]

A more detailed description of the anatomy of the hand and wrist complex can be found in other sources.[10,39,43,52,54,56,66,77,101,104]

SURFACE ANATOMY OF THE WRIST

Because the wrist consists of many small structures in close proximity, the clinician must pay special attention to identification of these structures. There are some guidelines that can be followed to help identify the clinically significant structures about the wrist. The reader can perform the following exercise:

The distal end of the radius is easily palpated. Notice how it flares distally. Palpate along its radial border to the styloid process; note the gap between the radial styloid and the carpals when the wrist and thumb are relaxed. Extend the thumb and notice how the abductor pollicis longus and extensor pollicis brevis tendons bridge this gap. The prominence on the dorsal aspect of the distal radius, Lister's tubercle, is easily palpated. Again, extend the thumb and follow the extensor pollicis longus tendon from this tubercle, about which it curves, down to the thumb.

With the thumb extended and the wrist slightly dorsiflexed, once again locate the abductor pollicis longus tendon. Now palpate ulnarly on the palmar aspect of the wrist, level with the radial styloid. The next prominent tendon is the flexor carpi radialis tendon. Palpate the radial pulse just radial to this tendon. Once again palpate in an ulnar direction. The next tendon, just ulnar to the flexor carpi radialis, is the palmaris longus tendon. The median nerve lies deep to this tendon, beneath the flexor retinaculum.

The distal end of the ulna is also easily palpated. Feel the interval between it and the distal radius. Notice how much smaller the distal ulna is compared with the radius. The ulnar styloid process is quite prominent on the dorsoulnar aspect of the distal ulna. Palpate to the end of the ulnar styloid and notice the gap between it and the carpals, which opens with radial deviation and closes with ulnar deviation. With the wrist in radial deviation, the ulnar collateral ligament can be felt bridging this gap.

From the ulnar styloid process dorsoulnarly, palpate distally to the next large prominence — the dorsal aspect of the triquetrum. From the dorsal aspect of the triquetrum, palpate around palmarly to the prominent pisiform situated in the palmoulnar corner of the palm. Grasp the pisiform with two fingers and notice how it can be wriggled back and forth with the wrist in flexion, but not with the wrist in extension. This is because of the increased tension on the flexor carpi ulnaris tendon that attaches to the pisiform. Palpate the flexor carpi ulnaris tendon proximal to the pisiform. Feel the pulse from the ulnar artery just radial to this tendon. The ulnar nerve is situated just deep to and between the ulnar artery and the flexor carpi ulnaris tendon. Once again, locate the dorsal aspect of the triquetrum, the large prominence just distal to the prominent ulnar styloid. Slide your palpating finger distally over the dorsal aspect of the triquetrum. Feel the small interval or "joint line" between it and the hamate. With the index finger over the dorsal aspect of the hamate, bring the thumb around palmarly at the same level. With the thumb, palpate the prominent "hook" of the hamate deep in the hypothenar eminence; it is usually slightly tender to palpation. Between the hook of the hamate and the pisiform, beneath the

pisohamate ligament, is the tunnel of Guyon. The ulnar nerve and artery pass through this tunnel.

Now imagine a line running dorsally from the base of the middle finger to Lister's tubercle. At the midpoint of this line, or just radial to it, the base of the third metacarpal can be felt as a prominence. The capitate lies just proximally to this prominence. With the wrist in neutral position, the dorsal concavity of the capitate can be palpated as a depression at the dorsum of the wrist. Just proximal to this depression is the lunate. If a palpating finger is placed over the lunate and capitate while passively flexing and extending the wrist, the distal end of the lunate can be felt to slide into the depression in the capitate on extension and out on flexion.

In the deepest portion of the anatomical snuff box the dorsoradial aspect of the scaphoid bone can be palpated. It is most easily felt with the wrist in ulnar deviation. Just distal to the scaphoid you can feel the trapezium. You should be able to identify the trapezium–first metacarpal articulation. The trapezoid is easily palpated as a prominence at the base of the second metacarpal.

BIOMECHANICS OF THE WRIST

The wrist is composed of three joints: the distal radioulnar joint, the radiocarpal joint, and the midcarpal joint. With this description it is understood that the radiocarpal joint includes the articulation between the disk and the carpals, since the disk acts as an ulnar extension of the distal radial joint surface. From a functional standpoint, however, it is best to speak of an ulnomeniscotriquetral joint in addition to the three joints listed above. In this way the movements of the ulna and the carpals can be better considered in relation to the disk. (Refer to Appendix A for a description of the movements that occur at these joints and the arthrokinematic motions that accompany these movements.)

Movements among the many bones of the wrist are, indeed, complex. The clinician must have a basic knowledge of the major interarticular movements to be successful in evaluating painful conditions affecting the wrist and in restoring movement when it is lost.

FLEXION–EXTENSION

The primary axis of movement for wrist flexion–extension passes through the capitate. The wrist close-packs in full dorsiflexion, since it must assume a state of maximal intrinsic stability in order to allow one to transmit pressure from the hand to the forearm. In functional activities such force transmission usually occurs with the wrist in dorsiflexion, for example, when pushing a heavy object or walking on all fours. As with any synovial joint, the close-packed position at the wrist is achieved by a "screw home" movement — a movement involving a conjunct rotation (see Chapter 2). The carpus, on dorsiflexion, moves in a supinatory rotation. This is easily observed by watching your own wrist as it passes from neutral to full extension. The reason for this rotation is that the scaphoid moves in a manner that differs from the movement of other proximal carpal bones.[72] As the wrist moves from a position of flexion to neutral, the distal row of carpals remains relatively loose-packed with respect to the proximal row, and the proximal row remains loose-packed with respect to the radius. Disk movement occurs at both the radiocarpal joint and the midcarpal joint. At about the neutral position, or just slightly beyond, as the wrist continues into dorsiflexion, the distal row of carpals becomes close-packed with the scaphoid but not with the other proximal carpals (lunate and triquetrum). Because of this close-packing, the scaphoid moves with the distal row of carpals as the wrist moves into full dorsiflexion. During this final stage of dorsiflexion, then, movement must occur between the scaphoid and lunate as the distal row continues to dorsiflex against the lunate and triquetrum. Looking at it another way, the scaphoid moves more with respect to the radius than do the lunate and triquetrum. This asymmetry of movement results in a supinatory twisting with the carpus that twists capsules and ligaments to close-pack the remaining joints at full dorsiflexion (Fig. 12–18).

As in any joint, the bones forming the wrist are most susceptible to fracture or dislocation when in the close-packed position. Most frequently fractured are the scaphoid and the distal end of the radius. The most common dislocations are a palmar dislocation of the lunate relative to the radius and remaining carpals and a dorsal dislocation of the carpals with respect to the lunate and the radius. The common mechanism of injury for all the above injuries, as would be expected, is a fall on the dorsiflexed hand.

RADIAL–ULNAR DEVIATION

The axis of movement for radial-ulnar deviation also passes through the capitate. Ulnar deviation occurs over a much greater range of movement than radial deviation. This is because radial deviation is limited by contact of the scaphoid tubercle against the radial styloid process, whereas the triquetrum easily clears the ulnar styloid process, which is situated more dorsally and is less prominent than the radial styloid process. Both radial and ulnar deviation involve movements at the radiocarpal and midcarpal joints.[116] The associated arthrokinematic movements are not pure, but rather involve rotary movements between proximal row and radius, and between distal row and proximal row. As described by Kapandji, the proximal row tends to move into pronation, flexion, and ulnar glide during radial deviation with respect to the radius and disk (Fig. 12–19).[53] At the same time, the distal row moves into supination, extension, and ulnar glide with respect to the proximal row. The opposite movements occur during ulnar deviation (Fig. 12–20). This can be easily observed on a cadaver and seems to be due entirely to the shapes of the joint surfaces rather than the capsuloligamentous influences. Radial deviation involves close-packing of primarily the midcarpal joint.

FUNCTION AND ARCHITECTURE OF THE HAND

The hand is a complex machine. It may be used as a means of expression, a tactile organ, and a weapon. The study of the hand is inseparable from that of the wrist and forearm, which function as a single physiological unit, with the wrist being the key joint. In pronation–supination the movement of the radius in relation to the ulna is in fact the movement of the hand around its longitudinal axis.[50,104] The entire upper limb is subservient to the hand.

FUNCTIONAL ARCHES OF THE HAND

For grasping objects the hand must change its shape. Cupping of the hand occurs with finger flexion, and flattening of the hand occurs with extension. Cupping improves the mobility of the hand for functional usage, and flattening is used for release of objects. Structurally, the hand and wrist conform to three basic physiological functional arches, which are concave palmarly. Usually three transverse arches (two carpal and one metacarpal arch) and one longitudinal arch are described (Fig. 12–21). To these the oblique arches of opposition between the thumb and each of the fingers may also be added.[53,54] These arches allow coordinated synergistic digital flexion and thumb–little finger opposition. Usually the distal phalanges flex toward the scaphoid tubercle or obliquely. Only the index ray flexes in a sagittal plane. Full thumb–little finger opposition usually

Fig. 12–18. Flexion of the wrist showing neutral position (A), dorsiflexion with carpus moving palmarly and in supinatory rotation (B), and palmar flexion with carpus moving dorsally (C).

achieves parallel pulp-to-pulp contact of the distal phalanges of these two digits.

The longitudinal arch (or arches, since each ray with its corresponding metacarpal and adjacent carpal forms its own arch) is centered about the metacarpophalangeal articulations, whose thick anterior

glenoid capsules and volar plates prevent hyperextension. The long finger ray and the capitate are the focal point.[91]

Two transverse carpal arches may be considered the proximal and distal carpal arch (see Fig. 12–21). The proximal arch is more mobile than the distal

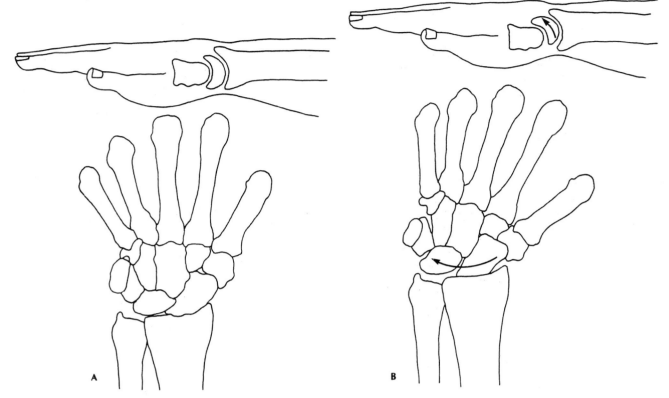

Fig. 12-19. Radial deviation of the wrist. *(A)* The wrist is shown in neutral position. *(B)* With radial deviation, the proximal row of carpal moves into dorsal and ulnar glide.

carpal row because of its connections to the radius and the distal row. The scaphoid, lunate, and triquetrum that make up this row have their own distinct movements.

The transverse arch of the distal row originates basically at the central carpus, specifically at the capitate, which moves with the fixed metacarpals. The trapezium, trapezoid, and hamate also make up this distal row.

The metacarpal arch is formed by the metacarpal heads (see Fig. 12-21). The long axis of the carpal gutter traverses the lunate, the capitate, and the third metacarpal bones. This arch is endowed with a great deal of adaptability because of the mobility of the peripheral metacarpals. It is relatively flat when the hand is at rest but demonstrates considerable curvature with strong clenching of a fist or with thumb–little finger opposition.

Pathologic conditions may destroy the arches of the hand and cause severe functional disability by flattening the transverse arches and flattening or reversing the longitudinal arch.

LENGTH–TENSION RELATIONSHIPS

Flatt[34] states that "In the normal limb, the placing of the hand is largely controlled by the multi-axial wrist joint." The wrist provides a stable base for the hand, and its position controls the length of the extrinsic muscles to the digits. The muscles that control wrist motion serve two important functions. They provide the fine adjustment of the hand into its functioning position, and, once this position is achieved, they stabilize the wrist to provide a stable base for the hand.

As the fingers flex, the wrist must be stabilized by the wrist extensor muscles to prevent the long finger flexor muscles from simultaneously flexing the wrist and allow for optimal length–tension in the long finger muscles. As the wrist position changes, the effective functional length of the finger flexors change and hypothetically the magnitude of force should also change. As grip becomes stronger, synchronous wrist extension lengthens the extrinsic flexor tendons across the wrist and maintains a favor-

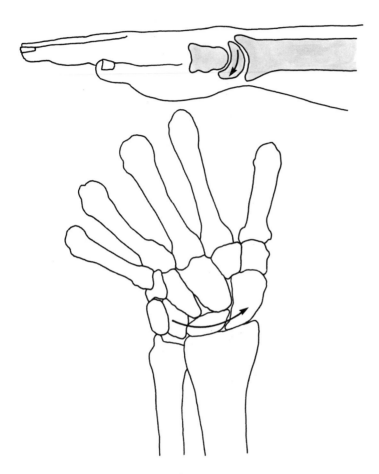

Fig. 12–20. Ulnar deviation of the wrist. The proximal row of carpals moves into palmar and radial glide.

able length of the musculotendinous unit for a strong contraction. Hazelton and associates[42] investigated the peak force that could be exerted at the interphalangeal joints of the finger during different wrist positions. Their study found the greatest interphalangeal flexion force occurred with ulnar deviation of the wrist (neutral flexion–extension). The wrist position in which the least force is generated is volar flexion. For strong finger or thumb extension, the wrist flexor muscles stabilize or flex the wrist so the long finger extensors can function more efficiently.

When the wrist is extended, the pulp (soft cushion on the palmar aspect of distal phalanges) of the thumb and index finger are passively in contact; when it is in flexion, the pulp of the thumb reaches the level of the proximal interphalangeal joint of the

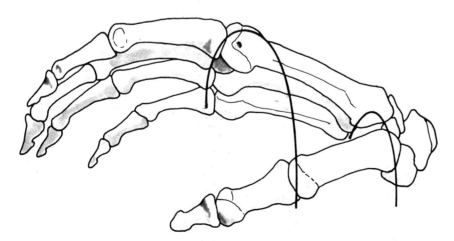

Fig. 12–21. The longitudinal and transverse arches of the hand, side view.

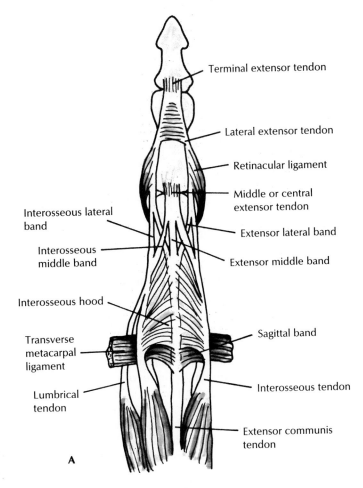

Terminal extensor tendon

Lateral extensor tendon

Retinacular ligament

Middle or central
extensor tendon

Interosseous lateral
band

Extensor lateral band

Interosseous
middle band

Extensor middle band

Interosseous hood

Sagittal band

Transverse
metacarpal
ligament

Lumbrical
tendon

Interosseous tendon

Extensor communis
tendon

Fig. 12–22. The main insertions of the extensor
apparatus: dorsal view *(A)* and lateral view *(B)*.

A

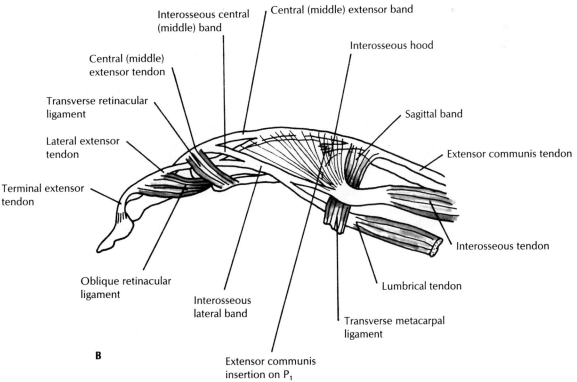

Interosseous central
(middle) band

Central (middle) extensor band

Central (middle)
extensor tendon

Interosseous hood

Transverse retinacular
ligament

Lateral extensor
tendon

Sagittal band

Terminal extensor
tendon

Extensor communis tendon

Interosseous tendon

Oblique retinacular
ligament

Lumbrical tendon

Interosseous
lateral band

Transverse metacarpal
ligament

B

Extensor communis
insertion on P_1

index finger. The position of the wrist has important repercussions on the position of the thumb and finger. Movements of the wrist are usually in reverse of movements of the fingers and reinforce the action of the extrinsic muscles of the fingers.

Extensor Mechanism

The extensor mechanism, also called the dorsal finger mechanism or extensor apparatus, is a subject of great interest and complexity (Fig. 12–22). The extensor tendons have the advantage of running almost entirely extrasynovial, which facilitates repair, but because they are also thin they tend to become rapidly adherent to the underlying bones and joints. Excursion of the extensor tendons of the hand is considerably less than that of the flexors, and thus it is more difficult to compensate for a loss of length.[104]

The extensor tendons are discrete and obvious at the level of the dorsal forearm, wrist, and hand. At the level of the metacarpophalangeal joint it is proper to speak of the dorsal tendinous structures as the extensor mechanism or apparatus. The extensor mechanism is a broad, flat aponeurotic band composed of extrinsic extensor tendon and the lateral bands formed by the tendons of the interosseous and lumbrical muscles (see Fig. 12–22). It is important to understand that the extrinsic tendons exert their primary force at the metacarpophalangeal joints. An isolated contraction of the extensor digitorum produces clawing of the fingers (metacarpophalangeal hyperextension with interphalangeal flexion from passive pull of the extrinsic flexor tendons).

The intrinsic tendons are primary extensors of the interphalangeal joints of the fingers. The intrinsic tendons lie volar to the axis of motion of the metacarpophalangeal joints and are actually metacarpophalangeal flexors. They lie dorsal to the axis of motion of the proximal and distal interphalangeal joints and are, therefore, extensors of those joints.[81] Proximal and distal interphalangeal extension occurs concurrently and can be caused by the lumbrical or interosseous muscles through their pull on the extensor hood (see Fig. 12–22) (a flattened portion of the communis tendon just distal to the metacarpophalangeal joint). There must be tension in the extensor digitorum.

The thumb has a similar anatomical situation but with one important exception. The thumb has an extrinsic extensor (extensor pollicis longus) that exerts it force on the distal phalanx. Forceful hyperextension of the interphalangeal joint is prevented and thumb extension reduced with the loss of this tendon.[81]

Prehension

The major musculoskeletal function of the hand lies in its abilities to grip objects. Prehension is seen in all forms of the animal world. According to Rabischong,[88] forms of prehension may be divided into four types: organs that pinch (i.e., pincers of the lobster), encircle, push, and adhere. Usually an animal can use only one of these forms of prehension. Only in humans has it obtained perfection. This is largely due to opposition of the thumb, which brings it into contact with each finger.[52,53] Since this requires the hand to function as a unit, prehension can never be fully measured in terms of movement of an individual joint. Many classifications of these movements were used until Napler divided them into two categories: power grip and precision grip.[80]

Power Grip. Power grip is a forceful act resulting in flexion at all fingers: the thumb, when used, acts as a stabilizer to the object held between the fingers and the palm (Fig. 12–23). This typically involves clamping an object with partially flexed fingers against the palm of the hand, with counterpressure from the adducted thumb. The fingers assume a position of sustained (isometric function) flexion that varies in degree with the weight, size, and shape of the object. The ulnar two fingers flex across toward the thenar eminence. In the final posture the hypothenar and the thenar eminences are used as buttresses as the fingers flex around the object to be grasped.[19] With all power grips the hand is kept stable and the power movements are produced by either radial or ulnar deviation of the wrists, as in the action of hammering, by supination and pronation of the wrist, and by extension of the elbow. Varieties of power grip include cylindrical grip, spherical grip, hook grip, and lateral prehension.[71]

A crude form of this grip (cylindrical) is used while gripping a heavy object as a hammer and forcefully driving a nail, with the thumb providing stability and power. An example of a more refined power grip is an ulnar grip, which is used when a lighter object lying across the palm is gripped mainly by the two ulnar fingers and the thumb is used for control.[19]

Power grip is the result of a sequence of (1) opening the hand, (2) positioning the fingers, (3) approaching the fingers to the object, and (4) maintaining a static phase, which actually constitutes the grip.[63]

Precision Grip. With precision grip the first three steps of the power grip sequence are shared. However, precision grip does not contain a static phase. The first three steps are followed by dynamic movement rather than a static phase, and *precision han-*

Fig. 12-23. Modes of power grip. Drawings of a hand in spherical *(A)* and in cylindrical *(B)* grip positions.

dling may be a better term. The muscles primarily function isotonically.[63] The object has to be picked up and manipulated by the fingers and thumb (Fig. 12-24). The object is not in contact with the palm of the hand but is manipulated between the opposing thumb and against the fingers—mainly against the next two fingers or the index finger.

The sensory surface of the digits is used for maximum sensory input to influence delicate adjustments. Varieties of precision grip include (1) palmar pinch, in which the pad of the thumb is opposed to the pad of one or more fingers—this is used for picking up and holding an object; (2) lateral pinch or opposition, in which the palmar aspect of the pad of the thumb presses on the radial surface of the first phalanx of the index—this occurs when one holds a coin or a sheet of paper; and (3) tip prehension, in which the tips of the pads or even the edges of the nails of the thumb are opposed to the tip of the index finger (or middle finger)—it allows one to hold a thin object or pick up a very fine object such as a

pin.[52,53] Tip prehension is the finest and most precise grip and is easily upset by any disease of the hand since it requires a whole range of movements and fine muscle control.

It is of interest that the various functions of the digits can be related to the patterns of the nerve supply. Opening the hand depends on the radial nerve. The muscles of the thumb required of opposition are innervated by both the median and ulnar nerves. Flexion and sensation of the radial digits, important in precision grip, are controlled chiefly by the median nerve, whereas flexion and sensation of the ulnar digits depend on the ulnar nerve.

FUNCTIONAL POSITIONS OF THE WRIST AND HAND

The functional position of the wrist and hand is that which is naturally assumed by the hand to grasp an object or the position from which optional function

Fig. 12–24. Modes of prehension: palmar *(A)*, tip *(B)*, and lateral *(C)*.

is most likely to occur.[53,82] From this position it is possible to grasp an object with minimal effort. The functional position is one in which (1) the wrist is slightly extended (20°) and ulnarly deviated (10°); (2) the fingers are slightly flexed at all their joints, with the degree of flexion increasing somewhat from the index to the little finger; and (3) the thumb is in

midrange opposition with the metacarpophalangeal joint moderately flexed and the interphalangeal joints slightly flexed (Fig. 12–25). It is not necessarily the position in which a hand should be immobilized. The preferred position for immobilization depends on the disability. However, this position is often the position of choice since other positions

Fig. 12–25. The functional position of a hand.

may result in serious functional sequelae. For example, if a finger is immobilized in extension it may become ankylosed.

EXAMINATION

The wrist structures are innervated primarily from C6 through C8. Lesions affecting structures of similar segmental derivation may refer pain to the wrist, and, conversely, lesions at or about the wrist may refer pain into the relevant segments. Since the wrist is located distally, and pain is more commonly referred in a proximal to distal direction than in a retrograde direction, pain from lesions at or about the wrist is fairly well localized. Symptoms experienced at the wrist or hand, however, must always be suspected as possibly having a more proximal origin. Common lesions that often refer pain to this region include lower cervical pathologic processes (*e.g.,* spondylosis, disk disease), tendinitis or capsulitis at the shoulder, thoracic outlet syndrome, and tennis elbow. If subjective findings do not seem to implicate a local problem, a scan examination of the neck and entire extremity may be warranted before proceeding with an in-depth evaluation of the wrist (see Chapter 19, The Cervical–Upper Extremity Scan Examination).

HISTORY

A structured line of questioning should be pursued, as set out in Chapter 4, Assessment of Musculoskeletal Disorders.

Common lesions at or about the wrist vary in onset from insidious (carpal tunnel syndrome, de Quervain's tenosynovitis, rheumatoid arthritis) to those in which an incident of trauma is definitely recalled (Colles' fracture, scaphoid fracture, lunate dislocation, or capsuloligamentous sprains). Again, the clinician must be prepared to direct the line of questioning to elicit information concerning more proximal regions, especially if the onset is insidious. If a traumatic event is cited, the examination should attempt to determine the exact mechanism of injury. Since rheumatoid arthritis is not uncommon at the wrist, inquiry might be made about possible bilateral problems and problems with the metacarpophalangeal joints and joints of the feet.

PHYSICAL EXAMINATION

I. **Observation**
   A. *General appearance and body build*
   B. *Functional activities.* Observe the way the person shakes hands, noting the firmness of grasp and temperature and moisture of the hand. Note during dressing activities whether one hand tends to be favored. Observe for fumbling with fasteners or small objects — a problem typical of carpal tunnel syndrome or neurologic dysfunction of more proximal origin. Note whether the patient willingly puts pressure through the wrist, as when standing up from a chair.
   C. *General posture and positioning of body parts.* Note how the arm and hand are carried and especially whether they swing naturally when walking. The person with a sympathetic reflex dystrophy, not an infrequent complication following healing of a Colles' fracture, invariably walks in with the elbow flexed and the forearm held across the upper abdomen.

II. **Inspection**
   A. *Bony structure and alignment.* This is especially important following a fracture of the distal radius. The most common complication following Colles' fracture is healing of the fragments in a malaligned position, resulting in a "dinner fork" deformity (Figs. 12–26 and 12–27). In such a deformity the distal end of the radius is displaced and angulated dorsally, foreshortened, and often rotated into supination. Such a deformity must be considered when determining treatment goals, since normal range of motion can never be obtained in such cases.
      1. Note structural alignment of head, neck, shoulder girdle, arm, and forearm.
      2. Note carefully the structural alignment

Fig. 12-26. Dorsal and lateral view of a Colles' fracture, showing extension fracture of the lower end of radius.

Fig. 12-27. Lateral and dorsal view of the characteristic "dinner fork" deformity resulting from a Colles' fracture.

and relationships of the distal end of the radius and ulna, the carpals, and the metacarpals (see section on the surface anatomy).

3. Note any structural deformities of the hands and fingers such as boutonnière or swan-neck deformities, ulnar drift, claw hand, or ape hand.

B. *Soft tissue*

1. Muscle contours
   a. Note especially any atrophy of the thenar muscles (this may accompany carpal tunnel syndrome), the hypothenar muscles (suggestive of an ulnar nerve lesion), and intrinsics.
   b. Note any generalized atrophy of the arm or forearm (this invariably occurs with immobilization but may be masked by edema).
   c. Note any localized atrophy about the shoulder girdle and rest of limb, which may suggest neuromuscular involvement of related segments.

2. Joint regions
   a. Inspect for effusion of any upper extremity joints.
   b. Notice other periarticular swellings: Herberden's nodes about the distal interphalangeal joints are characteristic of osteoarthrosis of those joints.
   c. Small pea-sized ganglia are commonly found on the dorsal or palmar aspect of the wrist and are usually of little significance.
   d. Large nodules about the wrist, extensor surface of the forearm, and elbow are characteristic of rheumatoid arthritis.

3. General soft tissue inspection
   a. Generalized edema of the distal extremity is invariably present following immobilization in all but younger patients.
   b. Localized edema over the dorsum of the hand suggests an infection involving any part of the hand.
   c. If swelling or edema is present, volumetric measurements and girth measurements should be taken for documentation of a baseline.

C. *Skin*

1. Color
   a. Redness with inflammation
   b. Often cyanotic in reflex sympathetic dystrophy
   c. Colorless with severe neurologic deficit

2. Texture (see under palpation)
3. Moisture (see under palpation)
4. Scars, blemishes

D. *Nails*

1. Splitting, ridging (typical in reflex sympathetic dystrophy)
2. Clubbing (may suggest cardiopulmonary disorder)
3. Hollowing

III. Selective tissue tension tests. Both tendon excursion (active range of motion) and joint motion (passive range of motion) are evaluated with a computation of total active motion (TAM) and total passive motion (TPM), as recommended by the Clinical Assessment Committee of the American Society for Surgery of the Hand. This method is used for measuring and recording finger and thumb motions.[3] If joint stiffness is present, closely examine the end feel of each joint before measuring passive range of motion with a goniometer.

A. *Active movements.* Record range of motion, pain, and crepitus.

1. Wrist flexion–extension and radioulnar deviation and forearm pronation and supination. Active radial and ulnar deviation performed with the thumb held in a fist under the other fingers may be helpful in distinguishing de Quervain's tenovaginitis from osteoarthrosis of the trapezium–first metacarpal joint (both of which are common lesions).
2. Include shoulder and elbow movements, especially after immobilization and when reflex sympathetic dystrophy is suspected.

B. *Passive movements.* Record range of motion, pain, crepitus, and end feel.

1. Same movements as above
2. Also ask patient to place the hand flat on a table with wrist dorsiflexed and elbow extended and to lean forward so as to transmit body weight through the forearm and wrist.

C. *Resisted movements.* Record as strong or weak, painful or painless.

1. Resist all wrist, forearm, finger, and thumb movements.
2. If referred pain from more proximal re-

gions is suspected, include resisted elbow and shoulder movements.

D. *Joint-play movements.* Record mobility and irritability (pain or muscle guarding)
   1. See Chapter 6, Peripheral Joint Mobilization Techniques, for joint-play movements at wrist and hand
   2. Special intercarpal movements should be performed if an intercarpal ligament sprain is suspected. The therapist may use his or her knowledge of surface anatomy to move any of the carpal bones against its neighbors.

IV. **Neuromuscular tests** (see Chapter 4 for relevant tests)
   A. Strength, sensation, reflex, and coordination testing should be performed at this point if neuromuscular involvement is suggested by findings thus far in the examination. Gross grip strength can be measured by a dynamometer. Force generated by the normal man is about 46 kg and that by the normal woman is about 23 kg.[99,118] If the subject is not able to grip the dynamometer, a sphygmomanometer may be used, with which the normal male grip is usually greater than 300 mm and the female grip is about 300 mm.[106] A pinch meter is used in testing pinch strength.

   The status of the motor system can be further described in terms of muscle tone. Coordination can be tested by performing activities such as tracing a diagram or buttoning a button. Standardized tests such as the Jebsen Hand Function Test, the Minnesota Rate of Manipulation Test, the Purdue Pegboard Test, the Valpar Work Sample Series, and the O'Conner Dexterity Test are available for more detailed evaluation of manual dexterity and coordination.[6,31,47]
   B. A useful test for median nerve pressure at the carpal tunnel is to ask the patient to strongly flex the wrist while maintaining a strong three-jaw-chuck grasp. This position should be held for 1 minute. The onset of paresthesias into the first three or four fingers during this test is suggestive of a carpal tunnel syndrome.
   C. If carpal tunnel syndrome is suspected, percuss the median nerve where it passes through the carpal tunnel. Reproduction of paresthesias suggests nerve involvement at this level (Tinel's sign).
   D. Involvement of the cervical nerve roots and peripheral nerves may affect both muscle strength and sensation of the upper extremity. The level of cervical nerve root or peripheral nerves may be determined by identifying "key muscles" or joint actions and sensory areas, which are representative (see Chapter 4, Assessment of Musculoskeletal Disorders). Numerous tests have been described to evaluate the various sensory modalities of the hands. Two-point discrimination, vibratory threshold, temperature, and sudomotor activity may assist in lesion identification.[23,32,118]

V. **Palpation**
   A. *Skin*
      1. Moisture
      2. Texture
      3. Temperature
      4. Mobility
      5. Tenderness. Dysesthesias, such as burning on light palpation, suggest nerve root or peripheral nerve pathology, for example, pressure.
      6. A common condition following immobilization (especially after Colles' fracture) is the development of a reflex sympathetic dystrophy. The exact cause is unknown. Many believe it to be related to the development of edema during immobilization. Some believe it results from trauma to a nerve from the original injury, for example, contusion of the median nerve from the displaced distal fragment in Colles' fracture. Others believe psychological factors also play an important role. In early phases of the development of this disorder the skin may be dry, rough, and warm from decreased sympathetic activity. Later, increased sympathetic activity, with hyperhidrosis and vasoconstriction, seem to predominate. Skin palpation reveals several findings in this disorder.
         a. Hyperhidrosis
         b. Smooth, glossy skin
         c. Decreased temperature (cold, clammy hands)
         d. Hypersensitivity to normally non-noxious sensory stimuli; even light touch may be painful
         e. Loss of mobility of the skin in relation to subcutaneous tissues from interstitial fibrosis accompanying tissue edema
   B. *Soft tissues*

1. Tenderness. Palpate tendons and ligaments, especially for local tenderness.
2. Mobility, consistency. Soft tissues feel indurated and adherent in reflex sympathetic dystrophy from interstitial fibrosis, as well as atrophied, fibrotic muscle.
3. Edema and swelling (common with reflex sympathetic dystrophy)
4. Pulse, radial and ulnar arteries. This may be performed in conjunction with various maneuvers of the arm (hyperabduction), shoulder girdle (depression, elevation and retraction), and neck if thoracic outlet syndrome is suspected. The Allen test is usually performed to determine patency of the radial, ulnar, and digital arteries by asking the patient to pump the blood out of the hand and then maintain a fist while the examiner occludes both arteries at the wrist; when the hand is opened it will appear white, and arterial filling on the respective side can be observed as pressure is released from one artery at a time.[44]

C. *Bones*
1. Tenderness. The radial styloid process is often the site of referred tenderness from more proximal lesions usually within the C5 or C6 segment. It is usually also tender in de Quervain's tenosynovitis.
2. Relationships. Palpate for structural alignment and positioning of the various bony components of the wrist.

IV. **Special tests**
A. A test for *intrinsic tightness* has been described by Bunnell.[12] The intrinsic tightness test is performed by holding the patient's metacarpophalangeal joint in extension (stretching the intrinsics) and then passively flexing the proximal interphalangeal joint. The intrinsics are then relaxed by flexing the metacarpophalangeal joint. If the proximal interphalangeal joint can be passively flexed more with the metacarpophalangeal joint in flexion than when it is in extension, there is tightness of the intrinsics. Capsular or collateral ligament tightness of the proximal interphalangeal joint will limit proximal phalangeal motion, regardless of the position of the metacarpophalangeal joint. Loss of flexion at the distal interphalangeal joint can also be due to a joint contracture or to a contracture of the oblique retinacular ligament.[44,62]

B. Functional assessment of the patient with a hand disability is carried out most effectively through the use of a variety of testing methods.[2,3,93]

COMMON LESIONS

CARPAL TUNNEL SYNDROME

Carpal tunnel syndrome is a very common condition. Women present with this problem more commonly than do men. It rarely affects young people. The cause is variable. In certain instances it is due to some known disorder involving increased pressure within the carpal tunnel. Such situations include a displaced fracture of the distal radius, a lunar or perilunar dislocation, and swelling of the common flexor tendon sheath. In most cases, the cause is not readily determined. Some believe it to be a vascular deficiency of the median nerve at the carpal tunnel, while others believe direct pressure to the nerve to be the cause. Symptoms and signs accompanying this disorder are more suggestive of a pressure phenomenon.[20]

I. **History**
A. *Onset of symptoms*—Usually insidious unless, of course, following trauma resulting in fracture, dislocation, or swelling of the wrist
B. *Nature of symptoms.* The complaint is most often that of paresthesias (pins and needles) felt into the first three or four fingers of the hand. The patient is most troubled by being awakened at night, usually in the early hours of the morning, from paresthesias in the hand. Onset of paresthesias often occurs with activities involving prolonged use of the finger flexors, such as writing and sewing. Often the patient complains of clumsiness on activities requiring fine finger movements. At times a burning sensation is felt in the median nerve distribution of the hand as well. Subjective complaints of actual weakness are rare. The problem can be unilateral or bilateral. **Note:** C6 or C7 nerve root involvement and thoracic outlet syndrome often present as paresthesias in a similar distribution as that of carpal tunnel syndrome. In the case of nerve root involvement, however, the patient is rarely awakened by paresthesias and use of the hand does not bring on symptoms. Differentiation from thoracic outlet syndrome, based on subjective find-

ings, is more difficult, since these patients are usually awakened at night with paresthesias and parethesias may come on with certain activities involving use of the upper extremity. In thoracic outlet syndrome, paresthesias are more likely to involve the entire hand (although often the patient is not sure in just how many fingers paresthesias are felt) or perhaps just the more ulnar side of the hand from lower cord involvement only. The objective examination will help differentiate the two conditions in any case.

II. **Physical examination**

A. *Observation.* There may be some clumsiness with activities requiring fine finger movements, such as handling buttons or other fasteners.

B. *Inspection.* Some thenar atrophy may be noticed, but usually only in chronic cases.

C. *Selective tissue tensions tests.* Results are noncontributory, except perhaps some subtle weakness on resisted thumb movements.

D. *Neuromuscular tests.* Only in severe, chronic cases can true weakness of the first two lumbricals of the thumb be noticed. Substitution, overlapping innervation, or subtle involvement make motor testing unreliable.

  1. Careful sensory testing may reveal some deficit in the tips or dorsal ends of the first three or four fingers (usually the second or third). However, mild cases or early cases sufficient to cause significant symptoms may not present with a detectable sensory deficit.

  2. The special tests mentioned under "Neuromuscular Tests" will usually reproduce the paresthesias.

  3. Tinel's sign (reproduction of paresthesias by tapping the median nerve at the wrist) may be positive.

  4. Nerve conduction studies of the median nerve are the most reliable but are often unnecessary diagnostically.

E. *Palpation*—Usually noncontributory.

III. **Management**

These patients often do remarkably well simply by wearing a resting-splint for the wrist at night. The reason why this helps is not entirely clear, except that it maintains the wrist in a neutral position, the position of least pressure within the carpal tunnel. (For this reason it seems more likely that this disorder is a pressure phenomenon rather than a release phenomenon.)

The patient can be shown how to don the splint without impairing venous return from fastening straps or wraps too tightly. The splint may or may not include the fingers. It is usually not necessary to wear the splint during the day. However, if night use does not provide relief of symptoms, a several-day trial of continuous use of the splint followed by gradual weaning should be instituted. Whether the splint is worn continuously or at night only, after 1 or 2 weeks of relief from symptoms, use of the splint can gradually be decreased and eventually discontinued.

Only in persistent cases is surgery required to divide the flexor retinaculum and relieve the pressure.

LIGAMENTOUS SPRAINS

Ligamentous sprains are also quite common and often lead to chronic wrist pain unless treated appropriately. Most commonly involved, in our experience, are the lunate-capitate ligament, dorsally, and the radiocarpal ligament, palmarly. However, any other of the several ligaments about the wrist may conceivably be sprained.

I. **History**

A. *Onset of pain.* Ligamentous lesions are invariably of traumatic rather than degenerative onset. The patient usually recalls the traumatic event. A fall on the outstretched hand may rupture one or more of several ligaments about the wrist, but often one of the ligaments attached to the lunate is sprained. This is because of the tendency toward a lunar or perilunar dislocation with such an injury. In fact, at this point in the examination, such a dislocation cannot be ruled out. Because a fall on the outstretched hand tends to force the wrist into hyperextension, the palmar radiolunate and palmar lunocapitate ligaments tend to be sprained. However, if the lunate partially dislocates palmarly with spontaneous reduction, the dorsal radiolunate ligaments may also be sprained (Fig. 12–28).

Occasionally the fall is such that the person strikes the dorsum of the hand, forcing the wrist into extreme palmar flexion. This usually results in a sprain of one of the ligaments attached dorsally to the capitate. The ulnar collateral ligament is often sprained with a Colles' fracture.

B. *Site of pain.* The pain is usually well localized to a small area that corresponds well to the site of the lesion.

Fig. 12-28. Lunate dislocation. *(A)* The injury occurs when the radius forces the lunate in a palmar direction, resulting in dislocation *(B)*.

C. *Nature of pain.* The pain is felt with use of the wrist. Often a particular activity is cited as being most aggravating; the activity stresses the involved ligament. In the case of a dorsal radiocarpal sprain, often the activity that tends to reproduce the pain puts pressure down through the hand (as when doing pushups).

II. Physical examination

   A. *Observation*—Usually noncontributory

   B. *Inspection*—Usually noncontributory. Localized swelling following an injury to the wrist almost never accompanies a ligamentous injury only. Fracture or dislocation should be suspected.

   C. *Selective tissue tension tests*

   1. Active movements. Possibly (but not necessarily) some pain may be noted on the extreme of a movement that stresses the ligament.

   2. Passive movements

   a. It is quite possible for a ligamentous lesion to exist that is not stressed at the extreme of any passive anatomical movement.

   b. Often the only maneuver that reproduces the pain, other than some specific joint-play movement test, is having the patient lean forward, transmitting the body weight through the arm, forearm, extended wrist, and hand. This is most likely to reproduce pain from a lesion of the palmar radiolunate or dorsal lunocapitate ligaments.

   c. Also note that the dorsal radiocarpal ligament may be stressed on full passive pronation (applying the force through the hand and wrist to the forearm) and the palmar radiocarpal ligament may be stressed on full passive supination.

   3. Resisted movements. Strong and painless. **Note:** Resist pronation and supination at the distal forearm, not at the hand, to avoid stressing the radiocarpal ligaments.

   4. Joint-play movements

   a. The specific intra-articular movement that stresses the involved ligament is likely to reproduce the pain, but, again, joint-play movement in itself may not be sufficient to reproduce the pain.

   b. The most important movements to perform are dorsal-palmar glide of the capitate on lunate and lunate on radius.

   c. Some hypermobility of the lunate may be detected following partial dislocation and spontaneous reduction of the lunate with a fall on the dorsiflexed hand.

   d. Some hypermobility of the capitate may be detected following a fall on the palmarly flexed hand in which a lunocapitate or capitate–third metacarpal ligament may be ruptured

   D. *Neuromuscular tests.* Results are noncontributory.

   E. *Palpation.* Localized tenderness usually corresponds well with the site of the lesion.

III. **Management**

   A. Temporary restriction of activities that tend to stress the involved ligament

   B. Friction massage to the site of the lesion to increase mobility of the collagen fibers without longitudinally stressing the ligament. As an adjunct, ultrasound may be used to assist in the resolution of chronic inflammatory exudates.

AFTER COLLES' FRACTURE

In most outpatient settings, patients who have sustained a Colles' fracture comprise the largest proportion of those with wrist disorders. The term *Colles' fracture* is usually used to refer to fractures of the distal end of the radius, with or without an associated fracture at the distal ulna. This is one of the most common of all fractures. It affects primarily older people. Women are afflicted more often than men because of the prevalence of osteoporosis, especially in older women. These patients are often referred to physical therapists following the period of immobilization because of complications resulting in residual loss of function. The most common complications following these injuries are (1) malunion (*not* nonunion) of bony fragments and (2) development of a reflex sympathetic dystrophy. Pain and loss of movement are the major factors limiting function following immobilization of a Colles' fracture.

Mechanism and Nature of Injury

Colles' fracture invariably results from a fall on the outstretched hand in an older person. The patient lands with the wrist in dorsiflexion and the forearm in pronation. The lunate acts as a wedge to shear the distal 2 cm, or so, of the radius off in a dorsal direction. The momentum of the body weight causes the distal fragment to displace radially and rotate in a supinatory direction with respect to the proximal bone end (see Fig. 12–26). Because this metaphyseal area of bone is typically osteoporotic, the compression force often results in comminution and impaction of the distal fragment. The major fracture line runs transversely across the distal radius, usually about 2 cm proximal to the radiocarpal joint. The momentum that results in radial displacement may also cause a sprain of the ulnar collateral ligament and an avulsion fracture of the ulnar styloid process.[24]

The characteristic "dinner fork" deformity results from the wrist and hand being displaced dorsally with respect to the forearm (see Fig. 12–27). Often included in the deformity is radial displacement of the wrist and hand.

Management by the Physician

Closed manipulative reduction is usually carried out in an effort to bring the fragments back into anatomical alignment. Reduction is usually not so much of a problem as is maintenance of reduction. In unstable, comminuted fractures there is a tendency for the distal fragment to slip back into its postinjury position of dorsal, radial, and supinatory displacement. In an attempt to maintain anatomical reduction, the wrist is usually splinted in a position of flexion and ulnar deviation, with pronation. In some cases external fixation with a Roger Anderson device may be used. The elbow is usually left free. Note that since the elbow is left free, splinting in a position of excessive pronation may result in a force tending to pull the distal fragment into radial displacement and supination from tension on the brachioradialis with elbow extension. This would defeat the original purpose of positioning the part in pronation and ulnar deviation.

The plaster splint is left on for at least 4 weeks. Nonunion is rare since this fracture occurs in highly vascularized, metaphyseal bone.

Complications

Malunion.   It is rare for a Colles' fracture to heal without some residual malalignment. The radius invariably ends up foreshortened such that the radial styloid process no longer extends beyond the ulnar styloid process. The distal end of the radius also tends to be angulated and displaced dorsally; the distal radial articulation surface no longer faces 10° to 15° in a palmar direction. It should be realized that the malalignment described above will result in a permanent loss of full wrist flexion and ulnar deviation. In addition, there may be some residual malalignment of the distal fragment toward supination, resulting in a permanent loss of pronation. The distal fragment may also heal when displaced radially, but this would have little effect on motion.

Reflex Sympathetic Dystrophy. Reflex sympathetic dystrophy is not uncommon following Colles' fracture. In fact, in our experience this condition develops more often following Colles' fracture than after any other injury. Also, according to our experience, the majority of patients sent to physical therapy following immobilization of Colles' fracture have this condition to some degree (otherwise they probably would not require ongoing physical therapy).[13,25,79,97,98,115]

The pathophysiology of this condition is not well understood nor agreed on. It is generally agreed, however, that sympathetic dysfunction occurs as part of a vicious circle initiated reflexly by some alteration in afferent input from the periphery. Several different proposals have been offered as to the precipitating factor in this condition, including direct trauma to a peripheral nerve, edema from prolonged immobilization, pain, and psychological predisposition. The characteristic features of the disorder are hyperalgesia, edema, and capsular tightness of the joints of the hand, wrist, and often the shoulder (it is often referred to as shoulder–hand syndrome, although the shoulder is not always involved). The elbow occasionally stiffens as well. As mentioned in other than the early phases of this condition, there is usually increased sympathetic activity involving the distal part of the extremity, with vasoconstriction and hyperhidrosis. The vasoconstriction causes a cyanotic appearance and atrophy of the musculoskeletal tissues; the skin becomes glossy and thin; the nails, brittle; and the bones, osteoporotic. (Early osteopenia, seen on roentgenography, is often marked. This early bone atrophy is believed to be a result of hyperemia that is often present in the earlier stages; excessive blood flow to bone causes increased resorption).

Carpal Tunnel Syndrome. The median nerve may be traumatized at the time of injury. Prolonged pressure to the nerve may come about from malalignment of bony fragments, persistent edema involving the carpal tunnel, or both. (See section on carpal tunnel syndrome for discussion of symptoms and signs.)

Late Rupture of the Extensor Pollicis Longus Tendon. The extensor pollicis longus tendon normally takes quite a sharp turn around Lister's tubercle at the dorsum of the distal radius on its way to inserting at the thumb. Malalignment of bony parts following Colles' fracture may cause excessive friction to this tendon, which may result in fraying of the tendon and eventual rupture. Pain on active and passive thumb flexion or opposition along with pain on resisted thumb extension are suggestive of such a problem before actual rupture. Painless weakness of thumb extension, some time after injury, is characteristic of rupture of the tendon.

I. History

A. Determine the date of initial injury, subsequent treatment, the length of time the part was immobilized, and the dates of removal of splints. Inquire as to whether exercise and elevation activities were performed while the part was immobilized. Of course, a patient whose wrist had been immobilized for 8 weeks with no instruction in shoulder exercises and elevation activities and who has not used the part since removal of the splint 2 weeks ago will be expected to present with more dysfunction and disability than the patient who has just come out of the splint after having had the wrist immobilized for 6 weeks, during which time range of motion for the shoulder was carried out along with intermittent periods of elevation and active finger movements.

B. The standard questions relating to the patient's pain should be asked (see Chapter 4, Assessment of Musculoskeletal Disorders). Any acute inflammatory process, initiated at the time of injury, should have resolved during the period of immobilization. Considering this, any residual pain would be expected to be due primarily to stiffness and to be associated with use of the part. Complaints of pain at rest, pain that awakens the patient at night, and inability to use the part because of pain are suggestive of reflex sympathetic dystrophy in this case. Take note of any complaints of shoulder pain because of the possibility of stiffening of the shoulder from immobilization and perhaps shoulder–hand syndrome. Pain on use of the thumb may be suggestive of involvement of the extensor pollicis longus tendon. Complaints of burning pain or paresthesias into the median nerve distribution of the hand should lead one to suspect carpal tunnel syndrome.

C. Determine and document the patient's present functional status.

1. What specific daily activities cannot be performed with the involved hand that could be performed before the injury?
2. What activities can be performed but with some difficulty or pain?
3. Consider, especially, eating, grooming, dressing, household chores, occupational activities, and recreational activities.

II. Physical examination

A. *Observation.* Typically these patients walk into a room holding the hand and forearm out in front of them, across the chest or abdomen.

1. Is the arm used when rising from a chair?
2. Does the arm hang normally to the side and swing freely and normally when walking?
3. Does the patient use the hand and arm during dressing activities, or does he or she guard it carefully?
4. Observe the face for wincing during movement of the part.

B. *Inspection*

1. Skin and nails. Note especially trophic changes that are suggestive of a reflex sympathetic dystrophy: brittle, split nails; smooth, glossy skin; cyanotic appearance to skin in the distal part of extremity.
2. Subcutaneous soft tissue. Atrophy of the forearm musculature is invariably found but perhaps somewhat masked by edema, which is usually noticed most in the hand and forearm.
3. Bony structure and alignment. Some degree of malalignment is likely to be present. In the classic "dinner fork" deformity, the wrist and hand are offset dorsally with respect to the forearm. There is usually some displacement radially also. The radial styloid process may no longer extend further distally than the ulnar styloid process, as it should, because of impaction of the distal fragment.

C. *Selective tissue tension tests*

1. Active and passive range of motion
   a. The interphalangeal and metacarpophalangeal joints of the hand are usually restricted in a capsular pattern—the metacarpophalangeal joints being especially restricted in flexion, the interphalangeal joints especially restricted in extension.
   b. Wrist and forearm movements are restricted in all planes. Flexion, ulnar deviation, and pronation are likely to be restricted from bony malalignment; check for "bony end feel." Extension, radial deviation, and supination are likely to be limited because the hand is usually immobilized in a position opposite each of these movements (see above).
   c. All movements are likely to be painful at the extremes, especially in the presence of a reflex sympathetic dystrophy.
   d. Be sure to check shoulder range of motion for possible capsular tightening.
2. Resisted movements
   a. Pain on resisted thumb extension may suggest some involvement of the extensor pollicis longus tendon secondary to bony malalignment.
   b. Otherwise, resisted movements should be strong and painless.
3. Joint-play movements. Considerable restriction of all joint play movements of the wrist and hand is likely to be found.

D. *Neuromuscular tests.* Here concern is primarily with the function of the median nerve. The special test mentioned under carpal tunnel syndrome should be performed.

E. *Palpation*

1. Skin
   a. The skin is likely to feel cool, moist, smooth, and tight, especially in the presence of a reflex sympathetic dystrophy.
   b. Tenderness to light palpation of the skin is characteristic of a reflex sympathetic dystrophy.
2. Subcutaneous soft tissue. Pitting-type edema is very often present distally. The tissues may feel "tight" and bound down in the hand and forearm because of the fibrosis accompanying prolonged edema.
3. Bones. Careful bony palpation will reveal the extent of residual malalignment.

F. *Other.* A radiologist's report should be ordered so that the therapist can determine the degree of bony malalignment. This is helpful in setting treatment goals. Also, marked osteoporosis usually accompanies a reflex sympathetic dystrophy. It is often said that as much as 40% of bone resorption may take place before osteopenia shows on roentgenograms. If roentgenograms suggest considerable osteoporosis, techniques to regain range of motion must not be performed using forces applied over a long lever arm.

Management

Functional use of the part is lost or restricted primarily due to pain and loss of motion. As in any joint in which motion is lost from capsular tightening, much of the patient's pain may be due to joint stiffness; the joint capsule is stretched excessively during use of the part. However, these patients often complain of pain that is out of proportion to the extent of the dysfunction. Such an abnormal pain state is characteristic of a reflex sympathetic dystrophy. In such situations the patient may complain of severe pain to light touch or other normally non-noxious stimulation. This complaint may act as a considerable barrier to efforts to regain joint motion.

Pain Management.   If such an abnormal pain state is apparent, special care must be taken not to reinforce the patient's pain behavior and not to allow such reinforcement by family members, so as to avoid development of an operant pain problem. On the other hand, the patient's very real pain problem cannot be ignored. The patient must be advised that, while in no way is the pain imagined, the pain is not in this case serving a useful function by signaling potential harm to tissues.

Unless the problem is carefully explained to the patient, he or she cannot be expected to carry out home instructions that may well ask the patient to perform exercises and other activities that may be somewhat painful. The patient will also doubt the therapist's professional judgment if certain techniques that cause considerable discomfort are used unless the rationale of their use is carefully explained.

In addition to discussing the problem with the patient, the therapist must take some measures to try to make the treatment sessions as painless as possible. This is one disorder in which some modality or procedure might be used solely for its effect to reduce the patient's pain, so as to allow one to carry out other treatment procedures, such as joint mobilization. A whirlpool bath during, or just before, mobilization procedures may act as a counterirritant, as well as increasing blood flow to the part. The part may be kept in the water for application of ultrasound in preparation for mobilization procedures.

Restoration of Joint Motion.   These patients require an intensive mobilization program. All the joints of the extremity, with the possible exception of the elbow, are likely to be restricted in the case of reflex sympathetic dystrophy. It is usually desirable to have the patient come in for treatment at least three times a week for passive mobilization. Treatment should include ultrasound to help increase the extensibility of capsular tissue, followed by specific joint mobilization techniques. Such techniques are especially indicated because they are performed with forces applied over very short lever arms.

A home program of active and active-assisted range of motion exercises should be instituted. Take care to show the patient exercises that do not involve forces applied over long lever-arms, especially when working on finger flexion and extension. These patients usually have some degree of tissue edema that contributes to the restriction in range of motion. Frequent elevation of the part with activation of the muscle pump should be included in the home program. Encourage use of the part for dressing, grooming, and light activities.

Simple strengthening exercises for finger, wrist, and shoulder muscles should be instituted. Strengthening the rotator cuff is especially important because of the important role these muscles play biomechanically. Exercises should be kept simple, and the number of exercises should be kept at a minimum. The patient who becomes confused or exhausted with a home program is likely to abandon the program completely. This is an important consideration here because these patients need to perform range of motion exercises for most of the upper extremity joints, in addition to strengthening exercises and elevation activities. Whenever possible, exercises should be designed that incorporate strengthening range of motion and elevation so as to keep the program simple and concise.

In cases in which a marked or persistent reflex sympathetic dystrophy presents a major obstruction to rehabilitation, the patient may undergo a series of sympathetic blocks. In such a program the patient may be admitted to the hospital or to ambulatory surgery. The stellate ganglion is injected with an anesthetic in an attempt to reduce sympathetic activity to the part and to break up the cycle. Typically, a series of five injections are given on a daily basis. Such a program in no way precludes continuation of the normal physical therapy program. In fact, the ideal situation is for the patient to be seen in physical therapy each day following the block for mobilization procedures. Obviously, close communication and cooperation among orthopaedics, anesthesiology, and physical therapy is an important factor here.

In our experience, the active phase of a reflex sympathetic dystrophy following a Colles' fracture tends to resolve over a period of several months. However, a patient may be left with some residual disability. Some residual loss of motion is not unlikely because of the often extensive fibrosis of joint capsules as well as extra-articular structures. Goals, in these cases, should be set toward restoration of *functional* motion, not necessarily *physiological* motion. In older persons, the two are less likely to coincide. Of more significance, however, is the tendency toward development of a chronic pain state. Operant management at this point may be indicated over, or in addition to, continued physical treatment. The possibility of psychological consultation should be discussed with the physician.

All too often these patients continue to come in for treatment over a prolonged period of time without demonstrable improvement in function. While vigorous treatment is indicated in the early phase after immobilization, once improvement plateaus for, say, a 2-week or 3-week period, treatment should gradually be discontinued in favor of a progressive home program. Keep in mind, however, that improvement is rarely linear in such cases, and some fluctuation between spurts of improvement and periods of plateauing can be expected. Until satisfactory, functional use of the part is regained, intermittent follow-up visits should be arranged for reassessment and progression of the home program. As usual, improvement should be based primarily on objective findings and subjective reports of increased function (not on subjective reports of decreased pain).

DE QUERVAIN'S TENOVAGINITIS

De Quervain's tenovaginitis is a relatively common condition. It is generally believed to be an inflammation and swelling of the synovial lining of the common sheath of the abductor pollicis longus and the extensor pollicis brevis tendons where they pass along the distal-radial aspect of the radius.

   I. **History.** Pain is felt over the distal-radial aspect of the radius, perhaps radiating distally into the thumb or even proximally up the forearm. The onset is usually insidious. The patient notes pain primarily with activities involving thumb movements, such as wringing or grasping activities.
  II. **Physical examination.** This condition must be differentiated from osteoarthrosis of the trapezium–first metacarpal joint, which is also a fairly common disorder. In osteoarthrosis, *A.*

and *B.* below are negative, and joint play movements at the trapezium–first metacarpal joint will be restricted and painful.
   A. Pain on resisted thumb extension and abduction
   B. Pain on ulnar deviation of the wrist with the thumb held fixed in flexion. On this movement the tendons and the sheath are placed on a stretch.
   C. Tenderness to palpation over the tendon sheath in the region of the radial styloid process.
 III. **Management**
   A. The physician may elect to inject the sheath with a corticosteroid preparation or a local anesthetic. Surgical incision of the sheath is occasionally performed.
   B. If injection is not contemplated or if it is unsuccessful, a trial of ultrasound and friction massage over a 1-week or 2-week period on a basis of three to five times per week is warranted. The rationale of this program is to maintain and increase mobility of the tendons within the sheath and to help resolve the chronic inflammatory process. In more severe or persistent cases, temporary restriction of thumb movements with a small opponens splint should be considered, to prevent continued irritation to the inflamed sheath process.

SCAPHOID FRACTURE AND LUNATE DISLOCATION

In the older person, a fall on the outstretched hand results in a Colles' fracture, since the proximal carpals are jammed into the weak osteoporotic radius. However, in the younger person, in whom the radius is strong and healthy, the scaphoid may fracture on impact, or the radius may force the lunate palmarly, resulting in lunate dislocation in a palmar direction (see Fig. 12–28).

A lunate dislocation may be detected on a standard anteroposterior roentgenogram by the lunate's appearing triangular rather than quadrangular and, in a lateral view, by its abnormal position. In any event, the therapist should always palpate for lunate positioning in patients referred to physical therapy after a fall on the outstretched hand.

A scaphoid fracture is not always so obvious. Often a fracture here will not show on standard roentgenograms. A key clinical sign is localized bony tenderness in the anatomical snuff box on palpation. When this is found in a patient referred following a fall on the outstretched hand, the therapist should suspect a scaphoid fracture and also consult the physician. A rather high incidence of avascular necrosis of the proximal fragment of the scaphoid occurs with this fracture because the blood supply to the scaphoid often enters only from the distal aspect of the bone. The fracture, then, cuts off the blood supply to the proximal fragment. It is generally agreed that strict, prolonged immobilization of the wrist and thumb is necessary to minimize the possibility of avascular necrosis and nonunion.

SECONDARY OSTEOARTHRITIS OF THE THUMB

The carpometacarpal joint of the thumb is particularly liable to osteoarthrosis. Women are more predisposed to the development of this disorder than are men, and it can occur without evidence of osteoarthrosis in any other joint.[13,14] Typically it is bilateral, although it can be unilateral and may occur following prolonged overuse or trauma. It is a frequent finding following Bennett's fracture.[118]

The key structures in the trapeziometacarpal joint are the palmar or ulnar ligaments, which hold the beak of the thumb metacarpal down to the ridge on the trapezium, and the intermetacarpal ligaments, which hold the first to the second metacarpal (see Fig. 12–8).[83] In normal flexion and extension these ligaments undergo very little stress. However, in opposition and power pinch the joint surfaces twist one on the other and are prevented from coming apart by these ligaments.[61] Unequal stresses over time, an incongruency resulting from injured joint surface or ligamentous disruption, can result in osteoarthrosis (as the initial stage) with the ultimate development of osteoarthritis.[68]

Initially, erosion of the joint surfaces causes pain. After a time, the joint commonly subluxates because of degenerative changes, causing a gradual proximal travel of the metacarpal base of the saddle of the trapezium, together with an adduction deformity.[16] A secondary hyperextension deformity of the metacarpophalangeal joint may develop with attempted abduction, resulting in weakness and loss of function.

I. History

The patient's first complaints are usually of pain aggravated by use. Advice is often sought long before destructive changes take place. Typical symptoms include the following:

A. Pain on extremes of movement of the thumb or when gripping or holding tools for long periods. The pain is usually localized to the base of the thumb just anterior and distal to the anatomical snuff box.

B. Marked instability and weakness of the hand with a tendency to drop things and difficulty guiding or manipulating tools

C. Occasional subjective complaints of numbness of the thumb and stiffness

D. Deep-seated grinding which is particularly uncomfortable.

E. Occasional swelling

II. Physical examination

A. In later stages the patient may present with an adduction deformity and hyperextension of the metacarpophalangeal joint.

B. Active range of motion will often reveal crepitus and increased motion.

C. Passive backward stretching of the thumb in abduction brings on the pain.

D. Joint-play motions, particularly axial rotation, reproduce the pain. Later instability of the joint is evidenced by the prominence of the metacarpal base and hypermobility.[68]

E. Resisted motions are painless. Pinch strength will progressively decrease.

F. Tenderness is well localized over the joint on its anterior aspect. Osteophytes are sometimes palpable anteriorly.

III. Management

A. In the early stages the physician may elect to use corticosteroid injections. In advanced cases intra-articular silicone is often effective and for this reason arthroplasty and arthrodesis are required less often than formerly.[21] If arthritis clearly involves other trapezial joints, arthrodesis of the trapeziometacarpal joint will give only limited relief of symptoms, as will arthroplasty of that joint. Excision of the trapezium may be necessary, and good results have been reported from this procedure alone.[16,22,37] If the joint remains unstable, replacement of the excised trapezium by rolled tendon[76] or fascia[114] or with a Silastic prosthesis is increasingly practiced.[27,30,67,87,100]

B. In the early stages, osteoarthrosis or traumatic arthritis respond well to friction massage.[21] At any point, relief can be provided by fitting the patient with a splint. Patients often find it useful to continue to use the splint for many months or even years while undertaking heavy work. Mobilization techniques, when indicated, and isometric exercises are useful. Patient education should include emphasis on avoiding positions of stress and activities that provoke the symptoms.

THE STIFF HAND

Stiffness and capsular restriction at the wrist and hand proper are common clinical problems seen by physical therapists. Whether due to fracture immobilization, soft-tissue contractures (Dupuytren's disease), burns, reflex sympathetic dystrophy, postoperative reconstructive hand surgery, complications of mastectomy, joint disease, peripheral nerve injury, or constriction by a cast or poorly applied dressing, stiffness of the fingers and hand proper (metacarpals) that may result can be ruinous. Mobility is essential in normal function, and it can be disastrous when roentgenographic results of a fracture of the hand are normal but the patient is left with a stiff "frozen" hand.[118]

The major contributor to the stiff or frozen hand is edema. Postoperative or post-traumatic edema of the hand has been shown to be a normal physiological response to injury. Edema is reversible; the degree and rapidity of reversibility determine its deleterious effect. If edema can be controlled early, subsequent scar formation is minimized in comparison with scar that forms if edema is prolonged and brawny. Persistence of edema may lead to joint stiffness and reflex sympathetic dystrophy. The measures against persistent post-traumatic or postsurgical edema merit particular attention. Edema is usually the result of an impairment of the microcirculation combined with the release of vasodilatating substances such as histamine and kinins, which also increase the vascular permeability.[78] Vascular dilatation evoked by pain receptors also play a role. Abnormal autonomic reflexes are believed to be a major contributor in the early and later stages of reflex sympathetic dystrophy, in which edema is the most constant physical finding (see "Colles' Fracture"). As time passes, the swelling worsens rather than improves.[64] Later motion is further inhibited by joint stiffness and brawny edema.

The sequence of events following edema has been described by Bunnell.[8,12]

> When a hand remains swollen, from whatever cause, the moveable parts are bathed in serofibrinous exudate. Fibrin is deposited between the various tissue layers and the folds of the joint capsules, between the tendons and their sheaths, throughout the ligamentous tissue itself and between and within the muscles. While soaked in the exudate, all of these tissues swell with edema and become shorter and thicker. The fibrin seals them in this condition and soon as the fibroblastic growth transforms all to connective tissue, ligaments become shorter and thicker. The folds of synovial membrane, the capsules of the joints, the plicae of tendon sheaths and the tendons and their sheaths become plastered together with organized adhesions.

Typically in the hand proper, edema is localized to the dorsum of the hand, where the tissues are most easily distended. The swelling of the dorsal aspect causes metacarpophalangeal joint extension, which predisposes to stiffness, scar formation, and contractures. Then fibrosis ensues, and a vicious circle begins.

Finger joints may stiffen after injury even though the insult was distant. Tendency toward stiffness of the fingers is greatest in adults and the aged but varies among individuals. Some persons have a tendency to form scar tissue in the periarticular tissues, while others form keloids in the skin.[105] Anatomical factors that can cause limitations of motion include joint or capsular restriction, scar contraction of the skin (burns), contracted muscle, or an adherent tendon and a bony block or exostosis. All tissues can contract or become adherent: subcutaneous tissue, fascia, nerves, vessels, and cartilaginous and bony structures.

Stiffness of the hand resulting from edema, scar formation, muscle contraction, or a combination of these problems renders the hand stiff by interfering with either joint mobility or power gliding of the musculotendinous unit. The effects of edema on tendon gliding result in fluid collection in the layered paratenon, causing increased work to effect tendon gliding and a decrease in longitudinal paratenon gliding. Consequently, edema forming even after a minor injury may restrict gliding even though the joints exhibit a near-normal range of motion.[112] Full passive extension of the joints may not be possible because the swollen paratenon restricts gliding of the flexor tendons. The degree of joint impairment is more dependent on the anatomy of the joint, its supporting structures, and the position of the joint when the cicatrix was forming and maturing. Scar formation is particularly disabling in regard to tendon gliding because no matter what the position of the tendons, tendon gliding is impaired. Scar forms not only at the site of the lesion but also at many sites far removed. For example, a tendon lacerated in the fibro-osseous tunnel may evoke scar formation in the paratenon of the flexor tendons proximal to the wrist.[112]

Involvement of muscle compounds functional

loss. Muscles may become involved by internal or external cicatrix formation or by myostatic contracture. Muscle imbalance in nerve palsy can result in contractures combined with the effects of edema and cicatrix reaction to the initial injury.[112]

EXAMINATION

History

The patient presents with a primary complaint of loss of hand function due to stiffness following post-traumatic or postsurgical immobilization or lack of immobilization. Stiffness alone is usually not painful, but in some cases may be. The existence of pain poses a diagnostic problem. Nonunion of a fracture, neuroma, or degenerative arthritis must be considered. Once these causes have been eliminated, the distinction is made between pain occurring during mobilization, which appears to be due to traction at the gliding planes or irregularities of the articular surfaces, or pain presenting in the absence of mobilization. The latter may be related to sympathetic dystrophy.

Inspection

A stiff hand may restrict the normal swinging movement of the arm as the hand is held stiffly by the side. Some swelling may be present and may be intra-articular or extra-articular. Synovitis of the metacarpophalangeal and proximal interphalangeal joints bulges into the looser tissues on the extensor surface of the hand. Its shape is determined by the synovial attachments around the joints, which tend to spread on either side of the tendon in a proximal direction. Synovitis produces a diffuse swelling and can be easily differentiated from traumatic swelling of the joint structures, which usually forms a localized swelling on one side of the joint.

Extra-articular swelling may be either localized or diffuse. Diffuse swelling of a digit produces a sausage-shaped deformity. Localized swelling may involve the soft tissues around a joint and tendon sheath. In the palm and fingers it usually involves the flexor tendon sheath and may then be associated with nodule formation and triggering of the thumb or finger.[16,19,68]

Localized swelling may be due to ganglia or cystic swellings associated with Heberden's nodes.

Selective Tissue Tension and Neurologic Tests

Assessment of range of motion, strength, sensibility, and the patient's ability to perform activities of daily living completes the evaluation. Knowledge of the causes of joint stiffness is essential before evaluation of the range of motion of the chronically stiff hand. Testing for skin tightness is routinely done.[2,3,93]

The capsular and extracapsular structures contributing to joint stiffness will be discussed according to the position of stiffness of the joint.

METACARPOPHALANGEAL JOINT

The initial response following trauma to a hand is an increase in tissue fluid, either lymph, hemorrhage, or both. Fluid increases in the tissues of the joints. The fluid in the tissue of the capsule and collateral ligaments tends to produce an effective shortening of the structures. Fluid in the joint distends the capsule, and the joint assumes a position of maximum capacity. The anatomical positions are greatest in the metacarpophalangeal joints, and these joints are the key to the resultant negative hand: metacarpophalangeal extension, interphalangeal flexion, and wrist flexion.[111] Left in this attitude, certain peri-articular changes occur and contractures develop.

Stiffness in Extension

Stiffness in extension can be due to contraction of the dorsal skin, extensor apparatus, capsular restriction (dorsal aspect), contraction of the collateral ligaments, or lesions of the joint structures. The joint factors that contribute to stiffness of the joint include capsular restriction, pannus formation in the volar synovial pouch, and articular surface erosions with or without pannus invasion.

Extracapsular factors that can contribute to stiffness of the metacarpophalangeal joint in extension include skin contractures, extensor tendon adhesions at the dorsum of the wrist, unopposed extension (loss of active metacarpophalangeal flexion), and forearm extensor muscle contractures.

Stiffness in Flexion

Capsular factors that can contribute to stiffness of the metacarpophalangeal joints in flexion include deformities of the metacarpophalangeal joints, contractures or binding of the proximal sinus of the volar plate, contraction of the collateral or accessory collateral ligaments, and erosion of the articular surfaces with or without fusion.[105,112]

Extracapsular factors contributing to metacarpophalangeal joint stiffness in flexion include contractures of the palmar skin and fascia, adhesions or contractures of the flexor tendons, and intrinsic muscle contractures.

PROXIMAL INTERPHALANGEAL JOINT

At the proximal interphalangeal joint, the flexor superficialis comes into contact with the distal portion of the volar plate and may become adherent to it. The same is true of the flexor profundus at the distal interphalangeal joint. The fibrous sheath of the flexor tendons extend from the proximal interphalangeal joint to the metacarpophalangeal joint. It inserts on the volar plate and on the phalanges but not on the metacarpal. This explains the important role it may play in stiffness in flexion of the proximal interphalangeal joint but not in stiffness of the metacarpophalangeal joint.[105] Other problems limiting extension of the proximal interphalangeal joints include adherence of the retinacular ligament to the collateral ligaments, adherence of the collateral ligaments, a bony block or exostosis, scarring of the skin on the volar surface of the finger and contraction of the superficial fascia or forearm musculature, and contraction of the fibrous portion of the fibro-osseous tunnel.

Abnormalities limiting flexion of the proximal interphalangeal joints include scar contracture of the dorsal skin of the finger, an adherent extensor tendon, capsular restriction, adherence of the collateral ligaments or retinacular ligament to the lateral capsular ligament or of the volar capsular ligament to the proximal phalanx, interosseous or lumbrical tendon adherence, intrinsic muscle contracture exostosis, a bony block, or articular surface erosion or pannus formation.[105]

MANAGEMENT

An understanding of the capsular and extracapsular factors responsible for normal joint stability and the factors responsible for the development of stiff joints is required in post-traumatic and postoperative mobilization of stiff joints. It is obviously better to prevent stiffness from occurring than to have to treat it. One of the most important aspects is the prevention of edema, which is done as soon after the injury or elective surgery as possible. Active motion, elevation, massage, anti-inflammatory medications, the use of a continuous passive motion device,[90] intermittent compressive therapies, ice immersions, compressive wrapping or gloves, elastic tape for wrapping of individual fingers, and string wrapping may be considered.[15,17,45,86] Placement of the hand in a protective position by means of a functional resting splint (secured with a figure-of-eight elastic wrap to help distribute pressure over a wide area) should be considered when severe edema is present.[75]

Active Mobilization

The mainstay of the therapeutic program is active exercise. Early active mobilization should be started as soon as the lesions allow, but two extremes must be avoided: prolonged immobilization and excessive painful mobilization. The need for active use of the hand in mobilizing stiff joints cannot be overemphasized. Voluntary exercises and the use of the hand by the patient throughout the day is far superior in results to forceful passive range of motion applied for brief periods of times per day. Daily forcing of the fingers joints causes reactive pain and swelling and is equivalent to spraining them daily, according to Bunnel.[8] Correct motions of the fingers and wrist are more important than strength of motion. Co-contraction of the agonist and antagonist should be prevented. The use of biofeedback is often helpful in preventing unwanted muscle activity. Certain activities such as precision tasks can be done in elevation. Active exercises should include full range of motion to the elbow and shoulder of the involved arm.

Modification of Scar Tissue

The most accepted clinical method of accelerating the modification of scar tissue is the application of stress to the scar. Treatment by mobilization is based on concepts that were initially empirical but that have more recently been proved by laboratory studies.[9,73,85,113] Slight persistent tension is capable of remodeling the collagen within scar tissue. Active mobilizations can be profitably combined with massage to increase suppleness and prevent contractures.[105] Direct application of stress to the scar tissue can be accomplished in a number of ways: (1) direct pressure by massage or bandages, (2) serial or dynamic splints, (3) joint mobilization techniques in the presence of capsuloligamentous tightening or adherence (see Chapter 6), and (4) passive range of motion or stretching techniques.

Massage

According to Wynn-Parry,[118] massage has no place in hand therapy to reduce muscle spasm, relieve pain, or improve circulation. Ice and active mobilization are the best means of reducing spasm. Pain is more efficiently and less expensively relieved by analgesia or other methods of modulation. Active exercises are infinitely better at increasing circulation than massage. Massage (soft-tissue mobilization) finds its most effective role in breaking down adhesions and fibrosis; mobilizing scar tissue; stretching restricted fasciae, skin, joint capsules, and ligaments; and helping to reduce edema. The use of massage not only applies compressive and distractive forces directly to the scar but also helps to alter the fibrotic process and reduce any edema that may be present. Deep friction massage is particularly useful in the management of tenosynovitis and for decreasing adhesions that form at ligaments after a sprain (see Chapter 8, Friction Massage).[21] Joint massage has been found to be a valuable adjunct in treating degenerative joints whose chief complaint is stiffness or pain and stiffness.[84] Connective tissue massage often can provide gentle stretch of the capsule without traumatizing the joint structures.[28,103] A common problem in the management of the hand is overstretching of the capsules in the small joints of the fingers. These joints need to be stretched gently. Forceful stretching can only cause reactive pain and swelling, with the joints becoming stiffer than ever. A variety of soft-tissue mobilization techniques have been taught and used effectively through the years to stretch abnormal fibrous tissue and to increase flexibility and range of motion.[4,49,69]

Splinting

Between physical therapy sessions, when retraction is marked, serial splints as advocated by Wynn-Parry and dynamic or static splints can be used to provide a prolonged pull or traction on the scar tissue.[118] In long-standing contractures, elongation by slow traction will be necessary. Continuous mild traction provides a light prolonged stretch on the restraining tissue until, by cell multiplication, they actually grow longer, so that lengthening is permanent.[60,92] It is important that dynamic splints be well adapted to the patient. If evaluation reveals that limitation in the range of motion is strictly related to soft-tissue contracture around a particular joint, a splint must be designed to apply traction to that specific joint. Traction must act perpendicular (at a right angle to the treatment plane) to the involved phalanx. When evaluation reveals that restrictions in active range of motion are due to a combination of joint contracture and muscle tightness, a two-stage splinting program is required.[75] Initially a splint is designed to increase the passive range of motion of the involved joint. Later, when normal joint mechanics have been restored, the splinting program is directed at providing stretch to the involved intrinsic or extrinsic musculature.

Joint Mobilization

Free joint play within a useful or functional range of motion is necessary to avoid joint trauma. If joint play is restricted, joint-mobilizing techniques should be used (see Chapter 6, Peripheral Joint Mobilization Techniques).[51] When pain is the dominant factor, grade I and II mobilization techniques are appropriate. If these techniques are successful and pain-free active motion increases, treatment is taken further into the range. Chronically, these stretching techniques can be vigorous as long as pain and irritation are avoided. Before initiating stretching techniques to muscle or inert tissue, there should be normal gliding of the joint surfaces in order to avoid joint damage. It is important that both joint dynamics and muscle strength and flexibility be balanced as the hand is restored to functional usage.

Passive Range of Motion and Stretching Techniques

In vitro research has shown that prolonged low-intensity stretching at elevated tissue temperatures maximizes permanent lengthening of connective tissue and minimizes deterioration in tensile strength.[5,7,35,36,38,46,60,65,92,107,109,110] When employing this principle of combining heat and stretch to a stiff hand, McEntee suggests that an elastic tape be applied to the involved finger or fingers in the direction in which increased motion is desired to maintain a prolonged stretch.[75] Once the hand is stretched with the tape, it can be dipped in paraffin or placed under a hot pack for the desired time.[75] Active exercises should follow immediately for the best results. As an adjunct to prolonged stretch, manual passive range of motion or stretching techniques may be used. The complexity of the joints and multijoint muscles of the fingers requires careful evaluation and management. Fingers should always be stretched individually, not grossly. When stretching the extrinsic muscles (which are multijoint muscles), elongation over all the joints, simultaneously, should be avoided. Stretching in this manner can result in joint compression and damage to the smaller or less stable joints. Gently distract the joints to avoid compression of the segments being mobilized. Use short levers whenever possible and apply the stretch force in a gentle, slow, and sustained manner. Hold the patient in the stretched position for at least 15 to 30 seconds or longer. Muscles are more amenable to stretch when they are preceded by some form of warm-up exercise. The best and most specific warm-up exercise is contraction against resistance. Successive techniques of isometric contractions, relaxation and stretching (contract-relax method) followed by stimulation of the antagonist helps to relax the muscles so they are more easily stretched.[29,41,48,58,59,74,102,108,117]

Therapy is more effective if it is supplemented by frequent self-stretching. In general, the more frequent the stretching, the more moderate the intensity. The principle of moving the body in relationship to the stabilized extremity affords an excellent stretch and allows for a greater degree of pain-free movement (see Chapter 7, Automobilization Techniques of the Extremities). For example, to stretch the long finger flexors, have the patient (in a standing position) rest the palm of the involved hand on a table. Using his other hand he extends the joints from distal to proximal in succession or he actively extends them, unassisted, when possible. When the joints are extended, he fixates or maintains this position with his other hand as he actively moves his trunk forward, which brings his arm (with the elbow extended) up over his hand, resulting in wrist extension.[57] Motion is taken to the point of discomfort and maintained. Motion is progressed as the length improves.

Reverse stretching techniques can also be used. for example, to stretch the extensor digitorum communis, the patient is instructed to maximally flex the elbow and then actively flex the fingers to their maximum range, beginning with the most distal joint first and progressing proximally until the wrist is simultaneously flexed. Once all the slack is taken up in the hand, the elbow is straightened. As a result, the stretch is primarily directed at the muscle belly rather than the tendons and joint structures of the hand.

Resistive Exercise

Joint motion without adequate muscle support can cause additional trauma to the joints as functional activities are resumed. Initially isometric exercises are recommended to increase strength when there is a loss of joint play and when there is significant pain. Once joint play is restored, resistive isotonic exercises are recommended within the available range.[57] This does not imply that normal range of motion need be present but that joint play, within the available range, be present. Graded resistive activity progressing from manual resistive exercises that employ proprioceptive neuromuscular facilitation techniques to progressive resistive exercises that employ weights, the resistance of an elasticized tension cord (isoflex exercises), or self-resistance, and activities such as woodworking can be selected to help increase strength of the hand.

Squeezing activities, such as squeezing a rubber ball or a bit of putty, should be forbidden since they prevent full range of flexion, which is one of the goals of treatment. Full range of motion is the primary target. Therapeutic and functional activities, as well as early return to work, are preferred to increase strength, endurance, and active motion of the chronically stiff hand. Acceptance of the hand by the patient, motivation, re-education, and preparing the patient to return to a former job and activities are all the responsibilities that the hand care team must assume.

Management of the postsurgical hand goes beyond the scope of this book. Details of preoperative and postoperative care are readily available in the literature.[1,8,16,22,27,30,37,67,70,76,87,100]

REFERENCES

1. American Academy of Orthopedic Surgeons: Symposium on Tendon Surgery in the Hand. Philadelphia, CV Mosby, 1975
2. American Society for Surgery of the Hand: The Hand-Examination and Diagnosis. Aurora, CO, 1978
3. American Society for Surgery of the Hand: The Hand: Examination and Diagnosis. New York, Churchill Livingstone, 1983
4. Bajelis D: Myofascial release: IV. Management of sport injuries presented at a course on physical therapy management of the extremities, Seattle, July 1986
5. Barcroft H, Edholm OG: The effect of temperature on blood flow and deep temperature in the human forearm. J Physiol 102:5–20, 1943
6. Baxter PL, Ballard MS: Evaluation of the hand by functional tests. In Hunter JM, Schneider LH, Mackin EJ, Bell JA (eds): Rehabilitation of the Hand. St. Louis, CV Mosby, 1984
7. Becker AH: Traction for knee-flexion contractures. Phys Ther 59:1114, 1979
8. Boyes JH (ed): Bunnell's Surgery of the Hand. Philadelphia, JB Lippincott, 1970
9. Brand PW: Hand rehabilitation management by objectives. In Hunter JM, Schneider LH, Mackin EJ, Bell JA (eds): Rehabilitation of the Hand. St. Louis, CV Mosby, 1978
10. Brand PW: Clinical Mechanics of the Hand. St. Louis, CV Mosby, 1985
11. Brown CP, McGrouther DA: The excursion of the tendon of the flexor pollicis longus and its relation to dynamic splintage. J Hand Surg 9(A):787–791, 1984
12. Bunnell S: Ischaemic contracture, local, in the hand. J Bone Joint Surg 35(A):88–101, 1953
13. Cailliet R: Reflex sympathetic referred pain. In Cailliet R: Shoulder Pain, 2nd ed, pp 108–124. Philadelphia, FA Davis, 1981
14. Cailliet R: Hand Pain and Impairment, 3rd ed. Philadelphia, FA Davis, 1982
15. Cain HD, Liebgold HB: Compressive centripetal

wrapping technic for reduction of edema. Arch Phys Med 48:420–423, 1967

16. Campbell-Reid DA, McGrouther DA: Surgery of the Thumb. Boston, Butterworths, 1986

17. Carter PR: Common Hand Injuries and Infections: A Practical Approach to Early Treatment. Philadelphia, WB Saunders, 1983

18. Cornacchia M: Considerazioni sulla meccanica articolare del pollice. Chir Organi Mov 33:137–153, 1949

19. Corrigan B, Maitland GD: Practical Orthopaedic Medicine. Boston, Butterworths, 1985

20. Cyriax J: Textbook of Orthopaedic Medicine. Diagnosis of Soft Tissue Lesions. 8th ed, vol 1, pp 182–199. Philadelphia, Ballière Tindal, 1984

21. Cyriax J: Textbook of Orthopaedic Medicine, Treatment by Manipulation, Massage and Injections. 11th ed, vol 2, pp 127–139. Philadelphia, Ballière Tindal, 1984

22. Dell PC, Brushart TM, Smith RT: Treatment of trapeziometacarpal arthritis: Results of resection arthroplasty. J Hand Surg 5:243–249, 1978

23. Dellon AL: Evaluation of Sensibility and Re-education of Sensation in the Hand. Baltimore, Williams & Wilkins, 1981

24. De Palma F: The Management of Fractures and Dislocations: An Atlas, 2nd ed. Philadelphia, WB Saunders, 1970

25. deTakas G: Nature of painful vasodilatation in causalgic states. Arch Neur Psychiatry 50:318–326, 1943

26. Eaton RG: Joint Injuries of the Hand. Springfield, IL, Charles C Thomas, 1971

27. Eaton RG: Replacement of the trapezium for arthritis of the basal articulation: A new technique with stabilization by tenodesis. J Bone Joint Surg 61(A):76–83, 1979

28. Ebner M: Connective Tissue Manipulations, Therapy and Therapeutic Application. Malabar, FL, Robert E. Knieger Publishing Co., 1985

29. Evjenth O, Hamberg J: Muscle Stretching in Manual Therapy: A Clinical Manual — The Extremities, vol I. Alfta, Sweden, Alfta Rehab Forleg, 1984

30. Ferlic DC, Busbee GA, Clayton ML: Degenerative arthritis of the carpometacarpal joint of the thumb: A clinical follow-up of eleven Niebauer prostheses. J Hand Surg 2:212–215, 1977

31. Fess EE, Harmon KS, Strockland JW, Streichen JB: Evaluation of the hand by objective measurement. In Hunter JM, Schneider LH, Markin EJ, Bell JA (eds): Rehabilitation of the Hand. St. Louis, CV Mosby, 1978

32. Fess EE, Moran CA: Clinical assessment recommendations. Aurora, CO, American Society of Hand Therapists, 1981

33. Flatt AE: The pathomechanics of ulnar drift. Final Report Social and Rehabilitation Services. Grant RD, ed. Washington, DC, Department of Health Education and Welfare, 1971

34. Flatt AE, Fischer GW: Stability during flexion and extension at the metacarpophalangeal joints. In La Main Rhumatoide, Monographie du GEM, pp 51–61. Paris, L'Expansion Scientifique Francaise, 1967

35. Flax HJ, Miller RV, Horvath SM: Alterations in peripheral circulation and tissue temperature following local application of short wave diathermy. Arch Phys Med Rehabil 3:630–637, 1949

36. Gersten JW, Wakin KG, Herrick JF, Krusen FH: The effect of microwave diathermy on the peripheral circulation and on tissue temperature in man. Arch Phys Med Rehabil 30:7–25, 1949

37. Gervis WH: A review of excision of the trapezium for osteoarthritis of the trapeziometacarpal joint after 25 years. J Bone Joint Surg 55(B):56–57, 1973

38. Glazer RM: Rehabilitation. In Happenstall RB (ed): Fracture Treatment and Healing. Philadelphia, WB Saunders, 1980

39. Grant JCB, Basmajian JV: Grant's Method of Anatomy, 7th ed. Baltimore, Williams & Wilkins, 1965

40. Hakstian RW, Tubiana R: Ulnar deviation of the fingers: The role of joint structure and function. J Bone Joint Surg 49(A):299–316, 1967

41. Haugen P, Stern-Knudsen O: The effect of a small stretch on latency relaxation and the short-range elastic stiffness in isolated frog muscle fibres. Acta Physiol Scand 112:121–128, 1981

42. Hazelton FT, Smidt GL, Flatt AE: The influence of wrist position on the force produced by the finger flexors. J Biomech 8:301–306, 1975

43. Hollinshead WH: Anatomy for Surgeons, Vol 3, The Back and Limbs, pp 437–562, 3rd ed. New York, Harper Medical, 1982

44. Hoppenfeld S: Physical Examination of the Spine and Extremities. New York, Appleton-Century-Crofts, 1976

45. Hunter JM, Schneider LH, Mackin EJ, Bell JA (eds): Rehabilitation of the Hand. St. Louis, CV Mosby, 1984

46. Jackman RV: Device to stretch the Achilles tendon. J Am Phys Ther Assoc 43:729, 1963

47. Jebson RH, Taylor N, Trieschman RB, Trotter MJ, Howard LA: An objective and standardized test of hand function. Arch Phys Med Rehabil 5:311–319, 1969

48. Jenkins RB, Little RW: A constitutive equation for parallel-fibered elastic tissue. J Biomech 7:397–402, 1974

49. Johnson G: Functional Orthopedics II: Advanced techniques of soft tissue mobilization for evaluation and treatment of the extremities and trunk. Presented at a course by the Institute of Physical Arts. San Francisco, 1985

50. Johnson RK, Shrewsbury MM: The pronator quadratus in motions and in stabilization of the radius and ulna at the distal radioulnar joint. J Hand Surg 1:205–209, 1976

51. Kaltenborn FM: Mobilization of the Extremity Joints, 3rd ed. Oslo, Olaf Norlis Bokhandel, 1980

52. Kapandji IA: Biomechanics of the interphalangeal joint of the thumb. In Tubiana R (ed): The Hand, vol I. Philadelphia, WB Saunders, 1981

53. Kapandji IA: The Physiology of the Joints, Vol I, Upper Limb. New York, Churchill Livingstone, 1970
54. Kapandji IA: Biomechanics of the thumb. In Tubiana R (ed): The Hand, vol I. Philadelphia, WB Saunders, 1981
55. Kaplan EB: The participation of the metacarpophalangeal joint of the thumb in the act of opposition. Bull Hosp Joint Dis 27:39–45, 1966
56. Kauer JMG. Functional anatomy of the carpometacarpal joint of the thumb. Clin Orthop 220:7–13, 1987
57. Kisner C, Colby LA: Therapeutic Exercise: Foundations and Techniques. Philadelphia, FA Davis, 1985
58. Knott M, Voss DE: Proprioceptive Neuromuscular Facilitation, Patterns and Techniques. New York, Hoeber & Harper, 1956
59. Knutsson E: Proprioceptive neuromuscular facilitation. Scand J Rehabil Med Suppl 7:106–112, 1980
60. Kottke FJ, Pauley DL, Ptak KA: The rationale for prolonged stretching for correction of shortening of connective tissue. Arch Phys Med Rehabil 47:345–352, 1966
61. Kuckynski K: The thumb and saddle. Hand 7:120–195, 1975
62. Landsmeer JMF: The anatomy of the dorsal aponeurosis of the human finger and its functional significance. Anat Rec 104:31–453, 1949
63. Landsmeer JMF: Power grip and precision handling. Ann Rheum Dis 22:164–197, 1962
64. Lankford LL: Reflex sympathetic dystrophy. In Green LL (ed): Operative Hand Surgery, vol I, chap 13. New York, Churchill Livingstone, 1982
65. Lehmann JF, DeLateur BJ, Silverman DRT: Selective heating effects of ultrasound in human beings. Arch Phys Med Rehabil 47:331–339, 1966
66. Lewis OJ, Hamshere RJ, Bucknill TM: The anatomy of the wrist joint. J Anat 106:539–552, 1970
67. Lister GD, Kleinert HE, Kutz JE, Atasoy E: Arthritis of the trapezial articulations treated by prosthetic replacement. Hand 9:117–129, 1977
68. Lister GD: The Hand: Diagnosis and Indications, 2nd ed. New York, Churchill Livingstone, 1984
69. Little KE: Toward more effective manipulative management of chronic myofascial strain and stress syndromes. J Am Osteopath Assoc 68:675–685, 1969
70. Littler JW: The hand and upper extremity. In Converse JM (ed): Reconstructive Plastic Surgery. Philadelphia, JB Lippincott, 1977
71. Long C, Conrad DW, Hall EA: Intrinsic-extrinsic muscle control of the hand in power grip and precision handling. J Bone Joint Surg 52(A):853–867, 1970
72. MacConaill MA: Mechanical anatomy of the carpus and its bearing on surgical problems. J Anat 75:166–175, 1941
73. Madden JW, de Vore G, Arem AJ: A rational postoperative management program for metacarpophalangeal joint implant arthroplasty. J Hand Surg 2:358–366, 1977
74. Markos P: Ipsilateral and contralateral effects of proprioceptive neuromuscular facilitation techniques on hip motion and electromyographic activity. Phys Ther 59:1366–1373, 1979
75. McEntee PA: Therapist's management of the stiff hand. In Hunter JM, Schneider LH, Mackin EJ, Bell JA (eds): Rehabilitation of the Hand. St. Louis, CV Mosby, 1984
76. Menon J, Schoene H, Hohl J: Trapeziometacarpal arthritis: Results of tendon interpositional arthroplasty. J Hand Surg 6:442–446, 1981
77. Milford LW: Restraining Ligaments of the Digits of the Hand: Gross and Microscopic Anatomic Study. Philadelphia, WB Saunders, 1968
78. Mittelbach HR: The Injured Hand: A Clinical Handbook for General Surgeons. New York, Springer Verlag, 1979
79. Moberg E: Shoulder–hand–finger syndrome. Surg Clin North Am 40:367–373, 1960
80. Napler JR: The prehensile movements of the human hand. J Bone Joint Surg 38(B):902–913, 1956
81. Newmeyer WL: Primary Care of Hand Injuries. Philadelphia, Lea & Febiger, 1979
82. Norkin C, Levangie DK: Joint Structure and Function: A Comprehensive Analysis. Philadelphia, FA Davis, 1983
83. Pagalidis T, Kucznski K, Lamb DW: Ligamentous stability of the base of the thumb. Hand 13:29–35, 1981
84. Paris SV: The Spinal Lesion. Christ Church, New Zealand, Pegasus Press, 1965
85. Peacock EE: Some biomechanical and biophysical aspects of joint stiffness: Role of collagen synthesis as opposed to altered molecular bonding. Ann Surg 164:1–12, 1966
86. Perry JF: Use of a surgical glove in treatment of edema in hand. J Am Phys Ther Assoc 54:498–499, 1974
87. Poppen N, Niebauer J: "Tie in" trapezium prosthesis: Long-term results. J Hand Surg 3:445–450, 1978
88. Rabischong P: Les problèms fondamentaux du rétablissement de la préhension. Ann Chir 25:927–933, 1971
89. Rosse C: The Hand. In Rosse C, Clawson DK (eds): The Musculoskeletal System in Health and Disease, p 227. Philadelphia, Harper & Row, 1980
90. Salter RB: Textbook of Disorders and Injuries of the Musculoskeletal System, 2nd ed. Baltimore, Williams & Wilkins, 1983
91. Sandzen SC: Atlas of Wrist and Hand Fractures. Littleton, MA, PSG Publishing Co, 1979
92. Sapega AA, Quedenfeld TC, Moyer RA, Butler RA: Physiological factors in range-of-motion exercises. Phys Sports Med 9:57–65, 1981
93. Schamber D: Simply Performed Tests of the Hand. New York, Vantage Press, 1984
94. Simmons BP, De La Caffiniere JF: Physiology of flexion of the fingers. In Tubiana R (ed): The Hand, vol I, Philadelphia, WB Saunders, 1981
95. Smith EM, Juvinall R, Bender L, Pearson J: Role of

the finger flexors in rheumatoid deformities of the metacarpophalangeal joints. Arthritis Rheum 7:467–480, 1964

96. Spinner M: Kaplan's Functional and Surgical Anatomy of the Hand. Philadelphia, JB Lippincott, 1984

97. Steinbrocker O, Argyros TG: The shoulder–hand–syndrome: Present status as a diagnostic and therapeutic entity. Med Clin North Am 42:1533–1553, 1958

98. Steinbrocker O, Spitzer N, Friedman NH: The shoulder–hand syndrome in reflex dystrophy of the upper extremity. Ann Intern Med 29:22–52, 1948

99. Swanson AB, Goran-Hagert C, Swanson G: Evaluation of impairment of hand function. In Hunter JM, Schneider LH, Mackin EJ, Bell JA (eds): Rehabilitation of the Hand. St. Louis, CV Mosby, 1978

100. Swanson AB, Swanson G, Watermeier JJ: Trapezium implant arthroplasty: Long-term evaluation of 150 cases. J Hand Surg 6:128–141, 1981

101. Taleisnic J: The ligaments of the wrist. J Hand Surg 1:110–118, 1976

102. Tanigava MC: Comparison of the hold-relax procedure and passive mobilization on increasing muscle length. Phys Ther 52:725–735, 1972

103. Tappan F: Healing Massage Techniques: A Study in Eastern and Western Methods. Reston, VA, Reston Publishing Co, 1978

104. Tubiana R: Examination of the Hand and Upper Limb. Philadelphia, WB Saunders, 1984

105. Tubiana R: The Hand, vol I. Philadelphia, WB Saunders, 1981

106. Wadsworth CT: Wrist and hand examination and interpretation. J Orthop Sports Phys Ther 5:108–120, 1983

107. Wakim KG, Krusen FH: Influence of physical agents and of certain drugs on intra-articular temperature. Arch Phys Med Rehabil 32:714–721, 1951

108. Wallin D, Ekblom B, Grahn R, Nordenborg T: Improvement of muscle flexibility: A comparison between two techniques. Am J Sports Med 13:263–268, 1985

109. Warren CG, Lehmann JF, Koblanski JN: Elongation of rat tail tendon: Effect of load and temperature. Arch Phys Med Rehabil 52:465–474, 1971

110. Warren CG, Lehmann JF, Koblanski JN: Heat and stretch procedures: An evaluation using rat tail tendon. Arch Phys Med Rehabil 57:122–126, 1976

111. Watson HK: Stiff joints. In Green DP (ed): Operative Hand Surgery, vol I. New York, Churchill Livingstone, 1982

112. Weeks PM, Wray RC: Management of Acute Hand Injuries. St. Louis, CV Mosby, 1973

113. Weeks PM, Wray R, Kuxhaus M: The results of nonoperative management of stiff joints in the hand. Plast Reconstr Surg 61:58–63, 1978

114. Wilson J: Arthroplasty of the trapeziometacarpal joint. Plast Reconstr Surg 49:143–148, 1972

115. Woolf D: Shoulder–hand syndrome. Practitioner 213:176–183, 1974

116. Youm Y, McMurtry RY, Flatt AB, Gillespie TE: Kinematics of the wrist: I. An experimental study of radioulnar deviation and flexion-extension. J Bone Joint Surg 6(A):432–434, 1978

117. Wright V, Johns R: Physical factors concerned with stiffness of normal and diseased joints. Bull Johns Hopkins Hosp 106:215–231, 1960

118. Wynn-Parry CB: Rehabilitation of the Hand. Toronto, Butterworths, 1973

119. Zancolli EA: Structural and Dynamic Basis of Hand Surgery. Philadelphia, JB Lippincott, 1979

120. Zancolli EA, Ziadenberg C, Zancolli E: Biomechanics of the trapeziometacarpal joint. Clin Orthop 220:14–26, 1987

13 *The Hip*

Randolph M. Kessler and Darlene Hertling

REVIEW OF FUNCTIONAL ANATOMY

OSTEOLOGY

The acetabulum is formed superiorly by the ilium, posteroinferiorly by the ischium, and anteroinferiorly by the pubis. The acetabulum faces laterally, anteriorly, and inferiorly (Fig. 13–1A). It is deepened by the fibrocartilaginous acetabular labrum, allowing it to enclose slightly more than half a sphere. The bony, fibrocartilaginous labrum and cartilaginous constituents of the acetabulum are interrupted inferiorly by the acetabular notch (Fig. 13–1B). This notch is traversed by the transverse ligament of the acetabulum (Fig. 13–1C).

The head of the femur constitutes about two thirds of a sphere. Slightly below and behind the center of the articular surface of the head is a roughened indentation termed the *fovea*, to which the ligament of the head of the femur attaches (see Fig. 13–1B). The neck of the femur connects the head and shaft of the femur. In the frontal plane, the angle formed by the neck and shaft of the femur is about 125° in the adult but closer to 150° in the young child. This is often termed the *angle of inclination* (Fig. 13–2). In the transverse plane, the neck forms an angle of about 15° with the transverse axis of the femoral condyles, such that with the transverse axis of the condyles lying in the frontal plane, the neck of the femur is directed about 15° forward (Fig. 13–3). This is referred to as the *angle of torsion* or *angle of declination* of the hip. Note, then, that in the anatomical position, both the acetabulum and the neck of the femur are directed anteriorly. Because of this, in the normal standing position, a large area of the articular surface of the head of the femur is exposed anteriorly and the effective weight-bearing surface of the head is confined to a relatively small area on the posterosuperior aspect of the head.

An increase in degrees of the normal inclination angle is referred to as *coxa valgum;* a decrease in the angle is called *coxa varum* (see Fig. 13–2). When an increased torsion angle is present, we speak of an *anteverted hip*, whereas a hip in *retroversion* is one in which there is less than a normal torsion angle (see Fig. 13–3). Clinically, it should be apparent that a patient with an anteverted hip will appear to lack external rotation, and a patient with a retroverted hip will appear to lack internal rotation. Also, the person with an anteverted hip will tend to walk with a toe-in gait; with retroversion, a toe-out gait is characteristic.

The greater trochanter is a prominence projecting laterally and superiorly from the junction of the neck and shaft of the femur. It serves as an area for attachment of many of the muscles controlling movement at the hip. Situated posteromedially to the junction of the neck and shaft is a smaller prominence, the lesser trochanter; it also provides an area of insertion for muscles controlling the hip (see Fig. 13–1A).

Trabeculae

The trabecular patterns of the upper femur reflect the normal stresses sustained by the hip; they correspond to the normal lines of force in this area (Fig. 13–4). The main system of trabeculae consists of two sets of trabeculae. The arcuate bundle resists a bending moment or a tendency for the weight of the body to shear the head and neck inferiorly with respect to the shaft of the femur; this bending moment is brought about by the lever arm created by the medially projecting neck of the femur. The vertical bundle resists vertical compressive forces through the head of the femur. The arcuate bundle runs from the lateral cortex of the shaft of the femur, just inferior to the greater trochanter, upward and medially to the middle and inferior cortical region of the head of the femur. The vertical bundle is contiguous with the medial cortex of the shaft of the femur, running straight upward to the superior cortex of the head.

Another trabecular system runs from the medial

(Text continues on p. 276.)

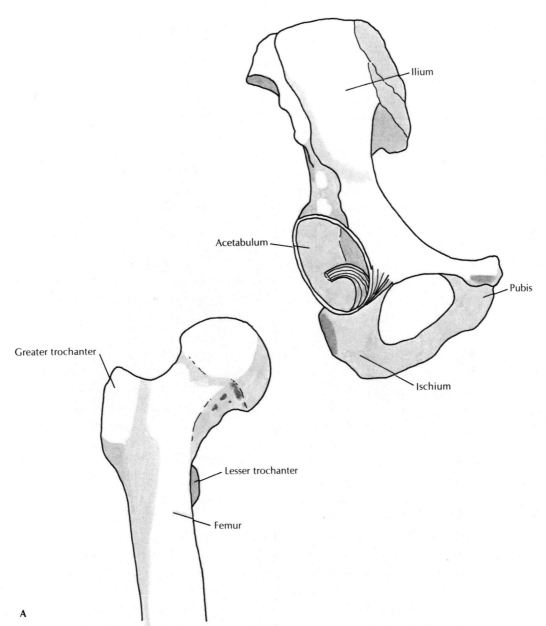

Fig. 13–1. Components of the right hip joint, showing the relationship of the acetabulum to the femur *(A)*, the acetabular fossa to the proximal femur *(B)*, and the ligaments of the acetabulum *(C)*.

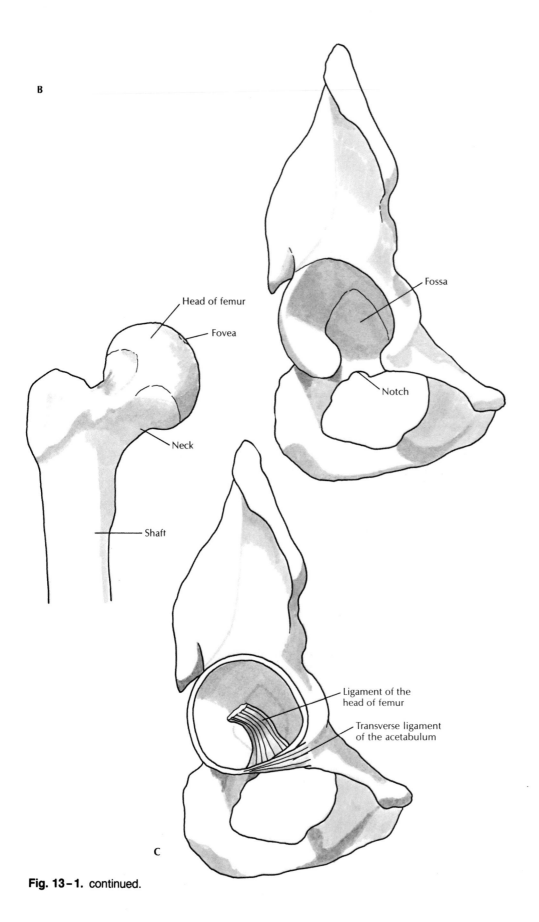

B

Head of femur

Fovea

Neck

Shaft

Fossa

Notch

Ligament of the
head of femur

Transverse ligament
of the acetabulum

C

Fig. 13-1. continued.

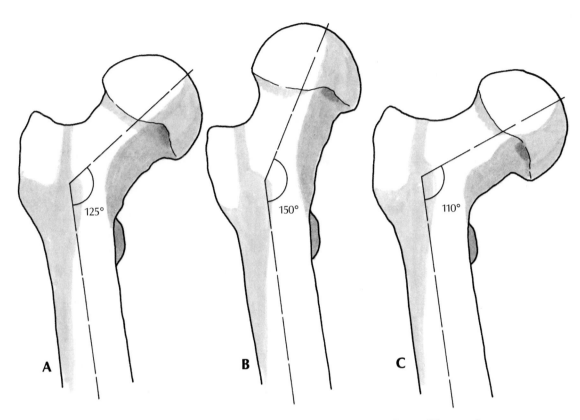

Fig. 13-2. Angle of inclination of the femur: *(A)* coxa varum; *(B)* coxa valgum; *(C)* normal angle.

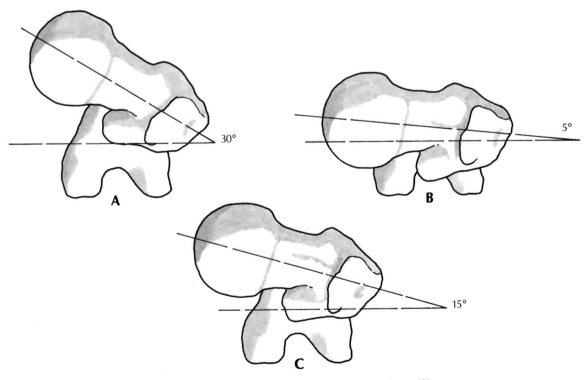

Fig. 13-3. Angle of torsion or declination of the femur in the transverse plane: *(A)* anteversion; *(B)* retroversion; *(C)* normal angle.

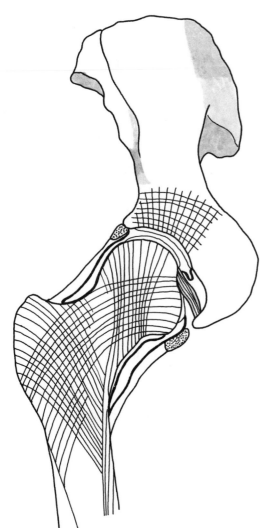

Fig. 13-4. Trabecular patterns of the upper femur.

cortex at the base of the neck, upward laterally through the greater trochanter. These trabeculae resist the tensile forces from the muscles attaching to the trochanter.

The areas where the vertical bundle and the trochanteric bundle intersect the arcuate bundle are areas of particular strength. The intervening region is an area of relative weakness, made weaker by osteoporosis in older people. This region is often the site of femoral neck fractures.

ARTICULAR CARTILAGE

The area of the acetabulum covered by articular cartilage is a horseshoe-shaped region. The area not covered by articular cartilage corresponds to the total sweep of the ligament of the head of the femur when the hip is moved through a full range of movement in all planes. This nonarticular portion is the acetabu-

lar fossa and is lined by a fat pad (see Fig. 13-1B). The entire head of the femur is covered by articular cartilage except for the small fovea where the ligament of the head attaches.

LIGAMENTS AND CAPSULE

The joint capsule of the hip joint is thick and strong and is reinforced by strong ligaments. Its fibers run longitudinally, parallel to the neck of the femur (Fig. 13-5). The capsule runs from the rim of the acetabulum and labrum to the intertrochanteric line anteriorly and to about 1 cm proximal to the intertrochanteric crest posteriorly. Much of the neck of the femur, then, is intracapsular. Some deep fibers of the joint capsule run circularly around the neck of the femur, forming the zona orbicularis.

The iliofemoral ligament is one of the strongest ligaments in the body. It is sometimes referred to as the Y ligament of Bigelow, since it resembles an inverted Y. It attaches proximally to the lower portion of the anterior-inferior iliac spine and to an area on the ilium just proximal to the superior and posterosuperior rim of the acetabulum. The ligament, as a whole, spirals around to overlie the anterior aspect of the joint, attaching to the intertrochanteric line. The more lateral fork of the Y attaches to the anterior aspect of the greater trochanter, whereas the more medial fibers twist around to attach just anterior to the lesser trochanter (see Fig. 13-5A).

This ligament primarily checks internal rotation and extension. It allows a person to stand with the joint in extension using a mimimum of muscle action; by rolling the pelvis backward, a person can "hang" on the ligaments. Note that the ligament prevents excessive movement in the direction toward the close-packed position of the hip joint. Looking at it in another way, with movement toward the close-packed position, this ligament becomes taut and twisted upon itself, causing an approximation of the joint surfaces and a "locking" of the joint. Some of the lateral fibers of the iliofemoral ligament probably pull tight on adduction.

The ischiofemoral ligament attaches proximally to an area of the ischium just posterior and posteroinferior to the rim of the acetabulum. Its fibers run upward and laterally to attach to the posterosuperior aspect of the neck of the femur, where the neck meets the greater trochanter (see Fig. 13-5B). The ischiofemoral ligament also pulls tight on extension and internal rotation of the hip.

The pubofemoral ligament runs from the pubis, near the acetabulum, to the femur, just anterior to the lesser trochanter. It tightens primarily on abduc-

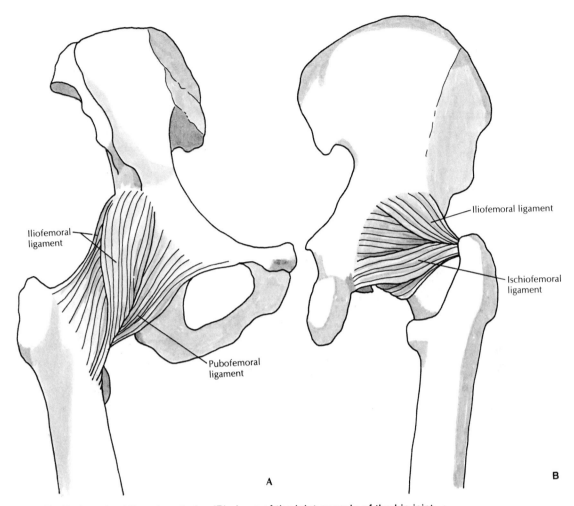

Fig. 13–5. Anterior *(A)* and posterior *(B)* views of the joint capsule of the hip joint.

tion but also helps check internal rotation of the hip (see Fig. 13–5*A*).

The ligament of the head of the femur (ligmentum teres) attaches to the roughened nonarticular area of the acetabulum inferiorly near the acetabular notch, to both sides of the notch, and to the transverse ligament that traverses the notch. It lies in the nonarticular acetabular fossa as it runs up and around the head of the femur to the fovea (see Fig. 13–1*C*).

Although it pulls tight on adduction of the hip, its mechanical function is relatively unimportant. Of more significance is its role in providing some vascularization to the head of the femur and perhaps in assisting with lubrication of the joint. The ligament of the head of the femur is lined with synovium. It is believed that this ligament may act somewhat similarly to the meniscus at the knee by spreading a layer of synovial fluid over the articular surface of the head of the femur as it advances to contact the opposing surface of the acetabulum.

As mentioned, the transverse ligament crosses the acetabular notch to fill in the gap. It converts the notch into a foramen through which the acetabular artery (from the obturator artery) runs, eventually becoming the artery of the ligament of the head of the femur (see Fig. 13–1*C*).

SYNOVIUM

The synovial membrane of the hip joint lines the fibrous layer of the capsule. It also lines the acetabular labrum and, inferiorly, continues inward at the acetabular notch to line the fat pad in the floor of the acetabular fossa and to cover the ligament of the head of the femur. From the femoral attachment of the capsule at the base of the neck, the synovium reflects backward proximally to line the neck of the femur.

The synovial "cavity" of the joint often communicates anteriorly with the iliopectineal bursa. It does

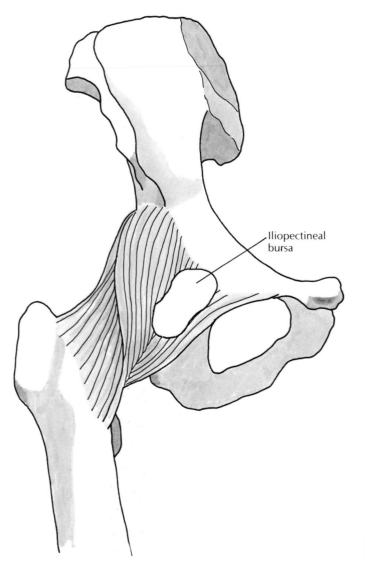

Iliopectineal
bursa

Fig. 13-6. Anterior aspect of the hip joint showing the iliopectineal bursa.

so through a gap between the pubofemoral ligament and medial portion of the iliofemoral ligament.

BURSAE

The rather large iliopectineal bursa overlies the anterior aspect of the hip joint and the pubis and lies beneath the iliopsoas muscle as it crosses in front of the hip joint. This bursa often communicates with the hip joint anteriorly through a space between the pubofemoral and iliofemoral ligaments. This may be a factor in the characteristic anterior pain experienced by patients with hip joint disease (Fig. 13-6).

One or more trochanteric bursae overlie the greater trochanter, reducing friction between it and the gluteus maximus, which passes over the trochanter, and the other gluteals, which attach to the trochanter. This bursa is most extensive posterolaterally to the trochanter, where it underlies the gluteus maximus. It is important clinically because of the prevalence of trochanteric bursitis.

BLOOD SUPPLY (Fig. 13-7)

The blood supply to the head of the femur is of particular importance because of its significance in common pathologic conditions at the hip, including fractures and osteochondrosis of the femoral head (Legg-Perthes disease). The head of the femur receives its vascularization from two sources, the artery of the ligament of the head of the femur and the arteries that ascend along the neck of the femur. The importance of the artery of the ligament of the head of the femur is variable, but for the most part it sup-

Medial circumflex artery

Lateral circumflex artery

Fig. 13-7. Blood supply to the head of the femur.

plies only a small area adjacent to the fovea. In as many as 20% of persons it fails to anastomose with the other arteries supplying the head of the femur.

The primary blood supply to the head of the femur, then, is derived from the arteries that ascend proximally along the neck of the femur to pierce the head of this bone just distal to the margin of the articular cartilage. These are branches of the medial and lateral femoral circumflex arteries. The medial circumflex artery passes around posteriorly to give off branches that ascend along the posteroinferior and posterosuperior aspects of the neck of the femur. The lateral circumflex artery crosses anteriorly to give off an anterior ascending artery at about the level of the intertrochanteric line. The ascending arteries pierce the joint capsule near its distal attachment to the femur and run proximally along the neck of the femur intracapsularly. They run deep to the synovial lining of the neck. Because of their relationship to the neck, they are subject to interruption in the case of a femoral neck fracture. Also, since they are intracapsular, it is believed that increased intracapsular pressure caused by joint effusion may stop flow. This is believed to be a factor in osteochondrosis and in some cases of idiopathic avascular necrosis of the head of the femur. The circumflex vessels give off extracapsular branches to the trochanteric regions of the femur. This area also receives vascularization from the superior gluteal artery and a perforating branch of the profunda.

NERVE SUPPLY

Innervation to the hip joint is supplied by branches from the obturator nerve, the superior gluteal nerve, and the nerve to the quadratus femoris and by branches from the femoral nerve, both muscular and articular. These nerves represent segments L2 through S1.

BIOMECHANICS

The hip joint, being a ball-and-socket joint, exhibits three degrees of freedom of motion. In this respect it is analogous to the glenohumeral joint. Unlike the shoulder, however, the hip is intrinsically a very stable joint. This is due, in part, to the fact that the acetabulum forms a much deeper socket than the glenoid cavity; the head of the femur comes closer to forming a full sphere than does the head of the humerus. The acetabulum, with its labrum, is able to enclose over half a sphere and to grasp passively the head of the femur to maintain joint integrity; it is difficult to pull the head from the acetabulum without removing or tearing the acetabular labrum. Coaptation of joint surfaces is also maintained, in part, by atmospheric pressure. Because of the relatively large surface area of contact between joint surfaces, the atmospheric pressures holding the joint surfaces together may be as much as 25 kg. This is sufficient to maintain coaptation of the joint with all soft tissues about the joint removed and the limb hanging freely. It is only when the vacuum created between the joint surfaces (by the close fit) is released by, say, drilling a hole through the acetabulum, that the limb will drop free. Intrinsic stability at the joint is further enhanced by the strong ligamentous support at the hip. Since the major ligaments at the hip pull taut and are twisted on themselves with extension, the hip joint is particularly stable in the standing position. As mentioned, the twisting of the capsule that occurs with movement toward the close-packed position effects a type of "screw home" movement at the hip in which the joint surfaces become tightly approximated. As with any joint, the close-packed position at the hip (extension–abduction–internal rotation) is the position of maximal congruence of joint surfaces.

Because the acetabulum and the neck of the femur are both directed anteriorly, their respective mechanical axes are not coincidental. There are two positions of the hip in which these axes are brought into alignment. One position is attained by flexing the hip to about 90°, abducting slightly, and rotating slightly externally. The other position is one of extension, abduction, and internal rotation. Note that the former position is the one that the hip would assume in a quadruped situation, and the latter is the close-packed position of the joint. As mentioned, in the upright position, a considerable portion of the articular cartilage of the head of the femur is exposed anteriorly. During normal use of the joint, as in walking, there is a relatively small contact area between the acetabulum and the femoral head. This may be a factor in the prevalence of degenerative hip disease in humans; stresses of weight-bearing are born by a small surface area of cartilage, and a relatively large area of cartilage may not undergo the intermittent compression necessary for adequate nutrition (see Chapter 2, Arthrology). It should be apparent that the smaller the torsion angle at the hip (the less it is anteverted), the greater the stability of the bone, since the axes of the acetabulum and neck of the femur are closer to being in alignment. A smaller torsion angle also favors an increase in the effective contact area between joint surfaces, for the same reason.

Because of its intrinsic stability, the normal hip joint rarely dislocates when compared with, say, the shoulder or elbow. The shoulder, elbow, or any other joint for that matter, usually dislocates when a force is applied over the joint when it is in its close-packed position. This is not true at the hip, which will usually only dislocate when its capsule and major ligaments are lax and its joint surfaces and bony axes are out of congruence. From this and the above discussion one might predict that the hip is most prone to dislocation when in a position of flexion (ligaments lax), abduction, and internal rotation (noncongruence). Dislocation usually occurs with a force driving the femur backward on the pelvis with the hip in this position, for example, striking the knee on the dashboard of a car in a head-on collision. With such an injury, the head of the femur is driven posteriorly through the relatively weak posterior capsule.

Since the hip is freely movable in all vertical planes, it is not subject to capsuloligamentous strain from horizontal forces applied to it in most positions, even though, due to the length of the leg, these forces acting over a long lever arm are potentially quite large. However, since the hip is a weight-bearing joint, it is subject to vertical loading that must be born by its bony and cartilaginous components. In the case of a person bearing equal weight through both legs, the vertical force on each femoral head is equal to half the weight of the body minus the weight of the legs. When standing on one leg, however, the weight-bearing femoral head must support more than the weight of the body. This is because the center of gravity (at about S2) is located some distance medially to the supporting femoral head. This lever arm through which the force is acting causes a rotary moment about the supporting femoral head with a tendency for the opposite side of the pelvis to drop. This rotary movement must be countered by the hip abductor muscles, primarily the gluteus medius, gluteus mimimus, and tensor fascia lata, on the weight-bearing side. The point of application of this counterforce provided by the abductor pull is at the greater trochanter, which is considerably closer to the fulcrum (femoral head) than is the center of gravity line that represents the force produced by the body weight. Since the distance from femoral head to trochanter is about one half of the distance from the femoral head to the center of gravity line, the abductors must pull with a force equal to two times the superincumbent body weight in order to prevent the pelvis from dropping to the non-weight-bearing side. The total force acting vertically at the femoral head is equal to the force produced by the pull of the abductors plus the force produced by the body weight, or up to *three times the body weight*.[21,25,44] Note that in this case "body weight" is actually the total body weight minus the weight of the supporting leg.

During stance phase of the normal gait cycle, the vertical forces acting at the femoral head are substantial. If the abductors are not strong enough to counter the forces tending to rotate or tilt the pelvis downward to the opposite side, an abnormal gait pattern results. Either the pelvis will drop noticeably to the opposite side of the weakness, usually resulting in a short swing phase on that side, or the person will lurch toward the side of weakness during stance phase on the weak side. The effect of the lurch is to shift the center of gravity toward the fulcrum (femoral head), reducing the moment-arm about which the forces from the body weight may act, thereby reducing the necessary counterpull by the abductors. In fact, a marked lurch may actually shift the center of gravity lateral to the fulcrum, allowing gravity to substitute for the hip abductors, thus preventing the pelvis from dropping to the opposite side. This lurching gait is often referred to as a "compen-

sated gluteus medius gait." It is usually seen in patients with painful hip conditions, such as degenerative joint disease, in which there is some weakness of the abductors and in which it is desirable to reduce compressive forces acting at the joint for relief of pain. It is also seen in patients with abductor paralysis.

The "abductor lurch" may be prevented by providing an external means of preventing the pelvis from dropping toward the uninvolved side during stance phase on the involved side. This external force may be provided by use of a cane on the uninvolved side. An upward force is transmitted from the ground through the cane to counter the weight of the body tending to rotate the pelvis downward on that side. The forces acting through the cane do so about a moment arm even longer than that about which the force of gravity on the body weight acts, since the point of contact of the hand on the cane is farther from the supporting femoral head than is the center of gravity line. For this reason, a relatively small force applied through the cane is required to compensate for the abductors and relieve the vertical forces acting at the involved hip. Note that the forces acting upward through the cane must be transmitted to the pelvis through contraction of the lateral trunk muscles, shoulder depressors, elbow extensors, and wrist flexors on the side of the cane.

It should be clear from the above discussion that forces of muscle contraction contribute significantly to compressive loading at the hip. This is not only true in a weight-bearing situation. Studies in which strain gauges have been inserted into prosthetic hips suggest that supine straight-leg raising causes a compressive force to the hip that is greater than the body weight.[44] This is an important consideration in the early management of patients who have undergone an internal fixation for a hip fracture.[31]

EVALUATION

HISTORY

The hip joint is derived from segments L2 through S1. Clinically, however, pain of hip joint origin is primarily perceived as involving the L3 segment. Typically, the patient with hip joint disease complains first of pain in the midinguinal region. As the process progresses, or as the painful stimulus intensifies, pain is likely to be felt into the anterior thigh and knee. At this point pain may also be described in the greater trochanteric region and buttock as well. In some instances (and not uncommonly) pain is felt most in the knee, and the patient may actually believe the knee is at fault. In general, pain in the trochanteric region spreading into the lateral thigh is more suggestive of trochanteric bursitis. Pain in the buttock spreading into the lateral or posterior thigh is more suggestive of pain of lower spinal origin.

Because of its freedom of movement in all planes and its great stability, the hip is seldom afflicted by disorders of acute traumatic origin. The hip is a common site, however, of degenerative joint disease and, to a lesser extent, rheumatoid arthritis. The clinician should ask whether the patient suffered any childhood hip disorders such as congenital dysplasia, osteochondrosis (Legg-Perthes disease), or slipped capital epiphysis, since these may predispose to early hip degeneration. Bursitis, either trochanteric or iliopectineal, is also fairly common at the hip.

The clinician must also determine whether the patient has a history of back problems. Low back disorders may mimic hip disease and vice versa because of the segmental relationships. Also, hip disease often leads to back problems because of the biomechanical relationships. (Refer to Chapter 4 for a complete list of questions to be included in the history.)

PHYSICAL EXAMINATION

I. Observation
A. Gait
1. A lurch to one side during stance phase is suggestive of hip pain or abductor weakness or both on the side to which the lurch occurs.
2. Dropping of pelvis on the opposite side of the stance leg is suggestive of abductor weakness (uncompensated) on the side of the stance leg.
3. Development of an excessive lordosis during stance phase may suggest hip flexion contracture on the side of the stance leg.
4. A backward lurch of the trunk during stance phase may suggest hip extensor weakness on the side of the stance leg or hip flexor weakness on the side of the swing leg.
5. A persistent inclination of the pelvis to one side during all phases of the gait cycle, combined with a lack of heel-strike on the side of inclination, suggests an adduction contracture on the side of the inclination.

B. Functional activities
1. Loss of hip motion may result in considerable difficulty removing and donning shoes, socks, and slacks.
2. The patient may "sacral sit" to compensate for a lack of hip flexion.
C. Note general posture and body build.

II. Inspection
A. Skin—Usually noncontributory in common hip disorders; observe for old surgical scars.
B. Soft tissue
1. Observe for atrophy about the hip and thigh. Document thigh atrophy by girth measurements.
2. Hip joint effusion is usually not visible due to heavy soft-tissue covering.
C. Bony structure and alignment. Measure and record deviations.
1. Use plumb bob to assess mediolateral and anteroposterior alignment in the standing position (including the spine).
2. Assess relative heights of the following structures:
   a. Navicular tubercles
   b. Medial malleoli
   c. Fibular heads
   d. Popliteal folds
   e. Gluteal folds
   f. Greater trochanters
   g. Anterior-superior iliac spines
   h. Posterior-superior iliac spines
   i. Iliac crests

Note: A vertical structural deviation arising from some abnormality at the hip joint or upper end of the femur is suggested if, from the floor upward, all of the above-mentioned landmarks are level up to the trochanters, but the anterior-superior iliac spines, posterior-superior iliac spines, and iliac crests are not. Be sure to note whether the relative levels of the anterior-superior and posterior-superior iliac spines on one side are the same as the levels on the opposite side. If not, the asymmetry may be due to a sacroiliac torsion rather than some abnormality at the hip joint or upper femur. If the trochanters are level and the anterior-superior and posterior-superior iliac spines and iliac crest on one side are lower by the same amount than their counterparts on the opposite side, one may suspect one of several possibilities: coxa vara on the low side, coxa valga on the high side, a shortened femoral neck on the low side or lengthened neck on the high side (rare), or cartilaginous narrowing from hip joint degeneration on the low side. The two most common of these are coxa vara and hip joint degeneration. Coxa vara is usually associated with a decreased angle of declination (torsion angle); hip joint degeneration sufficient to cause a clinically detectable vertical asymmetry will be accompanied by other symptoms and signs of degenerative joint disease (see Common Lesions).

Documentation of the extent of coxa vara, hip joint narrowing, or other cause of asymmetry may be made by assessing the position of the greater trochanter relative to a line drawn from the anterior-superior iliac spine to the ischial tuberosity (Nélaton's line). The "normal" trochanter should lie about on this line. This measurement is primarily useful in unilateral conditions in which it may be compared with the "normal" side. Documentation of total leg-length discrepancy should be made by measuring from the anterior-superior iliac spine to the medial malleolus of the same side.

III. Selective tissue tension tests

A. *Active movements.* The emphasis here should be on assessing functional activities involving use of the hip. Functional activities (in order of sequence) should include the following:

1. Gait
2. Sitting, bending forward to touch the toes, and crossing the legs
3. Going up and down stairs, one step at a time
4. One-legged standing (observe for dropping of the pelvis to opposite side— Trendelenburg's sign)
5. Running straight ahead
6. Running and twisting
7. Jumping

In the hip, the active movements commonly tested in standing are flexion and extension, since more information of the other motions of the hip can usually be obtained from tests of passive and combined movements. The normal range of hip flexion (knee bent) is 120°, but there is a wide variation.

B. *Passive movements.* Passive movements should be compared with the noninvolved side. The type of end feel should be noted and passive over pressure applied. Although the movement must be gentle, the examiner should apply passive over pressure at end range to find out the type of end feel, whether

there is any limitation of motion (hypomobility) or excessive range (hypermobility), and if it is painful.

1. Flexion–extension
   a. Joint motions are best assessed with a Mundale pelvic femoral angle measurement using the standardized side-lying position.[32] Draw a transverse line for the pelvis, connecting the anterior-superior and posterior-superior iliac spines (line *AB* in Figure 13–8A) with the hip in full flexion (with the knee flexed) or extension (with the knee straight). Construct a perpendicular line *CD* from this line to the most superior point of the greater trochanter; the angle between this line and the long axis of the femur, *DE*, is measured in full flexion and extension. By using the same landmarks the clinician can assess other hip positions, including weight-bearing flexion.

      Considering the ease of measurement, reliability, and reproducibility, the use of the prone extension test is recommended to measure hip extension in children with cerebral palsy and those with meningomyelocele. The Thomas test is recommended in the supine position as an alternative for nonspastic patients (see special tests).[2,48]

   b. Straight-leg raising. Measurement of hamstring flexibility can be determined by using the same sidelying positioning and landmarks as in Mundale's measurement (see **1.a**). It should be noted that between the lines CD and DE, an angle alpha exists in the resting position (see Fig. 13–8A). In maximum flexion an angle beta is obtained between the reference line (see Fig. 13–8B). In order to obtain the result of isolated coxofemoral flexion, alpha must be subtracted from beta. Once the angle alpha is determined, the subject is asked to perform maximal hip flexion without bending the knee. Abduction of the subject's leg is eliminated by supporting the leg on a powder board table. Instruct the subject not to perform movements of knee flexion, hip rotation, or movements of the ankle joint during hamstring mea-

A

B

Fig. 13-8. Reference lines for the measurement of hip extension *(A)* and in the position of maximal hip flexion with the straight leg *(B)* as described by Mundale and co-workers (1956).[32]

surement. Finally the angle beta is determined (see Fig. 13–8*B*).[50]

2. Abduction–adduction. When measuring, be sure to prevent internal-external hip rotation and lateral tilting of the pelvis. The pelvis must first be fixed by the examiner with one hand while the extended leg is then passively abducted with the other hand. When assessing abduction (supine), the leg to be tested should be close to the edge of the plinth so when full abduction of the extended leg is reached, the knee can be passively flexed to assess one-joint adduction, mainly pectineus and the adductors, versus two-joint adduction (namely gracilis, biceps femoris, semimembranosus and semitendinous).[22]

   Adduction of the hip is normally limited by one leg coming into contact with the other. One leg should be held in slight flexion so as to cross over the other leg.
   a. Capsular restriction will result in rather marked limitation of abduction and mild limitation of adduction.
   b. Full motion with pain at the extremes of adduction, abduction, or both may be present in cases of trochanteric bursitis.

3. Internal-external rotation. Passive hip rotation may be tested by three methods.
   a. Assess while the patient lies supine with the hip and knees extended. The examiner rapidly rotates the leg inward and outward via the ankle. In the early stages of hip disease, before hip deformity develops, a characteristic type of end feel due to loss of normal fluid type is perceived.[6] This test also becomes a useful mobilization technique.
   b. Measure sitting with hips and knees flexed.
   c. Measure prone with knee flexed (this is a more "functional" measurement since the hip is extended as in walking).
   d. Limited internal rotation and *excessive* external rotation suggest retroversion (decreased angle of declination). Limited external rotation and *excessive* internal rotation suggest increased anteversion (increased angle of declination). If internal rotation is

considerably limited and external rotation somewhat limited, capsular tightening is likely.

4. Combined hip flexion–adduction–rotation. This test uses the femur as a lever and stretches the posterolateral and inferior capsule and compresses the superior and medial portions of the capsule. With the patient supine, the examiner flexes the patient's knee and hip fully and then adducts the leg. As the knee is moved fully toward the patient's opposite shoulder, the examiner compresses the hip joint.
   a. The examiner should stabilize the pelvis and apply passive over pressure at the end of range. This test will also reveal tightness of the external rotators, particularly the piriformis.[22] If a tight piriformis is present, adduction and internal rotation range are decreased and painful. This test may produce pain in the buttock if a tight piriformis is impinging on the sciatic nerve or if an inflamed bursa is compressed beneath the stretched gluteus maximus. The distance of the knee from the chest is noted.
   b. The range and pain response to the adduction component should also be assessed with the hip in different positions of flexion and rotation.

5. On all passive movements, note the following:
   a. Range of motion. The capsular pattern of restriction is marked limitation of internal rotation and abduction, moderate limitation of flexion and extension, and some limitation of external rotation and adduction.
   b. Pain
   c. Crepitus
   d. End feel

C. *Resisted isometric movements*
1. Resist maximal isometric contraction of muscles controlling all major hip movements, allowing no motion of the joint. Resisted knee flexion and extension should be carried out as well as the six isometric tests of the hip:
   a. Flexion (supine) with the legs extended or with the hip and knee flexed to 90°. Resistance is applied above the knee. Painful weakness may indicate a

psoas tendinitis; a painless weakness may be due to rupture of the psoas or to an L2 nerve root lesion.[6]

b. Extension (supine) with an extended knee. Apply resistance at the heel. Pain in the upper part of the thigh may be due to a lesion of the origin of the hamstrings.

c. Adduction (supine) bilaterally. The knees are squeezed against the examiner's closed fist. Pain on resisted adduction suggests a lesion of the adductors, known as rider's sprain.[7]

d. Abduction (prone) with the opposite leg well stabilized. The hand around the patient's knee resists the patient's attempt to abduct the thigh. Resisted abduction can compress the gluteal bursa, as may passive abduction. A painful weakness may be due to a gluteus medius tendinitis.[6]

e. Internal and external rotation (prone) with a flexed knee. Resistance is applied at the ankle. Pain, on resisted rotation, is considered an accessory sign in gluteal bursitis.[7]

2. Tendinitis about the hip is very rare, but resisted hip flexion may reproduce pain in the presence of iliopectineal bursitis, and resisted hip abduction, or resisted hip extension and external rotation, may reproduce pain in trochanteric bursitis.

D. *Joint-play movement tests*

1. The same movements used for specific joint mobilization techniques are used as examination maneuvers. (see Chapter 6, Peripheral Joint Mobilization Techniques).

2. Assess

a. Amplitude of movement: hypomobile–normal–hypermobile

b. Irritability: pain–protective muscle spasm

IV. Neuromuscular tests

A. If a neurologic deficit is suspected at this point in the examination, it may be appropriate to perform sensory, motor, reflex, and coordination tests (see Chapter 4).

B. Most chronic joint conditions result in some weakness of muscles controlling the joint because of disuse and reflex inhibition. At the hip some muscle groups are so powerful that mild or even moderate weakness may not be detected by manual muscle testing.

Even if detected, manual testing does not permit documentation of the extent of weakness (or strength). For this reason, it is best to test each of the major muscle groups controlling the hip—abductors, adductors, flexors, and extensors—by determining the number of repetitions that can be performed against a constant load, for example, by determining the 10 RM (repetition maximum). This allows for comparison with a "normal" side or predetermined norm, and for documentation of a baseline.

V. Palpation

A. *Skin.* Palpate hip girdles and lower extremities (usually noncontributory in local lesions at or about the hip because of heavy soft-tissue covering).

1. Temperature

2. Moisture

3. Tenderness

4. Texture

5. Mobility

B. *Soft tissue*

1. Mobility and consistency

2. Swelling (joint effusion usually cannot be palpated at the hip)

3. Tenderness

a. There may be localized tenderness anteriorly if the iliopectineal bursa is inflamed or distended. It may be distended with joint effusion since it often communicates with the joint.[52]

b. There may be localized tenderness laterally if the trochanteric bursa is inflamed.

c. There may be areas of referred tenderness (so-called trigger points) in the related segments (L2–S1) if a lesion is affecting any of the deep somatic tissues at or about the hip.

C. *Bony structures* (see under Inspection)

VI. Special tests

A. *Assessment of common shortened muscle groups*

1. Hip flexors

a. The Thomas test detects a fixed hip flexion deformity in patients who have developed a compensatory lumbar lordosis that then masks the hip flexion.[49] With the patient supine, with the coccyx just over the edge of the plinth, the contralateral hip is flexed until the pelvis is tilted backward and the lumbar lordosis is eliminated. A flexed hip position shows shortening of the iliopsoas; tendency for simultaneous extension in the knee joint points to shortening of both the iliopsoas and the rectus femoris.

   b. Ely's test for the iliopsoas and rectus femoris.[17] The patient lies prone. If the iliopsoas is shortened, the hip remains in flexion. If passive flexion of the knee provokes a compensatory increase of flexion in the hip joint and hyperlordosis of the lumbar spine, the rectus femoris muscle is tight.

   c. Weight-bearing test with the patient assuming normal standing posture, using the pelvic femoral angle to assess the hip flexion angle in relationship to the floor[32]

2. The hamstrings (supine)

   a. 90°–90° straight-leg raise.[46] The patient flexes the hip to 90° and grasps behind the knee with both hands. The examiner then extends the knee through the available range. A measurement of 20° from full knee extension is within normal limits.

   b. Straight-leg raising test. The examiner flexes the hip so the knee is kept in extension. To avoid error, the lumbar spine should be monitored and kept flat on the plinth so there is no lordosis or kyphosis of the lumbar spine. When the hip flexors are shortened, the contralateral leg should be flexed at the hip and the knee joint passively or flexed with the sole of the foot on the plinth so the lumbar spine is kept flat.

3. Tensor fasciae latae (iliotibial band).

   a. A positive Ober test indicates a contracture of the iliotibial band.[35] It is performed in the side-lying position with the lower leg flexed at the hip and knee for stability and the pelvis well stabilized by the examiner. The examiner then passively abducts and extends the upper leg with the knee straight or flexed. Maintaining extension and neutral rotation of the hip, the leg is allowed to passively drop toward the plinth. If shortening is present, the leg will remain abducted. With the knee flexed the iliotibial band is slack and the flexibility of the tensor fascia latae muscle is revealed.[17] The move-

ment may reproduce pain associated with trochanteric bursitis or tendinitis at the tibial insertion of the iliotibial band.

B. *Other tests*

1. *Scouring.* This special test stresses the posterior and lateral hip capsule. It also reveals an abnormal end feel as the hip is rotated.[15,46] Normally the end feel is that of a smooth arc. In early joint changes, a clearly perceived bump in the arch will be noted. A grating sensation or sound may be elicited in the presence of an osteoarthritic hip. The test is carried out with a posterolateral force applied through the hip joint via pressure applied by the examiner, through the flexed knee. The femur is rotated repetitively in the acetabulum between the position of 90° of hip flexion (with full adduction) and 140°.

2. *Noble's compression test.*[34] This test is used to reveal a possible iliotibial band friction syndrome existing near the knee. With the patient supine and the knee and hip flexed to 90°, thumb pressure is applied lateral to the femoral epicondyle (or 1–2 cm proximal to it). While maintaining the thumb pressure, the patient's knee is slowly extended passively. Severe pain elicited at about 30° flexion indicates a positive test.

3. *Baer's sacroiliac point.* Baer's point is tender in the presence of a sacroiliac lesion or in the presence of iliacus flexor spasms. This point is located approximately 2 inches from the umbilicus on an imaginary line drawn from the anterior-superior iliac spine to the umbilicus.[30]

4. *Joint-clearing tests.* These are tests that take the joint(s) in question to end range and stretch the capsule or other soft tissues to reproduce symptoms. If no symptoms are reproduced and range is within normal limits, the joint is cleared from involvement in the problem being assessed. These tests are important since pain may be referred to the hip both from joints above and below the hip. For example, the lumbar spine may project pain via the sciatic or femoral nerve and knee pain may be projected up to the hip via the obturator nerve. Tests such as squatting and valgus–varus stress tests may be used to clear the knee. Full active flexion, extension, and lateral flexion may be used to clear the lumbar spine.

5. *Femoral torsion tests.* A variety of clinical tests (Craig's test or Ryder's method) have been proposed to assess the degree of hip anteversion.[27] Comparative ranges of internal and external hip rotation in the prone position may suggest increased retroversion or anteversion. In weight bearing, the appearance of the patellae will often suggest excessive femoral torsion when the patient is requested to stand with the knees in full extension and the feet aligned so they are pointing straight ahead. In excessive anterversion, the patellae face inward (squinting patellae). When the hips are externally rotated until the patellae are facing to the front, the feet and legs will be pointed outward.

6. *Assessment of leg-length equality.* A number of anatomical (a decrease in the vertical dimensions of bony structure) and functional (a right-left asymmetry in joint position) methods have been proposed for assessing true and apparent leg-length discrepancies.[5,9,20,53] From a clinical standpoint, limb-length assessment should be done with the patient in a weight-bearing position with measurements determined by placing a calibrated block under the sole of the foot to level the pelvis. A gravity goniometer or level placed between the posterior-superior iliac spines can be used to assess when the pelvis is level. Discrepancy is determined by the height of the calibrated blocks needed for correction. Assessment should be accompanied by palpation and additional tests, if indicated, to determine the source of discrepancy (*i.e.,* foot, ankle, knee, sacroiliac and lumbar spine tests).

   a. Cartilagenous narrowing. Compare clinical to roentgenographic findings.

   b. Coxa vara/coxa valga. Malleoli, fibular heads, and trochanters are level. Posterior-superior and anterior-superior iliac spines and iliac crests are lower on the varus side and higher on the valgus side. Coxa vara is often associated with retroversion; coxa valga is usually associated with increased anteversion. In coxa vara, the trochanter lies above Nélaton's line; in coxa valga, it lies below. Compare clinical findings to roentgenograms.

   c. Short femoral shaft. Malleoli, fibular heads, and popliteal folds are level. The greater trochanter and pelvic landmarks are lower on the short side.

   d. Short tibia. The malleoli are level. The popliteal folds, fibular heads, and tibial tubercle are lower on the short side.

   Note: Dynamic evaluation should include a gait analysis and assessment of shoe wear.

COMMON LESIONS

DEGENERATIVE JOINT DISEASE (OSTEOARTHROSIS)

Degenerative joint disease (DJD) at the hip often progresses to a point at which it results in significant disability. This is true at the hip more so than at any other joint. Clinically, persons with DJD of the hip frequently present to outpatient health care services because of pain and disability. DJD is the most common disease process affecting the hip. Primary DJD is distinguished from secondary DJD by the elimination of predisposing factors and is considered a result of aging alone, whereas *secondary osteoarthritis* is the term used when the condition follows previous damage by disease or by mechanical disorders.

The etiology of DJD of the hip varies from patient to patient. In a considerable number of patients with this problem, the etiology is not entirely clear. While age is an important factor, the pathologic process of DJD is not a result of tissue changes with aging *per se.* In fact, the cartilaginous changes occurring with normal aging are seen first in the "nonarticular" areas of cartilage, whereas changes found in DJD are seen first in those areas of cartilage undergoing most frequent contact, for example, during weight bearing.[1,3,10,11,29,31,42,51] DJD is a disease of older persons, because it takes a considerable length of time to cause the fatigue of tissue, such as fibrillation of articular cartilage, that is characteristic of the disease.[28]

The asymptomatic changes occurring with normal aging of articular cartilage probably result from a nutritional deficiency; the areas of cartilage not undergoing frequent intermittent compression do not undergo the absorption and squeezing out of synovial fluid necessary for adequate nutrition. This is especially true in older persons, because they tend to use their joints less frequently and through smaller ranges of movement.

The degenerative tissue changes that occur with primary DJD are usually reactions to increased stress to the joint over time.[10,11,28,31,33,40] The tissue changes may be of a "compensatory" hypertrophic nature, such as the bony proliferation that typically occurs at the joint margins and subchondral bone or capsular fibrosis. They may also be of an atrophic nature, such as the fatigue of cartilaginous collagen fibers or the degradation of cartilage ground substance (proteoglycan). Perhaps the most disputed issue with respect to pathogenesis is whether the first tissue changes occur in the subchondral bone or in the articular cartilage. It is generally accepted, however, that regardless of which tissue changes take place first, they take place first and foremost in the regions undergoing greatest stress with normal activities and changes in subchondral bone will, over time, result in changes in articular cartilage, and vice versa.[42,47] It must be emphasized at this point that normal attenuation of forces applied to a joint is dependent on the elastic properties of subchondral bone as well as those of articular cartilage. If stresses are not normally attenuated in one of these tissues, the other will undergo increased stresses.[39,40] Thus, with subchondral bony sclerosis, the overlying articular cartilage undergoes increased stress as the subchondral bone becomes stiffer and less elastic. With fibrillation and softening of articular cartilage, increased stress is transmitted to the subchondral bone. Such abnormal stresses will inevitably lead to progression of the process (see Chapter 2, Arthrology). It is interesting to note the difference in eventual reaction to increased stress between subchondral bone and articular cartilage; subchondral bone becomes more dense (sclerotic), whereas articular cartilage breaks down. This difference reflects the differences in vascularity and regenerative capacities of the two tissues.

If one accepts that in many, if not most, cases of DJD the pathogenesis is closely related to increased stress to joint tissues over time (or fatigue) then conditions that may predispose the joint to increased stresses must be considered as possibly contributing to the etiology of DJD. Perhaps the most important condition at the hip to consider in this regard is congenital hip dysplasia.[3,13,19,31] A deficient acetabular roof and increased femoral anteversion angle are common sequelae of this condition. The resultant decrease in effective weight-bearing surface area at the joint predisposes the posterosuperolateral femoral head and superolateral acetabulum to early degenerative changes. Residual structural changes in joint components that may follow osteochondrosis or slipped femoral capital epiphysis—both of which affect younger persons—may have similar effects.

It is also suggested that leg-length disparity may be a factor in predisposing to unilateral DJD of the hip on the side of the longer leg.[12,14] In the standing position, the pelvic obliquity produced by the leg-length discrepancy would cause the long limb to assume a position of relative adduction with respect to the acetabulum. The increased adduction angulation on weight-bearing results in an increased joint incongruence, causing greater stress to the lateral roof of the acetabulum. In addition, the center of gravity is shifted toward the short-leg side, increasing the moment-arm about which the force of the superincumbent body weight acts at the supporting femoral head on the long-leg side (see section on biomechanics). A greater pull by the abductors on the long side then is required to prevent the pelvis from dropping to the short side during stance on the long side. This would increase the vertical compressive force acting at the femoral head during weight bearing on the long-leg side.

Another condition that demands concern regarding its potential to contribute to the acceleration of hip degeneration is capsular tightness.[3,26,38] Traditionally, capsular tightness has been regarded to be more a *result* of than a *cause* of hip degeneration. While this is undoubtedly so, the clinician must consider the role that capsular tightening may play in accelerating the progression of the disease and in some cases in actually initiating the degenerative process. The hip, unlike the shoulder, is a joint that is continually brought close to its close-packed position during normal functional activities, such as walking. With every step, at push-off, the hip is brought into a position of extension, internal rotation, and abduction, taking up most of the slack in the joint capsule by twisting the capsule on itself. The twisting of the capsule effects a compression of the joint surfaces. The compression force is normally in addition to, but acts after, the peak vertical compressive force of weight-bearing. In other words, the peak compressive loading due to capsular twisting is normally not superimposed on that of weight-bearing, but rather these forces are successively applied to the joint during the stance phase.[31,38] This is in accordance with the viscoelastic property of articular cartilage, which favors gradual loading over time as opposed to quick "shock-loading" with respect to its ability to attenuate compressive forces.[39-41] If, however, for whatever reason, the hip joint capsule loses extensibility, the slack will be taken up in the joint capsule sooner and the joint surfaces will become *prematurely* approximated during walking. This premature approximation causes the peak compressive loading from capsular twisting to become closer to being superimposed on the peak compressive loading of weight-bearing. It causes a greater magnitude of compressive forces to be applied to the articular cartilage over a shorter period of time, approximating a situation of shock-loading. Certain studies suggest that shock-loading, even more than loss of normal lubrication, is one of the most important factors in fatigue of articular cartilage.[41] It should also be recognized that symptoms of pain on weight-bearing in the presence of hip DJD are not due to compressive forces *per se* but result from strain to the capsuloligamentous structures as they pull prematurely tight with each step (recall that articular cartilage is aneural). Such capsular pain is enhanced by the low-grade capsular inflammation that tends to develop as the disease progresses.[3] Studies in which compressive forces have been calculated in degenerated hips before surgery and then determined after total hip arthroplasty suggest that such surgery does reduce the "flexor moment" acting at the hip from a tight capsule.[38] This may explain the often dramatic symptomatic improvement enjoyed by these patients soon after operation. In view of the above discussion, it seems that a major goal of conservative management in the earlier stages of hip DJD should be prevention and reduction of capsular tightening of the joint. Such an approach, in addition to providing symptomatic improvement, may help to slow the acceleration of the degenerative process; the effective weight-bearing surface area of cartilage is increased, and shock-loading is decreased.

Long-standing obesity may also be a contributing factor in accelerated degenerative changes at the hip. Because of the moment-arm about which the force of gravity on the body weight acts at the femoral head during stance phase, *an additional 3 pounds* may act at the supporting femoral head for each added pound of body weight.

I. History

   A. *Onset of symptoms.* The patient is usually a middle-aged or older person who describes an insidious onset of groin or trochanteric pain. The pain is first noticed after use of the joint, such as long periods of walking, hiking, or running. The patient may relate some childhood hip problem or an old injury, but more often does not.

   B. *Site of pain.* The pain is typically felt first in the groin area. As the problem progresses, the pain is more likely to be referred farther into the L2 or L3 segment, to the anterior thigh and knee. Later, other segments may become involved, with pain felt laterally and posteriorly. An occasional patient presents with a primary complaint of knee pain. This is because both the knee and the hip are largely derived embryologically from the same segment. Rarely is pain referred below

the knee in a person with only hip joint disease.

   C. *Nature of pain.* The pain is noticed first at the end of the day, after considerable use of the joint; relief is obtained by rest. Later, as some low-grade inflammation develops, the patient notices some morning stiffness. At this point, pain and stiffness are noticed when getting up from sitting; the pain largely subsides after several steps (after "getting the joint loosened up"), then returns again after walking a certain distance. As the degeneration becomes more advanced, some constant aching may be noticed. The pain is increased by any amount of walking, and the patient is frequently awakened with pain at night.

     With progressive capsular tightness, the patient first notices some difficulty squatting, for instance, when picking up an object from the ground. Gradually, it becomes more difficult to put on stockings and tie shoes. The ability to climb stairs may be lost in the later stages, and the patient may be able to ambulate only with the assistance of canes or crutches. Some discomfort with sitting may develop as hip flexion becomes restricted.

II. Physical examination

   A. *Observation*

     1. The patient may hesitate or have difficulty rising from sitting and initiating ambulation.

     2. An abduction or antalgic gait, a swinging type of gait if the hip is stiff, a lurching of the trunk toward the affected side if there is any shortening of the limb, or a Trendelenburg gait if any weakness of the abductors is present may be noted.

     3. The patient may have some difficulty removing shoes, socks, and slacks.

     4. Note use of aids.

   B. *Inspection*

     1. Some localized (abductor or gluteal) or generalized atrophy may be noticed on the involved side. Document thigh girth, if appropriate.

     2. If significant adduction and flexion contractures are present, the patient may tend to stand with the heel raised, the hip laterally rotated, and the pelvis elevated on the involved side.

     3. If a flexion contracture and adduction contracture are present, and the patient stands with both feet flat and knees extended, the lumbar spine will be in some hyperlordosis, the pelvis will be shifted laterally toward the involved side (noticed in plumb-bob alignment), and the spine will be functionally scoliotic so as to bring the upper trunk back to the midline.

4. Assess levels of bony landmarks for leg-length equality. If this is unequal, attempt to determine the source of the discrepancy.

C. *Selective tissue tension tests.* The capsular pattern of restriction of the hip is one in which the greatest loss is that of abduction, flexion, and internal rotation. These motions are always limited, although the order of restriction may vary. The one exception is the medial type of osteoarthritis in which the head of the femur is displaced into the deepened acetabular cavity, so that rotation, in both directions, and abduction tend to be most limited.[6]

1. Active movements
   a. Assess functional activities
      i. Squatting—Usually unable to perform in moderate to advanced cases
      ii. One-legged stance. Pelvis will drop to opposite side if abductors are significantly weak (positive Trendelenburg sign).
      iii. Stair climbing—May be restricted in advanced cases
      iv. Sit and bend forward—Usually painful or restricted
   b. Note ability to perform, pain, and crepitus.
2. Passive movements
   a. Limited in a capsular pattern of restriction
      i. May be limited by pain and spasm—acute.
      ii. May be limited by soft-tissue restriction and discomfort—chronic
   b. Note pain, crepitus, range of motion, and end feel.
3. Resisted movements—Strong and painless
4. Joint-play movements
   a. Hypomobility of all joint-play movements
   b. Note whether they are restricted by pain and spasm or by soft-tissue restriction.

D. *Neuromuscular tests*
   1. If at this point a possible coexistent spinal lesion is suspected, motor, sensory, and reflex testing, in addition to other tests, may be warranted.
   2. Assess the patient's "balance" (*e.g.,* one-legged standing with eyes closed), since this is often affected owing to alteration in afferent input from the joint capsule receptors and controlling muscles.[8]
   3. Mild to even moderate muscle weakness of the large muscle groups controlling the hip must be tested by heavy, repetitive loading. Weakness, especially of the abductors, will be found in all but minor cases.

E. *Palpation*
   1. Often noncontributory
   2. Possibly some warmth noted anteriorly
   3. Usually some tenderness anteriorly, over trochanter and buttock. Possibly some "trigger points" of referred tenderness elsewhere in the thigh.

F. *Other*
   1. Compare roentgenographic findings with clinical findings. However, early DJD can be detected clinically before roentgenograms show positive findings and rather extensive changes may show on roentgenograms in the absence of significant symptoms.
   2. Because of the loss of hip extension that is characteristic of DJD and the compensatory hyperlordosis that develops when standing, these patients are predisposed to the development of back problems. A back evaluation may be warranted.

III. **Management.** The approach to management of patients with hip DJD will, of course, depend on the stage of the disease as determined by the extent of the lesion and the degree of disability. For the sake of discussion early and advanced cases are distinguished as follows:

Early
—Pain is noticed only with fatigue.
—There is only mild limitation of internal rotation, extension, and abduction associated with pain at the extremes of these movements.
—The patient walks with little or no limp.

Advanced
—There is some constant aching; the patient is

often awakened at night; there is considerable morning stiffness.
—Motion is markedly limited in a capsular pattern.
—Ambulation is performed with a marked limp or with the use of aids (canes or crutches).

The above criteria, of course, reflect the two extremes; many patients presenting with symptoms and signs fall somewhere between these. Note also that information from roentgenograms is not included as a criterion, since it cannot be reliably correlated to symptoms, signs, degree of disability, or prognosis.

The major difficulty facing the physical therapist with respect to management of these patients is that rarely is the patient with *mild* DJD of the hip seen—and this is the patient to whom therapists ultimately have the most to offer. The reason for this is twofold: (1) considerable progression of the disease may ensue before the patient experiences sufficient pain or disability to warrant seeking medical help and (2) physicians often do not refer patients with symptoms and signs of early DJD to physical therapists because therapists in the past have not met their potential in managing these patients. Too often the patient is issued a cane and advised to return if the condition worsens, at which time surgical intervention may be indicated.

A. *Management in the early stages of DJD*
  1. Goals
    a. Restoration of normal joint mechanics
    b. Prevention of further progression of the disease—capsular tightness or other possible causes of increased stress to the joint.
  2. Therapeutic procedures
    a. Restore normal capsular mobility with joint mobilization and active and active-assisted range of motion program. Ultrasound should be helpful in increasing capsular mobility when used during or prior to mobilization procedures.
    b. Restore normal muscle strength with progressive-resistive exercise program. Emphasize especially abductor strengthening.
    c. Range of motion exercises to be done indefinitely, instruction in appropriate levels, and other measures to minimize compressive stress to the hip

  d. Attempt to determine if there is some underlying biomechanical or constitutional factor that may predispose the joint to abnormal stresses
    i. Obesity. For each additional pound of body weight, an additional 3 pounds is applied to each hip joint during stance phase of normal walking. Although few physical therapists are qualified to institute a weight-loss program, the patient can be directed to the appropriate services, on agreement by the physician. A general conditioning program may be supervised by the therapist as an adjunct to a weight-loss program. The patient must be shown simple exercises to help maintain hip range of motion to be done indefinitely on a regular basis.
    ii. Leg-length disparity. As mentioned, inequality of leg length may be a factor in development of DJD on the long-leg side. Gradual, serial elevation of the heel and sole on the uninvolved (short) side, by 1/4 inch at a time, may be indicated, along with regular range of motion exercises.
    iii. Congenital hip dysplasia and epiphyseolysis (slipped capital epiphysis). These conditions both result in permanent structural abnormalities that often lead to increased stress to joint surfaces at the superolateral aspect of the hip joint. Some increased congruity of joint surfaces may be achieved by elevating the heel and sole of the shoe on the uninvolved side in unilateral cases. This places the involved hip in a relative position of abduction as well as automatically shifting the center of gravity line closer to the involved hip so as to reduce the moment-arm about which it acts during stance phase on the involved side.

    Since these patients are more or less permanently predisposed to accelerated degenerative changes, they should be encouraged to avoid activities that may be particularly stressful to the hip. Jogging and long-distance walking should be abandoned in favor of swimming and non-weight-bearing exercises. For patients whose regular activities involve considerable walking, alternative modes of travel and perhaps use of a cane should be encouraged.

These patients especially must maintain good strength and motion at their hips for maximal stabilization and maximal distribution of weight-bearing forces over joint sufaces.

B. *Management in moderate to advanced stages.* Unfortunately, the patient is often given the impression that he or she must simply wait until the disease progresses to a point at which surgery is indicated. Accordingly, the patient is often not referred to rehabilitative services, again because therapists have not demonstrated in the past that they have much to offer these patients. When these patients are referred to physical therapy, it is often simply for instruction in the use of a cane.

The approach to management of these patients must be more comprehensive and more vigorous. Surgery becomes inevitable unless appropriate measures are taken in the early or moderate stages of the disease. Even so, one may simply be delaying a potentially inevitable event. But one must also consider that these patients are usually middle-aged or older and that if progression of the disease can be retarded and a satisfactory level of function maintained, the patient may very well live out his or her life without undergoing major surgery.

1. Goals
   a. Restoration of function to optimal level
   b. Restoration of joint mechanics to optimal level
2. Therapeutic procedures
   a. Instruct the patient in the use of the appropriate walking aid to reduce compressive loading at the hip, to relieve pain on ambulation, and to increase ambulation endurance.
   b. A raised toilet seat may be desirable.

   c. The patient may be made aware of special adaptations in shoe fasteners and devices to assist in putting on and taking off shoes and socks. In this regard, an occupational therapist can be of assistance.
   d. The use of other adaptive aids and devices should be instituted insofar as they may assist the patient in the ability to perform daily activities with less pain or difficulty.
   e. Primary considerations in regard to improving joint mechanics include increasing capsular extensibility and increasing the strength of the muscles controlling the hip. The basic program is outlined above under management in the early stages. In moderate or advanced stages, however, the joint is likely to be more "irritable," in that motion will tend to be limited more by pain and muscle spasm than by a pure capsular restriction. For this reason, progression of the mobilization program must often proceed more slowly. In addition, at some point in more advanced cases, motion in some planes may reach a point at which it is restricted by bony impingement because of the bony hypertrophic changes that are characteristic of the disease.

In most respects, the approach to management of these patients should closely resemble that of patients with a frozen shoulder, the primary differences being the functional considerations and the concern for reduction of compressive forces in patients with hip disease. However, there is no reason not to proceed with an intensive mobilization and strengthening program in cases of capsular hip restriction, as is done routinely with patients with capsular tightness at the shoulder. Remember that it is the tight capsule in cases of DJD at the hip that is a primary source of the patient's pain; it is a chief factor in intensifying and localizing compressive forces at the hip joint during walking.

Surgery should be considered in patients with severe degree of pain or disability or who fail to respond to conservative treatment. Total hip replacement is the treatment of choice in older patients while a femoral osteotomy may still have a role in surgical management.[6]

TROCHANTERIC BURSITIS

Trochanteric bursitis is one of the few other common musculoskeletal disorders affecting the hip region for which patients are often referred to physical therapy.[45]

I. **History**
  A. *Onset.* The onset is usually insidious. Occasionally an acute onset is described in association with a particular activity, such as getting out of a car, during which a "snap" is felt at the lateral or posterolateral hip region. Presumably such an incident involves a snapping of a portion of the iliotibial band over the trochanter, with mechanical irritation of the intervening bursa.
  B. *Site of pain.* The pain is felt primarily over the lateral hip region. It tends to radiate distally into the L5 segment; the patient describes pain over the lateral aspect of the thigh to the knee and occasionally into the lower leg. Some patients also experience pain referred into the lumbosacral region on the side of involvement. This pain pattern closely resembles that of an L5 spinal lesion, which is a more common disorder than trochanteric bursitis and which must be differentiated by means of careful examination.
  C. *Nature of pain.* The pain is aggravated most by ascending stairs—the strongly contracting gluteus maximus causes compression of the inflamed bursa—and by rolling onto the involved side at night. Indeed, the greatest complaint is often that of being awakened at night with pain. The pain is a deep, aching, "scleratogenous" pain rather than the sharp, lancinating, dermatomal pain characteristic of L5 nerve root irritation.

II. **Physical examination**
  A. *Observation.* Usually noncontributory. The lesion is not severe enough to cause a limp.
  B. *Inspection.* Usually noncontributory. If the iliotibial band is tight, the patient may stand with the pelvis shifted laterally, away from the involved side on mediolateral plumb-bob assessment, with perhaps some increased valgus of the knee on the involved side.

  C. *Selective tissue tension tests*
    1. Active movements. No functional limitations
    2. Passive movements
      a. Full passive abduction may cause pain from squeezing of the bursa between the trochanter and the lateral aspect of the pelvis.
      b. Placement of the hip into full passive flexion combined with adduction and internal rotation compresses the inflamed bursa beneath the stretched gluteus maximus.
      c. An Ober test may reveal iliotibial band tightness.
    3. Resisted movements
      a. Resisted abduction will reproduce the pain by squeezing the bursa beneath the strongly contracting gluteals.
      b. Resisted extension and resisted external rotation may cause pain if the bursa underlying the gluteus maximus is involved.
    4. Joint-play movements. Mobility is normal and painless.
  D. *Neuromuscular examination.* Results are noncontributory.
  E. *Palpation.* A discrete point of tenderness will be found over the site of the lesion, usually over the posterolateral aspect of the greater trochanter. Other areas of referred tenderness are often found elsewhere in the L5 segment, usually over the lateral aspect of the thigh. No increased temperature can be detected.

III. **Management**
  A. *Goals*
    1. Resolution of the chronic inflammatory process
    2. Prevention of recurrence
  B. *Techniques*
    1. Temporarily avoiding continued irritation to the bursa
      a. Arranging pillows so as to avoid rolling onto the painful side
      b. Avoiding climbing stairs and long walks
      c. Ultrasound to the site of the lesion. This is a condition for which ultrasound is often dramatically effective over a course of three to six sessions. The increase in blood flow apparently assists in the resolution of the inflammatory process.

2. A tight iliotibial band may be the cause of or the result of the disorder.[45] Full mobility of the iliotibial band should be restored as the condition resolves. Be sure that good muscle strength of the gluteals is restored, since they may weaken in long-standing cases.

ILIOPECTINEAL BURSITIS

Iliopectineal bursitis is somewhat more rare than trochanteric bursitis. It presents in a similar manner, but resisted hip flexion and full passive hip extension reproduce the pain. The onset is insidious. The pain is felt most in the groin, with a tendency toward radiation into the L2 or L3 segment. Since this bursa often communicates with the joint, ascertain whether involvement of the bursa is a manifestation of hip joint effusion by checking for a capsular pattern of pain or restriction.

Management of patients with iliopectineal bursitis should follow the same approach as outlined for trochanteric bursitis.

MUSCLE STRAINS

Strains may be defined as damage of some part of the contractile unit caused by overuse (chronic strain) or overstress (acute strain). Strains are graded as mild (first degree), moderate (second degree), and severe (third degree).[36] In severe strains, there is a loss of function of the muscle, tendon, or its attachment caused by a complete tear. The strain will occur at the weakest link of the muscle–tendon unit. Under stress, the muscle may tear, the musculotendinous junction may give way, or the tendon or its bony attachment may be damaged.

The most commonly strained muscles of the hip are the hamstrings, adductor longus, ilopsoas, and rectus femoris.[43,45] Resisted isometric muscle contraction will reproduce the pain as well as passive stretch (except in a complete tear). In order to have a definitive diagnosis of the lesion, it is important to isolate muscles one at a time. The involved structures will be tender to palpation.

Treatment follows a common pattern. In acute strains this includes rest, anti-inflammatory agents, and physical methods. Initially ice and compression may be indicated. Up to 5–7 days following the injury, the muscle remains very vulnerable to reinjury because of the loss in loading capabilities and the risk of intermuscular hemorrhage.[24] Warm-up, stretch, resistive exercise, and gradual resumption of activity follow. To prevent random alignment of new collagen fibers, deep friction massage should be used.

With chronic strains, prevention is more important than cure. Gradually building up activities so that the muscle–tendon unit is able to withstand a heavier work load is a key component of rehabilitation.

CONCLUSION

The lumbar spine, sacroiliac, and hip joint function as a mechanical unit and should not be assessed or treated in an isolated fashion. Much abnormality presenting apparently simply as joint pain may be the expression of a comprehensive imbalance of the musculoskeletal system—articulations,[2,4,16,18] ligaments, muscles, fascial planes[30] and intermuscular septa, tendons and aponeuroses together with defective neuromuscular control.[23] The iliopsoas is usually the first contracture to develop and can affect the lumbar spine, pelvis, and hip. The inhibitory effect of a tight postural muscle is evidenced when weakness of the gluteus maximus accompanies tightness of the iliopsoas.

Many patients with a lateral pelvic tilt of 1 to 2 cm will present with early degenerative changes of the hip on the longer side as well as low back and sacroiliac problems.[15,16,37]

REFERENCES

1. Barnett CH: Effects of age on articular cartilage. Residue Rev 4:183, 1963
2. Bartlett MD: Hip flexion contractors: A comparison of measurement methods. Arch Phys Med Rehabil 64:521, 1983
3. Cameron HU, MacNab I: Observations on osteoarthritis of the hip joint. Clin Orthop 108:31–40, 1975
4. Chadwick P: The significance of spinal joint signs in the management of groin strain and patellofemoral pain by manual techniques. Physiotherapy 73:507–513, 1987
5. Clarke GR: Unequal leg length: An accurate method of detection and some clinical results. Rheumatol Phys Med 11:385–390, 1972
6. Corrigan B, Mailand GD: Practical Orthopedics. Boston, Butterworths, 1985
7. Cyriax JH, Cyriax PJ: Illustrated Manual of Orthopedic Medicine. Boston, Butterworths, 1983
8. Dee R: Mechanoreceptors of the hip joint capsule and

their reflex contribution to posture. In Symposium on Osteoarthritis, pp 52–65. St. Louis, CV Mosby, 1976

9. Fisk JW, Balgert ML: Clinical and radiological assessment of leg length. NZ Med J 81:477–480, 1975

10. Freeman MAR: The fatigue of cartilage in the pathogenesis of osteoarthritis. Acta Orthop Scand 46:323–328, 1975

11. Gofton JP, Trueman GE: Studies in osteoarthritis of the hip: I. Classification. Can Med Assoc J 104:679–683, 1971

12. Gofton JP, Trueman GE: Studies in osteoarthritis of the hip: II. Osteoarthritis of the hip and leg length disparity. Can Med Assoc J 104:791–799, 1971

13. Gofton JP, Trueman GE: Studies in osteoarthritis of the hip: III. Congenital subluxation and osteoarthritis of the hip disparity. Can Med Assoc J 104:911–915, 1971

14. Gofton JP, Trueman GE: Studies in osteoarthritis of the hip: IV. Biomechanics and clinical considerations. Can Med Assoc J 104:1007–1011, 1971

15. Grieve GP: The Hip. Physiotherapy 69:196–204, 1983

16. Grieve GP: Common Vertebral Joint Problems. Edinburgh, Churchill Livingstone, 1981

17. Gruebel-Lee DM: Disorders of the Hip. Philadelphia, JB Lippincott, 1983

18. Gunn CC, Milbrandt WE: Bursitis around the hip. Am J Acupuncture 5:53–60, 1977

19. Hoagland FT: Osteoarthritis. Orthop Clin North Am 2:3–19, 1971

20. Hoppenfield S: Physical examination of the hip and pelvis. In Hoppenfield S: Physical Examination of the Spine and Extremities. New York, Appleton-Century-Croft, 1976

21. Inman VT: Functional aspects of abductor muscles of the hip. J Bone Joint Surg 29(A):607–619, 1947

22. Janda V: Muscle Function Testing. Boston, Butterworths, 1983

23. Janda V: Muscles, central nervous motor regulation and back problems. In Knorr I (ed): The Neurobiologic Mechanisms in Manipulative Therapy. London, Plenum Press, 1978

24. Krejci V, Koch P: Muscle and tendon injuries in athletes. Chicago, Year Book Medical Publishers, 1979

25. LeVeau B: In Lissner HR, Williams M: Biomechanics of Human Motion, 2nd ed. pp 100–102. Philadelphia, WB Saunders, 1977

26. Lloyd-Roberts GC: The role of capsular changes in osteoarthritis of the hip joint. J Bone Joint Surg 35(B):627–642, 1953

27. Magee DJ: Orthopedic Physical Assessment. Philadelphia, WB Saunders, 1987

28. Mankin HJ: Biochemical and metabolic aspects of osteoarthritis. Orthop Clin North Am 2:19–31, 1971

29. Mankin HJ: Biochemical changes in articular cartilage in osteoarthritis. In Symposium on Osteoarthritis, pp 1–23. St. Louis, CV Mosby, 1976

30. Mennell JB: Physical Treatment, Movement, Manipulation, and Massage. Philadelphia, Blakiston, 1947

31. Morris JM: Biomechanical aspects of the hip joint. Orthop Clin North Am 2:33–55, 1971

32. Mundale MO, Hislop HJ, Rabideau RJ, Kottke FJ: Evaluation of extension of hip. Arch Phys Med Rehabil 37:75–80, 1956

33. Murray RO, Duncan C: Athletic activity in adolescence as etiological factor in degenerative hip disease. J Bone Joint Surg 53(B):406–419, 1971

34. Noble HB, Hajek MR, Porter M: Diagnosis and treatment of iliotibial band tightness in runners. Phys Sports Med 10:67–74, 1982

35. Ober FB: The role of the iliotibial and fascia lata as a factor in causation of low-back disabilities and sciatica. J Bone Joint Surg 18(A):105–110, 1936

36. O'Donoghue DH: Treatment of Injuries to Athletes, 4th ed. Philadelphia, WB Saunders, 1984

37. Patriquinn D: Differential diagnosis of lateral hip, inguinal and proximal anterior thigh pain. Proceedings of the 7th International Congress on Physical Medicine and Rehabilitation, Stockholm, 1980

38. Paul JP: Forces transmitted at the hip and knee of normal and disabled persons during a range of activities. Acta Orthop Belg [Suppl] 41:78–88, 1975

39. Radin EL, Paul IL: Does cartilage compliance reduce skeletal impact loads? Arthritis Rheum 13:139–144, 1970

40. Radin El, Paul IL: The mechanics of joints as it relates to their degeneration. In Symposium on Osteoarthritis, pp 34–44. St. Louis, CV Mosby, 1976

41. Radin El, Paul IL: Response of joints to impact loading. Arthritis Rheum 14:356–362, 1971

42. Reiman I, Mankin HJ: Quantitative histological analysis of articular cartilage and subchondral bone from osteoarthritic and normal human hips. Acta Orthop Scand 48:63–73, 1977

43. Renstram P, Peterson L: Groin injuries in athletes. Br J Sports Med 14:30–36, 1980

44. Rydell N: Forces acting on the femoral head prosthesis: A study on strain gauge supplied prostheses in living persons. Acta Orthop Scand (Suppl) 88:1–132, 1966

45. Sammarco G: The hip in dancers. Med Probl Performing Artists 2:5–14, 1987

46. Saudek CE: The hip. In Gould JA, Davies GJ (eds): Orthopedic and Sports Physical Therapy. St. Louis, CV Mosby, 1985

47. Sokoloff LS: The general pathology of osteoarthritis. In Symposium on Osteoarthritis, pp 23–34. St. Louis, CV Mosby, 1976

48. Staheli LT: Prone hip extension test: Method of measuring hip flexion deformity. Clin Orthop 123:12–15, 1977

49. Thomas HO: Diseases of Hip, Knee, and Ankle Joints, with Their Deformities (Treated by New and Efficient Method), 2nd ed. Liverpool, Dobb, 1876

50. Van Roy P, Borms J, Haentjens A: Goniometric study

of the maintenance of hip flexibility resulting from hamstring stretches. Physiother Pract 3:52–59, 1987

51. Vignon E, Arlot M, Meunier P, Vignon G. Quantitative histologic changes in osteoarthritic hip cartilage. Clin Orthop 103:269–278, 1974

52. Warren R, Kaye JJ, Saluiati EA: Arthrographic demonstration of an enlarged iliopsoas bursa complicating osteoarthritis of the hip: A case report. J Bone Joint Surg 57(A):413–415, 1975

53. Woerman AL, Binder-MacLeod SA: Leg length discrepancy assessment: Accuracy and precision in five clinical methods of evaluation. J Orthop Sports Phys Ther 5:230–236, 1984

14 *The Knee*

Darlene Hertling and Randolph Kessler

REVIEW OF FUNCTIONAL ANATOMY

OSSEOUS STRUCTURES

The distal end of the femur consists of two large condyles, separated posteriorly by the very deep intercondylar notch and anteriorly by the patellar groove in which the patella glides. The anterior condylar surface is referred to as the *trochlear surface* of the femur.

Looking anteriorly (Fig. 14–1), the medial condyle extends farther distally than does the lateral condyle, so that when standing with the distal surfaces of the condyles level, the femur and tibia form a valgus angle of about 10°. Both condyles have epicondyles extending from their sides. Medially, the adductor tubercle lies just superior to the medial epicondyle. The articular cartilage extends farther superiorly on the anterior surface of the lateral condyle than it does on the same aspect of the medial condyle.

Looking inferiorly (Fig. 14–2), the articular surface of the distal femur forms a ∪ about the deep intercondylar notch. The lateral condyle extends considerably farther anteriorly than does the medial condyle, helping to prevent lateral dislocation of the patella caused by the horizontal component of the direction of quadriceps pull. The medial condyle angles backward and medially. The lateral condyle lies in the sagittal plane.

Looking medially or laterally (Fig. 14–3), the condyles do not describe part of a circle, but rather their radius gradually decreases from anterior to posterior. The medial condyle is longer anteroposteriorly, with a more gradual change in radius from back to front. The small lateral condyle tends to flatten sooner, as one follows the curvature from back to front. The difference in the two condyles plays a part in the length rotation and locking mechanism of the knee, as discussed in the section on biomechanics.

The upper end of the tibia (Fig. 14–4) consists of two large condyles with joint surfaces superiorly for articulation with the femur. Both condyles are offset posteriorly to overhang the tibial shaft. They are also angulated 5° to 10° downward anteroposteriorly. The medial tibial condyle is larger; its superior surface is concave in all directions. The smaller lateral tibial condyle is actually convex anteroposteriorly. However, the lateral meniscus forms a concave articular surface for articulation with the convex lateral femoral condyle. Posterolaterally on the lateral tibial condyle is an articular facet for the head of the fibula, which faces somewhat downward. At the anteroinferior junction of the tibial condyles is the tibial tuberosity, an eminence onto which the patellar tendon inserts. Superiorly, between the condyles, is the roughened intercondylar area. The medial and lateral intercondylar tubercles, or eminences, lie centrally in the intercondylar area.

The patella (Fig. 14–5) is a triangular sesamoid bone, its apex lying inferiorly, embedded in the back of the quadriceps tendon. The posterior surface of the patella is cartilage-covered for articulation in the patellar groove of the femur, between the femoral condyles. The patellar articular surface consists of a lateral facet, a medial facet, and a small odd medial facet. The patella gives extra purchase to the quadriceps tendon in producing knee extension, especially toward the limits of extension.

MENISCI

The medial meniscus is semicircular, being larger posteriorly than anteriorly. Its anterior horn inserts onto the intercondylar area of the tibia, in front of the attachment of the anterior cruciate ligament, and its posterior horn inserts in front of the attachment of the posterior cruciate ligament. Peripherally, it is attached to the joint capsule, the short capsular fibers of the medial collateral ligament, and to the outer margin of the superior aspect of the medial

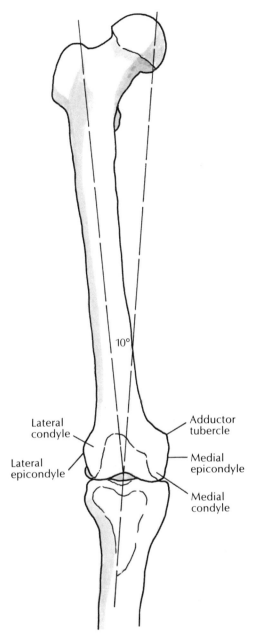

Lateral
condyle

Lateral
epicondyle

10°

Adductor
tubercle

Medial
epicondyle

Medial
condyle

Fig. 14–1. Anterior view of the right femur.

tibial condyle by the coronary ligament. The coronary ligament constitutes the inferior aspect of the joint capsule (Fig. 14–6).

Whereas the medial meniscus forms part of a larger circle, the lateral meniscus forms almost all of a smaller circle. Its two horns attach quite close to each other, just in front of and just behind the intercondylar eminence. The periphery of the lateral meniscus attaches to the tibia, the capsule, and a coronary ligament, but not to the lateral collateral ligament. The lateral meniscus is more mobile than the medial meniscus, owing to its shape and less ex-

tensive peripheral attachments. A ligament usually runs from the posterior aspect of the lateral meniscus to the medial condyle of the femur. This meniscofemoral ligament runs behind the posterior cruciate, while another may run in front (Fig. 14–7). The popliteus tendon also attaches to the lateral meniscus; this attachment is said to assist in posterior movement of the meniscus during knee flexion.[123] Usually a transverse ligament connects the two menisci anteriorly. In recent years the meniscus, formerly considered to be an unimportant appendage within the knee, has been recognized as one of the prime protectors of knee use and function.[120] The menisci serve several functions in the knee. They act as shock absorbers, spreading the stress over the joint surface and decreasing cartilage wear. They aid in the lubrication and nutrition of the joint, reduce friction during movement, and improve weight distribution by increasing the area of contact between the condyles. They are vascular in their cartilaginous inner two thirds and are partly vascular and fibrous in their outer one third.[9] Because most recent literature indicates that removal of the total meniscus can lead to early degeneration of the joint,[55,127,172,180] most surgeons today remove only the torn portion of the meniscus rather than the entire structure.

LIGAMENTS

The medial collateral ligament is a long, flat band attached above to the medial epicondyle and below to the medial aspect of the shaft of the tibia, about 4 cm below the joint line (Fig. 14–8). Its fibers run somewhat anteriorly, from top to bottom. Older descriptions often refer to *deep, shorter fibers* and *posterior oblique fibers* of the medial collateral ligaments. These are both considered part of the joint capsule (see below) in the more recent literature.[93,216] The deep capsular fibers are attached to the medial meniscus.

The medial collateral ligament becomes tight on extension of the knee, abduction of the tibia on the femur, and outward rotation of the tibia on the femur. Some of the anterior fibers become tight on knee flexion. The medial collateral ligament also helps prevent anterior displacement of the tibia on the femur.

The lateral collateral ligament is a shorter, round bundle of fibers running from the lateral epicondyle to the fibular head (Fig. 14–9). It does not attach to the lateral meniscus. The popliteus tendon runs underneath the ligament between it and the meniscus. The lateral collateral ligament is largely covered by the tendon of the biceps femoris. The lateral collat-

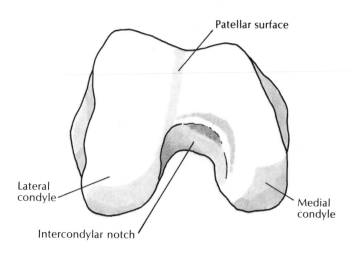

Patellar surface

Lateral condyle

Medial condyle

Intercondylar notch

Fig. 14-2. Inferior aspect of the distal end of femur.

eral ligament runs slightly posteriorly from top to bottom and is tight on extension of the knee, adduction of the tibia on the femur, and outward rotation of the tibia on the femur.

The anterior cruciate ligament runs from the anterior intercondylar area of the tibia backward, upward, and laterally to the medial aspect of the lateral femoral condyle in the intercondylar notch (see Fig. 14-7). It acts primarily to check extension of the knee, forward movement of the tibia on the femur, and internal rotation of the tibia on the femur. Because the anterior cruciate ligament pulls tight on internal tibial rotation and as the knee extends, some have proposed that this ligament guides the tibia into outward rotation during knee extension.[181]

The posterior cruciate ligament runs from the extreme posterior intercondylar area of the tibia forward, medially, and upward to the lateral aspect of the medial femoral condyle in the intercondylar notch (see Fig. 14-7). It primarily checks backward movement of the tibia on the femur and helps check internal rotation of the tibia on the femur. It also tightens on full knee extension, although some fibers may be tight throughout the range of flexion–extension of the knee. It is aided by the popliteus muscle in checking forward sliding of the femur on the tibia when squatting.

The patellofemoral ligament is a thickening of the patellar retinaculum. It passes from the adductor tubercle of the femur to the medial aspect of the pa-

A

B

Fig. 14-3. *(A)* Medial and *(B)* lateral aspects of distal end of the right femur.

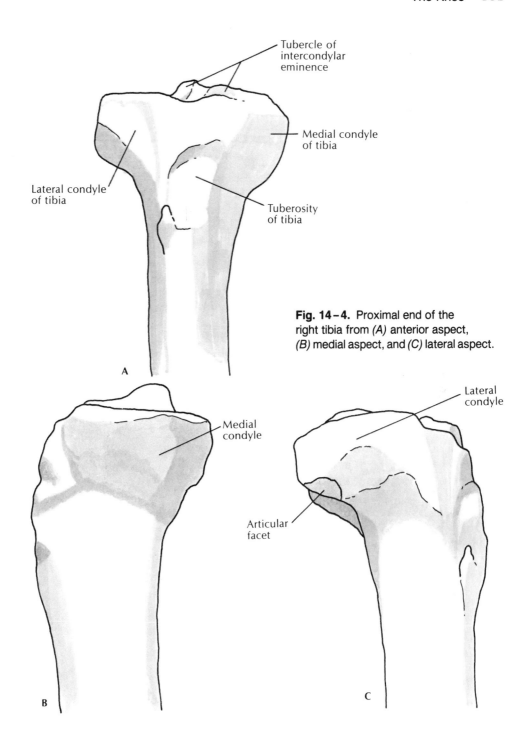

Tubercle of
intercondylar
eminence

Medial condyle
of tibia

Lateral condyle
of tibia

Tuberosity
of tibia

A

Fig. 14-4. Proximal end of the
right tibia from *(A)* anterior aspect,
(B) medial aspect, and *(C)* lateral aspect.

Medial
condyle

Lateral
condyle

Articular
facet

B

C

tella. Its femoral attachment often becomes irritated and tender in cases of patellofemoral tracking dysfunction.

A fibrous capsule surrounds the knee joint, attaching at the margins of articular cartilage. The superior aspect of the capsule runs from the articular margin of the femur to the periphery of the menisci. The inferior fibers run a short distance from the menisci to the tibia. The inferior capsule is often called the *coronary ligament*.

The fibrous capsule receives extensive passive and dynamic reinforcement (see Figs. 14-8 and 14-9). Passive reinforcement is provided by the above-mentioned ligaments and by what are referred to in older texts as the *deep layer* and *posterior oblique fibers* of the medial collateral ligament. These are

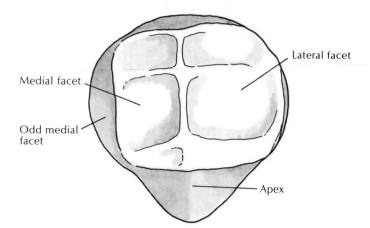

Fig. 14–5. Posterior aspect of the right patella.

thickenings of the medial and posteromedial aspects of the joint capsule that provide added stabilization against valgus and external rotatory stresses. The posterior oblique fibers are now referred to as simply the *posteromedial capsule*. The short capsular fibers deep to the medial collateral ligament are attached to the medial meniscus. There are also some thickenings of the capsule posteriorly, referred to as the *oblique* and *arcuate popliteal ligaments*.

Dynamic capsular reinforcement is provided to all aspects of the joint capsule. Anterior reinforcement is provided by the patellar tendon, inferiorly, and quadriceps tendon, superiorly. These can be said to constitute the anterior capsule, because a fibrous capsule *per se* is absent anteriorly. Anteromedial and anterolateral reinforcement are provided by the medial and lateral patellar retinacula, which are superficial to, and may blend with, the fibrous capsule. These help stabilize the patellofemoral joint during loaded knee extension.

The distal aspect of the iliotibial band provides anterolateral reinforcement. This stabilizes against excessive internal rotation of the tibia on the femur and thus works in conjunction with the cruciates.

The pes anserinus tendons (semitendinosus, gracilis, and sartorius) and the semimembranosus tendon give medial and posteromedial reinforcement. These help prevent abnormal external rotation, abduction, and anterior displacement of the tibia on the femur. In doing so they dynamically reinforce the medial collateral ligament, the posteromedial capsule, and, to a certain extent, the anterior cruciate ligament.

Posterolateral support comes from the biceps femoris tendon. This helps check excessive internal rotation and anterior displacement of the tibia on the femur, providing reinforcement to the functions of the cruciates. It also may assist the lateral collateral ligament in preventing adduction of the tibia on the femur.

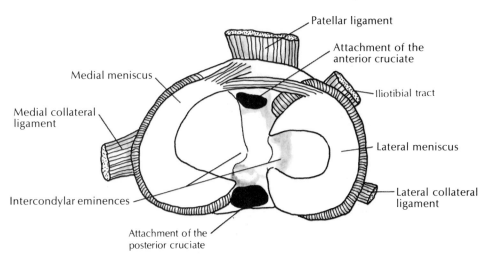

Fig. 14–6. The superior aspect of the right tibia, showing the menisci and tibial attachments of the cruciate ligaments.

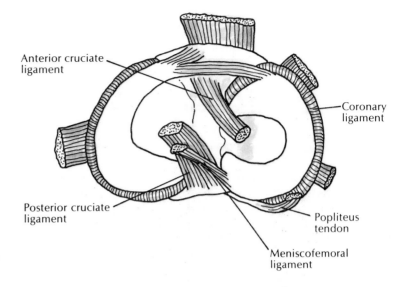

Fig. 14–7. Superior aspect of the right tibia, showing the ligaments.

Fig. 14–8. Medial aspect of the right knee.

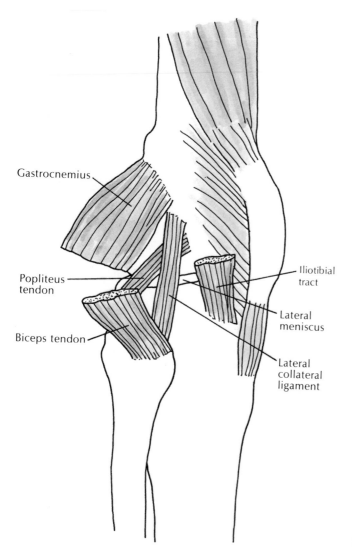

Gastrocnemius

Popliteus tendon

Biceps tendon

Iliotibial tract

Lateral meniscus

Lateral collateral ligament

Fig. 14–9. Lateral aspect of the right knee.

Finally, posterior reinforcement is provided by the insertions of the gastrocnemius muscles and from the popliteus muscle. The popliteus helps check external rotation of the tibia on the femur and backward displacement of the tibia on the femur.

BURSAE, SYNOVIA, AND FAT PADS

The synovium of the knee joint, in addition to lining the fibrous capsule, forms several large recesses (Fig. 14–10). Anteroinferiorly, it extends inward to line the back of the infrapatellar fat pad. The medial and lateral aspects of this lining unite centrally to form the ligamentatum mucosa that extends into the joint to attach to the intercondylar notch of the femur. Anterosuperiorly, the synovium runs from the superior aspect of the patella upward beneath the quadriceps tendon, then folds back on itself to form a pouch, and inserts on the distal femur above the condyles. This suprapatellar pouch is part of the joint cavity and provides sufficient slack in the synovium to allow full knee flexion. Posteriorly, the synovium invaginates into the intercondylar notch to pass in front of the cruciate ligaments. In this way the cruciates are intracapsular but extrasynovial.

In addition to the suprapatellar pouch, which also serves as a bursa, there are three additional major bursae anteriorly. The prepatellar bursa lies over the patella, and may become inflamed with prolonged kneeling activities ("housemaid's knee"). A bursa also lies between the patellar tendon and the tibia (deep infrapatellar bursa) and between the patellar tendon and skin (superficial infrapatellar bursa).

Posteriorly, a main bursa lies between the semimembranosus tendon and the medial origin of the gastrocnemius muscle. This bursa often communi-

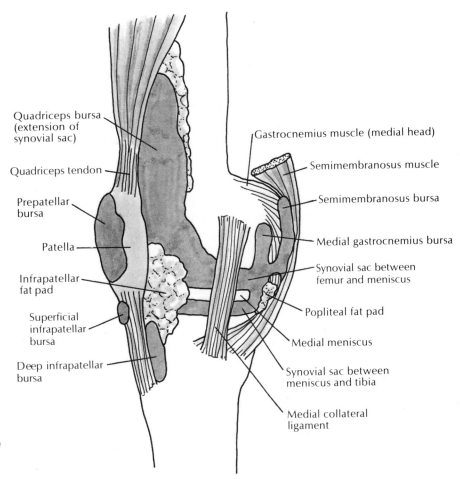

Quadriceps bursa
(extension of
synovial sac)

Quadriceps tendon

Prepatellar
bursa

Patella

Infrapatellar
fat pad

Superficial
infrapatellar
bursa

Deep infrapatellar
bursa

Gastrocnemius muscle (medial head)

Semimembranosus muscle

Semimembranosus bursa

Medial gastrocnemius bursa

Synovial sac between
femur and meniscus

Popliteal fat pad

Medial meniscus

Synovial sac between
meniscus and tibia

Medial collateral
ligament

Fig. 14–10. Medial aspect of the knee, showing the synovia and bursae.

cates with the joint and may become swollen with articular effusion, in which case it may be referred to as *Baker's cyst.* This bursa may also extend between the gastrocnemius and the capsule, or a separate bursa may be situated here.

Bursae may also exist beneath the tendons of the pes anserinus and the iliotibial band, just proximal to their insertions. These can become irritated with high levels of activity. There may also be other bursae about the knee joint, but these are of little clinical significance.

The large infrapatellar fat pad is situated deep to the patellar tendon and in front of the femoral condyles. When the knee is flexed, it fills the anterior aspect of the intercondylar notch. With the knee extended, it occupies the patellar groove and covers the trochlear surface of the femur. The back of the fat pad is lined with synovium. It is thought that as the fat pad sweeps across the condyles during knee flexion and extension, it helps to spread a lubricating layer of synovial fluid over the joint surface of the femur prior to contact with the tibia.

BIOMECHANICS OF THE FEMOROTIBIAL JOINT*

STRUCTURAL ALIGNMENT

Because the medial femoral condyle extends farther distally than does the lateral condyle, there is usually a slight valgus angulation of about 5° to 10° between the tibia and the femur. With the transcondylar axis of the femur in the frontal plane the patella faces straight forward. In this position, the neck of the femur is directed about 20° forward as a result of the normal internal torsion of the femoral shaft with respect to the femoral neck. Also in this position, the transmalleolar axis at the ankle is rotated outward about 25° as a result of the normal external torsion of the tibial shaft, and the long axis of the foot is directed 5° to 10° outward.

* See the section on patellofemoral joint dysfunction in this chapter for a discussion of patellofemoral biomechanics.

MOVEMENT

The knee is normally biaxial; it flexes and extends around an axis that is horizontally oriented in the frontal plane in the standing position, and it rotates about a vertical axis. Knee flexion–extension is polycentric, the axis of movement shifting backward along a curved centroid as the knee moves from extension into flexion.

Flexion–Extension

Osteokinematics. The total range of knee flexion–extension in the healthy knee is from about 5° to 10° of hyperextension to 140° to 150° of flexion. Flexion is limited by soft-tissue approximation of the calf and posterior thigh. Extension is terminated by locking of the joint in its close-packed position as the capsules and ligaments draw tight and become twisted. As the knee approaches full extension, it also assumes a valgus angulation because the medial femoral condyle extends farther distally than the lateral condyle.

Arthrokinematics. The femorotibial joint is markedly incongruent in positions of flexion, but becomes progressively more congruent as the knee extends. In the flexed position, the small convex radius of the posterior femoral condyles contacts a relatively large radius on the tibial condyles. In fact, the lateral tibial condyle is actually a convex surface. Because the radius of curvature of the femoral condyles progressively increases anteriorly, the joint becomes more congruent as the contacting area on the femur moves anteriorly during knee extension (Fig. 14–11).

The fibrocartilaginous menisci reduce joint surface incongruency. Their mobility and deformability allow them to conform to the shape of the contacting femoral joint surfaces. The anterior segments of the menisci are somewhat mobile, whereas the posterior horns are comparatively fixed. Thus, as the knee extends and the contacting radius of the femoral condyle increases, the anterior aspects of the menisci glide forward. Conversely, as the knee flexes, the anterior segments of the menisci recede to conform to the smaller radius of curvature of the contacting femoral condyles (Fig. 14–12). By reducing joint surface incongruency, the menisci help distribute the forces of compressive loading over a greater area, thus reducing compressive stresses to the joint surfaces of the knee.

As indicated by the instant centers of motion, flexion and extension of the knee occur with a combination of rolling and sliding at the joint surfaces. The

Fig. 14–11. Diagram showing loci of normal instant centers and congruency during flexion and extension of the knee.

Fig. 14-12. *(A)* During extension, the menisci glide forward, while *(B)* during flexion, the menisci recede to conform to the radius of curvature of the connecting femoral condyles.

closer the instant center is to the contacting joint surfaces, the greater the amount of rolling that occurs at a particular point in the range of movement. An instant center that lies some distance from the contacting surfaces indicates considerable sliding between the surfaces. Because the normal axes of movement for flexion and extension of the knee lie within the condylar region of the femur — not on the joint surfaces or a long distance away — it follows that both sliding and rolling accompany the movement. It can be seen from the loci of normal instant centers that the axis of movement shifts farther away from the joint surface as the knee extends, indicating relatively more sliding occurring as extension takes place (see Fig. 14–11).[63,64] Considering the tibia moving on the fixed femur, the direction of sliding and rolling of the tibial joint surface is anterior during extension and posterior during flexion.

Transverse Rotation

Because the femorotibial joint surfaces are incongruent in all positions but full extension, and because the menisci are semimobile, the knee joint can undergo some rotation in the transverse plane. This rotary movement can easily be produced actively or passively with the knee flexed, and is important for attenuation of rotary forces acting on the knee during normal function.

There is also an automatic, or conjunct, rotation at the knee that accompanies flexion and extension of the joint. This occurs as an external rotation of the tibia relative to the femur during the final 15° to 20° of extension, and an internal tibial rotation during the initial 15° or 20° of flexion from a fully extended position. Because the knee undergoes rotation and the menisci tend to move with the femur, much of the movement occurs between the menisci and the tibia.

Several factors contribute to the occurrence of knee rotation during flexion and extension.[11,181,196,209] First, and perhaps most important, is the shape and orientation of the medial femoral condyle. Looking at the femur end on, we see that the medial condyle is curved and obliquely oriented, whereas the lateral condyle is situated in the sagittal plane (see Fig. 14–2). Also of significance is the fact that the articular surface of the medial condyle is longer, in an anteroposterior direction, than that of the lateral condyle. As the tibia moves into extension the lateral side of the joint completes its movement before the medial side, because of the difference in lengths of the respective femoral articular surfaces. When this occurs, the medial side of the tibia continues to move forward along the curved medial femoral condyle, while the lateral tibial joint surface undergoes a lateral spin. The net effect is an external rotary movement of the tibia on the femur. This movement reverses when the knee flexes from a fully extended position. It is believed that the cruciates also play a role in guiding rotary movement at the knee. The cruciates tighten as the knee extends and are twisted in a direction to rotate the tibia externally as they tighten.

PATHOMECHANICS

Structural Alterations

Frontal Plane. Although the knee joint normally assumes a valgus angulation, the line of application representing the weight-bearing force acting on the knee tends to bisect the joint. This is because the femoral head is offset medially from the shaft of the femur (Fig. 14–13). Excessive genu valgum causes the weight-bearing force to be shifted to the lateral side of the joint, whereas genu varum results in a medial shift of the weight-bearing force line. Such alterations in force distribution may lead to accelerated wear on one side of the joint.[59] Common factors contributing to genu valgum are iliotibial band tightness, abnormal foot pronation, and femoral anteversion. Femoral retroversion tends to result in genu varum.

Transverse Plane. In the case of increased femoral anteversion, the femoral condyles are rotated too far internally with respect to the femoral neck. Thus, with the hip joint in a neutral position, the condyles and patellae face inward, or, conversely, with the patellae and condyles facing forward, the hip joint assumes an externally rotated position. Since the tendency during gait is to maintain normal alignment of the hip joints, the individual with increased femoral anteversion tends to walk with the knee rotated inward. This inward rotation may be transmitted to the foot as a toe-in stance or as abnormal foot pronation. At the knee, inward rotation results in a valgus angulation when the knee is semiflexed, as it is during most of the stance phase of gait. In a similar manner, abnormal retroversion of the hip causes a tendency for the patella to face outward during gait, for the knee to assume a varus position, and for the feet to either toe-out or supinate. In some individuals with torsional deviations of the femur, compensatory structural rotation of the tibia will develop. Thus, the child with femoral anteversion may also develop increased external tibial torsion to achieve normal foot placement. Similarly, internal tibial torsion may develop in association with femoral retroversion. Such torsional compensation at the tibia seems to enhance valgus–varus deviations.

Fig. 14-13. Knee joint angulation showing *(A)* normal valgus angulation, *(B)* excessive valgus angulation, and *(C)* varus angulation.

Intrinsic Movement Abnormalities

Capsular Tightness. One of the most common causes of gross restriction of knee motion is capsular tightness. Fibrosis and subsequent loss of extensibility of the joint capsule frequently follow immobilization after trauma or surgery and usually accompany the progression of chronic joint diseases, such as degenerative joint disease or rheumatoid arthritis. Capsular tightness at the knee results in a characteristic pattern of restriction in which knee extension is limited by 20° to 30°, and flexion is possible to only 80° or 100°. The functional disability resulting from capsular restriction will vary with the individual's particular activity level, but ambulation is inevitably altered because nearly full knee extension is necessary for normal gait. The mean total range of flexion and extension required for some common activities has been studied by Laubenthal and co-workers with the following results:[124]

Activity	Mean Total Flexion–Extension Necessary
Stance phase of gait	21°
Swing phase of gait	67°
Stair climbing	83°
Sitting and rising	83°

Because capsular restriction at the knee typically allows only 50° to 80° of flexion–extension, some functional alteration is likely.

Of great significance during walking is the effect of reduced knee extension on the stresses imposed on the articular surfaces of the joint. Normally, during the stance phase of gait, peak weight-bearing forces are borne with the joint just short of full knee extension, a position in which the tibiofemoral contact area is greatest, and a position in which the joint capsule has not been drawn completely tight.[59,113] Since stress equals force/unit area, the compressive stress of weight-bearing is minimized by a relatively large tibiofemoral contact area. Furthermore, the joint is not "shock loaded" by having the slack in the joint capsule suddenly taken up as the knee moves toward extension. If, however, knee extension is lacking from capsular tightness, the joint is unable to move to a position of maximal tibiofemoral contact, and as the knee extends, the joint capsule suddenly pulls tight; stress to the joint surfaces is increased in magnitude and the joint is shock loaded. The long-term effect is likely to be accelerated wear of the joint surfaces.

Rotary Dysfunction. A more subtle yet common movement disorder affecting the knee is loss of normal rotary mechanics. The pathologic implications of rotary dysfunction at the knee have been theorized by Smillie and confirmed by Frankel and co-workers.[64,189] As mentioned, the nature and extent of rotation accompanying knee flexion and extension is governed by the shapes of the articular surfaces and is influenced by capsuloligamentous configurations. Alteration in normal rotary mechanics may reflect articular surface abnormalities or capsuloligamentous disorders. Similarly, the effect of rotary dysfunction is to produce abnormal stresses to the joint surfaces as well as capsuloligamentous structures. Smillie proposes that since normal rotary movement is small and occurs at the very limits of knee extension, full knee extension is possible in the absence of normal rotation, but at the expense of increased deformation to articular tissues. Thus, knee extension occurring without normal external tibial rotation results in abnormal stresses to the medial joint surfaces, which are oriented to move into rotation, and increased tensile stresses to the cruciates, which pull tight on extension and internal tibial rotation. Furthermore, the tibia must rotate externally as the knee approaches full extension in order to prevent the lateral side of the medial femoral condyle from contacting the medial edge of the anterior cruciate ligament.

Several types of disorders may cause altered rotary mechanics at the knee. Smillie cites meniscal displacements, such as those associated with meniscus tears, as a frequent causative factor. Because knee rotation, when combined with flexion or extension, requires meniscofemoral as well as meniscotibial movement, it is likely that alterations in structural configuration of the menisci would interfere with normal rotary mechanics. Another common cause of restricted external tibial rotation is reduced extensibility of the medial or posteromedial capsuloligamentous structures. This typically occurs following injury or surgery, in which the posteromedial capsule or medial collateral ligament may heal in an adhered or shortened state. Laxity of these same structures will also lead to abnormal rotary mechanics, because external tibial rotation may be excessive or premature.[110,187] This would especially be the case if a secondary external rotation contracture developed.

In recognition of the pathomechanics and pathologic implications of rotary dysfunction at the knee, Helfet has described a simple means of clinically detecting this problem.[84] In general terms the method involves comparing femorotibial rotary alignment in a semiflexed and fully extended position. Using this test, in addition to instant center analysis, Frankel and co-workers demonstrated a positive correlation between reduced femorotibial rotation and abnormal compression of the joint surfaces during terminal knee extension.[64] In most of the patients evaluated, meniscal derangement was the underlying cause. Arthrotomy revealed abnormal wearing in localized areas of the medial articular surfaces in 22 of 30 knees. These findings confirm the nature of the kinematic abnormality associated with altered rotary mechanics and also suggest that such disorders, over a long period, may predispose to progressive degenerative joint disease.

Smillie believes that kinematic disturbance resulting from rotary dysfunction at the knee may also lead to fatigue disruption and fraying of the anterior cruciate.[189] He supports this contention with surgical case studies of isolated anterior cruciate lesions associated with chronic meniscal derangements.

The significance of rotary dysfunction at the femorotibial articulation is becoming better appreciated as our knowledge of detailed knee biomechanics improves. Because the disturbance is subtle, it is not readily recognized unless femorotibial rotary function is carefully examined. This type of assessment should become a routine component of knee examination in the rehabilitation period following capsuloligamentous injury or internal derangement.

PATHOMECHANICS OF COMMON LOADING CONDITIONS

Trauma

Knee joint injuries are commonly of traumatic origin. This stems, in part, from the fact that the knee is freely movable in only the sagittal plane (flexion–extension). Thus, forces acting to move the knee in the frontal or transverse planes are largely attenuated by internal strain to the soft tissues about the joint. Furthermore, such forces may act over the relatively long lever arms provided by the femur and the tibia, thereby increasing the potential loading of the joint structures.

Valgus–External Rotation. Because of the exposure of the lateral side of the knee to external forces, compared with that of the protected medial aspect, traumatic valgus stresses are much more common than varus stresses. Usually such forces also involve components acting in the transverse and sagittal planes, thus causing rotary and flexion–extension displacements. The knee is usually in some position of flexion when acted upon by a force from the lateral aspect, and thus the direction of rotary movement is usually such that the tibia is rotated laterally with respect to the femur.

Valgus–external rotary injuries occur most frequently in contact sports—especially football—and skiing. The degree of loading of the joint is accentuated by the fixation of the foot to the ground, for example, by the cleated shoe, and by forces acting over a long lever arm, such as a ski. This does not allow rotary forces to be attenuated by movement of the foot with respect to the ground, and more of the energy is absorbed as internal strain to joint structures. Because valgus and external rotation are primarily checked by the posteromedial capsule and the capsular and superficial fibers of the medial collateral ligament, it is these structures that are most commonly damaged. The menisci, especially the medial meniscus, may be injured because of the rotary stress component. With marked separation of the medial side of the joint, the anterior cruciate ligament may be torn as well. Specifically, it has been demonstrated experimentally that, with progressive force in a valgus–external rotation direction, structures are torn in the following sequence: (1) the deep capsular fibers of the medial collateral ligament, (2) the long superficial fibers of the medial collateral ligament and the posteromedial capsule, and (3) the anterior cruciate ligament. A torn medial meniscus would complete the so-called terrible triad of O'Donoghue.

Hyperextension. Because the knee is used in a position close to its physiological limits of extension for most functional activities, hyperextension injuries also affect the knee quite commonly. Again, the individual involved in violent contact sports and the skier are particularly vulnerable to such injuries. Experimental studies suggest that forced hyperextension of the knee results in tearing first of the posterior capsule, followed by the anterior cruciate, then the posterior cruciate ligaments.[112]

Anteroposterior Displacement. Forces producing a pure translatory movement between the tibia and femur in an anteroposterior direction are somewhat less common than the above-mentioned injuries. Of these, perhaps the "dashboard injury" occurs most frequently. In such cases the victim, in a suddenly decelerating automobile, is thrust forward, striking the tibial tubercle of the bent knee on the dashboard. The tibia is forced posteriorly on the femur, stressing the posterior cruciate ligament, often to the point of rupture.

Isolated anterior cruciate tears, resulting from forces in the opposite direction, are rare. In fact, there is much controversy over the frequency of isolated anterior cruciate lesions. When they do occur, the mechanism of injury is more likely to be a force stressing the tibia into internal rotation on the femur.[112,215]

Rotation. Forced external rotation of the tibia on the femur tends to stress the collateral ligaments and the posteromedial capsule. As mentioned above, these forces usually occur in conjunction with valgus stresses, and therefore typically affect the medial stabilizing structures.

Internal rotation of the tibia on the femur is checked by the cruciate ligaments. It is believed that forced internal rotation is the primary mechanism in isolated anterior cruciate ligament injuries.[112,215]

Forced rotation may also injure the menisci.[154] The medial meniscus, being less mobile by virtue of its attachment to the capsular fibers of the medial ligament, is much more frequently injured than the lateral meniscus. The menisci are particularly stressed when the knee is forced into rotation in an improper direction during flexion or extension. Thus, when the tibia, which is supposed to rotate internally during initial knee flexion, is forced externally as the knee goes into flexion, the menisci are caught between trying to move into flexion with the tibia and into rotation (in the wrong direction) with the femur. The result is often excessive deformation and tearing of a meniscus. If, as typically occurs, there is a valgus component to the rotary force, the medial meniscus is additionally stressed through its attachment to the medial ligament. Rotary stresses sufficient to produce meniscal damage do not necessarily require external forces. Often the victim simply twists suddenly on the weight-bearing leg. This usually occurs during athletic endeavors, but may also take place with less vigorous activities.

Occupations or activities involving rotation of the fully flexed knee, such as wrestling or mining in cramped quarters, particularly predispose to meniscus tears. This is because when the knee is fully flexed the menisci reach their limit of posterior excursion. Rotation, which involves posterior movement of one condyle and simultaneous anterior movement of the other, may further stress one meniscus posteriorly or cause the condyle to grind over the relatively fixed meniscus.

Most traumatic medial meniscus tears affect the posterior segment of the meniscus, with the tear running in a longitudinal direction.[189] Successive injury to the same meniscus may cause the tear to extend sufficiently anteriorly to allow the lateral segment of the torn structure to flip centrally into the intercondylar region—a "bucket-handle" tear (Fig. 14–14). When this occurs, it produces a mechanical block to full knee extension, and the knee is "locked." At this point, full extension can only occur at the expense of further damage to the meniscus or excessive stretching of the anterior cruciate ligament.

EVALUATION

A broad variety of common lesions affects the knee joint. Traumatic injuries may be experienced by the athlete as well as by the more sedentary individual. Symptomatic degenerative disorders involving the knee are not uncommon in middle-aged or older individuals, and "overuse" fatigue syndromes may affect virtually any age group. The approach to evaluation of knee disorders must be sufficiently flexible to accommodate such a broad spectrum of disorders. Presented here is a relatively comprehensive assessment scheme that includes most of the evaluative procedures needed to perform a thorough clinical examination of virtually any patient presenting with a common knee disorder. Practically speaking, the therapist will rarely ever use all of the tests and procedures outlined here in any one examination. However, the clinician should become proficient in performing all tests, and must be cognizant of the

Fig. 14–14. A longitudinal tear of the medial meniscus.

rationale for each one in order to optimize efficiency in administering a knee examination.

HISTORY

The key to an efficient yet comprehensive physical examination of the knee is the patient interview. Information elicited from the patient in the interview is necessary to gain insight into the nature and extent of the physical problem so as to best select the appropriate objective evaluative procedures. Subjective data are also important in determining the degree of disability resulting from the presenting disorder and in documenting a baseline.

Follow the format of inquiry set out in Chapter 4, Assessment of Musculoskeletal Disorders, when conducting the subjective portion of the knee examination. In addition, there are some specific questions that should be directed to patients presenting with knee problems, which are dependent on the nature of the disorder. If the problem is of recent traumatic onset, the clinician should ask the following:

1. What was the exact mechanism of injury? Was a "pop" felt?
2. Did the knee swell? If so, how long after the injury did the swelling become noticeable and where was the swelling observed?
3. To what extent was it possible to continue activities immediately following the injury? Was it possible to walk? If the injury occurred during athletic activities was a litter or some other form of passive or assisted transport required?

If the problem is of a chronic nature, the following questions should be asked:

1. Does the knee click, grind, grate, or pop? If so, was the onset of these symptoms associated with the onset of the present problem?
2. Has the knee ever locked, buckled, or given way? If so, under what specific circumstances? Is there some particular activity that tends to cause it?
3. Is climbing stairs, either ascending or descending, a problem?
4. Is it possible to run? What is the effect of running backward, stopping quickly, or changing directions quickly?

INTERPRETATIVE CONSIDERATIONS

Site of Pain

The knee joint receives innervation from the L3 through S2 segments of the spinal column and, depending on the site of the pathologic process, pain from knee disorders may be referred into any of these segments. Most common knee problems affect the anteromedial or medial aspect of the joint, which is largely innervated by L3. Because the L3 segment usually does not extend much below the knee, it is rare for a patient with a common knee disorder to experience pain radiating farther distally than mid-leg. It is more common for pain originating at the knee to be referred proximally into the anterior or anteromedial thigh. Note that the anterior aspect of the hip joint is also innervated primarily by L3 and that referred pain of hip joint origin may be very similar in site to that arising from the knee. In fact, it is not unusual, especially in children, for a patient with a hip joint problem to complain of "knee pain."

In the patient with nontraumatic onset of pain about the knee, lesions situated elsewhere in the L3 through S2 segments must be ruled out. The two common sources of referred pain to the knee are the lumbosacral region and the hip region.

Pain felt over the posterior aspect of the knee is often secondary to effusion causing distention of the posterior capsule. Because the S1 and S2 segments, which innervate the posterior knee region, extend well down into the foot, posterior knee pain may be referred some distance distally.

— Pain of nontraumatic onset felt over a generalized region at the anteromedial aspect of the knee is most commonly from patellofemoral joint dysfunction. This is especially likely when the pain is aggravated most by descending stairs and prolonged sitting with bent knees.
— Localized anteromedial pain felt at the joint line, usually of sudden onset, is often related to meniscus injuries. The pain arises from the anteromedial coronary ligament. A sprain of the coronary ligament may be the sole lesion, or it may be associated with a tear of the body of the meniscus.
— Medial knee pain of traumatic onset following a valgus or rotary strain is usually of capsuloligamentous origin. A tear of the meniscus must also be ruled out.

Onset

Sudden, Traumatic Onset. Sudden injuries caused by trauma are common, especially from athletic activities involving contact or sudden changes in direction. A sudden twisting injury, in which the tibia is rotated externally on the femur without an external source of force, may tear either the capsular fibers of the medial collateral ligament (Grade I tear), the cor-

onary ligament (peripheral attachment of the meniscus), or the body of the medial meniscus. When some external force is involved, such as in contact sports, and the knee is also forced into valgus position, the posteromedial capsule, medial collateral ligament, or anterior cruciate ligament may also be damaged.

Valgus–external rotation injuries are the most common traumatic knee disorders. In other types of injuries the mechanism should be determined, when possible, in order to estimate the nature of the stresses and to identify which particular structure might have been traumatized.

Gradual, Nontraumatic Onset. In middle-aged and older patients, symptomatic degenerative joint disease (DJD) must be ruled out. Pain from DJD is typically noticed first near the end of the day or after long periods of walking. Later, pain and stiffness are felt on rising in the morning, easing somewhat after getting up and about.

Possible precipitating factors, such as recent immobilization, alteration in activities, past injuries, and previous surgeries, should be considered. Patellofemoral joint dysfunction, a very common knee problem, is frequently related to quadriceps insufficiency. This may include true quadriceps weakness, as from disuse, or some increase in loaded knee-extension activities in the presence of inadequately trained quadriceps muscles. Typical activities would be hiking, bicycling, or skiing.

Effusion. Articular effusion commonly follows traumatic injury to the knee joint. This may be the result of blood filling the joint or of overproduction of synovial fluid. The time frame of the onset of effusion often provides important insight into the nature of effusion. Hemarthrosis tends to develop over a relatively short period following injury, from several minutes to a few hours; synovial effusion occurs over a longer period of time, perhaps 6 to 12 hours before it is noticed. Synovial effusion causes a dull, aching type of pain from the distension of the joint capsule. Hemarthrosis may be associated with more severe discomfort caused by chemical stimulation of capsular nociceptors. Clinically, it is important to attempt to differentiate the nature of the effusion, since, in the case of hemarthrosis, an intra-articular fracture must be ruled out. Some relatively severe joint injuries, such as a complete rupture of the medial ligament, may not be followed by significant effusion because of leakage of fluid through the defect out from the confines of the joint capsule.

More subtle joint effusion may accompany chronic, nontraumatic knee disorders. The patient often describes posterior knee discomfort from posterior capsular distention.

Nature of Pain and Other Symptoms

Pain of Traumatic Origin. Pain secondary to trauma is typically felt immediately at the time of injury. It is important to realize that in the case of ligamentous injuries the severity of the pain and resulting immediate disability do not necessarily reflect the severity of the injury. A minor or moderate sprain of the medial capsule or ligament is often more painful and more disabling at the time of injury than a complete rupture of the medial collateral ligament.[163] This is because, in the case of a complete rupture, there are no longer intact fibers from which pain of mechanical origin can arise. Furthermore, later development of pain from joint effusion may not be significant because of leakage of fluid through the defect. Thus, after the initial pain from the ligament rupturing, the patient may feel relatively little pain, especially if involved in a highly motivating activity such as athletic competition.

Patellofemoral Joint Pain. Pain felt when sitting for long periods with the knee bent or when descending stairs is typical of patellofemoral joint problems.[15,76] These functions both involve high and prolonged patellofemoral compressive loading. Pain is felt more on descending than on ascending stairs because greater passive tension is developed in the quadriceps mechanism during eccentric contraction than during concentric contraction. Sitting is a problem because of prolonged patellofemoral compression. Bone, being viscoelastic, undergoes "creep" or continued deformation with prolonged loading.[65] Bone is also weaker, or more likely to yield, with slowly applied loads. Thus the likelihood of trabecular breakdown is greater with loading over a long period of time than with a similar load applied quickly.

Morning Pain. Pain that is present on wakening but subsides with initial use of the joint and then increases again after some period of use is typical of DJD.

Buckling or Giving Way. A joint that buckles or gives way is suggestive of structural instability or functional instability. The common structural disorder that causes giving way is loss of ligamentous integrity. In such circumstances the patient may cite a particular activity that is a problem, usually one that stresses the joint in a direction the involved ligament is supposed to check. Thus, persons with chronic medial collateral ligament ruptures find it a problem to turn abruptly away from the involved leg because of the valgus–external rotation stress imposed on the leg.[163,187] Similarly, persons with loss of cruciate integrity may have problems descending inclines or squatting.

Functional buckling occurs as a result of reflex muscle inhibition, presumably from abnormal joint receptor activity. A common cause is internal derangement from a meniscus tear or loose body. In such cases, an abnormality in arthrokinematics resulting from the mechanical derangement may reflexively incite a sudden inhibition of the quadriceps muscles, causing the joint to give way. The patient will usually not be able to attribute the incidence of buckling to any consistent situation or activity, but will claim that the joint gives way for no apparent reason.

PHYSICAL EXAMINATION

Observation

The clinician should record any functional deficits noted throughout the patient's visit. When possible, analyze and document the nature and extent of the deficit for future comparison. If the patient refers to a particular functional problem during the interview, he may be asked to attempt the particular activity or task in order to evaluate the problem more objectively. This is especially important for patients with relatively chronic problems who may not spontaneously demonstrate functional deficits during the evaluation. Specific functions to note for patients presenting with knee disorders would include the following:

Gait — Refer to Chapter 21, The Lumbar–Lower Extremity Scan Examination, for common gait abnormalities and possible causes. The ability to hop, run, change directions quickly, stop abruptly, and climb stairs might be specifically evaluated.

Function — In a joint of low irritability the patient may be asked to demonstrate the movements that produce the pain and the specific movement or action that produced the injury. To evaluate for asymmetry or pain, the following tests may be useful: With the patient squatting, note patellofemoral tracking. (Normally the patella should track freely and smoothly and describe a straight line over the second ray or midline of the foot.) Also check to see if both knees flex symmetrically.

Other useful maneuvers for patient evaluation include having the patient squat and bounce, and stand from a sitting position; observing the patient climb and descend steps; asking the patient to change direction quickly or stop abruptly during movement; observing the patient run forward or backward, hop, and so forth; and having the patient jump into a full squat.

Inspection

Examine and record specific alterations in bony structure or alignment, soft-tissue configuration, and skin status.

I. **Inspection of Bony Structure and Alignment.** The reader should refer to the section on assessment of structural alignment in Chapter 21, The Lumbar–Lower Extremity Scan Examination, for a complete discussion of this part of the examination. In many chronic knee problems, especially disorders of uncertain etiology, a complete structural assessment of the lower extremities and lumbosacral region should be carried out. In traumatic disorders of recent onset, the examination is often confined to the knee area. The following assessments are particularly relevant to examination of the knee:

A. *Standing examination*
  1. Frontal alignment. The patient is viewed from behind. Use a plumb line that bisects the heels. Vertical or horizontal asymmetries in the frontal plane are detected by determining the positions of the:

  —Navicular tubercles
  —Medial malleoli
  —Fibular heads
  —Popliteal folds
  —Gluteal folds
  —Greater trochanters
  —Posterosuperior iliac spines
  —Iliac crests

  Document vertical disparities (leg-length differences, see p. 288) or lateral shifts from a plumb line that bisects the heels. Note abnormal or asymmetrical valgus–varus angulations. Take care to differentiate tibial valgum or varum from genu valgum or varum; these are often confused. The knee is normally positioned in slight genu valgum, because the medial condyle extends farther distally than the lateral condyle.
    a. Excessive genu valgum may be documented by measuring the distance between the malleoli, with the medial femoral condyles in contact.
    b. Excessive genu varum is noted by measuring the intercondylar distance at the knee with the medial malleoli in contact.
    c. Vertical disparities are documented by measuring the distance from the lowest asymmetrical landmark to the floor.
    d. Horizontal deviations from the plumb line can be documented by measuring distances from the plumb line.
  2. Transverse rotary alignment. The patient is viewed from the front with the feet at a normal stance width and pointed outward 5° to 10° from the sagittal plane. Several structures are assessed.
    a. The intermalleolar line is normally rotated outward 25° to 30° from the frontal plane.
    b. The tibial tubercles should be in line with the midline or lateral half of the patellae.
    c. Patellae. With the feet in normal stance position, the patellae should face straight forward. A "squinting" patella may be indicative of medial femoral or lateral tibial torsion. The normal patellar posture for exerting deceleration forces in the functional position of 45° knee flexion places the patellar articular surface squarely against the anterior femur. A lower posture represents patella baja. A higher posture represents patella alta. Normally, the length of the patella and patellar tendon should be approximately equal. In patella alta, the patellar tendon is excessively long (Fig. 14–15A). When viewed from the side, a "camel" or double hump may be apparent, resulting from the uncovered infrapatellar fat pad.[96] Patella alta makes the patella less efficient in exerting normal forces, and lateral displacement occurs easily.[96,99]
    d. Q angle. The quadriceps angle (Q angle or patellofemoral angle) is formed by a line drawn from the center of the patella proximally toward the anterosuperior iliac spine, and a second line drawn from the center of the patella distally toward the tibial tubercle with the foot in the subtalar neutral position and the knee extended (weight-bearing). Normally the Q angle is 13° to

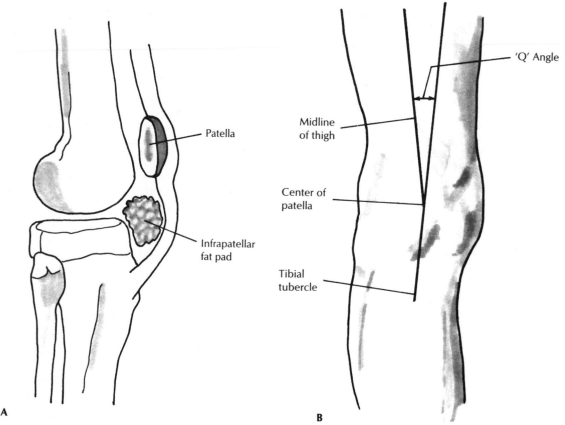

Fig. 14–15. Conditions predisposing the patient to recurrent subluxation of the patella. *(A)* The "camel" sign with a high-riding patella and uncovered fat pad. In a normal knee, the patella–patellar tendon ratio is approximately equal. *(B)* The quadriceps angle (Q angle) measures the divergence of the quadriceps from the sagittal plane. Normally, the Q angle should be 13° to 18° when the knee is straight and 0° in flexion.

18° (13° for males, 18° for females). An angle of greater than 14° indicates a tendency toward less patellar stability (Fig. 14–15B). An angle greater than 18° is often associated with patellar tracking dysfunction, subluxating patella, increased femoral anteversion, or increased lateral tibial torsion. (Hughston has advocated measurement of the Q angle with the patient sitting and the quadriceps contracted; if the quadriceps is contracted and the knee fully extended, the normal Q angle is 8° to 10° (with 10° or greater considered abnormal). If the patient is sitting and the quadriceps is relaxed [knee at 90°], the Q angle should be 0°.[96]

e. Anterosuperior iliac spines. A line drawn between the left and right anterosuperior iliac spines should be parallel to the frontal plane.

3. Anteroposterior alignment. The patient is viewed from the side. A plumb line facilitates assessment and measurement of deviations. In a relaxed standing position it is normal for the knee to assume a position of slight recurvatum. With the plumb line about 1 cm anterior to the lateral malleolus, the lateral femoral condyle should be slightly posterior to the plumb line. Abnormal angulation in the sagittal plane can be documented by measuring from some anatomical landmark to the plumb line.

B. *Sitting examination.* The patient sits with the legs hanging freely over the edge of the plinth. The following should be assessed:

1. *Femoropatellar alignment.* Assess the position and size of the patellae. They

should face straight forward, with the inferior poles of the patellae about level with the femorotibial joint line. A small, high-riding, outward-facing patella may predispose to a lateral patellar tracking disorder.

  a. A laterally facing patella suggests that the medial femoral condyle is considerably longer than the lateral condyle. This is likely to be associated with a valgus angulation when the knee is straightened.

  b. The inferior pole of the patella should be approximately level with the femorotibial joint line. A high-riding patella may be significant with respect to patellofemoral joint problems.[144]

2. *Femorotibial alignment.* The position of the tibial tubercles should be assessed with respect to the patellae in the sitting, knee-bent position. The tubercle usually lines up with the midline or lateral half of the patella. Of most importance here is symmetry.

  a. A tubercle that is positioned too far medially may represent posteromedial capsular tightness, as may occur with healing of a sprain or rupture of one of the cruciate ligaments.

  b. A tubercle that is situated too far laterally may suggest laxity (*e.g.,* rupture) of the posteromedial capsule or medial collateral ligament.

C. *Supine examination*

1. Legs straight

  a. Valgus–varus angulations may be measured with a goniometer.

  b. Leg-length disparities may be documented by measuring from the anterosuperior iliac spines to the medial malleoli.

2. Knees bent at 60° angle, feet flat on the plinth

  a. Tibial lengths can be compared by noting the heights of the tibial tubercles.

  b. Leg-length disparities of more proximate origin are detected by observing the lengths of the femurs. This is done by siting, from the side, a plane across the faces of the patellae.

  c. Anteroposterior femorotibial displacements are detected by compar-

ing the prominences of the tibial tubercles. This must be done before anteroposterior stability tests are carried out. In the presence of a posterior cruciate ligament rupture the tibia will sag back and the tibial tubercle will be less prominent. This will often be associated with a false-positive anterior drawer test for anterior cruciate damage.

  d. An excessively prominent tibial tubercle suggests previous osteochondrosis of the tibial apophysis (Osgood-Schlatter disease). This may lead to a high-riding patella.

II. Soft-Tissue Inspection

A. *Muscle contours*

1. Instruct the patient to maximally contract the quadriceps and calf muscle groups by fully extending the knees and plantar-flexing the ankle. Carefully assess the muscle contours for obvious atrophy or asymmetries. Often significant atrophy can be observed before it can be documented by girth measurements. When asymmetries can be measured, baseline values should be recorded so changes can be noted later.

2. Assess other muscle groups in a similar manner, including the hamstrings and the anterior and lateral compartments of the leg.

B. *Swelling.* If significant swelling exists, baseline girth measurements should be recorded when possible.

1. Generalized edema of the lower leg may accompany a variety of metabolic or vascular disorders. If occurring soon after a surgical procedure, it may indicate venous thrombosis, in which case a physician should be notified.

  Edema persisting some time after trauma or surgery may be associated with a reflex sympathetic dystrophy.

2. Localized swelling may be articular or extra-articular.

  a. Articular effusion is manifest as swelling of the suprapatellar pouch and loss of definition of the peripatellar landmarks. Often the posterior capsule becomes distended, causing mild popliteal swelling. This swelling may be localized at the semimembranosus bursa, even in the case of articular effusion, since this bursa often communicates with the synovial cavity. If there is sufficient intracapsular swelling, the knee will assume a flexed or resting position (15° to 25°).

   b. Extra-articular effusion is most often noted in the prepatellar bursa. This may swell after sudden or repeated trauma (*e.g.*, housemaid's knee). Occasionally the distal belly of a hamstring muscle will herniate through the superficial fascia when contracted. This may appear as a pronounced popliteal "swelling," but disappears when the muscle is made to relax.

III. Skin Inspection
   A. *Color*
   1. Localized erythema may suggest an underlying inflammatory process.
   2. Ecchymosis about the knee is most commonly associated with the following conditions:
      a. Contusion. The injury is usually over the lateral aspect.
      b. Ligamentous damage, in which the ecchymosis is usually noted medially.
      c. Recent patellar dislocation, in which the ecchymosis is seen medially.
   3. Cyanosis over the lower leg following trauma or surgery may be associated with a reflex sympathetic dystrophy.
   4. Scars. The cause should be determined. If surgical, the reason for the surgery should be discovered.
   5. Texture. In the presence of dystrophic changes, the skin of the lower leg becomes smooth and glossy.

IV. Selective Tissue Tension Tests
   A. *Active movements*
   1. Unilateral weight-bearing flexion–extension. If not contraindicated by recent trauma or significant disability, the patient should be asked to perform repeated one-legged half-squats. This yields some useful information concerning the functional capacity of the part. It is also a good method by which to compare the strength of the involved knee to a normal side, when possible; manual muscle testing is usually a poor test for quadriceps strength because the examiner may not be able to manually

overcome even a significantly weak muscle. Note the following:
      a. The patient's ability to perform the movement. Can the knee be fully extended? How many repetitions can be performed before tiring? (Compare this to the opposite leg.)
      b. Any tendency toward giving way of the knee.
      c. Patellofemoral or femorotibial crepitus. The examiner palpates at the medial and lateral patellar margins for the former, and at the femorotibial joint line for the latter. It is normal for a knee to "pop" or "snap" during this movement. A grinding similar to "sand in the joint" is more likely to indicate articular surface degenerative changes.
      d. Provocation of pain. If pain is experienced, determine the point in the range of movement at which it is felt.
   2. Non-weight-bearing flexion–extension. If the patient is unable to perform weight-bearing flexion–extension or is unable to do it through a full range of movement, flexion and extension in a supine position are assessed. For extension ask the patient to straighten the knee; then tell him to hold it extended and attempt to raise the leg against gravity (straight-leg raise). Then ask the patient to flex the knee as far as possible. The following should be noted:
      a. Range of motion. If the patient is unable to fully flex or extend the knee, apply some passive overpressure to determine whether the restriction is secondary to pain, weakness, or true tissue restriction. The amount of passive extension should be compared to extension maintained against gravity. The degree of any "extensor lag" should be documented.
      b. Crepitus during movement. If joint crepitus is present it should be determined whether it arises from the femorotibial or patellofemoral joint.
      c. The presence of pain and the point in the range at which it is felt.
      d. If a capsular restriction exists, flexion will be limited to 90° to 100° and extension will be lacking by 20° to 30°.
      e. Loss of knee extension in the pres-

ence of full flexion is most often caused by an internal derangement such as a bucket-handle mensicus tear.

f. Quadriceps lag. To complete the last 15° of knee extension, a 60% increase in force of the quadriceps muscles is required.[138] The loss of mechanical advantage, muscle atrophy, decreasing power of the muscle as it shortens, adhesion formation, effusion, or reflex inhibition may result in a quadriceps lag. This lag is usually associated with loss of accessory motion. To assess the inability to extend the knee fully; the following steps are recommended:

i. The patient lies supine with the heel supported on a small firm pillow or block so that the knee is allowed to sag into full extension.

ii. The patient is asked to lift the heel off the support. It should be possible to do this before the knee starts to lift. If a quadriceps lag is present, the knee will be observed to lift first.[40]

g. Dynamic tibial rotary function (Helfet test).[84] With the patient sitting, first assess the positions of the tibial tubercles, then passively extend each knee repetitively, over the final 25° of extension. Rotation of the tibia during extension is assessed by observing the tibial tubercle during the movement; normally the tubercle should be seen to rotate laterally through an angle of 10° to 15° during the final phase of extension. The involved side must be compared to the opposite knee. Loss of dynamic tibial rotation may be secondary to one of several factors:

i. The tibia may already be rotated at the starting position.

ii. Tightness or adhesion of the medial capsuloligamentous structures, such as may occur with immobilization during healing of a sprain

iii. An internal derangement such as a meniscus displacement or a cartilaginous loose body

h. Lateral and medial rotation of the tibia on the femur. With the patient seated and the knee flexed over the edge of the plinth, active axial rotation is assessed.

i. Range of motion: Medial rotation should be approximately 30° and active lateral rotation approximately 40°.

ii. Provocation of pain

iii. End feel: The end normal feel of this movement is tissue stretch.

B. *Passive movements*

1. Osteokinematic movements

a. Flexion–extension. The knee is passively flexed and extended, and the following parameters are noted:

i. Range of motion. If movement is limited, determine whether the pattern of restriction is capsular or noncapsular.

ii. Provocation of pain

iii. End feel

iv. Crepitus

b. Combined movement. Combined movements or quadrants can be tested. More information may be derived by testing passive range of motion in combination.

i. The flexion–adduction movements are the most helpful in eliciting pain.[139]

ii. Hyperextension.[40] With the patient lying supine, the examiner holds one hand over the patient's knee and uses the other hand to lift the lower leg at the foot; this is repeated with the resting hand held over the tibial condyle. Normally up to 15° passive hyperextension is possible. Once the range of hyperextension has been determined, the test can be used in combination with abduction and adduction.

iii. Compare both lower extremities; determine the range and pain response of performing combinations of flexion and extension.

c. Passive lateral and medial rotation (axial rotation). To test axial rotation, the patient should be sitting. The knee is first flexed to 90°, then is nearly fully extended. The normal end feel of rotation of the tibia on the femur is tissue stretch. An increased range with the knee flexed may be associated with a rotatory instability of the knee. Loss of motion occurs in many intrinsic knee disorders.[40] With the patient supine, the examiner uses a handhold at the foot, then rotates the tibia internally and externally on the femur, with the knee close to full extension.

   i. Hypermobility of external rotation suggests a medial ligament or posteromedial capsule rupture.

   ii. Pain on external rotation may be present with a sprain of the coronary ligament or medial collateral ligament. A valgus stress can be used to differentiate the two, because this will stress the medial collateral but not the coronary ligament.

   d. Hip range of motion, including straight-leg raising and flexibility testing of adduction and abduction. The Ober test should be used to assess iliotibial band tightness. The assessment for flexibility should include hip rotation, spine extension, and examination of the hamstrings, hip flexors, iliotibial band, and rectus femoris. To assess for tight hamstrings, have the supine patient flex the hip to 90°. While maintaining this flexion, see if the patient can fully extend the knee so the entire leg is straight. Lack of normal hamstring flexibility is shown as inability to extend the knee fully with the hip flexed to 90°.

   According to Janda, the first priority of treatment of motor imbalance is to lengthen the tight antagonist.[105] Tight muscles not only increase the work load of the agonists, but also (according to Sherrington's law of reciprocal innervation) act in an inhibitory way on their antagonists. This is an important factor in the quadriceps–hamstring relationship.[119,182,183]

2. Joint-play movements (stress tests). The status of the capsuloligamentous structures is assessed by performing the following passive movements. Note the provocation of pain or muscle guarding and whether the movement is hypomobile or hypermobile. The latter can best be determined by comparing to a "normal" side, but experience is also very helpful. The techniques for performing these movements are illustrated in Chapter 6, Peripheral Joint Mobilization Techniques.

Note: It is very important to take note of, and attempt to avoid eliciting, protective muscle guarding when performing the joint-play tests; false-negative results may mask a serious injury that warrants immediate attention.

   a. Anterior glide of the tibia on the femur (see Fig. 6–28).

   b. Posterior glide of the tibia on the femur (posterior drawer test) (see Fig. 6–27).

   c. Valgus–varus tilt (see Figs. 6–31 and 6–32).

   d. Internal and external rotation of the tibia on the femur (see Figs. 6–29 and 6–30).

   e. Patellar mobility
      i. Medial-lateral (see Fig. 6–33).
      ii. Superior-inferior (see Fig. 6–34).

   f. Distraction of the femorotibial joint (see Fig. 6–26). Compare with the unaffected side.

   g. Anterior-posterior glide of the proximal tibiofibular joint (see Fig. 6–35).

C. *Resisted isometric movements.* Lesions involving the muscles or tendons crossing the knee joint are not uncommon and are best detected by assessing the effect of maximal isometric contraction of the structure to be tested. Tendinitis most commonly affects the insertion of the iliotibial band, one of the pes anserinus tendons, or the insertion of the biceps femoris. The quadriceps are often contused in athletic activities, especially football.

   Provide manual resistance to the isometric contraction and determine whether the contraction is strong or weak and whether it is painless or painful. The most important movements to resist are the following:

Knee flexion—for the biceps femoris and pes anserinus tendons
Knee extension—for the iliotibial tendon and quadriceps muscles
External rotation of the tibia on the femur —for the biceps femoris tendon

Internal rotation of the tibia on the femur
—for the pes anserinus tendons

If lesions involving other muscles or tendons are suspected, the appropriate resisted movements should be tested. In cases of relatively chronic tendinitis brought on by repetitive minor trauma (*e.g.*, long-distance running), pain may not be elicited on resisted movement testing unless the patient has recently engaged in the provoking activity. To avoid false-negative findings, it may be helpful to have the patient perform the relevant activity just prior to testing. Also, testing repeated contractions of the suspected structure may increase the likelihood of eliciting discomfort in chronic cases.

V. **Ligamentous Instability Tests.** Because the knee, more than any other joint in the body, depends on ligaments to maintain its integrity, it is imperative that the status of the ligaments be tested. In assessing joint laxity in the anterior, posterior, medial, or lateral direction, the four primary restraints by the medial collateral, lateral collateral, anterior cruciate, and posterior cruciate ligaments are tested. The extent to which these four ligaments restrain their respective motions depends on the knee flexion angle. As the knee approaches extension, the participation of isolated ligaments lessens and the role of secondary restraints increases.[168]

When testing the ligaments of the knee, the examiner must watch for one-plane instabilities as well as rotational instabilities. Anterior and posterior motions of the tibia should be evaluated in varying degrees of rotation. The measurements obtained should always be compared to those from the normal knee.

It is important to grade the amount of laxity in a knee. In most clinical grading systems, grade I laxity represents up to 5 mm of motion; grade II, 6 mm to 10 mm; grade III, 11 mm to 15 mm; and grade IV, more than 15 mm.[168] However, instrumental measurements are challenging these concepts and more accurate classification systems are being adapted.[34,142,143,155]

A. *Straight instabilities*
   1. *Tests for anterior instability (one plane)*
      a. **Straight anterior drawer test** (see Fig. 6–28). The classic anterior drawer tests are done in the supine position

with the knee flexed 90° and the examiner sitting on the patient's foot to stabilize the tibia as described by Slocum[187] and Furman,[70] or with the patient supported in a semireclining sitting position (lower leg over edge of table) with the patient's foot stabilized between the examiner's legs to prevent rotation.[89] In either test, it is imperative that the hamstring muscles are relaxed. The examiner's hands are placed around the proximal tibia (over the gastrocnemius heads and hamstrings) with the thumbs over the tibial plateau and the joint line. The tibia is then drawn forward on the femur. The test is positive when the anterior displacement is more than 6 mm. If the test is positive with both tibial condyles displaced anteriorly, the usual mechanism is a tear of the posterolateral and posteromedial medial capsule and the medial and lateral capsular ligaments. This produces a combined anteromedial/anterolateral rotational instability. If the degree of subluxation is significant, the anterior cruciate is also ruptured.[157]

      b. **Lachman test.** The Lachman test described by Tory and associates[205] is considered the best indicator for injury to the anterior cruciate ligament, especially the posterolateral band.[107,108,168] It is essentially an anterior drawer test with the knee near full extension (flexed 15° to 20°). The test can be performed with the patient in a semisitting position (with the back supported) and the ankle stabilized between the examiner's legs or with the patient in supine. In the supine position one of the examiner's hands stabilizes the patient's femur while the proximal aspect of the tibia is moved forward with the other hand. The degree of anterior translation and the firmness of the end feel should be noted. The Lachman test is graded from 0 to 4+ (1+ = 5 mm; 2+ = 10 mm; 3+ = 15 mm; 4+ = 20 mm).[89] Fetto and Marshall[61] emphasize the importance of noting the type of end feel; for example, 1+

Lachman test with a soft end feel is diagnostic of an anterior cruciate tear. Positive results from the Lachman test may also reflect possible injury of the posterior oblique ligament and the arcuate–popliteus complex.

According to Henning and associates,[89] the Lachman test is positive in 92% of acute anterior cruciate ligament tears and in 99% of chronic tears. Positive results reflect anterior displacement, not reduction of a posteriorly displaced tibia.

2. *Tests for posterior instability (one plane).* Posterior cruciate instability is best measured by performing the posterior drawer test at 70° and 90° flexion.[168] When this ligament is torn, the examiner must carefully observe the profile of the knee from the lateral view during the drop-back test and should palpate the joint line during the posterior drawer test.

   a. Drop-back test (gravity drawer test) and Godfrey's chair test. Posterior tibial translation can be observed with the patient supine, the knee flexed 90° and the hip 45°, and the foot resting on a table; or with the heel supported on the seat of a chair with the hip and knee in 70° to 80° flexion (Fig. 14–16A and B).[57,74] The positions of the patella and the tibial tubercle are observed from the side. If the posterior cruciate is torn, the tibia will "drop back" or be displaced posteriorly on the femur.

       Next, with the patient's knees in full extension, elevate them by holding the great toes (Fig. 14–16C). Observe any external tibial rotation or recurvatum.[95] Compare one side with the other. Subtle degrees of hyperextension can be determined by holding the knee against the table and elevating the heel.[57] Measure the height of the heel above the table.

   b. *Posterior drawer tests*

     i. Passive posterior drawer test. The patient is placed in the same position as for the anterior drawer test with the hip flexed 45° and the knee 90°. The unaffected leg is examined first to determine the normal degree of laxity. The patient's foot is fixed in neutral rotation, and the examiner sits on the dorsum of the foot to stabilize it. The hands are used to push the tibia to and fro to reveal any backward movements of the tibia on the femur. This test is positive after disruption of the posterior cruciate ligament with a tear of the posterior capsular ligament.

     ii. Active posterior drawer test. For the 90° active drawer test, the patient is in the same position as for the passive drawer test, with the examiner holding the foot against the table.[168] The patient is instructed to contract the quadriceps and try to extend the knee by pushing the foot down toward the end of the table. Normally the tibia will either remain in neutral or move slightly posteriorly. In the presence of a torn posterior cruciate, the tibia will move forward because of the unbalanced force vectors of the quadriceps and patellar tendon.[168]

3. *Valgus stress test for medial instability (one plane).* Medial instability is secondary to disruption of the ligaments of the medial tibiofemoral compartment and results in a valgus subluxation of the tibia on the femur. Medial collateral ligament laxity is best evaluated by the valgus stress test performed at 30° flexion and 0°.[168]

With the patient supine and the knee flexed 30°, the examiner applies a valgus stress at the knee (pushes the knee medially) while the lower leg is hugged by the examiner to steady it (see Fig. 6–31). The test is repeated with the knee at 0°.

If the test is positive with the knee flexed 30° but negative with the knee fully extended, it implies that the medial collateral ligament has been damaged. If the test is positive with the knee at both 30° flexion and in full extension, this implies damage to both the medial capsular and cruciate ligaments.

If a stress roentgenogram is obtained when the test is performed in full exten-

Fig. 14-16. The sag signs. *(A)* Posterior sag sign. Note profile of the two knees: the left (nearer) sags backward compared with the normal right knee. *(B)* The Godfrey chair test also is used to identify posterior sag of the tibia. *(C)* The external rotation recurvatum test; apparent recurvatum and external tibial rotation demonstrate posterolateral rotatory instability.

sion, a 5-mm opening is indicative of a grade I injury; up to 10 mm, grade II injury; and more than 10 mm, grade III injury.[89,109,152]

4. *Varus stress test for lateral instability (one plane).* Lateral instability is caused by disruption of the lateral compartment and results in a varus subluxation of the tibia on the femur. The varus stress test is similar to the valgus stress test, but the hands are changed to apply a varus stress (*i.e.*, lateral push) to the knee (see Fig. 6–32). The test is done in 30° flexion and in full extension.

If the test is positive with the knee flexed to 30° but negative with the knee fully extended, the lateral collateral ligament probably has been injured to some degree. If it is also positive in extension, this implies damage to the cruciate and lateral capsule.

Laxity is graded the same as for the valgus stress test. When more than grade II laxity is present, there is a very high incidence of associated posterior and anterior cruciate ligament laxity.[53]

B. *Rotatory instability.* A variety of rotational instabilities can be present in an injured knee. There may be an isolated rotatory instability or one associated with other forms of straight instabilities. A rotary instability secondary to a ligamentous injury results in an excessive degree of rotation of the tibia on the femur. Typically, in such a case the patient presents with a history of the knee suddenly giving way without any warning. This may occur while walking down stairs or when a runner suddenly changes direction.

1. *Anteromedial rotatory instability.* Anteromedial instability was initially described by Slocum and Larson.[187] This is an anterior subluxation of the medial tibial condyle that also moves into external rotation on the femur. Anteromedial rotary instability is increased with a tear of the capsular ligament of the medial joint compartment, with loss of the anterior cruciate ligament, and/or the medial meniscus.[126]

This type of instability is diagnosed clinically in the presence of a positive anterior drawer test, which is performed while the tibia is held in external rotation.

2. *Anterolateral rotatory instability.* Anterolateral instability is caused by insufficiency of the anterior cruciate ligament.[71,72,186] The degree of instability is increased if the lateral capsular ligament is also torn. Anterolateral rotary instability results in anterior subluxation of the lateral tibial tubercle, which also moves into internal rotation on the femur.

Several tests have been described to diagnose this condition. Tests demonstrating translation of the tibia include the presence of a 90° positive anterior drawer while the tibia is held in neutral rotation[93,94] and the Lachman test with the knee in approximately 20° flexion.[205]

Tests demonstrating anterolateral rotatory laxity include a 90° flexion-rotation drawer test with the tibia rotated medially by 15°[31,159] and a variety of pivot shift tests. The pivot shift or jerk test, a confirmatory test of the anterior cruciate ligament, results in the tibia being subluxed anteriorly when the knee is straighter than 125°.[61,71,72,101,130,133] One or more of these maneuvers (pivot-shift test of MacIntosh and Galway, the Losee test, Slocum test, cross-over test, or Hughston's jerk test) designed to detect rotatory laxity, can be used.

a. Jerk test (lateral pivot–shift test). The patient is supine and the hip is flexed 45° and the knee 90°. The jerk test is elicited by the examiner grasping the patient's foot and fully internally rotating the tibia and applying a valgus stress to the proximal end of the tibia. The examiner then gradually straightens the knee (Fig. 14–17). At about 30° knee flexion, the lateral tibial condyle may subluxate or jerk forward suddenly. As the knee is further extended, the tibia returns to its former position.[93,94] This test has also been described as the lateral pivot–shift test.[71]

b. Losee test.[130,131] With the patient in a relaxed, supine position, the examiner's hand is placed palm down, with the fingers over the patient's patella and the thumb posterior to the fibular head. A valgus stress is ap-

Fig. 14–17. The "jerk test" or "lateral pivot–shift test." *(A)* Apply a valgus force with the hand near the fibular head and axial loading with internal rotation with the hand near ankle. *(B)* Simultaneously, slowly flex the knee. Whereas the pivot–shift is tested from extension to flexion, the jerk test is elicited while moving the knee from flexion to extension.

plied by the examiner, using his abdomen as a fulcrum, while the knee is extended slowly and the leg is allowed to internally rotate. The fibular head is pushed anteriorly with the examiner's thumb while the fingers push the femur posteriorly (Fig. 14–18). The test is positive if the tibial plateau subluxates anteriorly just short of full extension.

   c. Slocum's test. One advantage of the Slocum test over the previously described tests is that it allows hamstring and quadriceps relaxation.[152,186,187] The test is done with the patient lying on the unaffected side. The upper hip and pelvis of the involved limb are rotated posteriorly

until the weight is borne by the heel of the upper leg with the knee free of the table (Fig. 14–19). The examiner applies a valgus stress by pressing down on the tibia and femur while simultaneously flexing the knee from full extension to 30° flexion. The lateral condyle of the tibia will subluxate anteriorly as the knee is extended.

   d. Arnold and Coker have described a cross-over test in which, with the patient standing, the examiner fixes the foot of the patient's affected leg by standing on it.[10] The patient crosses the unaffected leg over the fixed foot and rotates the upper torso away from the fixed foot until it faces 90° in

Fig. 14–18. Losee test. *(A)* The knee is flexed 30° to 40° and, as the knee is slowly extended *(B)*, the fibular head is pushed forward.

Fig. 14–19. Slocum's anterolateral rotary instability (ALRI) test; the patient is supine and turned 30° toward the side opposite the involved knee.

the opposite direction. When this position is achieved, the patient contracts the quadriceps muscle. A positive test occurs when the patient describes the same symptoms as in the jerk test. This functional cross-over test reproduces the pivot–shift and is indicative of anterolateral rotatory instability.[7,204]

3. *Posterolateral rotatory instability.* Pos-

terolateral rotatory instability follows a tear of the arcuate ligament complex including the posterior cruciate ligament.[53,95] A number of tests can be used to identify its presence, which results in posterior subluxation and internal rotation of the lateral tibial condyle.

a. Reverse pivot–shift test. The primary test used to assess posterolateral rotatory instability is the reverse pivot–shift test.[100,152] The patient lies supine with the knees straight. The examiner places one hand around the patient's ankle and places the foot against the examiner's pelvis. Beginning at 80° flexion, with the foot externally rotated and a slight valgus force applied, the leg is slowly brought into extension (Fig. 14–20). If the test is positive, the lateral tibial plateau will suddenly move forward and internally rotate at approximately 20° flexion. This is the opposite of what happens in the true

A

B

Fig. 14–20. Reverse pivot–shift test to detect posterolateral instability. Beginning at 80° flexion with the foot externally rotated and a slight valgus force applied (A), the leg is slowly brought into extension (B).

pivot–shift, where the tibia subluxates in extension and reduces in flexion.[24]

b. Posteriolateral drawer test. Hughston described an alternate test for posterolateral rotatory instability.[95] The patient and examiner are in the same positions as for the previously described drawer tests, but the lower leg is slightly rotated externally. As the examiner pushes the tibia posteriorly, the lateral tibial condyle displaces posteriorly and the tibial tubercle displaces laterally.

c. External recurvatum test. The external recurvatum test is used to identify tears of the arcuate complex and the anteromedial and intermediate fibers of the anterior cruciate.[95] The patient lies supine with the knees straight, and the examiner lifts the legs by the toes to produce hyperextension at the knee. The test is positive when the tibia rotates externally with posterolateral displacement of the tibial tuberosity.

VI. Special Tests

A. *Tests for meniscal injury.* Clinical diagnosis of meniscal tears has been discussed by several authors, notably McMurray, Apley, Noble, Barry, Anderson, and Ricklin.[6,8,12,147,156,175] Most of these "meniscus signs" are known by the names of their initiators. The maneuvers can be very helpful in differentiating meniscus lesions from other knee joint lesions. Although these signs can help diagnose a meniscus lesion when they are positive, a negative test does not necessarily exclude the diagnosis of a torn meniscus. Most of these tests are quite similar, so any one can be used, although it is generally accepted that McMurray's is the best manipulative test.[6] Some of the better known meniscus signs are described below. (This list is by no means complete.)

1. *McMurray's test.* Nearly full range of knee flexion must be present in order to perform McMurray's test.[147] The knee is fully flexed and the tibia fully rotated either internally or externally. The examiner places the thumb and index finger over the medial and lateral femorotibial joint lines and, while maintaining rotation of the tibia, extends the knee to 90°. This test does not pertain to extension beyond 90°. Provocation of a painful area of movement and a palpable "click" elicited during the movement may indicate a positive test, although there is some question as to the reliability.[154]

2. *Apley's test.* The patient is prone with the knee bent to 90°.[8] Joint distraction or compression can be maintained to help differentiate between ligamentous injuries and injuries to the menisci or coronary ligaments. Pain elicited during external rotation with distraction suggests a collateral ligament injury. Pain on internal rotation with distraction may indicate a cruciate injury. Pain that is felt with rotation and compression, but not elicited when the joint is distracted, suggests a problem with a meniscus or a meniscal attachment (coronary ligament).[92]

3. *Steinmann's sign.* If localized tenderness is present along the anterior joint line, Steinmann's sign may be useful. In the presence of a possible meniscus tear, pain appears to move anteriorly when the knee is extended and posteriorly when the knee is flexed.[175] Rotating the tibia one way and then the other with the knee flexed 90° may localize pain to the joint line.

B. *Plica Tests.* A pathologic process affecting the synovial plica can mimic a meniscal injury and cause symptoms that are not unlike those of other common internal derangements of the knee; this makes differential diagnosis more difficult.[20,82] A symptomatic mediopatellar plica can often be palpated as a tender, bandlike structure paralleling the medial border of the patella. A palpable and sometimes audible snap is present during flexion and extension.

With the patient supine, the clinician should check for the presence of a pathologic synovial plica by passively flexing and extending the knee from 30° to 90° flexion. The examiner produces pressure on the patella medially with the heel of the hand while palpating the medial femoral condyle with the fingers of the same hand. The

Fig. 14–21. *(A)* Passive patellar tilt of $^+15°$, and *(B)* passive lateral glide test, demonstrating a patella being subluxated laterally to half its width.

examiner then flexes the knee and medially rotates the tibia slightly. A tender fold may often be palpated that recreates the familiar, painful popping sensation that the patient feels.

C. *Patellar Stability Tests*

1. *Apprehension test.* Patellar stability can be judged with the apprehension test performed at 15° to 20° flexion.[92] Attempt to push the patella laterally, noting the reaction of the patient and the tendency toward subluxation (usually associated with medial patellar tenderness).

2. *Passive medial-lateral glide.* To determine the tightness of the medial and lateral restraints of the patellofemoral joint, passive glides are performed (see Fig. 6–33). The tests can be performed in full extension and various degrees of flexion.

3. *Passive patellar tilt test.* To assess patellar laxity when the lateral patellar edge is elevated from the femoral condyle, passive patellar tilt is produced. A 0° or negative patellar tilt angle usually reflects excessive lateral retinacular tightness (Fig. 14–21*A*).[168]

4. *Passive lateral glide test.* To estimate lateral patellar excursion, the width of the patella is divided into fourths. Longitudinally, lateral overhang in excess of

half the width of the patella usually indicates lax or torn medial patellofemoral restraints (Fig. 14–21B).[168]

A Q angle of greater than 14° indicates a tendency toward patellar instability.

VII. Neuromuscular Testing. Resisted isometric movements are used primarily to detect painful lesions of muscles or tendons and give only general information pertaining to muscle strength. If it is desirable to detect or quantify subtle losses in muscle strength—as may arise from disuse or segmental neurologic deficits—or strength increases resulting from training, repeated loading of the muscle to near-fatigue levels must be carried out. This is especially true for large-muscle groups such as the quadriceps and calf muscles. Various exercise equipment may be used for this purpose. A particularly convenient, though expensive, method is use of an isokinetic apparatus, which gives a torque–curve readout. A simpler but very useful method for the quadriceps and calf groups is to ask the patient to perform repeated half-squats and toe-raises, respectively, in a standing position.

Manual tests for smaller groups, used especially to detect myotomic weaknesses associated with nerve-root lesions, are described in Chapter 21, The Lumbar–Lower Extremity Scan Examination.

Most current literature supports a quadriceps to hamstring strength ratio of 3:2.[155] If indicated, manual muscle testing for other muscle groups to detect myotomic weakness associated with nerve-root lesions should be conducted.

A scan examination of the key sensory areas and reflexes should be carried out, and the patellar (L3–L4) and medial hamstring (L5) reflexes checked. Any differences in sensation should be noted; a stroking test and sensibility to pin prick also may be indicated (see Chapter 21, The Lumbar–Lower Extremity Scan Examination).

VIII. Palpation. Clinically, palpation is best carried out in conjunction with inspection and is organized similarly.

    A. *Bony structures and soft-tissue attachments.* Note any abnormalities in size, position, or integrity of bony structures; determine the existence of tenderness, especially at tendon and ligament attachments, keeping in mind that deep tenderness is often referred. With the patient sitting at the edge of the plinth, legs hanging freely, palpate the following:

    1. Patella

        a. Note size, shape, and position. A small, high-riding patella may be a predisposing factor in patellofemoral joint problems. The proximal lateral pole of the patella may be enlarged in the presence of bipartite patella.[79,164] The inferior pole of the patellar tendon is a common location for "jumpers knee." With the knee in extension, the fat pad is normally extruded to either side of the taut patellar tendon. Hoffa described tenderness on palpating the fat pad, which has become known as the "fat pad syndrome."[90]

        b. Palpate the superior and inferior poles, where the quadriceps and patellar tendons attach, for tenderness.

        c. Passively hold the knee extended, push the patella medially, and palpate the medial articular facets on the back side of the patella for tenderness.

    2. Femoral condyles

        a. Note the prominence of the anterior aspect of the lateral condyle.

        b. Palpate the adductor tubercle, a major site of attachment for the medial retinaculum, as well as the site of insertion for the adductor magnus.

        c. The area over the medial femoral condyle should be palpated for a snapping, tender medial patellar plica. Although a medial patella plica is present to some degree in nearly every knee, it is rarely symptomatic.

        d. Palpate the medial and lateral joint lines. Cysts of the lateral cartilage are felt as hard lumps and are prominent at 45° flexion but disappear at both full extension and at 90° flexion.

    3. Proximal tibia

        a. Palpate the area of insertion of the pes anserinus and medial collateral ligament.

        b. Palpate the tibial tubercle, where the patellar tendon inserts.

        c. Palpate the lateral tibial tubercle, where the iliotibial band inserts.

4. Fibular head. The lateral collateral ligament inserts at its apex.

B. *Soft-tissue palpation*

1. Muscles. Palpate the various muscle groups about the knee for the following:

a. Mobility. This is especially important after surgery or prolonged immobilization, which may lead to the development of adhesions between muscle planes or between muscles and other tissues.

b. Continuity. Occasionally, a severe trauma may cause palpable ruptures of muscles or tendons.

c. Consistency. Prolonged disuse and reflex sympathetic dystrophy predispose to "stringy," fibrotic muscles. Contusions of the quadriceps often resolve with heterotopic bone formation, which may be palpable.

2. Ligaments

a. Anteromedial coronary ligament (anteromedial border of the medial meniscus). This is palpated at the anteromedial joint line. It becomes more prominent here when the tibia is passively rotated internally with respect to the femur. This is a site of point tenderness following medial meniscus tears or isolated coronary ligament sprains.

b. Medial collateral ligament. The palpating finger follows the medial joint line from its anterior aspect a short distance posteriorly until it is felt to be obliterated by the anterior margin of the medial collateral ligament. The posterior margin of the ligament can be similarly palpated where it crosses the joint line. The examiner should estimate the course of the ligament and palpate along its extent. It cannot be distinguished as a discrete structure because of its flat configuration. Localized tenderness will usually correspond well with the site of medial collateral ligament injuries.

c. Lateral collateral ligament. This is best palpated with the patient's ankle crossed over the opposite knee. It is felt as a well-defined, round structure, crossing the lateral joint line between the femur and fibular head. This is one of the few sites at which a ligamentous rupture is palpable; however, at the lateral collateral ligament this is a rare occurrence.

3. Tendons

a. Patellar tendon. This is easily palpated from the inferior pole of the patella to its insertion on the tibial tubercle.

b. Iliotibial band. From its insertion on the lateral tibial tubercle, the blunt, posterior edge of the iliotibial band can be felt well up into the lateral thigh region. Tenderness to palpation over the lateral femoral condyle in association with a tight iliotibial band suggests an iliotibial band friction syndrome (see Chapter 13, The Hip).[156,174]

c. Popliteus tendon. Popliteus tendinitis is readily diagnosed by palpating the area of the fibular collateral ligament with the leg in the "figure four" position.[145]

d. Biceps femoris. This is a very prominent tendon, easily felt at the posterolateral corner of the knee, inserting into the fibular head.

e. Patellar retinaculum. This structure may be palpated for mobility and tenderness. The lateral patellar retinaculum is palpated while attempting to displace the patella medially. A tight lateral retinaculum has been described as an important factor causing patellar pain.[62] Tension in the medial retinaculum can be tested between the medial edge of the medial border of the patella and the edge of the medial condylar ridge. This area is often tender in cases of patellofemoral joint dysfunction.

f. Medial retinaculum. The retinaculum is flat and cannot be distinguished as a distinct structure. It is palpated in a generalized area between the adductor tubercle and the medial border of the patella. It is often tender in cases of patellofemoral joint dysfunction.

g. Pes anserinus tendons. The pes anserinus tendons join to give a flat tendinous insertion on the anterome-dial aspect of the proximal tibia 5 to 7 cm below the joint line.

    i. The semitendinosus tendon is easily felt as a prominent, cord-like structure at the posterome-dial corner of the knee.

    ii. The gracilis tendon is more diffi-cult to distinguish, but can be felt as a "piano wire" between the semitendinosus tendon, posteri-orly, and the sartorius tendon, anteriorly.

    iii. The sartorius tendon is a large, blunt structure crossing the pos-teromedial aspect of the knee, anterior to the semitendinosus and gracilis tendons.

  h. Gastrocnemius heads. These are pal-pated deep in the popliteal fossa.

4. The popliteal space. The popliteal artery can usually be palpated at the midpor-tion of the popliteal space. Comparison of the popliteal artery pulse to the dorsal pedia and the posterior tibial pulse are helpful in assessing popliteal entrap-ment syndrome.[132] Swelling of the semi-membranosus bursa, the so-called Baker's cyst, is best palpated with the knee fully extended.

5. Palpation for effusion. When a large vol-ume of fluid accumulates within the confines of the synovial cavity, it is easily seen and palpated at the medial and lat-eral patellar margins, and distention of the posterior aspect of the joint is noted. Smaller quantities of fluid may be de-tected by one of the following measures:

  a. Milking the fluid distally out of the suprapatellar pouch with one hand while palpating along the medial and lateral patellar margins with the other. Fluid will be felt to drain be-neath the palpating fingers, and the patella may be felt to float up off the femoral condyles. Compare to the opposite knee.

  b. After having milked the fluid distally, as described above, tap the patella posteriorly with the free hand. If fluid has caused the patella to "float," a "click" will be felt as it is pushed down onto the femoral condyles. Palpate for distention of the semi-

membranosus bursa, which often communicates with the joint.

C. *Skin palpation.* The skin about the knee area and the distal aspect of the leg should be palpated lightly with the back of the hand. The examiner should note:

  1. Temperature. Localized areas of in-creased temperature may signify under-lying inflammation. In reflex sympa-thetic dystrophy or other vascular problems, the leg may feel abnormally cool.

  2. Tenderness. Burning dysesthesias may be associated with neural disorders, such as nerve-root impingements, or they may arise as referred tenderness from deep somatic pathologies.

  3. Moisture. Hyperhidrosis is common with reflex sympathetic dystrophy. Ab-normalities in skin moisture may also be associated with other vascular or meta-bolic disorders.

  4. Mobility. Skin mobility is often impaired by adhesion following surgery or pro-longed immobilization, and especially with development of a reflex sympa-thetic dystrophy.

SUMMARY OF EVALUATION PROCEDURES

The knee evaluation presented here is lengthy when considered in the context of a busy clinical practice. The experienced examiner rarely administers all of the tests discussed, but chooses the appropriate ex-amination procedures based on the patient interview and the general nature of the problem. To improve efficiency when administering a knee examination, the clinician must organize the tests according to patient positioning; the standing tests are done first, then the sitting tests, the supine tests, and finally the prone tests. The conceptual scheme of organizing the exam presented here must be translated into a more practical scheme based on patient positioning. Therefore, for each position, the relevant observa-tions, inspection procedures, selective tissue tension tests, neuromuscular tests, and palpation proce-dures must be carried out before asking the patient to change positions. The following outline summa-rizes the knee evaluation according to patient posi-tioning. It can be used as a checklist when adminis-tering the exam and as the basis for devising a knee evaluation form tailored to a particular clinical set-ting.

I. **Standing**
   A. Observation
      1. Gait
      2. Special functions—running, stair climbing, abrupt stops, abrupt turns, hopping, squatting, and so forth
   B. Inspection
      1. Standing structure and alignment
      2. Soft-tissue contours
      3. Swelling
      4. Skin
   C. Selective tissue-tension tests—active weight-bearing flexion–extension
   D. Neuromuscular tests
      1. Repeated half-squats (L3) (same as weight-bearing flexion–extension)
      2. Repeated toe-raises (S1–S2)
II. **Sitting**
   A. Inspection
      1. Patellar alignment and positioning
      2. Femorotibial rotary alignment
      3. Muscle contours with maximal isometric contraction
      4. Skin
   B. Resisted isometric movements
      1. Knee extension
      2. Knee flexion
      3. Internal tibial rotation
      4. External tibial rotation
   C. Neuromuscular tests—resisted hip flexion (L2, L3); patellar reflex (L3–L4)
   D. Palpation
      1. Bony structures and soft-tissue attachments
      2. Tendons
      3. Ligaments
III. **Supine**
   A. Inspection
      1. Tibial lengths (knees bent)
      2. Anteroposterior tibial alignment (knees bent)
      3. Femoral lengths (knees bent)
      4. Leg-length measurement (anterosuperior iliac spine to medial malleolus)
      5. Valgus–varus angulation
      6. Swelling or atrophy (girth measurements)
      7. Skin
   B. Selected tissue-tension tests
      1. Non-weight-bearing (active–passive)
         a. Flexion–extension—measured with goniometer
         b. Lateral and medial rotation
      2. Joint-play movements
         a. Anterior-posterior glide
         b. Valgus–varus tilt
         c. Internal–external rotation
         d. Patellar mobility
         e. Superior tibiofibular joint play
         f. Distraction
      3. Ankle range of motion
      4. Passive hip flexion–extension, abduction–adduction, and straight-leg raise
      5. Special tests for:
         a. Ligamentous instability
         b. Meniscal tears
         c. Patellofemoral joint involvement
   C. Neuromuscular tests—resisted dorsiflexion (L5)
   D. Palpation
      1. Muscles
      2. Effusion
      3. Skin
IV. **Prone**
   A. Inspection
      1. Soft tissues
      2. Skin
   B. Selected tissue-tension tests
      1. Passive hip internal–external rotation
      2. Resisted knee flexion
   C. Neuromuscular tests—medial hamstring reflex (L5)
   D. Palpation
      1. Muscles
      2. Skin

It is important to bear in mind that examination of the knee is never done in isolation. The knee is only a single component of the closed kinetic chain, and pathologic processes may exist proximal or distal to the knee. Pelvic obliquity or leg-length inequality must be recognized, because these problems affect the knee. Abnormal foot function is not uncommon and causes a variety of knee ailments, including patellar tendinitis and lateral knee pain.[191] It is documented in many studies that increased pronation of the foot or a rigid, supinated configuration contributes to knee problems.[26,134–136,141] Failing to recognize a foot abnormality as a cause of a knee problem may markedly delay treatment and recovery.

A patient with knee problems should be evaluated frequently with a motion examination both on and off a treadmill (using various speeds). Very frequently, a foot that looks as though it is one configuration will actually function as the opposite when in motion.[137] Videotapes or films are also helpful in diagnosing difficult problems.[26]

BASIC REHABILITATION OF THE KNEE

The concept of knee injury and its treatment is in an evolutionary process. To remain current in handling such injuries is a challenge that those treating the knee must constantly face. Many changes in treatment have resulted from arthroscopic techniques.[120] It should always be kept in mind that the knee is just one part of the closed kinetic chain of the spine and lower extremity. Rehabilitation must always be directed toward the entire system as well as specific problems. Maintenance of optimal function as healing ensues is the cornerstone for rehabilitation. Unnecessary loss of strength and range of motion (ROM) must be minimized without imposing inappropriate stresses in the healing tissue. Throughout the entire program, appropriate warm-up and aerobic activities are performed to maintain cardiovascular fitness.

I. **Management of Acute Joint Lesions**
   A. *Pain and swelling.* Ice is generally applied to minimize hemorrhages and swelling. Various forms of electrical stimulation, such as high-voltage pulsed galvanic stimulation (HVPGS) and interferential current stimulators (ICS) are frequently used to decrease swelling.[153] A compressive bandage and/or splint is usually applied to provide rest and control swelling. A foam-rubber or felt pad over the specific area of tissue damage may be helpful. Frequent elevation of the part should be encouraged to prevent fluid stasis, which may increase or prolong the swelling. Commonly used methods to decrease pain include transcutaneous electrical stimulation and gentle joint-play oscillation techniques (grade I). After the acute phase, to further assist in the resolution of inflammation and to promote healing, a heating modality (hot packs, whirlpool, ultrasound) or contrast treatments (hot pack, ice pack, or ice massage–ultrasound) might be considered.
   B. *Prevention of deformity and protection of the joint*
      1. Often the approach is to place the patient on crutches on a non-weight-bearing status initially (24 to 48 hours). Later canes or a walker may be necessary to distribute forces through the upper extremities while walking.
      2. Minimize stair climbing, sitting in deep chairs, or other activities of daily living that require forceful quadriceps contraction.
   C. *Stiffness*
      1. If tolerated, perform grade 1 or 2 femorotibial distraction and joint-play motions with the joint in 15° flexion or near the resting position.
      2. Passive or active assistive ROM exercises are carried out several times a day. Wall slides are often helpful in increasing the range of knee flexion. The patient is positioned close enough to the wall that the involved foot remains in contact with the wall throughout knee range of motion. The patient gains active range of flexion by sliding the injured leg down the wall and using the normal extremity to return it to the starting position with the knee extended.[184]
   D. *Muscle atrophy and adhesions*
      1. Begin with quadriceps-setting exercises. To promote early quadriceps activity, an indirect approach that will facilitate overflow from uninvolved areas to the quadriceps may be appropriate; this helps to avoid pain, which may result in reflexive inhibition.[50] The effect of isometric exercises can be further enhanced through the use of the "cross-over effect." By vigorously exercising the uninvolved contralateral leg, a cross-over strengthening effect can be obtained on the involved side.[85-87] Up to fifty repetitions of quadriceps exercises are encouraged each hour the patient is awake, but not to the point of increasing joint irritability. The patient may be sitting or supine. The foot and toes are dorsiflexed and the heel pushed away from the body. This helps to initiate the vastus medialis obliquus contraction. The length of the contraction (6 to 10 seconds) has repeatedly been demonstrated to be of importance in developing a maximum isometric contraction.[17,151] A stronger contraction may be elicited by resisting dorsiflexion.
      2. Straight-leg raises (SLRs) represent a progression of isometric exercises to strengthen the quadriceps muscle when the patient can maintain the knee extended while lifting the extremity. Progress is limited, however, if the patient does not do the SLRs correctly. Optimal results will be obtained if the principles of Gough and Ladley are applied with an isometric quadriceps set maintained throughout the exercise.[78,128,177,184] The pa-

tient tightens the quadriceps, holds for 2 seconds, then tightens the quadriceps harder and lifts the leg until the heel is 6 to 12 inches off the supporting surface. The extremity is held in that position for 2 seconds and then lowered slowly. The emphasis is on slow lowering of the leg to facilitate eccentric work, which has been demonstrated to be of importance in increasing strength.[1,25,36,37,116-118] The most effective resistance to the quadriceps is during the first few degrees of SLR.

3. Hamstring-setting exercises are performed in long sitting with 50° to 60° knee flexion. The patient attempts to dig the heel down into the mat while pulling downward on the leg.

   Note: With progression of all isometric exercises it is important that the position of the knee be altered in several ways to enhance isometric strengthening of the appropriate muscle groups at different angles and lengths in the pain-free range. Both submaximal and maximal isometric exercises must be performed at several angles, because isometrics are angle-specific and overflow is only about 15° in either direction.[129]

4. Hip exercises for proximal muscle strength should include hip isotonic abduction strengthening (in sidelying), which contributes to lateral knee stability; hip isotonic extension (in prone, working from a flexed position to neutral); and hip adduction, performed isometrically by squeezing a towel roll between the legs. Clinically, patients are able to perform quadriceps-setting exercises better following isometric adduction exercises. This may be related to the fact that the vastus medialis obliquus has an attachment to the adductor muscle tendon.[87]

II. **Management of subacute and chronic joint problems**
A. *Stiffness.* To decrease the effect of stiffness from inactivity, instruct the patient to perform active ROM.
B. *Pain from mechanical stress*
   1. Continue use of assistive devices for ambulation if necessary.
   2. Strengthen the quadriceps femoris.
      a. Begin with isometric exercises with the knee fully extended, because there is less patellar compression in extension.

b. When tolerated, have the patient perform SLRs with resistance, using a short lever arm.
c. Short-arc quadriceps exercises, with the patient sitting and a firm pad under the knee to limit flexion to less than 45°, are added once the patient can tolerate resistive SLR. If motion is not painful, light resistance is added at the ankle, as tolerated.
   Caution: Resistance applied to knee extension at an angle greater than 45° flexion creates excessive patellofemoral compression forces.
C. *Function and strength.* To improve knee function and balance strength, there should be a gradual transition from isometric to isotonic work. As previously mentioned, eccentric work has been shown to be important in developing strength and is a good introduction to isotonic work.[54]
   1. Proprioceptive neuromuscular facilitation (PNF) patterns and techniques can be effectively used to increase isometric and eccentric control in the short range and to improve isometric and isotonic control of both the quadriceps and hamstrings. If activity in the vastus medialis is a specific goal, one of two patterns should be emphasized.[201]
      a. Diagonal 1 flexion (D1F) pattern—pelvic protraction combining movements of flexion, adduction, and external rotation of the hip.
      b. Diagonal 2 extension (D2E) pattern—pelvic depression combining movements of extension, adduction, and external rotation of the hip.
   2. To selectively train and strengthen knee flexors, active isotonic knee flexion may be performed, with the patient standing, using ankle weights or a weighted boot and exercising through a range of 0° to 90°.[114] With the patient prone, resistance can be applied with a wall pulley, a boot, or manually; inner and outer hamstrings can be selectively strengthened by working out of the cardinal plane in diagonal patterns. Balance of ratio between flexor and extensor strength should be obtained.[32,33] Normally knee flexion force is about 67% of knee extensor force.[196]
   3. Bilateral PNF patterns emphasizing knee control are most easily performed with the

patient sitting. Techniques should first emphasize strengthening in the short range of knee extension and then be applied through gradual increments of range until resistance through full range of knee extension can be accomplished. To emphasize phasic control following slow controlled movement through the range, quick reversal motions with minimal resistance can be used.

4. Isokinetic strength training. Because muscle strength varies with joint position and the speed at which the exercise is performed (subject to either considerable acceleration or deceleration), total muscle development is unpredictable. Thus, variable-resistance strength-training modalities have been developed. It is questionable how well these machines accomplish this goal, because muscle length tension ratios vary from person to person.[167]

When available, isokinetic strength training can be an integral component of the strength-training program. Isokinetic exercise can be introduced before or after isotonic work. The patellofemoral forces should be considered in any rehabilitation program. If extensor mechanism problems exist, further restraints are put on activities requiring flexion–extension of the knee. Exercises with low forces and high repetitions will help prevent patellofemoral irritation.[140]

5. Endurance training. It must be remembered that strength and power are only part of the rehabilitation process. Endurance and aerobic capacity training should also be included.[41] There are two types of endurance that need to be developed in the rehabilitation process—cardiovascular and muscular endurance. To augment isokinetic effects, a convenient modality is the use of a stationary bicycle. The seat can be lowered to decrease knee extension or raised to decrease knee flexion if motion limitations exist. Early on, endurance training can start with initiation of stationary cycling for the unaffected limb. To enhance endurance capabilities, cycling activities should be performed at the initiation of the exercise program as well as at the end and should be performed to exhaustion. Swimming and other activities (e.g., rowing machines) can also be initiated.

6. Functional and weight-bearing activities. The muscular support of the knee (as for any joint) depends on coordinated co-contraction of the muscles about the joint. With weight-bearing, unless the knee is in recurvatum, the quadriceps and hamstrings are the predominant muscles that must support the knee with dynamic co-contraction.[19] The tibia will shift neither posteriorly nor anteriorly but will be pressed to the femur, lessening the forces on the cruciate ligaments and secondary restraints. Co-contraction activities might include step-up exercises, bilateral sitting leg presses, or mini-squats (through 30° range of knee flexion). Active assistive (negative weights), free, or resistive activity (e.g., wall pulleys, latissimus exercise bars), may be included. Isometric control of the quadriceps may be enhanced by manual resistance applied to the pelvis and by PNF techniques such as alternating isometrics (AI) and rhythmic stabilization (RS), which will increase the difficulty by challenging the quadriceps to maintain the knee in extension against the proximally applied force.

7. Proprioception and balance. Normal proprioception and balance are lost with a major knee injury, immobilization, or a lower extremity pathologic process.[66,213,217] Minimizing the atrophy of this system can begin with isometrics, which stimulate the mechanoreceptors. These exercises are followed by limited weight-bearing activity using a balance board in sitting, then by assisted balance activities (using parallel bars) in standing. Eventually, one-foot balance with and without the eyes open is added, then standing balance on the toes with balance boards, and finally, full weight-bearing balance activities outside the parallel bars or without arm support.

8. Timing and dynamic control. For patients who hope to return to strenuous athletic events, procedures to improve the timing of the muscular activity are necessary. This can be done when the injured knee has achieved 80% of quadriceps and hamstring strength of the normal extremity on

Cybex® testing.[184] Although fast bursts of activity can be promoted by some mechanical devices, to stimulate the control needed for most athletic endeavors and to emphasize a specificity of training, timing exercises in weight-bearing postures are important. Fast-alternating, weight-bearing activities include running in place or on a treadmill or jogging on a trampoline. Quick changes in a variety of weight-bearing postures (*i.e.*, plantigrade, supine activities, bridging) and while running in place will further challenge the timing of the quadriceps activity with variation of the angle of knee flexion. In the plantigrade position, an excessive amount of knee flexion should be avoided because it may simulate the squat thrusting exercises that can overstress the knee.[201] To further simulate control needed for specific athletic events, sideward, backward, and rotational movements may be added.

D. *Range of motion*
   1. Restore soft-tissue mobility by soft-tissue mobilization (STM) techniques (*i.e.*, connective tissue massage, pump massage, myofascial release, and friction massage). Restoration of normal mobility of the connective tissue means that tissue will be allowed to move through a normal excursion without encroaching on the function of other adjacent tissues or producing painful stress.
   2. Restore ROM and joint play. As normal osteokinematic ROM and strength are regained, the therapist must also ensure that normal arthrokinematics are restored. Most importantly, one must determine, using the Helfet test, that normal femorotibial rotary function returns. Occasionally a patient regains knee extension without concurrent return of external rotation, presumably because of residual tightness or adherence of part of the medial joint capsule. This may be a source of persistent chronic knee pain or eventual degenerative changes following an otherwise benign traumatic disorder. If such rotatory restrictions are detected, joint mobilization procedures should be instituted to correct them (see Chapter 6, Peripheral Joint Mobilization Techniques).

   Loss of knee extension is a common se-
quela to knee injury or surgery. Although loss of motion in either direction affects normal knee kinematics and can lead to a progressive arthrosis, loss of more than 10° of extension produces comparatively more complaints and alteration in normal gait patterns than a loss of flexion.[170] The infrapatellar contracture syndrome (with patellar entrapment resulting in patella infera or patella baja) is becoming more recognized in patients with a history of knee inflammation and swelling secondary to surgery or trauma associated with quadriceps weakness and knee immobility. A key finding is significant loss of superoinferior glide of the patellofemoral joint, particularly superior glide.[170]

Joint pain may be an expression of comprehensive imbalance of the musculoskeletal system, including defective neuromuscular control. The inhibitory effect of tight hamstrings (postural muscle) may vastly influence the strength of the vastus medialis and lateralis, which have mainly dynamic (phasic) functions.[104] Neglect of the close relationships between joints, soft-tissue, muscles, and the nervous system lessens diagnostic as well as therapeutic possibilities.

The patient should be instructed in an isotonic home program to maintain strength levels over many months, and in proper warm-up and stretching techniques.

COMMON LESIONS

LIGAMENTOUS INJURIES

History

The patient will invariably recall the traumatic event; you should attempt to determine the exact mechanism of injury.

Onset. One of the most common mechanisms occurs when a football player is tackled from the side with the foot planted and the knee slightly flexed. The victim is usually struck while trying to turn or "cut away." The forces on the knee include a valgus stress, external rotation of the tibia on the femur, and usually an anterior movement of the tibia on the femur. With sufficient force, the medial capsule is torn first, followed by the medial collateral ligament, then by the anterior cruciate ligament.[110] The medial meniscus is invariably torn as well, completing the "terrible triad of O'Donoghue."

A minor medial ligament sprain is a common lesion that usually results from an external rotation strain of the tibia on the femur. An external force may or may not be involved.

A force against the anterior thigh, which can drive the femur backward on the tibia, while the knee is close to full extension, tends to stress the anterior cruciate ligament. This is especially true if the tibia is in a position—or forced into a position—of internal rotation with respect to the femur. In fact, forced internal rotation of the tibia on the femur in itself may tear the anterior cruciate ligament. Internal rotary strains are thought by some to be the primary cause of isolated anterior cruciate ligament lesions.[112,215] A force driving the tibia backward on the femur will stress the posterior cruciate ligament. This seems to be true regardless of whether or not the knee is flexed, because the posterior cruciate remains relatively taut in most positions of the knee. An example of such an injury is the previously described "dashboard injury."

In the case of a force driving the knee into hyperextension, the posterior capsule tends to give way first, then the anterior cruciate ligament, and finally the posterior cruciate ligament.[112]

It is not uncommon in cases of severe ligamentous injuries for the patient to attempt to continue activities (e.g., return to the field in a football game) immediately following the injury. This is especially true in the case of a complete rupture of the medial collateral ligament, since no fibers remain intact from which pain can arise. The pain often subsides after a few minutes if the patient is in a highly motivating situation. No effusion ensues because the capsule is usually torn, allowing the fluid to leak out of the joint cavity. In partial ligamentous injuries, the patient is less likely to continue activity because of persisting pain following the injury.

In severe injuries the patient may describe painful effusion occurring within a few minutes after injury; this is highly suggestive of hemarthrosis, and an intra-articular fracture must be ruled out by the physician.

Slower development of effusion (e.g., over several hours) suggests synovial effusion secondary to capsular irritation. This is common with mild and moderate ligamentous injuries.

Site of Pain. The patient usually will point to a localized area that corresponds well to the site of the tear as being the primary site of pain. The exception is an isolated tear of the anterior cruciate, which is relatively rare and may result in more generalized discomfort.

In the case of effusion, especially hemarthrosis, the entire knee area is likely to be painful; the patient is less able to localize the site of injury. Also, in severe injuries involving several structures, localization is less likely because of generalized pain.

The knee is largely innervated by the L3 segment, although it also receives contributions from L4 to S2. Referred pain into these segments is a possibility, although this does not seem to occur as frequently with acute ligamentous lesions as it does with chronic, degenerative problems.

Nature of Pain and Disability. In the absence of significant effusion, the pain is described as a continuous, deep, fairly localized pain, which is increased by any movement tending to further stress the ligament (partial tear). When considerable effusion exists, a more intense, aching, throbbing pain is described that is aggravated by weight-bearing and virtually any movement. Hemarthrosis is, as a rule, more painful than synovial effusion.

If a moderately severe tear or complete rupture is left to heal, the pain will largely subside. The patient may walk quite comfortably but is unable to perform some particular activity such as running, jumping, cutting, walking down stairs, or squatting without having the knee give way. If carefully assessed, the particular disabilities will correspond to activities that tend to move the knee into directions that the stretched or ruptured ligament is meant to check. Some examples include

1. Inability to turn quickly—medial or lateral collateral ligament.
2. Inability to run forward—anterior cruciate ligament.
3. Inability to go down stairs easily, squat, or run backward—posterior cruciate ligament or posterior capsule.

A medial collateral ligament rupture will usually result in considerable disability, whereas isolated cruciate tears may cause little or no disability if quadriceps muscle function is good.[189]

Physical Examination

In the acute stage, once joint effusion, considerable pain, and significant muscle guarding have developed, it may prove very difficult to carry out some of the evaluation procedures. In any case, the knee must be examined, sparing the patient as much discomfort as possible and ensuring that no harm is imposed by the tests. The value of immediate, on-the-spot examination prior to the onset of effusion cannot be overemphasized.

I. Acute Lesion with Effusion

    A. *Observation.* The patient may hobble into the office, perhaps using crutches. The knee is held slightly flexed with only toe-touch weight-bearing, if any. Removal of the shoe, sock, and trousers is carried out with difficulty.

    B. *Inspection.* Joint effusion is obvious, especially in the suprapatellar region. The patient stands with the leg held semiflexed, often unable to place the heel on the floor.

        1. The Helfet test cannot be administered because the knee cannot be fully extended.

        2. Girth measurements at the suprapatellar region are increased from effusion.

        3. Some redness of the skin over the knee may be noticed. The skin may be somewhat shiny from being stretched.

    C. *Selective tissue-tension tests*

        1. Active movement

          a. Weight–bearing flexion–extension is impossible.

          b. In the supine position, active movement is limited in a capsular pattern because of joint effusion, with pain especially at the extremes of both motions. Passive overpressure is met with a muscle-spasm end feel.

        2. Passive movements. Flexion–extension is limited in a capsular pattern (about 15° loss of extension and 60° to 90° loss of flexion) with no crepitus and a muscle-spasm end feel.

        3. Resisted movements

          a. These should be strong and painless, barring concurrent tendon injury.

          b. Quantitative determination of muscle strengths must be deferred because of the acute condition.

        4. Passive joint-play movements of the femorotibial joint may be hypermobile and painful. (Be aware of possible false-negative results from muscle guarding.)

          a. Anterior glide

          b. Posterior glide

          c. Valgus–varus tilt

          d. Internal–external tibial rotation

          e. Patellar mobility cannot be validly assessed if significant effusion is present.

          f. Superior tibiofibular joint. Joint-play movement here may be painful in the case of a lateral collateral ligament sprain.

    D. *Palpation*

        1. There is likely to be localized tenderness at the site of the tear. There may be referred tenderness in nearby areas as well.

        2. Effusion is easily confirmed by the tap test or by emptying the suprapatellar pouch while palpating at the lateral patellar margins. Posterior capsular distension may also be noted. Hemarthrosis may accompany (1) a cruciate tear, (2) a meniscus tear extending to the peripheral attachment, (3) a severe capsular tear, or (4) an intra-articular fracture.

        3. The joint is warm and slightly moist.

    E. *Ligamentous stability and special tests* (see Physical Examination, above)

II. Acute Lesion without Effusion. Although most ligament injuries at the knee are followed by the development of some effusion, this is not always the case. The absence of significant effusion does not necessarily mean that the injury is mild. On the contrary, complete medial capsular ruptures, usually with tearing of all or part of the medial collateral ligament, may not be followed by much joint effusion, since the fluid escapes the confines of the joint capsule through the defect.

The primary difference between a patient presenting with effusion and one presenting without are that in the absence of effusion, the following will be observed:

    1. The patient will present with less of a gait disturbance. The knee will not be maintained in as much flexion, and the patient may be able to walk without aids.

    2. The available range of motion will be greater.

Generally, the patient who does not develop much joint swelling has less pain and disability. The clinician must carefully assess joint-play movements to determine whether the absence of effusion reflects a minor lesion or a very severe injury. Information acquired during the patient interview will also be instructive.

If it is determined that significant instability is

present on one or more joint-play movements, a physician experienced in dealing with such injuries must be notified at once, because immediate surgery may be indicated.

III. **Chronic Ligament Ruptures.** Unfortunately, patients occasionally present with chronic ligament ruptures. The primary complaint is functional instability or giving way of the knee with particular activities. Objectively, the patient may walk in without a limp or obvious disability. The only significant findings may be the following:

1. Difficulty performing some specific function such as running, turning sharply, squatting, descending stairs, or running backward
2. Quadriceps muscle atrophy, especially if the joint was swollen or immobilized[50]
3. Hypermobility on one or more joint-play movements or ligmentous stability tests
4. A positive Helfet test

Laxity of one of the medial stabilizing structures—the medial capsule or medial collateral ligament—is most likely to result in some disability. Often this is combined with anterior cruciate rupture. The result is instability of anterior glide and external rotation of the tibia on the femur. Functionally, the patient is unable to turn away from the involved side without the leg giving way, a real problem for a young, active individual. The medial meniscus may be torn at the time of injury or some time later from abnormal joint mechanics. The meniscus tear will compound the instability and the tendency for the knee to buckle.

Management

The approach to management of ligamentous injuries depends on several factors, including the patient's age and desired activity level and the nature of the pathologic process. It is important to determine the severity of the injury and whether the lesion is acute or chronic. Traditionally the severity of ligamentous lesions have been graded as follows:

Grade I: Mild sprain, with no gross loss of integrity of the ligament fibers. On examination there is no joint-play hypermobility.
Grade II: Moderate tear, with partial loss of integrity of the ligament, manifested as mild joint-play instability.
Grade III: Severe tear or complete rupture of the ligament, resulting in moderate to marked joint-play hypermobility.

This classification is useful for general communication purposes, but it cannot be used as an absolute guide to clinical management; it does not adequately represent the broad continuum of ligamentous injuries, nor does it take into account other individual factors such as the patient's age, activity level, motivational status, or the stage of the lesion.

The stage of the lesion—how acute or chronic it is—is also somewhat of an arbitrary designation. For the sake of this discussion, we will base this classification on specific clinical criteria that may reflect the nature of the existing inflammatory process.

Acute lesion
—The patient is unable to bear weight without pain and a significant limp.
—There is significant loss of knee motion with a painful, muscle-spasm end feel.
—There is obvious swelling or effusion.

Chronic lesion
—The patient can walk with minimal pain and without a significant limp.
—Knee motion is relatively free, or, if restricted, is limited by stiffness (non-painful end feel).
—There is little or no swelling.

Subacute lesion
—Some combination of acute or chronic criteria.

Grade I and II Sprains. Following a mild to moderate knee ligament injury, the patient should be able to return to a normal level of activity. In first-degree sprains, the treatment is relatively unimportant and is designed mostly to prevent pain. In second-degree sprains, the critical factor in treatment is protection in order to allow healing. The rehabilitation program should be started early, with more progressive exercise techniques and functional activities added later (see Basic Knee Rehabilitation, above). The general strengthening exercises usually do not need to be modified, although for medial lesions, care must be taken to avoid valgus stress at the knee and for lateral lesions, varus stress should be avoided.

Friction massage at the site of the lesion, applied transversely to the direction of the ligament fibers with the knee in different degrees of flexion–extension, may help to prevent adherence of the healing ligament to adjacent tissues and help to align newly produced collagen along the normal lines of stress.[45] Care should be taken not to apply friction at the proximal attachment of the medial collateral ligament, because occasionally a periosteal disruption results here in the development of a bony outcropping (Pellegrini–Stieda syndrome).[210] (Although this is undoubtedly an inevitable result of the original injury, the use of massage may be held suspect should some medicolegal question develop.)

Medial Collateral Ligament Tear (Grade III Sprain). It is the current thinking that medial collateral ligament (MCL) tears do not usually require surgical repair.[18,58,83,91,178,194] The normal course for these injuries is re-examination under anesthesia followed by arthroscopy of the knee.[149] It is necessary, however, to prove that an isolated injury of the MCL is present, with no involvement of the meniscal or cruciate structures. The MCL has an excellent secondary support system. Weight-bearing forces tend to compress the medial side, thus aiding in stability, and the injury can be protected adequately with bracing.

Whether surgical repair is used or not, the knee is usually immobilized in a hinge cast or brace cast to minimize atrophy and prevent valgus stress.[81] Rehabilitation after most MCL injuries can progress fairly rapidly (2 to 8 weeks). A treatment program similar to that for second-degree sprain can be carried out. Weight-bearing with crutches is continued until knee extension to 10° is possible. Return to sport activities is not allowed until a normal gait pattern has been achieved.

Anterior Cruciate Ligament Tear (Grade III Sprain). Injuries of the anterior cruciate ligament (ACL) are most problematic. In the nonsurgical patient, after control of swelling and pain, treatment begins with isometrics of the hamstrings and quadriceps to encourage co-contractions. Range of motion is limited and protected. Based on the studies of Daniels and associates, Henning and associates, and Paulos and associates, the range is limited from 90° of flexion to 45° of extension.[47,48,88,89,167,170] A protected exercise program is allowed in this range. Isometric internal and external rotation exercises, which are added once the patient has 90° flexion, have been shown to decrease any abnormal tibial rotation.[187,188] Special emphasis is placed on hamstring exercises. During all phases of the exercise program, electrical stimulation with maximum contraction is desirable to maintain muscle integrity.[153,197] Functional knee braces have been suggested permanently for sport activities involving cutting or rotational stresses.[13,56,194,200,203] Presently, there are two constructive types and designs, featuring hinge posts with or without shells to encompass the thigh. Gait studies have shown that under low loading conditions, the majority of functional knee braces limit excessive anterior tibial translation. However, under conditions of high loading that more closely simulate high activity levels, little or no control of anterior tibial translation occurs.

Anterior Crucial Ligament Repair. ACL repair or reconstruction, like nonsurgical rehabilitation, typically demands a protocol that minimizes any quadriceps muscle activity that involves anterior translation of the tibia. This means using midrange quadriceps work, avoiding terminal knee extension, and emphasizing hamstring strengthening to provide active stabilization. The advanced phase of treatment features eccentric quadriceps exercise and the removal of the extension stop of the rehabilitative brace.[5,39,56,203]

The operative methods of stabilization are either intra-articular or extra-articular. In intra-articular procedures, the site has to undergo revascularization followed by reorganization of collagen.[30,38,161] These procedures therefore necessitate a slower and longer rehabilitation process.[29,30,160,169,170,195]

With the use of securely fixed, high-strength, isometric grafts, the progressive rehabilitation protocol includes early protected motion, neuromuscular rehabilitation, and patellofemoral joint mobilization. Rehabilitation following ACL reconstruction is very lengthy. An athlete with such an injury will usually require a year before returning to full activity.

New synthetic ligaments, which show great promise, have been used both experimentally and clinically. Only a few have been approved for general use at this time by the Food and Drug Administration, and no long-term reports regarding their safety or efficacy are available.[4,22,23,28,69] Whereas a patient with a biological repair must stay on crutches for about 12 weeks and can not resume athletic activities for about a year, it has been estimated that patients with a synthetic ligament, such as a Gore Tex® prosthesis (WL Gore & Associates, Flagstaff, AZ), can be off crutches in a week or so and can resume athletic activities after 6 months.[22,67,121]

Posterior Cruciate Ligament Tear—(Grade III Sprain). Isolated PCL disruptions often have a good prognosis when treated nonoperatively.[42,46,51,167] Their prognosis after direct surgical repair is somewhat better than ACL repair because of a more generous blood supply. Whereas the knee with a torn ACL usually has symptoms of instability, the knee with a torn PCL has symptoms of disability: medial compartment arthritis (60%), patellofemoral arthritis (70%), and swelling and pain related to activity.[167]

Posterior Cruciate Ligament Repair. Acute PCL repair with augmentation appears to have a better success rate than does delayed reconstruction.[149,168] Unless synthetic ligaments are used, early postoperative motion after PCL repair usually is not recommended. A period of 4 to 6 weeks of immobilization is advocated to allow healing of the bone grafts prior to initiating joint motion. The focus of rehabilitation for both surgical and nonsurgical patients is on quadriceps exercises. In conservative rehabilitation the hamstrings are omitted in the early exercise phase, because they may accentuate posterior subluxation. Eccentric quadriceps exercises are started as soon as the patient can tolerate them. A common surgical procedure for posterior cruciate ligament repair is repositioning of the origin of the medial gastrocnemius muscle.[111] This transfer acts dynamically during weight-acceptance and the push-off phases of gait. In this case both quadriceps and gastrocnemius muscles are of primary importance with respect to exercise. Once the quadriceps have achieved 80% of the strength of the normal leg on Cybex® (or a similar testing device), hamstring exercises are added.[184] The length of time to return to sports is about the same as for injury of the ACL.

In addition to hamstring training to prevent anterior subluxation for ACL injuries and quadriceps training to increase structural stiffness and knee strength for PCL injuries,[73,106,212] it is important to include dynamic joint control training.[43,98,212] Even if the hamstrings and quadriceps are strengthened, it is important that they function quickly and adequately during unexpected trauma by improving neuromuscular coordination. Training should consist of balance and proprioception activities, functional development of the feet to grasp the ground, stabilization of the stance position, and improvement of reactions to sudden additional forces applied by the therapist.[98]

Lateral Collateral Ligament Tears—(Grade III Sprain). The lateral collateral ligament (LCL) or fibular collateral ligament is in itself not a very important stabilizing structure and can be treated nonsurgically.[149,168] When the secondary restraints, lateral capsule and cruciates are torn, functional instability is common and surgical correction is usually required. Rehabilitation after repair follows the guidelines for PCL rehabilitation and for posterolateral rotatory instability. Athletes, or other individuals placing unusual demands on the functional capacity of the knee, must undergo a more rigorous retraining program. For these patients, especially, exercises should approximate the type of loading normally imposed on the joint. Most athletic activities, as well as routine activities of daily living, involve relatively high rate loading conditions. Isokinetic exercise equipment with variable speed adjustments is a convenient means of providing high speed resistant to various muscle groups, while at the same time monitoring the percent of maximal torque output. Such exercises not only result in

strengthening, but also optimize the training effect of the exercise program.

Running, jumping, and athletic activities must not be allowed until strength is near normal, range of motion is full, and normal femorotibial rotation has returned. Such activities must be very gradually progressed from straight-ahead jogging to straight-ahead running, then running with gentle turns, and finally running with abrupt stops and turns. It must be emphasized here that clinical signs of healing, such as restoration of strength and range of motion with no pain on stress testing, in no way signify return of normal strength to the injured ligament.[158] Restoration of ligamentous strength requires a maturation process of collagen aggregation and realignment that may take from several months to a year following injury.[3,162] Any advantages of returning to activities involving intermittent high loading of the knee must be weighed against the risk of the still-weakened structure giving way prematurely, possibly resulting in a more serious injury than that originally suffered. In making judgments of appropriate activity levels, the desires of the coach and the highly motivated young athlete must often take second priority to knowledge of the rate and mechanisms of tissue healing.

MENISCUS LESIONS

Meniscus lesions affecting the knee are common injuries, especially in athletes. Once it has been determined through examination that a meniscus lesion exists, it is important that the injury be classified as a tear confined to the periphery or a tear involving the body of the meniscus. Often arthroscopy or arthrography will assist the physician in making this distinction. Most tears involving the body of the medial meniscus are accompanied by an anteromedial coronary ligament sprain.

History

Onset. The menisci move with the tibia in flexion–extension and with the femur in rotation. If, during flexion, external tibial rotation is forced instead of the internal rotation that should normally occur, abnormal stresses are applied to the menisci with the possibility of a tear occurring. The same, of course, applies to the case of forced internal tibial rotation during knee extension. Similarly, flexion or extension taking place in the absence of the normal rotary movement that should accompany it may result in a meniscus tear. The medial meniscus, being less mobile, is more susceptible to injury. Because tibial rotation is not possible in the fully extended knee, the history is one of twisting on a semiflexed knee. Again, athletes, especially those wearing cleated shoes and involved in contact sports, are particularly prone to suffering meniscus injuries, occasionally in conjunction with ligament tears.

Meniscus tears may also occur with hyperflexion of the knee, especially during weight-bearing. In this position, the femoral condyles have rolled back to articulate with the posterior aspects of the tibial articular surfaces. The menisci, then, must recede backward during flexion, but can only recede to a certain point before capsuloligamentous attachments restrict further movement of the menisci. If further flexion is forced once the menisci have reached their limit of backward movement, the menisci are susceptible to being ground between the femoral and tibial joint surfaces. This is especially true if rotation is forced in hyperflexion, because a rotary movement entails further backward movement of one condyle. Certain occupations, such as mining, in which one must move about in a squatting position, may predispose to development of meniscal tears from this mechanism. In athletics, the wrestler is classically prone to this type of injury.

Site of Pain. The person will usually feel "something give" in the joint, often with an accompanying deep, sickening type of pain. If not masked by other injuries or extensive effusion, the patient will often be able to point to the spot on the joint line corresponding to the site of the tear where the coronary ligament has been sprained.

Nature of Pain and Disability. The onset is usually sudden with an immediate deep pain associated with giving way of the joint. If hemarthrosis occurs, the typical severe, generalized pain arising within minutes of the injury is reported. If a longitudinal tear of the medial meniscus extends anteriorly past the midpoint of the meniscus, the lateral portion may slip over the dome of the medial femoral condyle. This grossly interferes with normal knee mechanics, with a resultant immediate locking of the joint so that the last 20° to 30° of extension are lost. An injury involving such immediate locking is usually preceded by one or more previous minor incidences of giving way followed by effusion. Finally, the developing longitudinal tear extends anteriorly far enough to cause such locking.

The person sustaining a meniscus tear is very hesitant to resume activity immediately following the injury, unlike the person suffering a ligamentous sprain. Synovial effusion, causing a generalized pressure sensation, may arise within hours following injury. Effusion nearly always accompanies a medial meniscus tear. It does not always accompany a lateral tear.

In the case of an untreated meniscus tear the acute stage may completely subside with restoration of motion. The person may resume normal activities with little or no pain. The complaint, however, is one of intermittent buckling of the joint for no apparent reason, even during simple walking. Occasional or persistent "clicking" of the joint may be reported. Chronic or intermittent effusion may also occur, probably from altered joint mechanics resulting in undue stress to the joint capsule.

Physical Examination

I. **Acute Stage**
   A. *Observation*
      1. The patient may hobble in on crutches with the knee held slightly flexed and touching down only the toe.
      2. Obvious effusion may be present.
      3. The patient may have difficulty removing the shoe, sock, and trousers.
   B. *Inspection*
      1. Effusion may be noted, especially in the suprapatellar region.
      2. The patient stands with the knee held semi-flexed.
      3. The Helfet test may not be performed because of incomplete extension.
      4. The suprapatellar girth measurement may be increased from effusion.
      5. The skin may appear slightly red and shiny.
   C. *Selective tissue-tension tests*
      1. Active movements
         a. Weight-bearing flexion–extension is impossible.
         b. Flexion–extension in supine reveals the following:
            i. A capsular pattern if effusion is present
            ii. Considerable loss of extension if the knee is locked, causing a distorted capsular pattern if effusion is present, a non-capsular pattern if little or no effusion is present
         c. Passive overpressure reveals a muscle-guarding end feel at the extremes of flexion and extension.
         d. If the knee is locked, a springy-rebound end feel will be noted moving into extension.
      2. Passive movements

a. These are essentially the same as indicated above for active movement, with perhaps slightly greater range of movement.

b. McMurray's test may not be performed if considerable effusion restricts flexion, because it is only applicable from full flexion to 90°. If flexion is possible, a painful click may be elicited on combined external rotation and extension if a tear exists in the posterior portion of the medial meniscus, or on combined internal rotation and extension if a posterior lateral meniscus lesion exists.

3. Resisted isometric movements. These should be strong and painless unless a tendon or muscle has also been injured. Quantitative strength measurements cannot be made because of the acute condition.

4. Passive joint-play movements
   a. Rotation opposite the side of the lesion may be painful, especially during Apley's test with compression applied. Distraction with rotation should relieve the pain.
   b. Otherwise, these movements should be relatively normal unless a ligamentous injury also exists.

D. *Palpation*
   1. Tenderness will be present at the joint line where a sprain of the peripheral attachment has occurred. This usually corresponds quite well with the side and site of the tear.
   2. Effusion, as mentioned, nearly always accompanies a medial meniscus tear, but not always a lateral tear. The tap test and emptying of the suprapatellar pouch will confirm the presence of minor effusion.
   3. The joint is warm, and the skin somewhat moist.

II. Chronic Tear

A. *History.* The patient describes intermittent giving way of the joint, often followed by some effusion, especially if the medial meniscus is at fault. There may be a history of locking with manipulative reduction by the patient, a friend, or physician, followed by immediate relief of pain and restoration of extension. The younger, active person is usually suffering a longitudinal tear, beginning posteriorly and gradually extending anteri-

orly. The older person may have a "degenerative" horizontal tear, with sliding occurring between the upper and lower portions. Clicking is noted by the patient when the femoral condyle passes over a centrally protruding piece of a meniscus.

B. *Objective signs*
   1. Quadriceps atrophy, especially involving the vastus medialis.
   2. Full range of motion, but perhaps some difficulty or apprehension when performing weight-bearing flexion–extension.
   3. Possibly a positive Helfet test owing to altered joint mechanics.
   4. Possibly a positive McMurray test if the posterior segment of the meniscus is torn.
   5. Pain on forced extension if the anterior segment of meniscus is torn.
   6. A positive Apley test when the joint is compressed, but not when it is distracted.
   7. Tenderness to palpation at the joint line, usually corresponding to the site of the lesion.
   8. Perhaps some mild chronic effusion.
   9. Quantitative quadriceps weakness compared to the other leg.

III. Coronary Ligament Sprain

A. *History.* The patient usually describes a twisting injury followed by some minor swelling and pain over the anteromedial knee region. Rarely is the victim significantly disabled immediately following the injury, and he or she usually does not seek medical attention in the acute stage.

The acute symptoms usually subside within a few days. If the meniscus maintains good mobility during healing, the patient should have no further problems. However, often the coronary ligament becomes adhered to the anteromedial margin of the medial tibial condyle as it heals, resulting in reduced mobility of this part of the meniscus. In such cases, the individual develops a more chronic problem characterized by intermittent twinging of the pain when the adhered tissue is stressed, usually with activities involving external rotation of the tibia on the femur. It is the persistent nature of the problem that eventually prompts the individual to seek medical assistance even though the disorder is otherwise minor.

B. *Objective findings*
   1. Consistent findings on physical examination.

a. Point tenderness over the anteromedial joint line.
b. Pain on external rotation of the tibia on the femur, but no pain on valgus stress.
2. Occasionally forced extension hurts as well. Rarely is effusion present by the time the person is seen clinically. There may be some minimal quadriceps atrophy if the problem has been long-standing.

Management

Acute Tear of the Body of a Meniscus.   If an acute meniscus tear is suspected on examination, the referring physician should be consulted and notified of the positive findings. Usually following arthroscopic evaluation of the knee joint, if an isolated tear is encountered (*i.e.*, one without concomitant ligament damage) a decision must be made as to whether repair or removal is the best treatment. Meniscal repair is a growing trend in orthopaedics. Immobilization is necessary following meniscal repair. If the procedure proves successful, recovery is expected in about 6 months. The majority of meniscal injuries still require removal of the torn portion of the meniscus. Clearly, arthroscopy has been shown to be the most effective way of doing this.[52,149] If surgery is not planned, treatment in the acute stage is essentially the same as that discussed in this chapter for an acute, minor ligamentous sprain (see p. 340). Weight-bearing must not be allowed on a locked knee and should be restricted on a knee that cannot fully extend because of effusion. Extension must not be forced in the locked knee, because, if the displaced piece of meniscus does not slip back, extension may occur only at the expense of the anterior cruciate ligament or articular cartilage.

Chronic Tear of the Body of a Meniscus.   Again, the physician should be notified if this is suspected. If arthroscopic surgery is not contemplated, the goal is restoration of optimal joint mechanics: mobilization, strengthening, and instruction in appropriate activity levels are necessary. A particular motion, especially extension, must not be encouraged if the restriction is secondary to an intra-articular block, as from a displaced piece of meniscus. Throughout meniscal rehabilitation, it is important to minimize compressive loading of the joint until adequate muscular protection and joint reorganization have been developed.

Coronary Ligament Tear.   Persons with coronary ligament tears are generally seen in the chronic stage only, because the acute pain and disability are usually not severe. The persistent intermittent knee pain is the result of adherence of the anteromedial coronary ligament to the underlying tibia; the adhesion is broken with some sudden movement, then adherence recurs during healing.

The objective of treatment is to gradually restore mobility to this part of the meniscus. This is accomplished through the use of ultrasound and transverse friction massage applied directly to the site of the lesion. Five to ten minutes of massage, over three to four treatment sessions are usually sufficient. Attention should be paid to quadriceps weakness if present. The patient may be instructed in self-administered friction massage, to be applied before activity.

EXTENSOR MECHANISM DISORDERS

Of all the knee problems presenting to the physical therapist, the most common are disorders of the extensor mechanism. The term extensor mechanism encompasses several anatomic structures: the patella and its articular surface as well as the trochlear surface of the femur, the patellar tendon and its attachment to both patella and tibial tuberosity, all of the associated supporting soft tissues (such as retinaculum, peripatellar synovium, and the structures known as synovial plica), the various parts of the quadriceps musculature, and the quadriceps tendon attachment into the patella.

PATELLAR TRACKING DYSFUNCTION (Chondromalacia Patellae)

Disorders of the patellofemoral joint constitute a large percentage of chronic knee problems of nontraumatic origin. Unfortunately, nonacute patellofemoral joint dysfunctions tend to be referred to as "chondromalacia patellae," which literally means *softening of the articular cartilage of the patella.* Because articular cartilage is not a pain-sensitive structure, the term "chondromalacia" does not adequately describe the clinically significant features of the pathologic process, nor does it take into account etiologic considerations. In fact, surgical studies suggest that surface chondromalacia *per se* is a relatively normal characteristic of most adult patellae and probably has little relationship in cause or effect to symptomatic knee problems.[2,77,148,165,185,199]

Biomechanical Considerations

The patella is a triangular sesamoid bone receiving attachment from above by the quadriceps tendon, medially and laterally from the patellar retinacula,

Fig. 14–22. Pull of the patellar tendon during loaded knee extension, showing the Q angle, and longitudinal and lateral vectoral components.

the patella to be pulled laterally with respect to the long axis of the femur during loaded knee extension.

As the patella glides inferiorly and superiorly during knee flexion and extension, it should do so in line with the long axis of the femur. It is important then that excessive lateral patellar movement does not occur. Prevention of excessive lateral patellar movement during loaded knee extension depends on structural and dynamic mechanisms of patellar stabilization. Structural factors include the following:

1. *Lateral femoral condyle* which, because it is prominent anteriorly, provides some abutment against lateral patellar movement (see Fig. 14–2).
2. *Deep patellar groove of the femur*, in which the patella glides when the knee is in positions of flexion.
3. *Angle between the pull of the quadriceps and the pull of the patellar tendon.* When the knee is in positions of flexion, there is an angle between the pull of the quadriceps and the pull of the patellar tendon, projected onto the sagittal plane (Fig. 14–23). The result of these pulls, represented vectorially, is a patellofemoral compressive force that holds the patella tightly against the patellar groove of the femur, disallowing extraneous movement.

and inferiorly from the patellar tendon. The patella glides inferiorly with respect to the femoral condyles when the knee is flexed, and superiorly when the knee is extended.

Because the medial femoral condyle extends further distally than does the lateral condyle, most knee joints assume a slight valgus angulation in the standing position (see Figs. 14–1, 14–13, and 14–22). The direction of pull of the quadriceps musculature tends to be in line with the femur, whereas the pull of the patellar tendon is in line with the long axis of the tibia. The angle formed between the line of pull of the quadriceps muscle and the patellar tendon is the Q angle.

The vector that represents the pull on the patellar tendon during loaded knee extension can be resolved into a longitudinal component and a lateral component (see Fig. 14–22). The longitudinal component is in line with the direction of pull of the quadriceps and with the long axis of the femur. The lateral vectorial component causes a tendency for

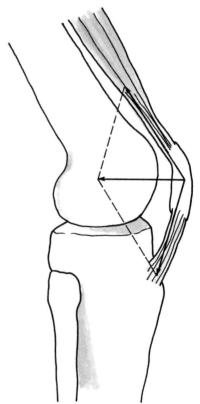

Fig. 14–23. Patellofemoral compression forces in the sagittal plane with the knee in a flexed position.

It should be noted that the structural stabilizing mechanisms mentioned here are primarily operational in positions of some knee flexion. As the knee approaches full extension, the patella begins moving superiorly out of the deep part of the patellar groove of the femur. In this position the sagittally projected angulation between the quadriceps muscle and patellar tendon decreases, thus reducing the patellofemoral compressive force that holds the patella firmly in the groove. As the knee moves into extension, especially when loaded, dynamic patellar stabilizing factors play an essential role.

The most important dynamic factor necessary to assure normal patellofemoral joint function is contraction of the vastus medialis obliquus (VMO) muscle. The distal fibers of the VMO originate from the medial aspect of the distal femur and run almost horizontally to insert on the medial aspect of the patella. They attach to the patella by way of the medial retinaculum. The horizontal orientation of these fibers of the VMO allows them to prevent excessive lateral movement of the patella during loaded knee extension (Fig. 14–24).

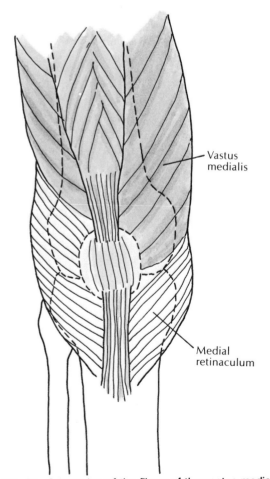

Fig. 14–24. Orientation of the fibers of the vastus medialis.

Vastus
medialis

Medial
retinaculum

Etiology

Chronic patellar tracking dysfunction is a condition in which the patella tends to be pulled too far laterally each time the knee is extended under load. Possible causes, both structural and dynamic, might include the following:

1. An increase in the valgus angulation between the quadriceps muscle and the patellar tendon, often referred to as an increased Q angle (see Fig. 14–22). Common causes are (1) increased femoral anteversion, (2) increased external tibial torsion, and (3) increased foot pronation.
2. A lateral femoral condyle that is not sufficiently prominent anteriorly. This results in a loss of the abutment effect normally provided by the lateral condyle (Fig. 14–25).
3. A small, high-riding patella, often called *patella alta*. The more superiorly the patella moves on the femur during knee extension, the less time it spends in the deep portion of the patellar groove, where it is better stabilized.

Dynamically, the most important cause of reduced lateral patellar stabilization is VMO insufficiency. This commonly occurs from disuse atrophy associated with immobilization or following injury to the knee. It may also occur when a person increases activities involving loaded knee extension, and the vastus medialis is not adequately conditioned to meet the added loads imposed on the extensor mechanism.

Pathologic Process

In order to best understand the clinical manifestations of patellar tracking dysfunction, we must first discuss the pathologic implications of excessive lateral patellar movement. As the patella moves against the femoral condyles, the contact area on the back of the patella varies with the position of the knee. During normal knee function, both the medial and lateral facets of the patellar articular surface receive compressive stresses from contact with the femur. The small odd medial facet, however, only makes contact at extremes of knee flexion, a position that the knee seldom assumes during normal daily activities (Fig. 14–26).[77] Thus, during normal use of the knee, the odd medial facet is nonarticulating and does not receive much compressive stress. Because of this, the subchondral bone is less dense, softer, and weaker at the odd medial facet, compared with that of the rest of the patella (Fig. 14–27).[173,206–208]

If the patella is pulled too far laterally during loaded knee extension, movement of the patella will

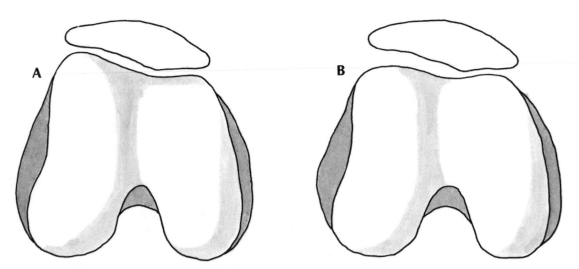

Fig. 14–25. Femoral condyles, showing *(A)* normal prominence of the lateral condyle and *(B)* insufficient prominence of the lateral condyle anteriorly.

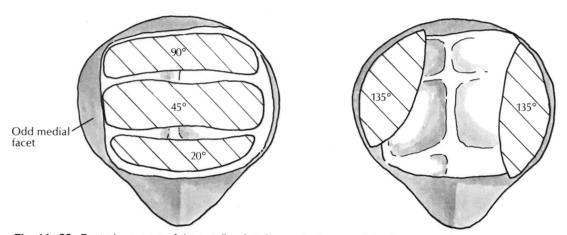

Fig. 14–26. Posterior aspect of the patella, showing contact areas of the facets during various degrees of flexion.

Fig. 14–27. Diagram of subchondral bone density of the patella. Density is reduced in the area of the odd medial facet.

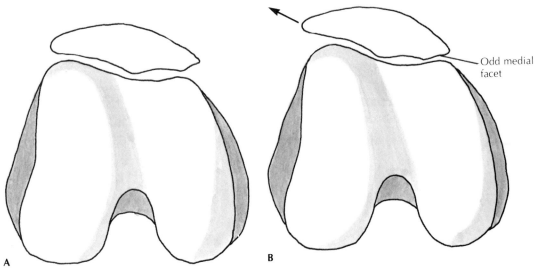

Fig. 14–28. *(A)* Position of patella during normal, loaded knee extension. *(B)* Abnormal lateral pull of the patella during loaded knee extension brings the odd medial facet into a contacting position.

follow the contour of the patellar groove of the femur. This causes the patella to undergo some rotation in the transverse plane, bringing the odd medial facet into a contacting position (Fig. 14–28). Under such conditions the relatively weak subchondral bone of the odd medial facet may not be able to withstand the loads imposed on it. This results in an increase rate of trabecular microfracturing, which may incite a low-grade, painful inflammatory response. Trabecular breakdown may be further enhanced by shear stresses between the soft odd medial facet and the stiffer medial facet during compressive deformation.[208] For a particular load, the odd medial facet would deform more than the medial facet, resulting in shearing when the two are compressed simultaneously. This would cause the pathologic process to progress into the medial facet of the patella.

Excessive lateral patellar movement during repeated knee extension may also cause abnormal tensile stresses to the medial retinaculum of the knee. This could also be a source of low-grade inflammation and pain associated with patellar tracking dysfunction.

Clinical Manifestations

The patient presenting with patellar tracking dysfunction usually demonstrates characteristic symptoms and signs consistent with the etiologic and pathologic factors mentioned. The consistent subjective complaints of a patient presenting with patellar tracking dysfunction include the following:

1. A gradual onset of pain. The patient often describes some recent increase in activities involving loaded knee extension or may report some knee injury or disuse preceding the onset of the problem.
2. Pain is felt primarily in a generalized area over the medial aspect of the knee and in the peripatellar regions.
3. The pain is aggravated by activities involving increased patellofemoral compressive stresses. These typically include walking down stairs and sitting with the knee bent for long periods of time. Slowly applied loads, such as those involved with sitting with the knees bent, are likely to cause more discomfort than high strain rate loading such as running or walking. This is because bone is stronger under fast strain rates for loads of equal magnitude.

The objective findings on physical examination of patients with patellar tracking dysfunction might include any of the following:

1. Some structural predisposing factor, such as an increased Q angle or a high-riding patella. Common causes of an increased Q angle include iliotibial band tightness, femoral anteversion, external tibial torsion, and increased foot pronation.

   To ascertain the weight-bearing status of the foot and detect any excessive pronation, determine the neutral position of the subtalar joint (see Chapter 15, The Ankle and Hindfoot). The normal weight-bearing foot should demonstrate a mild amount of pronation. If the patient is weight-bearing or running with the foot out of neutral position and near full pronation, an obligatory internal tibial rotation occurs and is actually prolonged, resulting in an increased force that is absorbed by the soft tissues of the knee.[102,103] Entities that will produce compensatory subtalar pronation include genu varum, triceps surae contractures, hindfoot varus, and forefoot supination.[27,99,102,103]

2. Other structural factors include marked tibia vara, especially when the varus is sharply localized to the tibia. If a lateral angulation of the tibia to the floor angle is greater than 10°, the extremity requires an excessive amount of subtalar joint pronation to produce a plantigrade foot. This can occur in both genu varum and tibia vara and may be a cause for peripatellar pain.[35]

3. Congenital recurvatum, which may be associated with patella alta and with generalized joint laxity with relative patellar hypermobility.[171,214] Leg-length discrepancy may result in hyperextension on the shorter side during single-leg stance and at the push-off phase of gait, which may accelerate extensor mechanism difficulties.[21,211]

4. Abnormal patellar tracking and patellofemoral crepitus during weight-bearing (if the tissue breakdown has spread to surface layers of articular cartilage). Abnormal patellar tracking may be observed in sitting as the patient flexes and extends the knee. The patella normally has 5 to 7 cm of longitudinal excursion with flexion and extension as it enters and exits the trochlear groove.[35] Normally there should be smooth longitudinal trajectory with a small amount of physiological rotation occurring.[122] Any abrupt or sudden movements at 10° to 30° flexion, as the patella enters or exits the femoral trochlea, is considered abnormal (i.e., abrupt lateral translations just before or at the end of extension, or a semicircular route of the patella as if it were pivoting around the lateral trochlear facet).[62] One other sign of abnormal position and tracking is the "grasshopper eye" patella. This is a combination of both high and lateral positions of the patella.[102]

5. Tightness of the lateral retinaculum noted when the patella is moved and when the retinaculum is palpated.[68]

6. Visible VMO atrophy when the patient is asked to strongly contract the quadriceps against resistance at 30°.

7. Discomfort when the patella is passively moved laterally (if the medial retinaculum is irritated) and tenderness to deep palpation of the back side of the medial patella and to palpation of the adductor tubercle, where the medial retinaculum attaches.

8. Alterations in stability (see Patellar Stability, p. 329).

9. Patellar discomfort elicited by provocation tests, which might include:
   a. Maintained inferior glide with an isometric contraction of the quadriceps.
   b. Resisted quadriceps contraction with the knee held at 30° to 45° flexion.

Management

Treatment of patellar tracking dysfunction must take into consideration etiologic and pathologic factors. The most important early measure is the reduction of activities involving high or prolonged patellofemoral compressive loads. This is necessary in order to prevent continued tissue trauma. The patient must understand the deleterious affects of such activities as descending stairs or bent-knee sitting, because these activities do not necessarily cause immediate pain.

Particular attention should be paid to strengthening the VMO. This may be necessary to correct VMO insufficiency or as an attempt to compensate for structural causes of patellar tracking dysfunction. In order to strengthen the VMO, it is often necessary to establish VMO control through techniques of neuromuscular facilitation (i.e., quick-stretch, cross-limb reversal; repeated contractions) and electrical stimulation.[176,193,202] Starting with quadriceps-setting exercises, progress to SLR, short-arc quadriceps (starting eccentrically), and finally to concentric contractions (as tolerated) with range limitation of 0° to 30° terminal knee extension. For training to be effective, the patient must not experience pain while exercising, because this will have a strong inhibitory effect on muscle function.[191,198] To enhance more normal tracking, the patella should be exercised during weight-bearing and it should be firmly taped in the direction of normal tracking during these exercises. The three components of the patella that must be assessed before taping are:

1. Rotation — The longitudinal axis of the femur and the patella should be in line with one another. To correct any alterations in alignment, firm taping from either the superior or inferior poles can be used. To correct external rotation of the inferior pole, tape from the middle inferior pole upward; for internal rotation of the inferior pole, tape from the middle superior pole downward.

2. Tilt—Most patients will present with a positive tilt sign (0° or less) because of tightness of the deep lateral retinacular fibers (Fig. 14–21A). Correction of this lateral tilt requires stretching and soft-tissue mobilizations. The patella should be firmly taped from the midline of the patella medially to lift the lateral border and provide a passive stretch to the lateral structures.
3. Glide—Most patients will require mobilization of the patella; usually, medial glide of the patella is most restricted.

Weight-bearing training is very important, because the knee primarily functions in a closed kinetic chain. Training in weight-bearing also places a major emphasis on eccentric control, thus facilitating muscle hypertrophy.[75,80] According to McConnell the following exercises have been found to be most useful:[146]

1. With the patient in a walk-stance position (symptomatic leg forward) and the knee flexed to 30°, the patient is instructed to contract the VMO and hold for a period of 10 seconds or so while the foot is supinated past subtalar neutral and then allowed to slowly return to partial pronation (slightly out of the resting position of pronation). This is repeated several times, then the knee is straightened and the exercise repeated. The object is to train the invertors of the foot, thus decreasing pronation.
2. The same exercise as above is repeated but with the knee flexed to about 70°. If the patient has difficulty achieving VMO control with either of these exercises, a slightly turned-out position may facilitate control. The patient should be instructed to relax the vastus lateralis and hamstrings as much as possible with both of these exercises. Pain-free progression may include half and three-quarter squats as greater control of the quadriceps is achieved.
3. Descending stairs is performed as an exercise to further facilitate eccentric and concentric quadriceps control. The leg to be exercised remains on the top step while the patient steps down and then back up slowly, with the leg remaining on the step contracting eccentrically and concentrically. Emphasis is again placed on proper alignment and normal tracking. Progression can be made by altering the height of the step or providing resistance.
4. Hamstring exercises are generally included, starting with hamstring sets and progressing to hamstring curls (as tolerated) with flexion limitations of 90°. To facilitate co-contractions, weight-bearing minisquats (up to 30° of knee flexion) and step-up exercises are most effective.

Assess the extensibility of the lateral retinaculum by noting the excursion of medial patellar movement with the knee close to full extension. If the lateral retinaculum appears tight, it should be stretched using the same technique as used to test its mobility. The effectiveness of stretching procedures may be enhanced by prior or simultaneous heating with ultrasound.

If the condition is associated with abnormal foot pronation and does not respond to the treatment measures mentioned, the clinician should consider stabilization of the foot to control pronation. This may be accomplished with various orthotic devices, such as a contoured arch support, or shoe modifications, such as a medial heel wedge or lateral sole wedge.

If a tight iliotibial band is found to contribute to functional valgus deviation at the knee, institute procedures to stretch the iliotibial band. A reverse Ober test may be used to manually stretch the entire band. This is best done passively with the patient lying on the involved side. The examiner sits behind the patient's pelvis to stabilize it against rolling backward. He or she positions the leg to be stretched with the hip in extension and neutral rotation and flexes the knee to about 90°. While providing support under the patient's knee and preventing hip rotation or knee extension, the therapist stretches the iliotibial band by adducting the extended hip away from the plinth. Mennell's selective stretching of various parts of the band and muscle belly may be used as well as other soft-tissue mobilization techniques.[150] Strong medial glide techniques with the patient in sidelying have proved to be most effective at stretching the tight lateral structures around the knee.[146] According to McConnell, this maneuver facilitates VMO training because patellar movements are no longer restricted.[146]

It is important to emphasize that tight hamstrings have long been recognized as a cause of various extensor mechanism disorders.[14,97] Efficient lengthening can be accomplished by gentle, nonballistic techniques (i.e., reciprocal inhibition of antagonists: contract–relax, hold–relax), prolonged static stretch, and soft-tissue mobilization techniques.[49,60,179,192,201] In the presence of leg-length discrepancy and a hyperextended knee, correction of the abnormal gait by a combination of a heel lift, gait training (employing a program of resistive pelvic training/PNF techniques), and quadriceps control exercises have been found to be effective.[115,211]

A final tool in the conservative management of patellar tracking dysfunction is some type of brace or external support. Generally it is recommended that taping or braces should be used with exercise and activity programs. Numerous knee braces are available.[125,166] These generally provide support for the knee, avoid direct pressure on the patella, prevent lateral subluxation, or create an uplift of the patella.

Shoe orthoses may be helpful in patients who have patellofemoral pain associated with pronated feet.[190]

There are few patients with patellar tracking dysfunction who do not respond satisfactorily to a well-designed and appropriately instituted conservative treatment program. Common causes of failure include (1) inadequate restriction of activities in the early stages of treatment or (2) inadequate or inappropriate quadriceps strengthening.

The rare patient who does not respond satisfactorily to a well-instituted conservative program may be a surgical candidate.[16,77,99] Surgery may involve loosening of a tight lateral retinaculum or reduction of the Q angle by moving the attachment of the patellar tendon medially. Occasionally the medial structures of the extensor mechanism are tightened as well.

THE PLICA SYNDROME

The medial synovial plica is found in 60% of normal knees.[168] Occasionally this plica may become thickened and fibrotic causing anteromedial knee pain and snapping. Conservative management using extensor mechanism rehabilitative techniques and ice massage may reverse conditions with mild inflammatory changes. If conservative treatment fails, arthroscopic excision may be undertaken to relieve symptoms. It is often necessary to continue work on the extensor mechanism through exercise and perhaps an external support.

PATELLAR TENDINITIS (Jumper's Knee)

Repetitive jumping in sports such as volleyball and basketball can create chronic inflammatory changes of the patellar or quadriceps tendon. These changes primarily are related to overuse. Pain is the key complaint and is associated with swelling and joint tenderness.

Patellar tendinitis rarely, if ever, occurs in knees without predisposing physical findings found in tracking problems (*i.e.*, patella alta, VMO dysplasia).[214] Many factors known to aggravate extensor mechanism disorders can accentuate the symptoms of patellar tendinitis (inflexibility of hamstrings or triceps surae). Traditionally, extensor mechanism

rehabilitation to deal with patellar tendinitis has been used. More recently, work on eccentric function of the quadriceps has been emphasized in dealing with this disorder. The basis of this program is to use activities that place maximal stress on the tendon in order to increase its tensile stress by performing variations of quick mini-squats.[44] Biomechanical linkage with ankle mechanics have demonstrated that most patients present with weakness of the ankle dorsiflexors. Again, good results have been obtained with a program of eccentric work.[97,214]

Flexibility training is important because not only does it increase elasticity of the muscle–tendon unit, but also it may increase the tensile strength of the tendon. Ice massage to the inflamed area and friction massage to the tendon are also helpful.

POPLITEAL AND SEMIMEMBRANOSUS TENDINITIS

Tendinitis of the popliteal or semimembranosus tendons follows overuse injuries, usually from long-distance running. Hyperpronation of the foot may result in either popliteal or bicipital tendinitis at the knee secondary to overuse.

In popliteal tendinitis the patient complains of localized pain over the lateral aspect of the knee. With the knee in the "figure-four" position, the lateral collateral ligament and popliteal tendon are stretched and can be palpated. When the popliteal tendon is inflamed, joint tenderness is noticed at its insertion on the femur anterior to the lateral condyle.[97]

Tendinitis of the semimembranosus can mimic a meniscal injury because of its proximity to the joint line. The semimembranosus functions synergistically with the popliteus to prevent excessive external rotation of the tibia. Therefore, hyperpronating problems of the foot can stress the insertion of the semimembranosus.

Treatment of these conditions consists of rest, ice for the first 72 hours, ultrasound, and flexibility/strengthening exercises. Proper training techniques and appropriate shoewear should also be addressed.

OSGOOD–SCHLATTER DISEASE

Osgood–Schlatter disease has in the past been considered a form of osteochondritis associated with a partial avulsion of the patellar tendon at its insertion into the tibial tubercle before this apophysis unites. More recent thinking views the process as one part of the spectrum of mechanical problems related to the extensor mechanism.[214] Almost all patients with this condition have some mechanical inefficiency of the extensor mechanism.

In fact, it is now felt that this is not really a "disease," but a form of tendinitis of the knee tendon. In young athletes, the tendon is attached to prebone, which is weaker than normal adult bone. With excessive stresses on the tendon from running and jumping, the structure becomes irritated and a tendinitis begins.

Objective findings include the following:

1. A tender swelling over the tibial tubercle
2. Pain is reproduced on resisting quadriceps extension. Squatting may also reproduce the pain.
3. Decreased flexibility. Most patients have significant restriction in the hamstrings, triceps surae, and quadriceps muscles.

With respect to treatment, the mechanical inefficiencies of the extensor mechanism should be treated by appropriate rehabilitative exercises. Inflexibility should be addressed through stretching and ankle dorsiflexion strengthening if weakness is found. This condition usually resolves without any significant additional treatment. Complete immobilization is neither necessary nor practical. Some sort of simple patellar support, such as a Neoprene® rubber knee sleeve, may be helpful.

REFERENCES

1. Abbott B, Bigland B, Ritche JM: The physiological cost of negative work. J Physiol 117:380–390, 1952
2. Abernathy PJ, Townsend PR, Rose RM, et al: Is chondromalacia patellae a separate clinical entity? J Bone Joint Surg 60(B):205–210, 1978
3. Adams A: Effect of exercise upon ligament strength. Res Q 37:163–167, 1966
4. Ahlfeld SK, Larson RL, Collins HR: Anterior cruciate reconstruction in the chronically unstable knee using an expanded polytetrafluoroethylene (PTFE) prosthetic ligament. Am J Sports Med 15:326–330, 1987
5. American Academy of Orthopaedic Surgeons: Knee braces: Seminar report. Chicago: American Academy of Orthopaedic Surgeons, 1985
6. Anderson AF, Lipscomb AB: Clinical diagnosis of meniscal tears: Description of a new manipulative test. Am J Sports Med 14:291–293, 1986
7. Andrews JR, Mc Leod WD, Ward T, et al: The cutting mechanism. Am J Sports Med 5:111–121, 1977
8. Apley G: The diagnosis of meniscus injuries. J Bone Joint Surg 29(A):78–84, 1947
9. Arnoczsky SP: The blood supply of the meniscus and its role in healing and repair. In American Academy of Orthopaedic Surgeons Symposium on Sports Medicine: The Knee, pp 94–110. St Louis, CV Mosby, 1982
10. Arnold JA, Coker TP, Heaton LM, et al: Natural history of anterior cruciate tears. Am J Sports Med 7:305–313, 1979
11. Barnett CH: Locking at the knee joint. J Anat 87:91–95, 1953
12. Barry OCD, McManus F, McCauley P: Clinical assessment of suspected meniscal tears. Ir J Med Sci 152:149–151, 1983
13. Beck C, Drez D, Young J, et al: Instrumental testing of functional knee braces. Am J Sports Med 14:253–256, 1986
14. Beck JL, Wildermuth BP: The female athlete's knee. Clin Sports Med 4:345–366, 1985
15. Bentley GL: Chondromalacia patellae. J Bone Joint Surg 52(A):221–232, 1970
16. Bentley GL: The surgical treatment of chondromalacia patellae. J Bone Joint Surg 60(B):74–81, 1978
17. Berger RA, Mathus DL: Movement time with various resistance loads as a function of pretensed and prerelaxed muscular contraction. Res Q 40:456, 1969
18. Bergfeld J: Functional rehabilitation of isolated medial collateral ligament sprains. Am J Sports Med 7:207–209, 1979
19. Blackburn TA: Rehabilitation of anterior cruciate ligament injuries. Orthop Clin North Am 16:141–269, 1985
20. Blackburn TA, Eiland WG, Brady WD: An introduction to the plica. J Orthop Sports Ther 3:171–177, 1982
21. Blustein M, D'Amico JC: Limb length discrepancy: Identification, clinical significance and management. Phys Ther 75:200–206, 1985
22. Bolton CW, Bruchman WC: The Gore-Tex expanded polytetrafluoroethylene prosthetic ligament: An *in vitro* and *in vivo* evaluation. Clin Orthop 196:202–213, 1985
23. Bonnarens FO, Drez D: Biomechanics of artificial ligaments and associated problems. In Jackson DW, Drez D (eds): The Anterior Cruciate Deficient Knee: New Concepts in Ligament Repair, pp 239–253. St Louis, CV Mosby, 1987
24. Bonnarens FO, Drez D: Clinical examination of the knee for anterior cruciate ligament laxity. In Jackson DW, Drez D (eds): The Anterior Cruciate Deficient Knee: New Concepts in Ligament Repair, pp 72–89. St Louis, CV Mosby, 1987
25. Bosco C, Komi PV: Potentiation of the mechanical behavior of the human skeletal muscle through prestretching. Acta Physiol Scand 106:467–472, 1979
26. Brody D: Techniques in the evaluation and treatment of the injured runner. Orthop Clin North Am 13:541–558, 1982
27. Brubaker CE, James SL: Injuries to runners. J Sports Med 2:189–198, 1974
28. Burri C, Henkemeyer H, Neugebauer R: Technique and results of alloplastic carbon fibre ligament substitution. Aktuel Probl Chir Orthop 26:135–147, 1983
29. Cabaud HE, Feagin JA, Rodkey WG: Acute anterior cruciate ligament injury and augmented repair. Am J Sports Med 8:395–401, 1980

30. Cabaud HE, Rodkey WG, Feagin JA: Experimental studies of acute anterior cruciate ligament injury and repair. Am J Sports Med 7:18–22, 1979
31. Cabaud HE, Slocum DB: The diagnosis of chronic anterolateral rotary instability of the knee. Am J Sports Med 5:99–104, 1977
32. Campbell D, Glenn W: Foot-pound torque of the normal knee and the rehabilitated post-meniscectomy knee. Phys Ther 59:418–421, 1979
33. Campbell D, Glenn W: Rehabilitation of knee flexors and extensor muscle strength in patients with meniscectomies, ligamentous repairs and chondromalacia. Phys Ther 62:10–15, 1982
34. Cannon WD: Follow-up of ACL reconstructions and studies with the knee laxity tester. Presented at the meeting of the Anterior Cruciate Ligament Study Group, Steamboat Springs, Colorado, March 16, 1984
35. Carson WG: Diagnosis of extensor mechanical disorders. Clin Sports Med 4(2):231–246, 1985
36. Cavagna GA, Dusman B, Margaria R: Positive work done by a previously stretched muscle. J Appl Physiol 24:21–32, 1968
37. Cavagna GA, Saibene FP, Margaria R: Effects of negative work on the amount of positive work performed by an isolated muscle. J Appl Physiol 20(1):157–158, 1965
38. Clancy WG, Nelson DA, Reider B, et al: Anterior cruciate ligament reconstruction using one-third of the patellar ligament augmented by extra-articular tendon transfers. J Bone Joint Surg 64(A):352–359, 1982
39. Colville MR, Lee CL, Ciullo V: The Lenox Hill brace: An evaluation of effectiveness in treating knee instability. Am J Sports Med 14:257–261, 1986
40. Corrigan B, Maitland GD: Practical Orthopaedic Medicine. Boston, Butterworths, 1985
41. Costill DL: Muscle rehabilitation after knee surgery. Phys Sports Med 5:71–74, 1977
42. Cross MJ, Powell JF: Long-term follow-up of posterior cruciate ligament rupture: A study of 116 cases. Am J Sports Med 12:292–297, 1984
43. Curt WW, Markey KL, Mitchell WA: Agility training following anterior cruciate ligament reconstruction. Clin Orthop 172:133–136, 1983
44. Curwin S, Stanish WD: Tendinitis: Its etiology and treatment. Lexington, Massachusetts, Collamore Press, 1984
45. Cyriax J: Textbook of Orthopaedic Medicine, 11th ed., Vol II, Treatment by Manipulation, Massage and Injections, pp 200–215. London, Bailliere Tindall, 1980
46. Dandy DJ, Pusey RJ: The long-term results of unrepaired tears of the posterior cruciate ligament. J Bone Joint Surg 64(B):92–94, 1984
47. Daniels DM: Instrumented measurement of anterior knee laxity. Presented at the meeting of the Anterior Cruciate Ligament Study Group, Steamboat Springs, Colorado, March 17, 1984
48. Daniels DM, Malcom LL, Losse G, et al: Instrumented measurement of anterior laxity of the knee. J Bone Joint Surg 67(A):720–726, 1985
49. Davis VB: Flexibility conditioning for running. In D'Ambrosia R, Drez D (eds): Prevention and Treatment of Running Injuries, pp 147–154. Thorofare, New Jersey, Slack, Inc. 1982
50. de Andrade JR, Grant C, Dixon A: Joint distension and reflex muscle inhibition in the knee. J Bone Joint Surg 47(A):313–321, 1967
51. Degenhardt TC: Chronic posterior cruciate ligament instability: Nonoperative management. Orthop Trans 5:486–487, 1981
52. DeHaven KE: Rationale for meniscus repair or excision. Clin Sports Med 4:267–273, 1985
53. DeLee JC, Riley MR, Rockwood CA: Acute straight lateral instability of the knee. Am J Sports Med 11:404–411, 1983
54. DeVries HA: Physiology of Exercise. Dubuque, Wm C Brown, 1974
55. Dixon A St J: Factors in the development and presentation of osteoarthritis of the knee. In Dixon A St J (ed): Progress in Clinical Rheumatology, pp 313–329. London, J & A Churchill, 1965
56. Drez D: Knee braces. In Jackson DW, Drez D (eds): The Anterior Cruciate Deficient Knee: New Concepts in Ligament Repair, pp 286–290. St Louis, CV Mosby, 1987
57. Drez D, Kinnard WH: Clinical examination. In Shahriaree H (ed): O'Connor's Textbook of Arthroscopic Surgery. Philadelphia, JB Lippincott, 1984
58. Ellsasser JC, Reynolds KC, Omohundro JR: The nonoperative treatment of collateral ligament injuries of the knee in professional football players. J Bone Joint Surg 56(A):1185–1190, 1974
59. Engin AE, Korde MS: Mechanics of normal and abnormal knee joint. J Biomechanics 7:325–334, 1974
60. Evjenth E, Hamberg J: Muscle Stretching in Manual Therapy: A Clinical Manual, Vol 1, The Extremities, pp 126–132. Alfta, Sweden, Alfta Rehab Forhaj, 1984
61. Fetto JF, Marshall JL: The natural history and diagnosis of anterior cruciate ligament insufficiency. Clin Orthop 147:29–38, 1980
62. Ficat RP, Philippe T, Hungerford DS: Chondromalacia patellae. Clin Orthop 144:55–62, 1979
63. Frankel VH, Nordin M: Basic Biomechanics of the Skeletal System, 2nd ed. Philadelphia, Lea & Febiger, 1980
64. Frankel VH, Burstein AH: Orthopaedic Biomechanics. Philadelphia, Lea & Febiger, 1971
65. Frankel VH, Burstein AH, Brooks DB: Biomechanics of internal derangement of the knee. J Bone Joint Surg 53(A):945–962, 1971
66. Freeman MAR, Dean MRE, Hanham IF: The etiology and prevention of functional instability of the foot. J Bone Joint Surg 47(B):678–685, 1965
67. Friedmann MJ, Ferkel RD, (eds): Prosthetic Ligament Reconstruction of the Knee. Philadelphia, WB Saunders, 1988

68. Fulkerson JP: Awareness of the retinaculum in evaluating patellofemoral pain. Am J Sports Med 10:147–149, 1982
69. Funk JF: Synthetic ligaments: Current status. Clin Orthop 219:107–111, 1987
70. Furman W, Marshall JL, Giris FG: The anterior cruciate ligament: A functional analysis based on post-mortem studies. J Bone Joint Surg 58(A):179–185, 1976
71. Galway HR, Beaupre A, Mac Intosh D: Pivot shift: A clinical sign of symptomatic anterior cruciate insufficiency. J Bone Joint Surg 54(B):763–764, 1972
72. Galway HR, MacIntosh DL: The lateral pivot shift: A symptom and sign of anterior cruciate ligament insufficiency. Clin Orthop 147:45–50, 1980
73. Glove TP, Muller S, Barreck EK: Non-operative treatment of the torn anterior cruciate ligament. J Bone Joint Surg 65(A):184–192, 1983
74. Godfrey JD: Ligament injuries of the knee. In Abstrom JP (ed): Current Practice in Orthopedic Surgery, Vol 5, pp 56–92. St Louis, CV Mosby, 1973
75. Goldberg A: Work-induced growth of skeletal muscle in normal and hypophysectomised rats. Am J Physiol 312:1193–1198, 1967
76. Goodfellow J, Hungerford DS, Woods C: Patellofemoral joint mechanics and pathology. Part 2: Chondromalacia patellae. J Bone Joint Surg 58(B):291–299, 1976
77. Goodfellow J, Hungerford DS, Zindel M: Patellofemoral joint mechanics and pathology: Functional anatomy of the patellofemoral joint. J Bone Joint Surg 58(B):287–290, 1976
78. Gough JV, Ladley G: An investigation into effectiveness of various forms of quadriceps exercises. Physiotherapy 57:356–361, 1971.
79. Green WR Jr.: Painful bipartite patellae. Clin Orthop 110:197–200, 1975
80. Gutman E, Schiaffino S, Hazlikova V: Mechanism of compensatory hypertrophy in skeletal muscles of the rat. Exp Neurol 31:451–464, 1971
81. Haggmark TN, Ericksson E: Cylinder or mobile cast brace after knee ligament surgery? Am J Sports Med 7:48–56, 1979
82. Hardarkerwt WT, Whipple TL, Bassett FH: Diagnosis and treatment of the plica syndrome of the knee. J Bone Joint Surg 62(A):222–225, 1980
83. Hastings DE: The non-operative treatment of collateral ligament injuries of the knee joint. Clin Orthop 147:22–28, 1980
84. Helfet A: Disorders of the Knee, 2nd ed. Philadelphia, JB Lippincott, 1982
85. Hellebrandt FA, Houtz SJ, Kirkorian AM: Influence of bimanual exercise on unilateral work capacity. J Appl Physiol 2:452–466, 1950
86. Hellebrandt FA, Houtz SJ, Partridge MJ, et al: Tonic neck reflexes in exercises of stress in man. Am J Phys Med 35:144–157, 1956
87. Hellebrandt FA, Waterland JC: Indirect learning: The influence of unimanual exercise on related muscle groups of the same and the opposite side. Am J Phys Med 41:45–55, 1962
88. Henning CE, Lynch MA, Glick K: An in vivo strain gauge study of elongation of the anterior cruciate ligament. Am J Sports Med 13:22–26, 1985
89. Henning CE, Lynch MA, Glick K: Physical examination of the knee. In Nicholas JA, Hershmann EB (eds): The Lower Extremity and Spine in Sports Medicine, Vol I, pp 765–800. St Louis, CV Mosby, 1986
90. Hoffa A: The influence of the adipose tissue with regards to the pathology of the knee joint. JAMA 43:795–796, 1904
91. Holden DL, Eggert AW, Butler JE: The non-operative treatment of grade I and II medial collateral ligament injuries to the knee. Am J Sports Med 11:340–344, 1983
92. Hoppenfeld S: Physical Examination of the Spine and Extremities. New York, Appleton–Century–Crofts, 1976
93. Hughston JC, Andrews JR, Cross MJ, et al: Classification of knee ligament instability, Part I. J Bone Joint Surg 58(A):159–172, 1976
94. Hughston JC, Andrews JR, Cross MJ, et al: Classification of knee ligament instability, Part II. J Bone Joint Surg 58(A):173–179, 1976
95. Hughston JC, Norwood LA: The posterolateral drawer test for posterolateral rotatory instability of the knee. Clin Orthop 147:82–87, 1980
96. Hughston JC, Walsh WM, Puddu G: Patellar Subluxation and Dislocation. Philadelphia, WB Saunders, 1984
97. Hunter SC, Poole RM: The chronically inflamed tendon. Clin Sports Med 6(2):371–388, 1987
98. Ihara H, Nakayama: Dynamic joint control training for knee ligament injuries. Am J Sports Med 14:309–315, 1986
99. Insall J, Falvo KA, Wise DW: Chondromalacia patellae: A prospective study. J Bone Joint Surg 58(A):1–8, 1976
100. Jakob RP: Observation on rotatory instability of the lateral compartment of the knee. Acta Orthop Scand (Suppl 191)52:1–32, 1981
101. Jakob RP, Staubli HU, Delalnd JT: Grading the pivot shift. J Bone Joint Surg 69(B):294–299, 1987
102. James SL: Chondromalacia patella: In Kennedy JC (ed): The Injured Adolescent Knee. Baltimore, Williams & Wilkins, 1979
103. James SL, Bates BT, Ostering LR: Injuries to runners. Am J Sports Med 6:40–50, 1978
104. Janda V: Muscles, central nervous motor regulation and back problems. In Korr I (ed): The Neurobiologic Mechanisms in Manipulative Therapy, pp 27–42. London, Plenum Press, 1978
105. Janda V: Treatment of Patients. Presented at the Fourth conference of the International Federation of Orthopedic Manipulative Therapists, Christchurch, New Zealand, 1980

106. Jones AL: Rehabilitation for anterior instability of the knee: Preliminary report. J Orthop Sports Phys Ther 3:121–128, 1982
107. Jonsson T, Alfhoff D, Peterson L, et al: Clinical diagnosis of ruptures of the anterior cruciate ligament. Am J Sports Med 10:100–102, 1982
108. Katz JW, Fingeroth RJ: The diagnostic accuracy of rupture of the anterior cruciate ligament comparing the Lachman test, the anterior drawer sign, and the pivot shift test in acute and chronic knee injuries. Am J Sports Med 14:88–91, 1986
109. Kennedy JC: The Injured Adolescent Knee. Baltimore, Williams & Wilkins, 1979
110. Kennedy JC, Fowler PJ: Medial and anterior instability of the knee. J Bone Joint Surg 53(A):1257–1270, 1971
111. Kennedy JC, Galpin RD: The use of the medial head of the gastrocnemius muscle in the posterior cruciate–deficient knee: Indication, technique, results. Am J Sports Med 10:63–74, 1982
112. Kennedy JC, Weinberg HW, Wilson AS: The anatomy and function of the anterior cruciate ligament, as determined by clinical and morphological studies. J Bone Joint Surg 56(A):223–234, 1974
113. Kettlekamp DB: Clinical implications of knee biomechanics. Arch Surg 107:406–410, 1973
114. Kisner C, Colby LA: Therapeutic Exercise: Foundations and Techniques. Philadelphia, FA Davis, 1985
115. Knott M, Voss D: Proprioceptive Neuromuscular Facilitation, 2nd ed. New York, Harper & Row, 1969
116. Komi PV: Measurement of the force–velocity relationship in human muscle under concentric and eccentric contractions. Med Sci Sport:8:224–229, 1973
117. Komi PV: Neuromuscular performance factors influencing force and speed production. Scand J Sports Sci 1:2–15, 1979
118. Komi PV, Bosco C: Utilization of stored elastic energy in leg extensor muscles by men and women. Med Sci Sports 10:261–265, 1978
119. Kottke FJ: Krusen's Handbook of Physical Medicine and Rehabilitation, 3rd ed. Philadelphia, WB Saunders, 1982
120. Larson RL: Overview and philosophy of knee injuries. Clin Sports Med 4:209–215, 1985
121. Larson RL: Future of prosthetic ligament reconstruction. In Friedman MJ, Ferkel RD (eds): Prosthetic Ligament Reconstruction of the Knee. Philadelphia, WB Saunders, 1988
122. Larson RL, Cabaud HE, Slocum DB: The patella compression syndrome: Surgical treatment by lateral retinacular release. Clin Orthop 134:156–157, 1978
123. Last RJ: The popliteus muscle and lateral meniscus. J Bone Joint Surg 32(B):93–99, 1950
124. Laubenthal KN, Smidt GL, Kettlekamp DB: A quantitative analysis of knee motion for activities of daily living. Phys Ther 52:34–42, 1972
125. Levine J, Splain S: Use of the infrapatellar strap in the treatment of patellofemoral pain. Clin Orthop 139:179–181, 1979
126. Levy IM, Torzilli PA, Warren RF: Effects of medial meniscectomy on anterior–posterior motion of the knee. J Bone Joint Surg 64(A):883–888, 1982
127. Lewis RJ: Degenerative arthritis. In Nickel VL (ed): Orthopedic Rehabilitation, pp 515–524. New York, Churchill Livingstone, 1982
128. Lieb F, Perry J: Quadriceps function: An electromyographic study under isometric contraction. J Bone Joint Surg 53(A):749–758, 1971
129. Logan GA: Differential applications of resistance and resulting strength measured at varying degrees of knee flexion. Ph. D. dissertation, University of Southern California, 1960
130. Losee RE: Concepts of the pivot shift. Clin Orthop 172:45–51, 1983
131. Losee RE, Johnson TR, Southwick WO: Anterior subluxation of the lateral tibia plateau. J Bone Joint Surg 60(A):1015–1030, 1978
132. Love JW, Whelan TJ: Popliteal artery entrapment syndrome. Am Med J Surg 109:620–624, 1965
133. Lucie RS, Wiedel JD, Messner DG: The acute pivot shift: Clinical correlation. Am J Sports Med 12:189–191, 1984
134. Lutter L: Injuries in runners and joggers. Minn Med 63:45–51, 1980
135. Lutter L: Cavus foot in runners. Foot Ankle 1:225–228, 1981
136. Lutter L: Running athlete in office practice. Foot Ankle 3:52–59, 1982
137. Lutter L: The knee and running. Clin Sports Med 4:685–698, 1985
138. Magee DJ: Orthopedic Physical Assessment. Philadelphia, WB Saunders, 1987
139. Maitland GD: Peripheral Manipulations. 2nd ed. Boston, Butterworths, 1987
140. Malone T, Blackburn TA, Wallace LA: Knee rehabilitation. Phys Ther 66:1553–1639, 1980
141. Mann R, Baxter D, Lutter L: Running symposium. Foot Ankle 1:190–224, 1981
142. Markolf, KL: Quantitative examination for anterior cruciate laxity. In Jackson DW, Drez D (eds): The Anterior Cruciate Deficient Knee: New Concepts in Ligament Repair, pp 90–101. St Louis, CV Mosby, 1987
143. Markolf K, Graff-Radford A, Amstutz H: *In vivo* knee stability: A quantitative assessment using an instrumented clinical testing apparatus. J Bone Joint Surg 60(A):664–674, 1978
144. Marks KE, Bentley G: Patella alta and chondromalacia. J Bone Joint Surg 60(B):71–73, 1978
145. Mayfield G: Popliteus tendon tenosynovitis. Am J Sports Med 5:31–36, 1977
146. McConnell J: The management of chondromalacia patellae: A long-term solution. Aus J Physiol 2:215–223, 1986
147. McMurray TP: The semilunar cartilage. Br J Surg 29:407–414, 1942
148. Meachim G, Emery IH: Quantitative aspects of patel-

lofemoral cartilage fibrillation in Liverpool necropsies. Ann Rheum Dis 3:39–47, 1974

149. Mellion MB: Office Management of Sports Injuries and Athletic Problems. St. Louis, CV Mosby, 1988

150. Mennell JB: Physical Treatment by Movement, Manipulation and Massage, 5th ed. Philadelphia, P Blakiston & Son, 1947

151. Muller EA, Rohmert W: Die Geschwindigkeit der Muskelkraftzunshme bei Isometricshes Training. Int Zeitschrift fur Angewandte Physiol 19:403–419, 1983

152. Muller W: The Knee: Form, Function and Ligament Reconstruction. New York, Springer–Verlag, 1983

153. Newton RA: Electrotherapeutic Treatment: Selecting Appropriate Waveform Characteristics. Clinton, NJ, JA Preston, 1984

154. Nicholas JA: Injuries to the menisci of the knee. Orthop Clin North Am 4(3):647–664, 1973

155. Nicholas JA, Hershman EB (eds): The Lower Extremity and Spine in Sports Medicine, Vol I. St Louis, CV Mosby, 1986

156. Noble CA: Iliotibial band friction syndrome in runners. Am J Sports Med 8:232–234, 1980

157. Norwood LA, Cross MJ: Anterior cruciate ligament: Functional anatomy of its bundles in rotary instability. Am J Sports Med 7:23–26, 1979

158. Noyes FR: Functional properties of knee ligaments and alterations induced by immobilization: A correlative biomechanical and histological study in primates. Clin Orthop 123:210–242, 1977

159. Noyes FR, Bassett RW, Grood ES, et al: Arthroscopy in acute traumatic hemarthrosis of the knee: Incidence of anterior cruciate tears and other injuries. J Bone Joint Surg 62(A):687–695, 1980

160. Noyes FR, Matthews DS, Mooar PA, et al: The symptomatic anterior cruciate deficient knee. Part II: The result of rehabilitation activity modification and counseling on functional disability. J Bone Joint Surg 65(A):163–174, 1983

161. Noyes FR, Mooar PA, Matthews DS, et al: The symptomatic anterior cruciate deficient knee. Part I: The long-term functional disability in athletically active individuals. J Bone Joint Surg 65(A):154–162, 1983

162. Noyes FR, Torvik PJ, Hyde WB, et al: Biomechanics of ligament failure. Part II: An analysis of immobilization, exercise, and reconditioning effects in primates. J Bone Joint Surg 56(A):1406–1418, 1974

163. O'Donoghue DH: Treatment of acute ligamentous injuries of the knee. Orthop Clin North Am 4(3):617–645, 1973

164. Ogden JA, McCarthy SM, Tokl P: The painful bipartite patella. J Pediatr Orthop 2:263–269, 1982

165. Outerbridge REE: The etiology of chondromalacia patellae. J Bone Joint Surg 43(B):752–757, 1961

166. Palumba PM: Dynamic patellar brace: Patellofemoral disorders: A preliminary report. Am J Sports Med 9:45–49, 1979

167. Parolie JM, Bergfeld JA: Long-term results of nonoperative treatment of isolated posterior cruciate ligament injuries in the athlete. Am J Sports Med 14:35–38, 1986

168. Paulos LE: Knee and leg: Soft-tissue trauma. In American Academy of Orthopaedic Surgeons: Orthopedic Knowledge Update 2, pp 414–425. Chicago, AAOS, 1987

169. Paulos LE, Noyes FR, Grood E, et al: Knee rehabilitation after anterior cruciate ligament reconstruction and repair. Am J Sports Med 9:140–149, 1981

170. Paulos LE, Payne FC, Rosenbery TD: Rehabilitation after anterior cruciate ligament surgery. In Jackson DW, Drez D (eds): The Anterior Cruciate Deficient Knee: New Concepts in Ligament Repair, pp 291–314. St Louis, CV Mosby, 1987

171. Paulos L, Rusche K, Johnson C, et al: Patellar malalignment: A treatment rationale. Phys Ther 60:1627–1632, 1980

172. Radin EL, de Lamotte F, Maquet P: Role of the menisci in the distribution of stress in the knee. Clin Orthop 185:290–294, 1984

173. Raux P, Townsend PR, Miegel R, et al: Trabecular architecture of the human patella. J Biomech 8:1–7, 1975

174. Renne J: The iliotibial band friction syndrome. J Bone Joint Surg 57(B):1110–1115, 1976

175. Ricklin P, Ruttmann A, Del Buno MS: Meniscus Lesions: Diagnosis, Differential Diagnosis and Therapy, 2nd ed. Stuttgart, Georg Thieme Verlag, 1983

176. Romero JA, Standford TL, Schroeder RV, et al: The effects of electrical stimulation of normal quadriceps on strength and girth. Med Sci Sports Exerc 14(3):194–197, 1982

177. Rosentswig J, Hinson MM: Comparison of isometric, isotonic and isokinetic exercises by electromyography. Arch Phys Med Rehabil 53:249–252, 1972

178. Sandberg R, Balkfors B, Nilsson B, et al: Operative versus non-operative treatment of recent injuries to the ligaments of the knee. J Bone Joint Surg 69(A):1120–1126, 1987

179. Schultz P: Flexibility: The day of the static stretch. Phys Sports Med 7:109–117, 1979

180. Seedhom BB: Load-bearing function of the menisci. Physiotherapy 62:223–228, 1976

181. Shaw JA, Eng M, Murray DG: The longitudinal axis of the knee and the role of the cruciate ligaments in controlling transverse rotation. J Bone Joint Surg 56(A):1603–1609, 1974

182. Shephard RJ: Physiology and Biochemistry of Exercise. New York, Praeger Press, 1982

183. Sherrington CS: The Integrative Actions of the Nervous System. New Haven, Yale University Press, 1906

184. Shields CL, Brewster CE, Morrissey MC: Rehabilitation of the knee in athletes. In Nichols JA, Hershmann EB (eds): The Lower Extremity and Spine in Sports Medicine, Vol 1. St Louis, CV Mosby, 1986

185. Shoji H: Chondromalacia patellae: Histological and biochemical aspects. NY State J Med 74:507–510, 1974

186. Slocum DB, James SL, Larson RL, et al: Clinical test

for anterolateral rotary instability of the knee. Clin Orthop 118:63–69, 1976

187. Slocum DB, Larson RL: Rotary instability of the knee: Its pathogenesis and a clinical test to determine its presence. J Bone Joint Surg 50(A):211–225, 1968
188. Slocum DB, Larson RL, James SL: Late reconstruction procedures used to stabilize the knee. Orthop Clin North Am 4(3):679–689, 1973
189. Smillie IS: Diseases of the Knee Joint, 2nd ed. New York, Churchill Livingstone, 1980
190. Sonzogni JJ: Physical Assessment of the injured knee. Emerg Med 6:74–92, 1988
191. Spencer J, Hayes K, Alexander I: Knee joint effusion and quadriceps reflex inhibition in man. Arch Phys Med Rehabil 65:171–177, 1984
192. Stanish WD: Neurophysiology of stretching. In D'Ambrosia R, Drez D (eds). Prevention and Treatment of Running Injuries, pp 135–146. Thorofare, New Jersey, Slack Inc, 1982
193. Steadman JR: Nonoperative methods for patellofemoral problems. Am J Sports Med 7:374–375, 1979
194. Steadman JR: Rehabilitation of first and second degree sprains of the medial collateral ligament. Am J Sports Med 7:300–302, 1979
195. Steadman JR: Rehabilitation of acute injuries of the anterior cruciate ligament. Clin Orthop 172:129–132, 1983
196. Steindler A: Kinesiology of the Human Body. Springfield, Charles C Thomas, 1955
197. Stillwell GK: Electrotherapy. In Kottke FS, Stillwell GK, Lehmann JF (eds): Krusen's Handbook of Physical Medicine and Rehabilitation, 3rd ed., pp 360–371. Philadelphia, WB Saunders, 1982
198. Stokes M, Young A: Investigation of quadriceps inhibition: Implications for clinical practice. Physiotherapy 70:425–428, 1984
199. Storigord J: Chondromalacia of the patella: Physical signs in relation to operative findings. Acta Orthop Scand 46:685–694, 1975
200. Stuller J: Bracing the unstable knee. Phys Sports Med 13:142–156, 1985
201. Sullivan PE, Markos PD, Minor MAD: An Integrated Approach to Therapeutic Exercise Therapy and Clinical Application. Reston, Virginia, Reston Pub Co, 1982
202. Surburg RR: Proprioceptive neuromuscular facilitation. Phys Sports Med 9:115–127, 1981

203. Teitz C, Larson R: Health Maintenance. In American Academy of Orthopedic Surgeons, Orthopaedic Knowledge Update 2, pp 6–7, Chicago, AAOS, 1987
204. Tibone J, Antich TJ, Fanton GS, et al: Functional analysis of anterior cruciate ligament instability. Am J Sports Med 14:276–283, 1986
205. Tory JS, Conrad W, Kalen V: Clinical diagnosis of anterior cruciate ligament instability in the athlete. Am J Sports Med 4:84–93, 1976
206. Townsend PR, Miegel RE, Rose RM, et al: Structure and function of the human patella: The role of cancellous bone. J Biomed Mater Res 7:605–611, 1976
207. Townsend PR, Raux P, Rose RM, et al: The distribution and anisotrophy of the stiffness of cancellous bone in the human patella. J Biomech 8:363–367, 1975
208. Townsend PR, Rose RM, Radin EL, et al: The biomechanics of the human patella and its implications for chondromalacia. J Biomech 10:403–407, 1977
209. Turner W (ed): Anatomical Memoirs of John Goodsir. Edinburgh, Adam & Black, 1968
210. Vaey FB: The painful knee. In Germain BF: Osteoarthritis and Musculoskeletal Pain Syndromes, pp 203–223. Hyde Park, New York, Medical Examination Pub Co, 1983
211. Walker HL, Schreck RC: Relationship of hyperextended gait pattern to chrondomalacia patellae. Physiotherapy 64:8–9, 1975
212. Walla DL, Albright JP, McAuley E, et al: Hamstring control and the unstable anterior cruciate ligament–deficient knee. Am J Sports Med 13:34–39, 1985
213. Wallace L: Balance as a predictor of knee injury in football. Presented at the annual meeting of the American Physical Therapy Association, Anaheim, California, June 19, 1982
214. Walsh WM: Office management of knee injuries. In Mellion MB (ed): Office Management of Sport Injuries and Athlete Problems. Philadelphia, CV Mosby, 1988
215. Wang YJB, Rubim RM, Marshall JL: A mechanism of isolated anterior cruciate ligament rupture: Case report. J Bone Joint Surg 57(A):411–413, 1975
216. Warren LF, Marshall JL: The supporting structures and layers on the medial side of the knee: An anatomical analysis. J Bone Joint Surg 61(A):56–62, 1979
217. Wyke B: The neurology of joints. Ann R Coll Surg Engl 41:25–50, 1967

15 The Ankle and Hindfoot

Randolph M. Kessler and Darlene Hertling

FUNCTIONAL ANATOMY OF THE JOINTS

OSTEOLOGY

The tibia flares at its distal end. As a result, the cross section of the bone changes from triangular, in the region of the shaft, to quadrangular in the area of the distal metaphyseal portion of the bone. Medially there is a distal projection of the tibia, the medial malleolus; located laterally is the fibular notch, which is concave anteroposteriorly for articulation with the distal end of the fibula. Along the medial side of the posterior surface is a groove for the passage of the tibialis posterior tendon. The term *posterior malleolus* is often used to refer to the distal overhang of the posterior aspect of the tibia (Fig. 15–1).

The lateral surface of the medial malleolus and the inferior surface of the tibia have a continuous cartilaginous covering for articulation with the talus. The articular surface of the inferior end of the tibia is concave anteroposteriorly. Mediolaterally, it is somewhat convex, having a crest centrally that corresponds to the central groove in the trochlear surface of the talus. This, then, is essentially a sellar joint surface. It is slightly wider anteriorly than posteriorly. The articular surface of the medial malleolus is comma shaped, with the "tail" of the comma being situated posteriorly (see Fig. 15–1).

The fibula, which is quite narrow in the region of its shaft, becomes bulbous at its distal end (Fig. 15–2). This distal portion of the bone, the lateral malleolus, is triangular in cross section. When viewed from a lateral aspect, the fibula is somewhat pointed distally. The lateral malleolus extends farther distally and is situated more posteriorly than the medial malleolus. The medial aspect of the lateral malleolus is covered by a triangular cartilaginous surface for ar-

ticulation with the lateral side of the talus. Above this surface, the fibula contacts the tibia in the fibular notch of the tibia. The apex of this triangular surface points inferiorly. There is a fairly deep depression in the posteroinferior region of the lateral malleolus termed the *malleolar fossa* that can be easily palpated. The posterior talofibular ligament attaches in this fossa. There is a groove along the posterior aspect of the lateral malleolus through which the peroneus brevis tendon passes.

The talus constitutes the link between the leg and the tarsus (Fig. 15–3). It consists of a body, anterior to which is the head. The body and head of the talus are connected by a short neck.

The superior surface of the body of the talus is covered with articular cartilage for articulation with the inferior surface of the tibia. This articular surface is continuous with the articular surfaces of the medial and lateral aspects of the talus. The superior surface is somewhat wider anteriorly than posteriorly. It is convex anteroposteriorly and slightly concave mediolaterally, corresponding to the sellar surface of the inferior end of the tibia mentioned previously. In this sense, the superior talar articular surface is trochlear, or pulley-like, and is often referred to as the trochlea.

The lateral aspect of the body of the talus is largely covered by articular cartilage for articulation with the distal end of the fibula (Fig. 15–4). This articular surface is triangular, with the apex situated inferiorly. Just below this apex is a lateral bony projection to which the lateral talocalcaneal ligament attaches.

The articular surface of the medial aspect of the talus is considerably smaller than that of the lateral side, and it faces slightly upward (Fig. 15–5). It contacts the articular surface of the medial malleolus on the tibia. It is comma shaped, with the tail of the comma being situated posteriorly. The roughened area below the medial articular surface serves as an attachment for the deltoid ligament. The medial and lateral talar articular surfaces tend to converge pos-

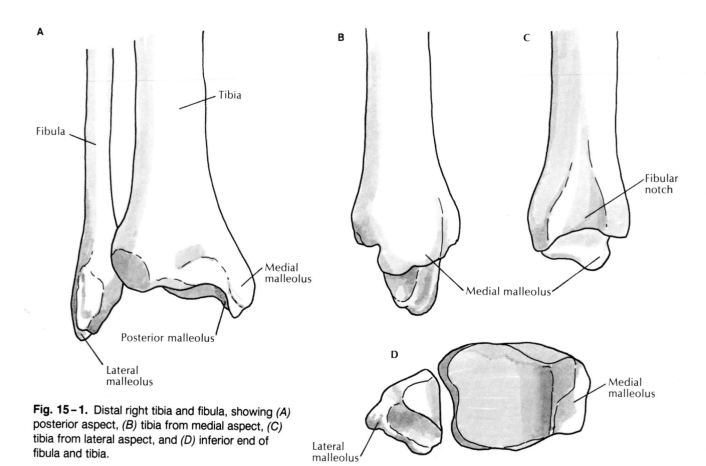

Fig. 15–1. Distal right tibia and fibula, showing *(A)* posterior aspect, *(B)* tibia from medial aspect, *(C)* tibia from lateral aspect, and *(D)* inferior end of fibula and tibia.

Fig. 15–2. Medial aspect of distal right fibula.

teriorly, leading to the wedge shape of the trochlea. It should be emphasized, however, that the lateral articular surface of the talus is perpendicular to the axis of movement at the ankle joint, whereas the medial surface is not. This has important biomechanical implications, which are discussed in the following section.

If one views the profiles of the lateral and medial sides of the trochlea, the lateral profile is seen as a section of a circle, whereas the medial profile may be viewed as sections of several circles of different radii; the medial profile is of smaller radius anteriorly than posteriorly.[47] More precisely stated, the contour medially is of gradually increasing radius anteroposteriorly, forming a cardioid profile. The importance of this is described in the section on biomechanics.

Posteriorly, the body of the talus is largely covered by a continuation of the trochlear articular surface as it slopes backward (Fig. 15–6). At the inferior extent of the posterior aspect is the nonarticular posterior process. The posterior process consists of a lateral and a smaller medial tubercle, with an intervening groove through which passes the tendon of the flexor hallucis longus. The posterior talofibular ligament

(Text continues on p. 363.)

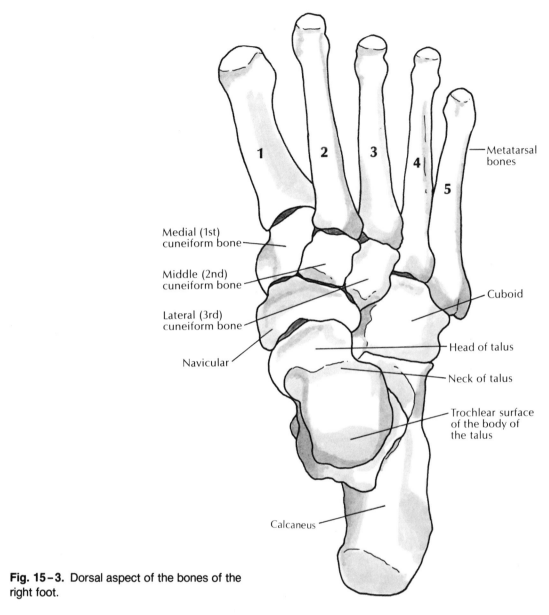

Metatarsal bones

Medial (1st) cuneiform bone

Middle (2nd) cuneiform bone

Lateral (3rd) cuneiform bone

Navicular

Cuboid

Head of talus

Neck of talus

Trochlear surface of the body of the talus

Calcaneus

Fig. 15–3. Dorsal aspect of the bones of the right foot.

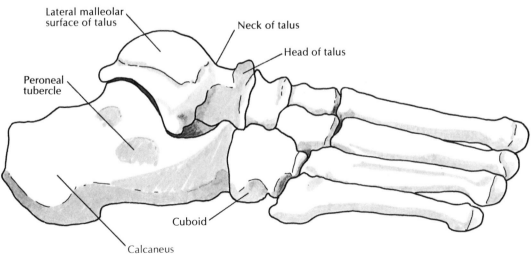

Lateral malleolar surface of talus

Neck of talus

Head of talus

Peroneal tubercle

Cuboid

Calcaneus

Fig. 15–4. Lateral aspect of the bones of the foot.

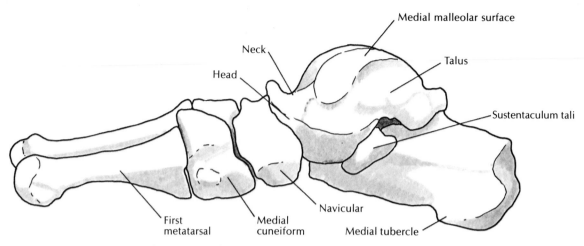

Fig. 15-5. Medial aspect of the bones of the foot.

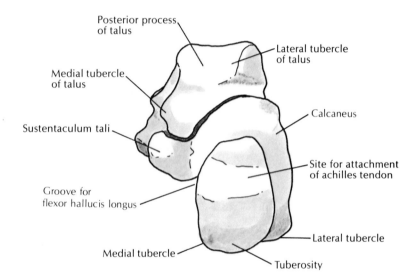

Fig. 15-6. Posterior aspect of calcaneus and talus.

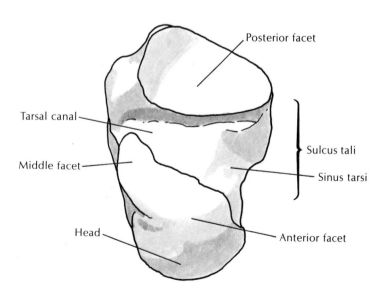

Fig. 15-7. Inferior surface of talus.

attaches to the lateral tubercle. The medial talocalcaneal ligament and a posterior portion of the deltoid ligament attach to the medial tubercle.

The neck and head of the talus are positioned anteriorly to the body. They are directed slightly medially and downward with respect to the body. The head is covered with articular cartilage anteriorly for articulation with the navicular and inferiorly for articulation with the spring ligament (plantar calcaneonavicular ligament).

The inferior surface of the talus has three cartilage-covered facets for articulation with the calcaneus (Fig. 15–7). The posterior facet, which is the largest of these, is concave inferiorly. The medial and anterior articular facets are continuous with each other and with the inferior articular surface of the head. Both the medial and the anterior facets are convex inferiorly and articulate with the superior aspect of the sustentaculum tali of the calcaneus. A deep groove, the sulcus tali, separates the posterior and medial facets on the inferior aspect of the talus. This groove runs obliquely from posteromedial to anterolateral. Where it is the deepest—posteromedially—it forms the *tarsal canal;* where it widens and opens out laterally it is referred to as the *sinus tarsi.* The interosseous talocalcaneal ligament and the cervical ligament occupy the sinus tarsi.

The calcaneus is situated beneath the talus in the standing position and provides a major contact point with the ground. It is the largest of the tarsal bones. The calcaneus articulates with the talus superiorly and with the cuboid anteriorly. Posteriorly it projects backward, providing considerable leverage for the plantar flexors of the ankle. The superior aspect of the calcaneus bears the posterior, medial, and anterior facets for articulation with the corresponding facets of the talus (Fig. 15–8). The posterior facet is convex, whereas the medial and anterior facets are concave. The medial and anterior facets are situated on the superior aspect of the sustentaculum tali, which is a bony projection of the calcaneus that overhangs medially. As with the corresponding facets on the talus, the medial and anterior facets of the calcaneus are usually continuous with each other. The medial and anterior facets are separated from the posterior facet by the *sulcus calcanei,* which forms the bottom of the sinus tarsi and tarsal canal, thus corresponding to the sulcus tali of the talus.

The posterior aspect of the large posterior projection of the calcaneus contains a smooth superior surface, which slopes upward and forward, and a rough inferior surface, which slopes downward and forward. The upper surface is the site of attachment

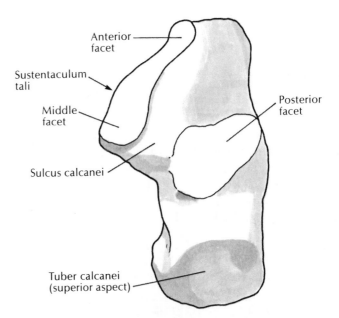

Fig. 15–8. Superior aspect of the calcaneus.

for the Achilles tendon (see Fig. 15–6). The lower surface blends inferiorly with the tuber calcanei, which is the point of contact of the calcaneus with the ground in the standing position.

The tuber calcanei on the inferior aspect of the calcaneus consists of a medial tubercle and a lateral tubercle, of which the medial is the larger. Anterior to the tuber calcanei is a roughened surface for the attachment of the long and short plantar ligaments (Fig. 15–9). At the anterior extent of the inferior surface of the calcaneus is the anterior tubercle, which also serves as a point of attachment for the long plantar ligament. On the inferior aspect of the medially projecting sustentaculum tali is a groove through which runs the flexor hallucis longus tendon.

The lateral aspect of the calcaneus is nearly flat. There is a small prominence, the peroneal trochlea, that is located just distal to the lateral malleolus (see Fig. 15–4). The peroneus brevis tendon travels downward and forward, just superior to this trochlea, while the peroneus longus tendon passes inferior to it. The calcaneofibular ligament attaches just posterior and slightly superior to the peroneal trochlea, at which point there may be a rounded prominence.

From the anterosuperior extent of the medial aspect of the calcaneus, the sustentaculum tali projects in a medial direction (see Fig. 15–8). The sustentaculum tali may be palpated just below the medial malleolus.

On the narrowed anterior aspect of the calcaneus

Plantar calcaneocuboid
ligament (short
plantar ligament)

Long plantar
ligament

Plantar calcaneonavicular
ligament

Sustentaculum tali

Groove for flexor
hallicus longus

Lateral tubercle
of calcaneus

Medial tubercle of
calcaneus

Tuber calcanei
(inferior aspect)

Fig. 15–9. Plantar surface of the foot.

is the cartilage-covered articular surface that contacts the cuboid bone. This is a sellar joint surface, being concave superoinferiorly and convex mediolaterally (see Fig. 15–3).

The remainder of the tarsus includes the navicular and cuboid bones, which contact the talus and calcaneus, respectively, and the three cuneiforms, which articulate with the first three metatarsals (Fig. 15–3). The cuboid extends distally to contact the remaining two metatarsals. (These bones will not be considered in detail here but will be referred to in the biomechanics section of this chapter).

LIGAMENTS AND CAPSULES

Inferior Tibiofibular Joint

The inferior tibiofibular joint is a syndesmosis and lacks articular cartilage and synovium. The distal fibula is situated in the fibular notch of the lateral aspect of the distal tibia and is bound to it by several ligaments (Figs. 15–10 and 15–11). The anterior and posterior tibiofibular ligaments pass in front of and behind the syndesmosis. They are both directed downward and inward to check separation of the two bones. The inferior transverse ligament is a thickened band of fibers that is closely related to the posterior tibiofibular ligament. It passes from the posterior margin of the inferior tibial articular surface downward and laterally to the malleolar fossa of the fibula. This ligament is lined inferiorly with articular cartilage where it contacts the posterolateral talar articular surface during extreme plantar flexion. The interosseous ligament is a continuation of the interosseous membrane of the tibia and fibula. It extends between the adjacent surfaces of the bones at the syndesmosis. The tibia and fibula are separated at the syndesmosis by a fat pad.

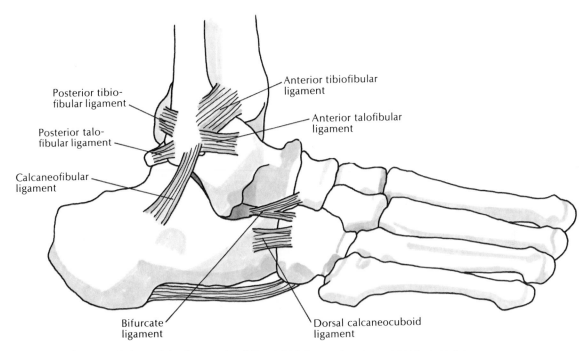

Fig. 15-10. Lateral view of the ligaments of the right talocrural and proximal tarsal joints.

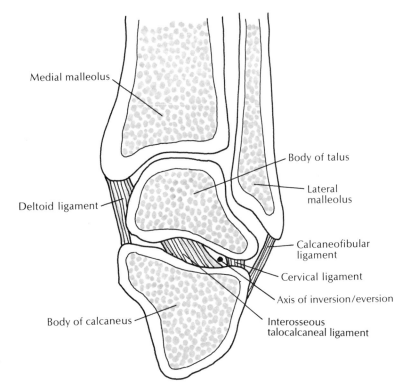

Fig. 15-11. Coronal section through the talocrural and subtalar joints.

The ligaments of the inferior tibiofibular articulation are oriented to prevent widening of the mortise. They are also important in preventing posterior displacement of the fibula at the syndesmosis, which tends to occur when the leg is forcibly internally rotated on the tarsus. It should be realized that complete sectioning of the inferior tibiofibular ligaments alone allows only a minimal increase in the intermalleolar space.[1] This is because the two bones are indirectly held together by their mutual connections to the talus, by way of the medial and lateral ligaments of the ankle. Significant diastasis, then, is usually accompanied by rupture of one or more of the talocrural ligaments, usually the deltoid ligament.

Ankle Joint (Ankle Mortise or Talocrural Joint)

The ankle joint is formed by the superior portion of the body of the talus fitting within the mortise, or cavity, formed by the combined distal ends of the tibia and fibula. The medial, superior, and lateral articular surfaces of the talus are continuous, as are those of the medial malleolus, the distal end of the tibia, and the lateral malleolus.

The fibrous capsule attaches at the margins of the articular surfaces of the talus below and to the tibia and fibula above, except anteriorly, where a portion of the dorsal aspect of the neck of the talus is enclosed within the joint cavity. The capsule extends somewhat superiorly between the distal ends of the tibia and fibula, to just below the syndesmosis. The fibrous capsule is lined by a synovial membrane throughout its entirety. The capsule is well supported by ligaments, especially medially and laterally.

The medial ligaments are collectively referred to as the *deltoid ligament* (Fig. 15–12). The anterior portion of the deltoid ligament consists of the tibionavicular ligament, superficially, and the deeper anterior tibiotalar fibers. The tibionavicular ligament blends with the plantar calcaneonavicular (spring) ligament inferiorly. The middle fibers of the deltoid ligament constitute the tibiocalcaneal ligament, with some tibiotalar fibers deep to it. The posterior tibiotalar ligament forms the posterior portion of the deltoid ligament. The deltoid ligament as a whole attaches proximally to the medial aspect of the medial malleolus and fans out to achieve the distal attachments described above. In this way, it is somewhat triangular, with the apex at its proximal attachment.

The lateral ligaments, unlike those of the medial side, are separate bands of fibers diverging from their proximal attachment at the distal end of the fibula (see Fig. 15–10). The anterior talofibular ligament—the most frequently injured ligament about the ankle—passes medially, forward and downward, from the anterior aspect of the fibula to the lateral aspect of the neck of the talus. The calcaneofibular ligament runs from the tip of the lateral malleolus downward and backward to a small prominence on the upper lateral surface of the calcaneus. It is longer and narrower than the anterior and posterior talofib-

Fig. 15–12. Medial view of the ligaments of the talocrural and proximal tarsal joints.

ular ligaments. The posterior talofibular ligament passes from the malleolar fossa medially and slightly downward and backward to the lateral tubercle of the posterior aspect of the talus.

It should be noted that the proximal attachments of both the medial and lateral ligaments of the ankle are near the axis of movement for dorsiflexion and plantar flexion. For this reason, these ligaments are not pulled tight to any significant extent during normal movement at the talocrural joint.[43] Also, the calcaneofibular ligament, which crosses both the talocrural and the talocalcaneal joints, runs parallel to, and inserts close to, the axis of movement at the subtalar joint. It, then, plays little or no role in restricting inversion at the subtalar joint. This is true in all positions of dorsiflexion and plantar flexion, since it maintains a parallel orientation to the subtalar axis throughout the range.

The ligaments about the talocrural joint primarily function to restrict tilting and rotation of the talus within the mortise and to restrict forward or backward displacement of the leg on the tarsus. The main exception to this is the tibiocalcaneal portion of the deltoid ligament, which is so oriented as to help check eversion at the subtalar joint as well as an "eversion tilt" of the talus in the mortise.

In the neutral position, the anterior talofibular ligament can check posterior movement of the leg on the tarsus and external rotation of the leg on the tarsus because it is directed forward and medially. With the foot in plantar flexion, the anterior talofibular ligament becomes more vertically oriented and is in a position to check inversion of the talus in the mortise. This ligament is the most commonly injured of the ligaments of the ankle, the mechanism of injury usually being a combined plantar flexion–inversion strain.

The calcaneofibular ligament is directed downward and backward when the foot is in the neutral position. When the foot is dorsiflexed, the ligament becomes more vertically oriented and is in a better position to check inversion of the tarsus with respect to the leg.

The posterior talofibular ligament is oriented so as to check internal rotation of the leg on the tarsus and forward displacement of the leg on the tarsus.

The deltoid ligament, considered as a whole, contributes to restriction of eversion, internal rotation, and external rotation, as well as forward and backward displacement of the tarsus. However, sectioning of the deltoid ligament alone apparently results primarily in instability into eversion of the tarsus on the tibia, the other motions being checked by other ligaments, as described previously.

Subtalar Joint

Functionally, the subtalar joint includes the articulation between the posterior facet of the talus and the opposing articular surface of the calcaneus, as well as the articulation between the anterior and medial facets of the two bones. These articulations move in conjunction with one another. Anatomically, the anterior and medial articulations are actually part of the talocalcaneonavicular joint; they are enclosed within a joint capsule separate from that of the posterior talocalcaneal articulation.

The joint capsules of the posterior portion of the talocalcaneal joint and the talocalcaneonavicular portion of the subtalar joint are separated by the ligament of the tarsal canal. This ligament runs from the underside of the talus, at the sulcus tali, downward and laterally to the dorsum of the calcaneus, at the sulcus calcanei. Since it is situated medially to the axis of motion of inversion–eversion at the subtalar joint, it checks eversion.[88] This ligament is often referred to as the *interosseous talocalcaneal ligament* (see Fig. 15–11).

More laterally, in the sinus tarsi, is the cervical talocalcaneal ligament. It passes from the inferolateral aspect of the talar neck downward and laterally to the dorsum of the calcaneus. It occupies the anterior part of the sinus tarsi. Since the cervical ligament lies lateral to the subtalar joint axis, it restricts inversion of the calcaneus on the talus.[88]

Also, within the lateral aspect of the sinus tarsi, bands from the inferior aspect of the extensor retinaculum pass downward, as well as medially, to the calcaneus. These bands are considered part of the talocalcaneal ligament complex. They help check inversion at the subtalar joint.

Talocalcaneonavicular Joint

The talocalcaneonavicular joint includes the articulation between the anterior and medial facets of the talus and calcaneus (described previously as part of the subtalar joint), the articulations between the inferior aspect of the head of the talus and the subjacent spring ligament, and the articulation between the anterior aspect of the head of the talus and the posterior articular surface of the navicular. The combined talonavicular and talo-spring ligament portion of this joint is essentially a compound ball-and-socket joint; the head of the talus is the ball, while the superior surface of the spring ligament and the posterior surface of the navicular form the socket. It should be noted that the superior surface of the spring ligament is lined with articular cartilage. The talonavicular portion of this joint constitutes the medial half of the transverse tarsal joint.

The talocalcaneonavicular joint is enclosed by a joint capsule, the posterior aspect of which traverses the tarsal canal, forming the anterior wall of the canal. The capsule is reinforced by the spring ligament inferiorly, the calcaneonavicular portion of the bifurcate ligament laterally, and the tibionavicular portion of the deltoid ligament medially (see Figs. 15–10 and 15–12).

The spring ligament passes from the anterior and medial margins of the sustentaculum tali forward to the inferior and inferomedial aspect of the navicular. As mentioned, its superior surface articulates with the underside of the head of the talus. This ligament maintains apposition of the medial aspects of the forefoot and hindfoot and in so doing helps to maintain the normal arched configuration of the foot. Laxity of the ligament allows a medial separation between the calcaneus and forefoot, with the forefoot assuming an abducted position with respect to the hindfoot. At the same time, the foot is allowed to "untwist," which effectively lowers the normal arch of the foot, and the talar head is allowed to move medially and inferiorly. Further discussion of the twisted configuration and arching of the foot is included in the section on biomechanics.

Calcaneocuboid Joint

The lateral portion of the transverse tarsal joint is the calcaneocuboid joint. The calcaneocuboid joint is a sellar joint in that the calcaneal joint surface is concave superoinferiorly and convex mediolaterally (see Figs. 15–3 and 15–4); the adjoining cuboid surface is reciprocally shaped. This joint is enclosed in a joint capsule distinct from that of the talocalcaneonavicular joint and constitutes the lateral half of the transverse tarsal joint. The joint capsule is reinforced inferiorly by the strong plantar calcaneocuboid (short plantar) ligament and the long plantar ligament. The short plantar ligament runs from the anterior tubercle of the plantar aspect of the calcaneus to the underside of the cuboid. The long plantar ligament runs from the posterior tubercles of the calcaneus forward to the bases of the fifth, fourth, third, and sometimes second metatarsals (see Fig. 15–9). Both of these ligaments support the normal arched configuration of the foot by helping to maintain a twisted relationship between the hindfoot and forefoot. Dorsally, the joint capsule is reinforced by the calcaneocuboid band of the bifurcate ligament (see Fig. 15–10).

SURFACE ANATOMY

Bony Palpation

Medial Aspect. The medial malleolus is easily palpated and observed as a large prominence medially. About 2 cm distal to the medial malleolus, the sustentaculum tali can be felt, especially if the foot is held in an everted position. The tibiocalcaneal portion of the deltoid ligament passes from the malleolus to the sustentaculum tali.

If the palpating finger is moved about 5 cm directly anterior to the sustentaculum, the *navicular tubercle* can be located as a prominence on the medial aspect of the arch of the foot. The tibionavicular portion of the deltoid ligament attaches just above the tubercle. Just superior, and perhaps slightly posterior, to the navicular tubercle, the medial aspect of the *talar head* can be palpated as a less prominent bony landmark. These two landmarks are important in assessing the structure of the foot with regard to the degree of twisting of the forefoot in relation to the hindfoot (the degree of "arching" of the foot).
Dorsal Aspect. At the level of the malleoli, the anterior aspects of the distal ends of the tibia and fibula can be felt. The junction of the two bones, at the syndesmosis, can usually be distinguished, although it is considerably obscured by the distal tibiofibular ligament that overlies it. With the foot relaxed in some degree of plantar flexion, the dorsal aspect of the talar neck can be felt just distal to the end of the tibia. With the foot held inverted and plantarly flexed, the anterolateral aspect of the articular surface of the talus can be easily felt just distal and somewhat lateral to the syndesmosis. Between the dorsal aspect of the talar neck and the most prominent aspect of the dorsum of the foot farther distally, which is the first cuneiform, is the navicular bone, the dorsal aspect of which can be palpated.
Lateral Aspect. The lateral malleolus lies subcutaneously and so is easily palpated. The fairly flat lateral aspect of the calcaneus also has little soft-tissue covering and can be felt throughout its extent. About 3 cm distal to the tip of the malleolus, a small prominence can be felt on the calcaneus. This is the peroneal tubercle (see Fig. 15–4). The peroneus brevis tendon passes superior to the tubercle, whereas the peroneus longus passes inferiorly. Occasionally a small prominence can be palpated just posterior to the peroneal tubercle; this is the point of insertion of the calcaneofibular ligament.

Just distal, and slightly anterior, to the malleolus, a rather marked depression can be felt if the foot is relaxed. This is the lateral opening of the sinus tarsi.

used

Traversing the lateral aspect of the sinus tarsi are the inferior bands of the extensor retinaculum and the cervical talocalcaneal ligament.

If the palpating finger is moved around dorsally and slightly superiorly from the sinus tarsi, the lateral aspect of the neck of the talus where the often-injured anterior talofibular ligament attaches can be felt.

Posterior Aspect.   At the posterior aspect of the heel is a prominent crest running horizontally between the upper and lower posterior calcaneal surfaces. The Achilles tendon gains attachment to the upper surface; the lower surface, covered by a fat pad, slopes forward to the medial and lateral tubercles on the inferior aspect of the calcaneus.

Palpation of the posterior aspect of the talus is obscured by the Achilles tendon, which overlies it prior to inserting on the calcaneus.

Inferior Aspect.   Palpation of the inferior aspect of the calcaneus is made difficult by the thick skin and fat pad that cover it. The weight-bearing medial tubercle can be vaguely distinguished posteriorly in most persons. Traction osteophytes (heel spurs) occasionally develop just anterior to the calcaneal tubercles where the long plantar ligament attaches.

Tendons and Vessels

Medial Aspect.   The tendons of the tibialis posterior, flexor digitorum longus, and flexor hallucis longus muscles cross behind the medial malleolus (Fig. 15–13A). The tibialis posterior is the most anterior of these and is best visualized or palpated when plantar flexion and inversion are performed against some resistance. Posterior to the tibialis posterior tendon is the flexor digitorum longus tendon, which is less prominent. Palpation of the flexor digitorum is facilitated by providing some resistance to toe flexion. The flexor hallucis longus tendon is deeper and runs farther posteriorly; it is not usually palpable. Between the flexor digitorum and flexor hallucis longus tendons runs the posterior tibial artery. Its pulse is palpable behind the malleolus. The tibial nerve, which usually cannot be palpated, runs deep and posterior to the artery.

Just anterior to the medial malleolus is the long saphenous nerve; it can usually be visualized and palpated.

Dorsal Aspect.   Running along the medial side of the dorsum of the ankle is the tendon of the tibialis anterior, which is the most prominent tendon crossing the dorsal aspect of the foot. It is made especially prominent by resisting inversion and dorsiflexion of the foot. It attaches to the medial aspect of the base of the first metatarsal.

Just lateral to the tibialis anterior tendon, the extensor hallucis longus tendon can easily be seen and palpated as the subject extends the big toe.

Running lateral to the extensor hallucis longus tendon, passing distally from where it emerges at the ankle, is the dorsalis pedis artery. Its pulse can best be palpated over the dorsum of the foot, at about the level of the navicular and first cuneiform bones.

Farther laterally, the common tendon of the extensor digitorum longus is seen and felt when the subject extends the toes (Fig. 15–13B). Its four branches can be distinguished where they develop, just distal to the ankle.

If the subject everts and dorsiflexes the foot, the tendon of the peroneus tertius is usually observable just proximal to its insertion at the dorsum of the base of the fifth metatarsal.

Lateral Aspect.   The peroneus longus and peroneus brevis tendons cross behind the lateral malleolus, with the brevis running more anteriorly. The brevis passes superior to the peroneal tubercle on the lateral aspect of the calcaneus; the longus passes inferior to the tubercle. Some resistance should be applied to the plantar flexion and eversion of the foot when palpating these tendons.

Posterior Aspect.   The Achilles tendon is quite prominent and is easily seen and felt proximal to its insertion on the calcaneus. Deep to the tendon, between the tendon and the upper surface of the posterior calcaneus, is the retrocalcaneal bursa. There is also a calcaneal bursa between the Achilles tendon and the skin. These bursae cannot be distinguished on palpation.

BIOMECHANICS

The structural relationships and movements that occur at the ankle and hindfoot are complex. From a clinical standpoint, however, it is important that the clinician have at least a basic understanding of the biomechanics of this region. The joints of the foot and ankle constitute the first movable pivots in the weight-bearing extremity once the foot becomes fixed to the ground. Considered together, these joints must permit mobility in all planes in order to allow for minimal displacement of a person's center of gravity with respect to the base of support when walking over flat or uneven surfaces. In this sense, maintenance of balance and economy of energy consumption are, in part, dependent on proper func-

Fig. 15–13. *(A)* Medial and *(B)* lateral views of the tendons and vessels of the dorsum of the foot.

tioning of the ankle–foot complex. Adequate mobility and proper structural alignment of these joints are also necessary for normal attenuation of forces transmitted from the ground to the weight-bearing extremity. Deviations in alignment and changes in mobility are likely to cause abnormal stresses to the joints of the foot and ankle, as well as to the other weight-bearing joints. It follows that detection of biomechanical alterations in the ankle–foot region is often necessary for adequate interpretation of painful conditions affecting the foot and ankle, as well as conditions affecting the knee, hip, or lower spine, in some cases.

STRUCTURAL ALIGNMENT

In the normal standing position, the patella faces straight forward, the knee joint axis lies in the frontal plane and the tibial tubercle is in line with the midline — or lateral half — of the patella. In this position, a line passing between the tips of the malleoli should make an angle of about 20° to 25° with the frontal plane.[5,42,47] This represents the normal amount of tibial torsion; the distal end of the tibia is rotated outward with respect to the proximal end. The lateral malleolus is positioned inferiorly with respect to the medial malleolus such that the intermalleolar line makes an angle of about 10° with the transverse plane.[47] The joint axis of the ankle mortise joint corresponds approximately to the intermalleolar line. With the patellae facing straight forward, the feet should be pointed outward about 5° to 10°.

If, when the feet are in normal standing alignment, the patellae face inward, increased femoral anteversion, increased external tibial torsion, or both, may be present. Clinically, the fault can be differentiated by assessing rotational range of motion of the hips and estimating the degree of tibial torsion by noting the rotational alignment of the malleoli with respect to the patellae and tibial tubercles. In the presence of increased hip anteversion, the total range of hip motion will be normal but skewed such that internal rotation is excessive and external rotation is restricted proportionally. Similar considerations hold for a situation in which the patellae face outward when the feet are normally aligned; femoral retroversion, internal tibial torsion, or both, are likely to exist.

With respect to the frontal plane, normal knee alignment may vary from slight genu valgum to some degree of genu varum. Since in most persons the medial femoral condyle extends farther distally than the lateral condyle, slight genu valgum tends to be more prevalent. At the hindfoot, the calcaneus should be positioned in vertical alignment with the tibia. A valgus or varus heel can usually be observed as a bowing of the Achilles tendon. A valgus positioning of the calcaneus on the talus is associated with pronation at the subtalar joint, whereas a varus hindfoot involves supination.

When considering the structure of the foot as a whole, it is helpful to compare it to a twisted plate (Fig. 15–14); the calcaneus, at one end, is positioned vertically when contacting the ground, whereas the metatarsal heads are positioned horizontally when making contact with a flat surface.[62] Thus, in the normal standing position on a flat, level surface, the metatarsal heads are twisted 90° with respect to the calcaneus.

To demonstrate this, a model can be constructed by taking a light rectangular piece of cardboard and twisting it so that one end lies flat on a table and the opposite end is perpendicular to the table top. Note the "arching" of the cardboard. This is analogous to the arching of the human foot. It should be realized that the term *arch* here applies to the configuration of the structure, which is dependent on the fact that it is twisted on itself. It does not refer to an arch in the true architectural sense, in which the arched configuration is dependent on the shapes of the component "building blocks." In the foot, both situations exist. On the medial side, there is little architectural arching and, therefore, little inherent stability of the medial arch. The medial arch is dependent almost entirely on the twisted configuration of the foot, which is maintained statically by the short and long plantar ligaments and dynamically by the anterior and posterior tibialis muscles. In contrast, the lateral side of the foot represents a true architectural arch (Fig. 15–15).[62] Here the cuboid, being wedged between the calcaneus and metatarsals, serves as the structural keystone. Only a small component of the lateral arch is a result of the twisted configuration of the foot.

Referring back to the cardboard model, notice that when the cardboard is allowed to untwist — by inclining the vertical end in one direction and keeping the other end flat on the table — the arch flattens. Inclining the vertical end in the opposite direction increases the twist and increases the arch. In the foot, inclination of the vertical component of the structure, the calcaneus, will result in similar untwisting or twisting; this results in a respective decrease or increase in the arching of the foot, if the metatarsal heads remain in contact with the ground (Fig. 15–16). The person who stands with the heel in a valgus position will have a relatively "flat" or untwisted foot, whereas a person whose heel is in a

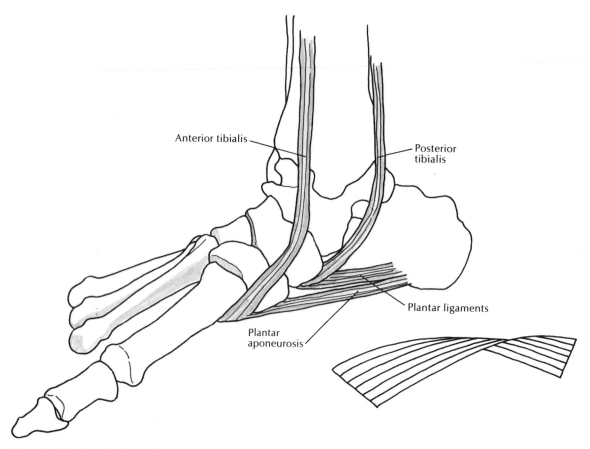

Anterior tibialis

Posterior tibialis

Plantar ligaments

Plantar aponeurosis

Fig. 15-14. The "twisted plate," which generates the medial arch.

varus position when standing will appear to have a "high" arch because of increased twisting between hindfoot and forefoot. The former situation is often termed a *pronated foot* or *flatfoot*, while the latter is termed a *supinated foot* or *pes cavus*. In the situation of the heel remaining in a vertical position but the metatarsal heads inclined on, say, an uneven surface, the effect will also be to twist or untwist the foot and, therefore, to raise or to lower the arch. For example, if the inclination is such that the first metatarsal head is on a higher level than the fifth, the forefoot supinates on the hindfoot, untwisting the foot and lowering the arch. Note that supination of the forefoot with the hindfoot fixed is the same as pronation of the hindfoot with the forefoot fixed; they both involve untwisting of the tarsal skeleton from motion at the subtalar, transverse tarsal, and tarsal-metatarsal joints.

Reference is often made to a *transverse arch* of the foot, distinguishing it from the *longitudinal arch*. The cardboard model should help to make it clear that some transverse arching results from the twisted configuration of the foot. This is simply a transverse component of the arch discussed previously. This transverse component will increase and decrease along with twisting and untwisting of the foot. There is also a structural component to the transverse arching of the foot, resulting from the contours and relationships of the tarsals and metatarsals. It must be realized, however, that at the level of the metatarsal heads in the standing subject, no transverse arch exists, since each of the heads makes contact with the floor.

ARTHROKINEMATICS OF THE ANKLE–FOOT COMPLEX

Ankle Mortise Joint

The superior articular surface of the talus is wider anteriorly than posteriorly, the difference in widths being as much as 6 mm.[5,47] The articular surfaces of the tibial and fibular malleoli maintain a close fit against the medial and lateral articular surfaces of the talus in all positions of plantar flexion and dorsiflexion. As the foot moves from full plantar flexion into full dorsiflexion the talus rolls backward in the

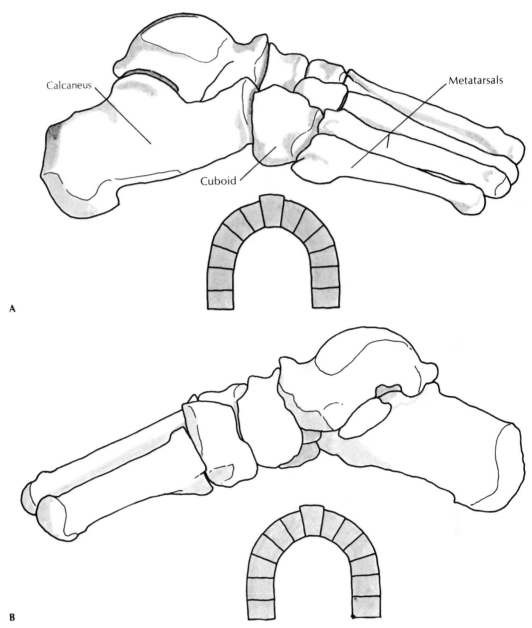

Fig. 15-15. (A) The lateral arch of the foot is a true arch. The calcaneus forms the ascending flank, the cuboid is the true keystone, and the fourth and fifth metatarsals are the descending flank. (B) The medial arch of the foot is not a true arch.

mortise. It would seem, then, that with ankle dorsiflexion the malleoli must separate in order to accommodate the greater anterior width of the talus. This separation could occur as a result of a lateral shift of the fibula, a lateral bending of the fibula, or both. However, it is found that the amount of separation that occurs between the malleoli during ankle dorsiflexion varies from none to only 2 mm, which is much less than would be expected considering the amount of wedging of the superior articular surface of the talus. There appears to be a significant discrep-

ancy between the difference in anterior and posterior widths of the trochlea of the talus and the amount of separation that occurs between the tibial and fibular malleoli with ankle dorsiflexion.

In understanding this apparent paradox, a closer look must be given to the structure of the trochlea and the type of movement the talus undergoes during ankle dorsiflexion. If both sides of the trochlea are examined it is evident that the lateral articular surface, which articulates with the fibular malleolus, is longer in its anteroposterior dimension than the

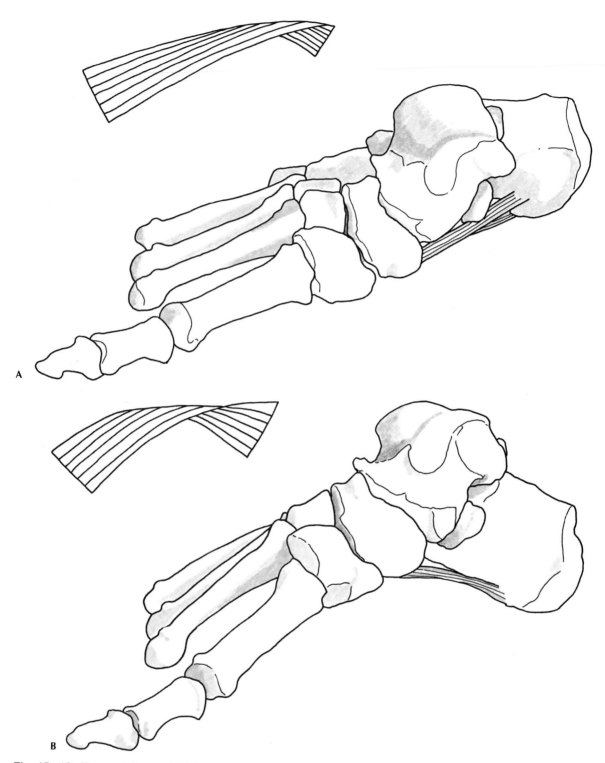

Fig. 15-16. The medial arch. *(A)* When it is allowed to "untwist," the arch flattens; *(B)* when the medial arch is "twisted," the arch increases.

medial articular surface. The reason for this is that the lateral malleolus moves over a greater excursion, with respect to the talus, during plantar flexion–dorsiflexion, than does the medial malleolus. This is partly because the axis of motion is farther from the superior trochlear articular surface laterally than medially. The corollary to this (and this is true of essentially all joints with sellar surfaces) is that the

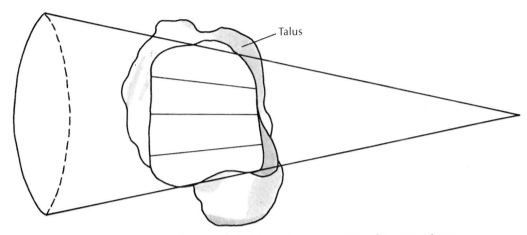

Fig. 15-17. Diagram to illustrate movement of the talus as a section of a cone, whose apex is situated medially, rotating within the mortise about its own long axis.

relatively trackbound movement that the talus undergoes on plantar flexion–dorsiflexion at the ankle is not a pure swing, but rather an impure swing; it involves an element of spin, or rotation, that results in a helical movement. Another way of conceptualizing this movement is to consider the talus as a section of a cone whose apex is situated medially rotating within the mortise about its own long axis, rather than a truly cylindrical body undergoing a simple rolling movement within the mortise (Fig. 15–17). As a result of this, the intermalleolar lines projected onto the superior trochlear articular surface at various positions of plantar flexion and dorsiflexion are not parallel lines. Therefore, the degree of wedging of the trochlea does not reflect the relative intermalleolar distances in dorsiflexion and plantar flexion of the ankle. The true intermalleolar distances are represented by the length of these nonparallel lines projected onto the superior trochlear surface. The projected line with the foot in plantar flexion is only slightly shorter, if at all, than that for dorsiflexion, and the necessary separation of the malleoli during dorsiflexion is minimal.[47]

Up to this point, the ankle mortise joint axis has been considered as a fixed axis of motion. This has been done for the sake of simplicity and convenience using the approximate center of movement as the joint axis. But, as mentioned in Chapter 2, Arthrology, no joint moves about a stationary joint axis. As indicated by instant center analysis of knee joint motion, this is true of the ankle mortise joint as well.[83] The surface velocities determined from the instant centers of movement show that when moving from full plantar flexion to full dorsiflexion there is initially a momentary distraction of the tibiotalar joint

surfaces, followed by a movement of combined rolling and sliding throughout most of the range, and terminating with an approximation of joint surfaces at the position of extreme dorsiflexion. These findings are consistent with the fact that the close-packed position of the ankle mortise joint is dorsiflexion; the tightening of the joint capsule that occurs with movement of any joint into its close-packed position produces an approximation of the joint surfaces.

Subtalar Joint

As discussed previously, this is a compound joint with two distinct articulations. From the outset, movement at this joint is somewhat difficult to conceptualize because the posterior articulation between the talus and calcaneus is concave superiorly on convex inferiorly, while the anteromedial articulation is convex on concave. Understanding talocalcaneal movement is perhaps facilitated by considering it analogous to movement at the proximal and distal radioulnar joints. The radioulnar joints, like the talocalcaneal joints, move in conjunction with one another and have only one degree of freedom of motion. The posterior calcaneal facet moving against the opposing concave talar surface can be compared with the radial head moving within the radial notch of the ulna. As this movement occurs, the anteromedial facet of the talus must move in relation to the concave anteromedial surface of the calcaneus, just as the head of the ulna must move within the ulnar notch of the radius at the distal joint of the forearm. In at least some persons, this type of movement at the subtalar joint is accompanied by a slight forward displacement of the talus during pronation and a backward displacement on supination, thus making the total movement a helical, or screw-like, motion.[66]

Neutral Position of a Joint

To facilitate arthrometric studies and to correlate function of the joints, it is necessary to assign to joints certain reference points called the neutral positions of those joints. By definition these neutral positions are purely reference points. They are, however, significant in that they make it possible to measure and define positional and structural variances.

The neutral position of the first ray is that position in which the first metatarsal head lies in the same transverse plane as the central three metatarsal heads when they are at their most dorsiflexed position.[81] From this neutral position, the first metatarsal can move an equal distance above and below the transverse plane of the lesser metatarsal heads when the first ray is moved through its full range.

Root and co-workers describe a neutral position of the subtalar joint that is that position of the joint in which the foot is neither pronated nor supinated.[81] Another way to state this is the position from which the subtalar joint could be maximally pronated and supinated. From this position, full supination of the normal subtalar inverts the calcaneus twice as many degrees as full pronation everts it. Subtalar neutral is two thirds from inversion and one third from eversion of the calcaneus.

Clinically this is important since the subtalar neutral position provides a foundation for meaningful and valid measurements and observations to take place with respect to the foot and entire leg. It is not only a basis for meaningful communication but is also the foundation for the application of precise therapy, such as the fabrication of an effective biomechanical orthotic device.[39] There is also a direct clinical correlation between the subtalar joint and the midtarsal joint. When the subtalar joint is held in its neutral position there is no longer the ability for the midtarsal joint to pronate. The midtarsal is unable to dorsiflex, evert, or abduct when the subtalar is in its neutral position. This position is termed the *normal locking position* of the midtarsal joint.

According to James, the talar head in a pronated foot can be palpated as a medial bulge; in a supinated foot the talar head bulges laterally. In the neutral position the talar head can be palpated equally on the medial and lateral aspects of the ankle.[50] The neutral position is usually present when the longitudinal axis of the lower limb and the vertical axis of the calcaneus are parallel. This method for establishing the subtalar neutral position is useful in both the open- and closed-chain positions.

A second method that is useful in the open-chain position involves visualizing and feeling the subtalar joint as it moves through its range of motion.[49] To begin, the examiner should place the ulnar surface of the thumb into the sulcus of the patient's fourth and fifth toes, moving the patient's foot from pronation to supination and back again. This movement is very similar in shape to that of a horse saddle, being very abrupt toward pronation and very flat and shallow toward supination (Fig. 15–18A). The bottom of this saddle is the neutral position of the subtalar joint. This can be confirmed visually by observing the lateral curves above and below the malleolus (Fig. 15–18B). If these curves are the same depth, this is the accurate neutral position. If the curve below the malleolus is deeper or shallower, then the foot is still in a pronated or supinated position and should be repositioned.

Transverse Tarsal Joints: Talonavicular and Calcaneocuboid Joints

Although perhaps some movement occurs between the cuboid and navicular bones, movement of these two bones is considered here as a unit with respect to the calcaneus and the talus. The configuration of the talonavicular articulation is essentially that of a ball-and-socket joint. Because of this configuration, it potentially has three degrees of freedom of movement, allowing it to move in all planes. However, because the navicular is closely bound to the cuboid bone laterally, its freedom of movement is largely governed by the movement allowed at the calcaneocuboid joint.[29] The calcaneocuboid joint, having a sellar configuration, has two degrees of freedom, each of which occurs about a distinct axis of motion. The axis of motion of most concern here is the axis of pronation and supination. This axis is similar in location and orientation to the subtalar joint axis, the major difference being that it is not inclined as much vertically. It passes through the talar head, backward, downward, and laterally. Such an orientation allows a movement of inversion–adduction–plantar flexion (supination) and eversion–abduction–dorsiflexion (pronation) of the forefoot. In the standing position, movement and positioning at the transverse tarsal joint occurs in conjunction with subtalar joint movement; when the subtalar joint pronates, the transverse tarsal joint supinates and *vice versa*. Pronation of the forefoot close packs and locks the transverse tarsal joint complex,

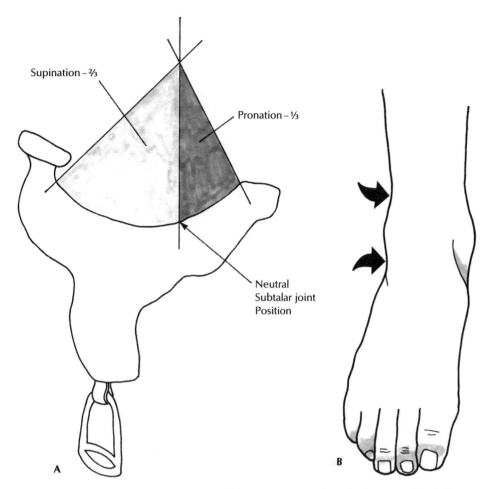

Fig. 15–18. Subtalar movement is very similar in shape to that of a horse saddle, being very abrupt toward pronation and flat and shallow toward supination. The bottom position is the neutral position of the subtalar (A), which can be visually confirmed by observing the lateral curves above and below the malleolus (B). These curves should be of the same depth.

whereas supination results in loose packing and a greater degree of freedom of movement.[62]

OSTEOKINEMATICS OF THE ANKLE–FOOT COMPLEX

Terminology

At this point, some terms related to movement and positioning of various components of the ankle and foot must be clarified. Throughout this chapter the following definitions will hold:

Inversion–Eversion—Movement about a horizontal axis lying in the sagittal plane. Functionally, pure inversion and eversion rarely occur at any of the joints of ankle or foot. More often they occur as a component of supination or pronation.

Abduction–Adduction—Movement of the forefoot about a vertical axis or the movement of the forefoot that results from internal or external rotation of the hindfoot with respect to the leg.

Internal-External Rotation—Movement between the leg and hindfoot occurring about a vertical axis. Pure rotations do not occur functionally but rather occur as components of pronation and supination.

Plantar flexion–Dorsiflexion—Movement about a horizontal axis lying in the plane corresponding to the intermalleolar line. Functionally, these usually occur in conjunction with other movements.

Pronation–Supination—Functional movements occurring around the obliquely situated subtalar or transverse tarsal joint axis. At both of these joints, pronation involves abduction, eversion, and some dorsiflexion; supination involves adduction, inversion, and plantar flexion of the distal segment on the proximal segment. This is because these joint axes are inclined backward, downward, and laterally. It must be appreciated that when the metatarsals are fixed to the ground, pronation of the hindfoot (subtalar joint) involves supination of the forefoot (transverse tarsal joint).

Pronated Foot – Supinated Foot — Traditionally, a pronated foot (in the standing position) is one in which the arched configuration of the foot is reduced; the hindfoot is pronated while the forefoot is supinated. In a supinated foot (standing) the arch is high, the hindfoot is supinated, and the forefoot is pronated.

Valgus – Varus — Terms used for alignment of parts. *Valgus* denotes inclination away from the midline of a segment with respect to its proximal neighbor, whereas *varus* is inclination toward the midline. At the hindfoot and forefoot, valgus refers to alignment in a pronated position and varus to alignment in a supinated position.

Orientation of Joint Axes and the Effect on Movement

In the normal standing position, the axis of movement for the knee joint is horizontal and in a frontal plane. With flexion and extension of the free-swinging tibia, movement will occur in a sagittal plane. The ankle mortise joint axis is directed backward mediolaterally about 25° from the frontal plane and downward from medial to lateral about 10° to 15° from horizontal. Movement of the free foot about this axis results in combined plantar flexion, adduction, and inversion or combined dorsiflexion, abduction, and eversion. Note that the above statements relate the movements at the respective joints to the orientations of the joint axes when the foot and leg are swinging freely. In this position, movements at one joint may occur independently of the other.

Therapists must be more concerned, however, with what happens when the foot becomes fixed to the ground and movement occurs simultaneously at the joints of the lower extremities. This is the situation during weight-bearing activities, or normal functional activities, involving the leg. The obvious question in this regard would be: How is it possible to move both the tibia and femur in the sagittal plane, such as when performing a knee bend with the knee pointed forward, when movement is occurring at the ankle and knee about two nonparallel axes? The heavy-weight lifter largely avoids the problem by pointing the knees outward, thus using external rotation and abduction at the hip. This brings the knee

and ankle axes closer to parallel alignment. The fact remains, however, that it is possible to perform a deep knee bend with the knee directed forward, and through a considerable range. Since the knee joint axis lies horizontally in the frontal plane, no problem would be expected there, since it is ideally oriented to allow rotation of the bones in the sagittal plane. It would seem, then, that by performing such a knee bend an internal rotatory movement must be applied to the ankle, since the ankle joint axis is externally rotated with respect to the frontal plane. Surely ankle mortise joints cannot be expected to withstand such stresses during daily activities. This apparent problem can be resolved by considering the orientation of the joint axis and associated movements at the subtalar joint.

The axis of motion for the subtalar joint is directed backward, downward, and laterally.[15,47,65,66] The degree of inclination and mediolateral deviation of the axis varies greatly among persons. The average deviation from the midline of the foot is 23°, whereas the average deviation from the horizontal is 42°. Because the axis of motion for the subtalar joint deviates from the sagittal plane and from the horizontal plane, movement at this joint involves combined eversion, dorsiflexion, and abduction or combined inversion, plantar flexion, and adduction. Note that pure abduction and adduction of the foot are movements that would occur about a vertical axis and that inversion and eversion occur about a purely horizontal axis. Since the subtalar axis is positioned about midway between horizontal and vertical, it follows that movement about this axis would include elements of adduction – abduction as well as eversion – inversion.

Now again consider a situation of simultaneous knee and ankle flexion in the sagittal plane with the foot fixed (*e.g.*, a deep knee bend). It was indicated that with such a movement an internal rotatory moment of the tibia on the talus would be applied to the ankle. Because the subtalar axis allows an element of movement about a vertical axis (rotation in the horizontal plane), this internal rotatory moment can be transmitted to the subtalar joint. Internal rotation of the tibia on the foot is, of course, equivalent to external rotation of the foot on the leg, which is referred to as abduction of the foot. Subtalar movement is essentially uniaxial, so that any movement occurring at the joint may occur only in conjunction with its component movements, that is, abduction can only occur in conjunction with eversion and dorsiflexion, the three together constituting pronation at the subtalar. Thus, with the foot fixed, simultaneous dorsiflexion of the ankle and flexion of the knee, keeping the leg in the sagittal plane, requires pronation at the subtalar joint. As a corollary to this, with such a movement, if pronation at the subtalar joint is restricted, an abnormal internal tibial rotatory stress will occur at the ankle mortise joint, an internal femoral rotatory stress will be placed on the knee, or both.[15] The need for subtalar movement can be reduced by moving the leg out of the sagittal plane (by pointing the knee outward), bringing the knee and ankle axes into closer alignment.

Similar considerations apply to the situation of a person rotating the leg over a fixed foot. Any rotation imparted to the tibia is transmitted to the subtalar joint (Fig. 15–19). For example, if one rotates the leg externally over a foot that is fixed to the ground, the subtalar joint undergoes a movement of supination. This is analogous to movement about a mitered hinge; movement of one component about a vertical axis is transmitted to the second component as movement about a horizontal axis. Supination causes the calcaneus to assume a varus position, which, since the metatarsals remain flat on the ground, increases the twist in the foot and raises the arch.[42] The opposite occurs with internal tibial rota-

tion; pronation of the hindfoot causes a relative supination of the forefoot; the foot untwists and the arch flattens. This can easily be observed if one attempts to rotate the leg with the foot fixed to the ground. With respect to the structural alignment, then, a person with excessive internal tibial torsion will tend to have a pronated hindfoot (calcaneus in valgus position) and a forefoot that is supinated with respect to the hindfoot. The resultant untwisting of the foot causes a flatfoot on standing. The person with excessive external tibial torsion will tend to have a varus heel and a high arch.

The degree of twisting and untwisting of the foot also varies with stance width.[62] When standing with the feet far apart, the heel tends to deviate into a valgus position with respect to the floor and the metatarsal heads remain flat; the metatarsals assume a position of supination with respect to the heel, thus untwisting the foot. The opposite occurs when standing with the legs crossed.

It should be noted that when standing with the hindfoot in pronation and the forefoot in supination, the medial metatarsals assume a position closer to dorsiflexion.[42] Since the joint axis of the first meta-

Fig. 15–19. (A) External rotation of the tibia over the fixed foot imparts a movement of supination to the foot, increasing the arch. (B) Internal tibial rotation flattens, or pronates, the fixed foot.

tarsal is obliquely oriented (from anterolateral to posteromedial), dorsiflexion of the first metatarsal involves a component of abduction away from the midline of the foot. Therefore, in a pronated foot, the first metatarsal is usually positioned in varus. On the other hand, a person with metatarsus primus varus, a condition in which the first metatarsal deviates into varus position, the foot will tend to assume a pronated position. This is because in order for the first metatarsal to be in a varus angle, it must also be in some dorsiflexion. This causes supination of the forefoot, which necessitates pronation of the hindfoot in order for the person to stand with the metatarsal head and calcaneus in contact with the ground.

Ankle and Foot During Gait

Clinicians must be concerned with the function of the joints of the ankle and foot during normal daily activities. The prime consideration here, of course, is walking. Again, because these are weight-bearing joints and because the foot becomes fixed to the ground during the stance phase, an understanding of the biomechanical interrelationships between these joints and the other joints of the lower extremity is necessary.

During the gait cycle, the leg progresses through space in a sagittal plane. In order to minimize energy expenditure, the center of gravity must undergo minimal vertical displacement. Minimization of vertical displacement of the center of gravity is largely accomplished by angular movement of the lower extremity components in the sagittal plane, that is, flexion–extension at the hip, knee, and ankle complex. The hip has no trouble accommodating such movement since it is multiaxial, allowing some movement in all vertical planes. The knee, although essentially uniaxial, allows flexion and extension in the sagittal plane because its axis of movement is perpendicular to this plane and horizontally oriented. The ankle mortise joint, however, cannot allow a pure sagittal movement between the leg and foot because its axis of motion is not perpendicular to the sagittal plane; it is rotated outward about 25°. During the normal gait cycle, however, movement between the foot and leg in the sagittal plane does occur. This is only possible through participation of another joint, the subtalar joint. Movement of the tibia in a parasagittal plane over a fixed foot requires simultaneous movement at the subtalar and ankle mortise joints. This is consistent with the fact that no muscles attach to the talus. Those muscles that affect movement at the ankle mortise joint also cross the subtalar joint, moving it as well.

In considering the various movements occurring at each of the segments of the lower extremity during gait, it is convenient to speak of three intervals of stance phase; these are (1) the interval from heel-strike to foot-flat, (2) midstance (foot-flat), and (3) the interval from the beginning of heel-rise to toe-off.

During the first interval, each of the segments of the lower extremity rotates internally with respect to its more proximal neighboring segment; the pelvis rotates internally in space, the femur rotates internally on the pelvis, and the tibia rotates internally on the femur (Fig. 15–20A).[56,58,84] It follows that the entire lower limb rotates during this phase and that distal segments rotate more, in space, than the more proximally situated segments. At the point of heel-strike, the foot becomes partially fixed to the ground, so that only minimal internal torsion between the heel and the ground takes place. Much of this internal rotation is absorbed at the subtalar joint as pronation (Fig. 15–20B).[91,99] Internal rotation of the leg with respect to the foot, occurring at the subtalar joint, makes the axis of the ankle mortise joint more perpendicular to the plane of progression. This allows the ankle mortise joint to provide for movement in the sagittal plane, which, of course, is the plantar flexion occurring at the ankle during this interval (Fig. 15–20C). Note that the foot tends to

A

Fig. 15–20.

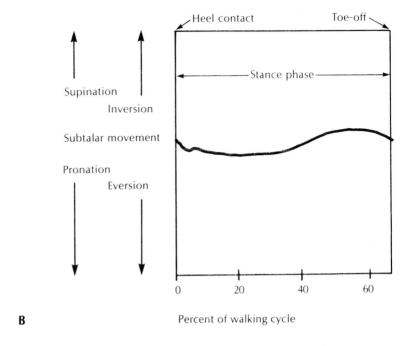

B   Percent of walking cycle

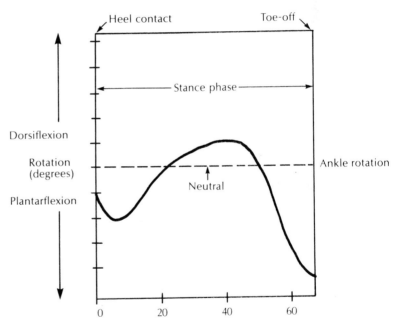

Fig. 15–20. The gait cycle. The composite
curves show (A) transverse rotations of the
pelvis, femur, and tibia (stance phase); (B)
subtalar rotation; and (C) ankle mortise
rotation (sagittal plane).

C   Percent of walking cycle

deviate slightly medially in this stage of stance phase.
This is because the obliquity of the ankle axis, in the
coronal plane, imposes a component of adduction of
the foot during plantar flexion.

At heel-strike, a moment-arm equal to the distance
between the point of heel contact and the ankle joint
develops. The reactive force of the ground acting on
the foot at heel-strike across this moment-arm will
tend to swing the tibia forward in the sagittal plane.

This results in some flexion at the knee, which is
consistent with the fact that the tibia is rotating internally with respect to the femur. Knee flexion, from
an extended position, involves a component of internal tibial rotation.

Note that at heel-strike, the hindfoot moves into
pronation while the tibialis anterior muscle contracts to bring the forefoot into supination. This
causes the foot to untwist, the transverse tarsal joint

to unlock, and the joints to assume a loose-packed position. The foot at this point is in a position favorable for free mobility and is, therefore, at its greatest potential to adapt to variations in the contour of the ground.[29,99]

Once the foot becomes flat on the ground, movement at the ankle mortise joint changes abruptly from plantar flexion to dorsiflexion.[75,78] Through the early period of foot-flat, during which most of dorsiflexion occurs, the segments of the lower extremity continue to rotate internally. This rotation is transmitted to the joints of the ankle, since the foot is now fixed to the ground. Some internal rotation of the tibia automatically occurs at the ankle mortise joint during dorsiflexion with the foot fixed, since the joint axis is inclined about 15° from horizontal, downward and laterally. However, most of the internal rotation takes place at the subtalar joint as a component of pronation.[15,99]

Throughout most of the period during which the foot is flat on the ground, the segments of the lower extremity rotate externally; the more distal segments rotate externally to a greater degree than their proximal neighbors.[59] Again, because the foot is fixed to the ground, the tibia rotates externally with respect to the foot. This occurs as supination at the subtalar joint. The change during foot-flat, from internal rotation to external rotation, takes place after most of ankle dorsiflexion is complete.

Because the forefoot is fixed to the ground, the inversion occurring at the subtalar joint imposes pronation at the transverse tarsal joint, causing a close-packing or locking of the tarsus. Consistent with this, the peroneus longus muscle contracts, maintaining a pronated twist of the metatarsals and bringing the foot as a whole toward its twisted configuration. The foot at this point is being converted into an intrinsically stable lever capable of providing for the thrust of pushing off.

During the final interval of stance phase, from heel-rise to toe-off, the segments of the lower limb continue to rotate externally. This external rotation of the tibia is again transmitted to the subtalar joint as supination of the hindfoot. With contraction of the calf muscle, the ankle begins plantar flexion, creating a thrust for push-off. This again creates a moment-arm acting on the knee, this time moving the tibia into extension with respect to the femur. Note that this is consistent with the external rotation of the tibia occurring during this phase, since knee extension involves a component of external tibial rotation.

The extension of the metatarsophalangeal joints, occurring with heel-rise, causes a tightening of the plantar aponeurosis through a windlass effect, since the distal attachment of the aponeurosis crosses the plantar aspect of the joints (Fig. 15–21).[43] This tightening of the aponeurosis further raises the arch and adds to the rigidity of the tarsal skeleton.

It should be emphasized that during this final phase of stance, the joint movements that occur automatically convert the foot into a stable lever system and require little, if any, muscle contraction in order to accomplish this.

In summary, then, the transverse rotations of the segments of the lower extremity that occur during stance phase of the gait cycle are transmitted to the ankle joints. This is because during the stance phase the foot is relatively fixed to the ground so that rotation between the foot and the ground is minimal. The ankle mortise axis is inclined slightly vertically (about 15° from the horizontal axis) while the subtalar joint axis is situated about midway between horizontal and vertical. Both joints are able to "absorb" rotatory movements transmitted to the ankle because of the vertical inclination of the joint axes. With the foot fixed to the ground, the tibia rotates slightly internally at the ankle mortise during dorsiflexion and externally during plantar flexion. Internal rotation of the talus with respect to the calcaneus occurs as pronation, while external rotation results in supination at the subtalar joint. Also, once the foot becomes flat on the ground, the metatarsal heads become fixed and the twisting and untwisting of the foot becomes dependent on the position of the hindfoot. At heel-strike, the tibia rotates internally, pronating the hindfoot, while the tibialis anterior contracts to supinate the forefoot; this results in an untwisted foot. During midstance, as the tibia rotates externally and the subtalar joint gradually supinates, the foot becomes twisted. This twisting is further increased by tightening of the plantar aponeurosis. The twisted configuration results in maximal joint stability with minimal participation of the intrinsic foot muscles. It is the twisted foot, then, that is best suited for weight-bearing and propulsion. During midstance there is little activity of the intrinsic muscles in the normal foot because the twisted configuration confers a passive, or intrinsic, stability on the foot. However, in the flatfooted person, considerably more muscle action is required since the foot is relatively untwisted.[62] The flatfooted person must rely more on extrinsic stabilization by the muscles. An untwisted configuration is desirable in situations in which the foot must be mobile, such as in adapting to surface contours of the ground. Consistent with this is the fact that at heel-strike, the foot assumes an untwisted state in preparation for conformation to the contacting surface.

Fig. 15-21. *(A)* The foot is flat. *(B)* Toe standing causes the aponeurosis to tighten. Tightening the plantar aponeurosis raises the arch and adds to the rigidity of tarsal skeleton.

A relatively common condition that illustrates the biomechanical interdependency of the weight-bearing joints is femoral anteversion. A person with femoral anteversion must stand with the leg internally rotated in order to position the hip joint in normal (neutral) alignment. Conversely, if the leg is positioned in normal alignment with the patella facing straight forward, the hip joint assumes a position of relative external rotation. External rotation at the hip decreases the congruity of the joint surfaces. During stance phase, as the femur externally rotates on the pelvis, the hip of the person with femoral anteversion will tend to go into too much external rotation. As the slack is taken up in the part of the joint

capsule that pulls tight on external rotation, the joint receptors sense the excessive movement. To avoid excessive joint incongruity and to prevent abnormal stress to the joint capsule, the person with femoral anteversion must *internally* rotate during stance phase. This internal rotation is transmitted primarily to the subtalar joint, which is best oriented to accommodate transverse rotations. Internal rotation at the subtalar joint causes pronation of the hindfoot; the foot untwists and the arch flattens. Thus, femoral anteversion predisposes to pronation of the foot. Also, because of the internal rotatory movement transmitted through the knee, femoral anteversion may also be a causative factor in certain knee disorders. For example, internal rotation imposed on a semiflexed knee causes the knee to assume an increased valgus position. This may predispose to patellar tracking dysfunction (see Chapter 14, The Knee). Since there is a tendency for the person with femoral anteversion to walk with increased hip joint incongruity, the force of weight-bearing is transmitted to a smaller area of contact at the articular surface of the hip. The result may be accelerated wear of the hip joint surfaces, perhaps leading to degenerative hip disease.

Femoral anteversion provides a good example of how a structural abnormality in one region may lead to localized biomechanical disturbances as well as altered mechanics at joints some distance away. This, again, is especially true of the lower extremity and should emphasize that when evaluating many patients with foot disorders it may be appropriate, if not necessary, to examine the structure and function of the knee, hip, and lower back. Conversely, foot or ankle dysfunction may precipitate disturbances in more proximal joints.

EXAMINATION

The L4, L5, S1, and S2 segments contribute to the ankle and foot. Symptoms arising in the more proximal regions of these segments may refer to the ankle and foot, the most common of which might be paresthesias arising from lumbar nerve root irritation. Actual pain of more proximal origin is rarely felt in the foot. Rather, foot and ankle pain usually arises from local pathologic processes. Pain arising from tissues of the foot or ankle may be referred a short distance proximally but almost never to the knee or above.

The common lesions affecting the ankle are of acute, traumatic onset, whereas those affecting the foot are more likely to be chronic disorders resulting from stress overload. Because of the biomechanical interdependency of the weight-bearing joints, attention must often be directed to the structure and function of more proximally situated joints during examination of patients with chronic or subtle foot disorders. Similarly, examination of the foot may well be in order in patients with disorders affecting more proximal regions.

HISTORY

A patient interview designed to elicit specific information related to the patient's pain, functional status, and other associated symptoms, as set out in Chapter 4, Assessment of Musculoskeletal Disorders, should be carried out. The following are general concepts that apply to information that may be elicited when a therapist interviews patients with common foot or ankle disorders.

—If the disorder was of an acute, traumatic onset, an attempt can be made to determine the exact mechanism of injury. Plantar flexion–inversion strains are more likely to result in capsuloligamentous injury, whereas forces moving the foot into dorsiflexion and external rotation (abduction) are more likely to produce a fracture.

—If the disorder is of a more chronic nature and of insidious onset, the therapist can attempt to determine whether a change in activity level or footwear may be associated with the onset of the problem. Also inquire about the effect of changing footwear. For example, a therapist might determine the effect of variations in heel height, including whether the problem is affected, for better or for worse, by going barefoot.

—Chronic stress overload (fatigue) disorders may be classified as (1) those due to high levels of activity in which the frequency or high rate of tissue stress is such that the body is unable to keep up with the increased rate of tissue microtrauma (the rate of tissue breakdown exceeds the rate of repair and the tissue gradually fatigues) and (2) those that occur with normal activity levels and are due to some structural or biomechanical abnormality that subjects the affected tissue to mildly increased stresses over a long period of time. Such stresses may produce pain on an intermittent basis and, over a long period of time, may induce tissue hypertrophy. Since these are mild stresses acting over a long period, the body is able to respond by laying down an excessive amount of tissue in an attempt to strengthen itself against these abnormal stresses. Tissue hypertrophy such as corns and calluses may, in itself, lead to pain by allowing localized areas of stress concentration.

Patients incurring tissue damage from high stresses acting over a relatively short time period are typically persons who have increased their activity level significantly. Often, but not always, the patient will blame a particular activity for contributing to the onset of the problem. Keep in mind that in such instances the patient may or may not be correct; the particular disorder may have been developing over some period of time, perhaps as a result of a biomechanical abnormality, and may simply be aggravated by a particular activity. By evaluating the mechanical effects of activities that reproduce the pain, the examiner can often find important clues as to the nature of a particular disorder.

Shoes tend to provide support for the twisted or arched configuration of the foot to varying degrees. A high heel causes the toes to dorsiflex when standing with the feet in contact with the ground. This raises the arch by tightening the plantar aponeurosis that crosses the plantar surface of the metatarsophalangeal joints (Fig. 15–21). Heels also reduce the passive tension on the Achilles tendon and gastrocnemius–soleus group and, by effectively reducing the toe lever-arm of the foot, reduce the active tension developed in the gastrocnemius–soleus muscle–tendon complex. Most shoes also provide some contoured base of support for the "arch" of the foot. This maximizes the contacting surface area of the foot and, therefore, distributes the stresses of weight-bearing over most of the sole of the foot. Proper contouring of a shoe also minimizes the amount of tension that needs to be developed in the plantar aponeurosis, long and short plantar ligaments, tarsal joint capsules, and intrinsic muscles to maintain a normal twisted configuration to the foot. When a person walks barefoot, the effects of the heel and contoured support are lost. This usually creates no problem in a person with good bony alignment and ligamentous support. However, in a person with a tendency toward pronation (untwisting of the foot) the added tension to the plantar ligaments may lead to pain. Or, if the ligaments are already lax, increased intrinsic muscle activity will be necessary. If such prolonged muscular activity is necessary, pain may also arise from muscular fatigue. These persons are often more comfortable wearing shoes than going barefoot. Even persons with normal foot structure may experience some foot pain with lower heel heights if they are accustomed to wearing a shoe with a heel. Lowering the heel reduces the support provided by the plantar aponeurosis, putting more tension on the plantar ligaments and joint capsules and calling for increased activity of the intrinsic muscles of the foot. This is why flat-soled shoes, especially, must have well-contoured "arch supports."

Shoes also provide an interface for shear and compressive stresses. Foot pain arising from localized pressure concentration, from shear stresses between the skin and an exterior surface, or from shearing between skin and subcutaneous tissue may be alleviated by going barefoot. This is primarily true in cases in which such stresses occur over all but the soles of the feet. Pain from pressure concentration over the sole of the foot, as frequently occurs over the head of the second metatarsal, may be reduced by wearing shoes, since the contouring of the shoe may serve to distribute the pressures of weight-bearing over a broader area.

Complaints of cramping of the foot may accompany muscular fatigue usually associated with some biomechanical disturbance. Cramping may also accompany intermittent claudication from arterial insufficiency. Claudication should always be suspect when the patient relates a history of pain or cramping of the feet, and usually of the lower leg, after walking some distance, but the pain is relieved with rest. Cramping may accompany disk protrusions, presumably from altered conduction of fibers subserving motor control or muscle reflexes. This cramping is noticed more often at night.

PHYSICAL EXAMINATION

I. Observation
 A. *General appearance and body build.* Weight-bearing stresses will be increased in the presence of obesity.
 B. *Activities of daily living.* Dressing, grooming, gait, and transfer activities (see gait analysis discussion under Lumbar–lower extremity scan examination). With localized foot or ankle disorders, usually only the gait is affected. Observe the patient walking with and without shoes. An antalgic gait associated with foot or ankle lesions is typically one in which heel-strike or push-off, or both, are lacking. This results in a shortened stride on the affected side, which is accentuated at faster paces. Chronic disorders may produce no obvious gait disturbances. However, look carefully for more subtle gait deviations, indicating a possible biomechanical abnormality of one or more of the weight-bearing joints that may be related to a foot problem. It is of primary importance to observe for abnormal rotatory movements of the weight-bearing segments; to assess rotations of the hindfoot into pronation and supination, look at the following:
  1. The patellae to judge rotary movements of the femur.
  2. The position of the malleoli with respect to each other or the tibia.
  3. The position of the calcanei.
  4. The degree of toeing-in or toeing-out.
  5. The degree of motion in ankle dorsiflexion and plantar flexion.
  6. The angle and base of gait. Normally, this angle does not exceed 15° from the midline of the body.[81]
  7. Point of heel contact. The position of the calcaneus in either eversion or inversion during heel-strike.[69]
  8. The approximate time of pronation.

Normally, pronation will occur 15% to 20% into the contact phase of gait.[82,86]

9. The approximate time of supination. Normally this will occur in the last half of stance.[81,86]

10. For the foot, the critical periods to identify during gait include[45]:
    a. Contact (heel- or rear foot-strike to foot-flat).
    b. Midstance.
    c. Lift-off (heel-rise to toe-off).

    The patient's gait should be reviewed during both walking and running. Very frequently a foot that looks as though it is one configuration will actually function as the opposite in motion.[7] Videotape or film analysis with slow motion and the use of a treadmill, if available, are invaluable in diagnosing difficult problems.[61] The practical advantage of a treadmill is control of speed.

II. Inspection

A. *Skin and nails*
1. If areas of abnormal callosities, redness or actual skin breakdown are noted, suggesting excessive shear or compression forces, document the size of the involved area to serve as a baseline measurement. This can easily be done by tracing the perimeter of the involved area on a piece of acetate (such as old roentgenographic film).
2. Excessive dryness or moisture may suggest abnormal vascularity or abnormal sympathetic activity to the part, or both.
3. Note the site and size of hypertrophic skin changes, such as corns and calluses. These suggest mildly increased shear or compression forces acting over a longer period of time than those that might produce localized inflammation or actual breakdown. Keep in mind that a painful callus is one in which the underlying tissue is in the process of breaking down.
4. Diffuse ecchymosis may be associated with common ankle sprains as well as more serious trauma.
5. Inspect the toe nails for splitting, overgrowth, inappropriate trimming, and inflammation of the nail beds.

B. *Soft tissue*
1. Swelling (see under palpation)
2. Wasting of isolated or generalized muscle groups

3. General contours

C. *Bony structure and alignment*
1. Note toe deformities such as claw toes, hammer toes, and varus–valgus deviations.[71]
    a. Claw toes are usually associated with a pes cavus deformity and may accompany certain neurologic disorders. The metatarsophalangeal joints are positioned in extension and the interphalangeal joints in flexion. Contracture of the long toe-extensors causes extension of the toes, which increases the passive tension on the long toe-flexors. The intrinsic muscles are overbalanced, both actively and passively, by these muscle groups.
    b. Hammer toes are a result of capsular contracture of the proximal or distal interphalangeal joints. The involved joint or joints are fixed in some degree of flexion.
    c. A valgus deformity of the first metatarsophalangeal joint is a common disorder. It may be associated with a varus deviation of the first metatarsal, a pronated foot, or both. The toe may be rotated, with the toe nail pointed inward.
2. Assess the length of the metatarsals. A line across the metatarsal heads should form a smooth parabola, with the second metatarsal being the longest. A shortened first metatarsal may lead to increased weight-bearing by the second and sometimes the third metatarsal, resulting in tissue hypertrophy, pain, or both.
3. Navicular tubercle. An imaginary straight line passes from the medial malleolus to where the head of the first metatarsal meets the ground. The navicular tubercle should be within one third of the perpendicular distance between this line and the ground.
4. The calcanei should be positioned vertically with little or no inward or outward bowing of the Achilles tendon.
5. The general configuration of the foot should be assessed in standing and sitting positions.
    a. When standing, an untwisted foot is one in which the hindfoot is in pronation and the forefoot in supination. The calcaneus will be in valgus position and the navicular tubercle will be

sunken and often prominent. The talar head also becomes prominent medially, and the forefoot often assumes an abducted position with respect to the hindfoot. There is often an associated valgus deformity of the first metatarsal-phalangeal joint.

With excessive twisting of the foot (pes cavus) the calcaneus assumes a varus position and the medial arch is well formed, with the navicular tubercle positioned well superiorly. There is often a tendency toward clawing of the toes in a cavus foot.

  b. When sitting, the foot should relax into a position of plantar flexion, inversion, and adduction. A "supple" or "mobile" flatfoot will take on a more normal configuration in sitting with the force of weight-bearing relieved. A "fixed" or "structural" flatfoot will maintain its planus (untwisted) state.

6. Perform a complete structural examination of the remainder of the lower extremities, the pelvis, and the lower back, as discussed in Chapter 21. Any structural deviations or asymmetries should be noted, and the possible effects on the biomechanics of the foot considered.

7. Inspect the shoes, inside and out, for wear patterns that may offer clues as to the presence of persistent biomechanical disturbances and localized areas of pressure. Also inspect for other possible sources of pain arising from the shoe, such as nails protruding through the insole and prominent seams.

  a. On the outer sole, the wear pattern should be displaced somewhat laterally at the heel. Over the front sole, the wear pattern should be spread fairly evenly across the area corresponding to the level of the first, second, and third metatarsophalangeal joints, with less wear laterally. There should be an even wear pattern across the rest of the medial side of the sole. Areas of localized excessive wear should be noted as well as abnormal wear patterns.

  b. The upper portion of the shoe should show a gently curved transverse crease line at the level of the metatarsophalangeal joints. Excessive curling of the vamp of the shoe and the front part of the sole may occur in a shoe that is too long, too narrow, or both. A crease line that runs obliquely, from forward and medial to backward and lateral, may arise from a stiff first metatarsophalangeal joint.

Localized prominences of the vamp commonly occur medially in the presence of hallux valgus or dorsally with hammer toes or claw toes. Such prominences should be noted.

Inspect for excessive overhanging of the upper shoe with respect to the sole. This is likely to be observed medially in shoes of patients with pronation of the hindfoot.

When viewed from behind, the cup formed by the counter of the shoe should rise vertically and symmetrically from the sole. Inclination of the counter medially, with bulging of the lateral lip of the counter, will be seen in shoes of patients with pronated feet.

Areas of excessive scuffing of the upper shoe should be noted. Scuffing of the toe of the shoe may occur with weak dorsiflexors or restriction of motion toward dorsiflexion.

  c. When inspecting the inside of the shoe, feel along the inner surface of the seams for prominent areas that may give rise to pressure concentration. Also feel along the entire surface of the inner sole for prominent areas that might be caused by protruding nails.

The wear pattern on the inside of the shoe should also be examined. There should be evidence of an even distribution of pressure over the medial and lateral sides of the heel counter, over the inner sole at the heel, and over the inner sole at the metatarsal heads.

III. **Selective tissue tension tests**
  A. *Active movements (functional movements)*
   1. Barefoot walking
     a. Normal gait
     b. On toes. If unable to do so, determine whether it is because of pain, weakness, or restriction of motion. The heel should invert and the arch should rise.
     c. On heels. If unable to do so, determine whether it is because of pain, weakness, or restriction of motion.
   2. Standing with feet fixed
     a. Externally rotate the leg with respect to the foot. This should cause some

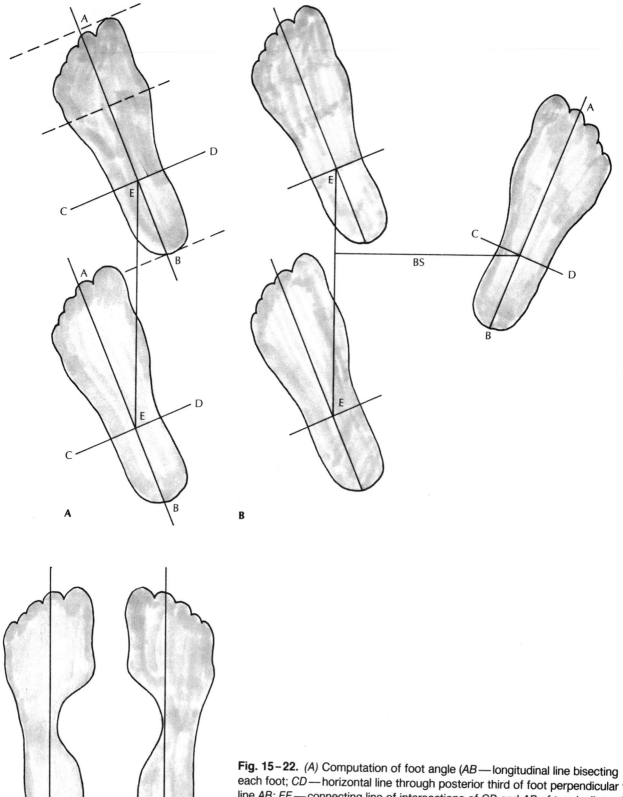

Fig. 15-22. *(A)* Computation of foot angle (*AB*—longitudinal line bisecting each foot; *CD*—horizontal line through posterior third of foot perpendicular to line *AB*; *EE*—connecting line of intersections of *CD* and *AB* of two ipsilateral feet [line of progression]; resulting angle is foot angle). *(B)* Computation of the base of support (*BS*—line drawn from intersection of *CD* and *AB* of contralateral foot perpendicular to line *EE*). *(C)* Computation of dynamic angle and base of walking template.

varus deviation of the heels and raising of the arches. Compare one foot to the other.

   b. Internally rotate the legs on the feet. This should result in some valgus deviation of the heels and flattening of the arches. Compare one foot to the other.

3. Standing, keeping knees extended
   a. Evert the feet by standing on medial borders of feet.
   b. Invert the feet by standing on lateral borders of feet.

4. Sitting, with legs hanging freely. Compare range of motion of one foot to the other. Assess pain, range of motion, and crepitus.
   a. Dorsiflexion
   b. Plantar flexion
   c. Inversion
   d. Eversion
   e. Toe movements

B. *Passive physiological movements*

1. Standing, before measurements are taken, determine the dynamic angle and base of walking using the patient's own line of progression as a reference.[70] A paper walkway (approximately 20 to 24 feet long) on which the patient's footprints can be recorded (after walking in a normal fashion) is most convenient.[9,70,87] Using the line of progression as a reference, select one left and one right footprint from the middle of the progression to use to construct a paper template of the footprints adjacent to each other. The dynamic foot angle and the distance between the middle of each heel are maintained (Fig. 15–22).
   Note: The paper walkway recording can be used for additional data collection such as stride length, velocity, and cadence in the gait analysis.
   a. With a felt-tipped marking pen, bisect the middle one third of the posterior calcaneus.[81] Extend the bisection line plantarly to the base of the supporting surface and from the middle one third of the calcaneus superiorly approximately 1 inch; the point of bifurcation is located at the junction of the proximal and middle one third of the bisected calcaneus.
   b. Next, bisect the distal one third of the

lower extremity just proximal to the malleoli. Extension of this line superiorly should bisect the knee joint within the popliteal space. Calipers may be used to determine the center of the most proximal point of the lower one third of the leg and at the level of the malleoli. With a felt-tipped marking pen, these two points are then connected to form the bisector of the lower one third of the leg.

   c. Measurement of neutral calcaneus stance (a relaxed foot with the subtalar joint allowed to pronate) (Fig. 15–23).
      i. Have the patient stand in a normal angle and base of gait (see **B.1.** above) and facing away from the examiner.[81] Using a goniometer or protractor, place the straight arm along the supporting surface (transverse plane). The center point of the goniometer or protractor is placed at the apex point of the angle created by the calcaneal bisection and the supporting surface (frontal plane). Rearfoot valgus is then measured to the nearest degree.
      ii. The normal weight-bearing foot should demonstrate a mild amount of pronation but should still allow for additional pronation.[12] If the patient is bearing weight or walking with the foot out of neutral position and near full pronation, an obligatory internal tibial rotation occurs and is prolonged, resulting in an increased force that is absorbed by the soft tissues of the knee.[49,50]

   d. Measurement of tibia varum (tibiofibular varum). If a lateral angulation of the tibia-to-floor angle is 10° or greater, the extremity requires an excessive amount of subtalar joint pronation to produce a plantigrade foot (Fig. 15–24).
      i. Have the client stand in a normal angle and base of gait. With the feet in a resting calcaneal stance position, recheck the bisections of the calcaneus and lower leg. When the bisections are acceptable, measure the frontal plane relationship

Fig. 15–23. Measurement of neutral calcaneus stance (a relaxed foot with the subtalar joint allowed to pronate).

Fig. 15–24. Measurement of tibia varum in the resting calcaneal stance position.

of the tibia to the transverse plane (or level ground). If a gravity goniometer is used, the angle between the bisection of the leg and vertical is read on the face of the goniometer. Tibia varum is present when the distal end of the bisection line of the leg is closer to the midsagittal plane than the proximal end. Tibia valgum is present if the leg is angulated in the opposite direction.

Note: Tibia varum (tibiofibular varum) measurements can also be performed with the foot positioned in subtalar neutral by palpating for talar congruency as the patient rotates the trunk to the left and right, allowing the tibia to externally and internally rotate, thus supinating and pronating the subtalar joint. Once subtalar neutral is reached, the subject is then asked to maintain this position while measurements are recorded. According to McPoil and co-workers the best patient position for clinical measurement of tibiofibular varum is the neutral calcaneal stance position. It would appear that the measurement of true tibia varum cannot be done without obtaining roentgenograms of the lower extremities taken during weight-bearing.[70]

e. Measurement of great toe extension can be made while the person is standing. The great toe is extended actively and assisted passively without dorsiflexing the first ray. Forty-five degrees has been found to be adequate for general ambulation.[64]

2. Passive range of motion. The patient sits with legs hanging freely. Compare range of motion of one foot to the other. Note the presence of pain or crepitus. Note abnormalities or asymmetries in range of motion. Note the presence of pathologic end feels.

a. Hindfoot
   i. Plantar flexion
   ii. Inversion
   iii. Eversion

b. Transverse tarsal

i. Plantar flexion
ii. Pronation (eversion)
iii. Supination (inversion)
iv. Abduction
v. Adduction
3. Supine
   a. Hip flexion–extension
   b. Knee flexion–extension
   c. First ray: position and mobility
      i. Place the foot in a neutral subtalar position (see Fig. 15–18). Load the forefoot (see **4.c.i** below). While maintaining the foot in neutral position, grasp the metatarsal heads (between the thumb and forefinger) with the loading hand. Grasp the first metatarsal head with the other hand.
      ii. Assess the position of the first metatarsal head in relationship to its neutral position and assess the end range position of the first metatarsal head in relationship to the second metatarsal head.[82]
      iii. While maintaining the foot in neutral subtalar position, manually plantar flex and dorsiflex the first ray. Assess the motion of the first ray in relationship to its neutral position and assess the end-range position of the first metatarsal head in relationship to the second metatarsal head.
      iv. Limited range may result from a combination of biomechanical factors such as excessive pronation or a short tendon or from restriction of the joint proper.[34]
4. Prone, with the feet over the edge of the table.
   a. Hip internal and external rotation with the knees flexed to 90°.
   b. Supination and pronation of the calcaneus. The amount of supination and pronation that is available can be measured by lining up the longitudinal axis of the lower limb and vertical axis of the calcaneus (Fig. 15–25).[50,82] Passive movement of the calcaneus into inversion (amount of supination) is normally 20°.[82] Conversely, the amount of eversion (pronation) is normally 10°.[82]
   c. Forefoot valgus–forefoot varus. The subtalar should be positioned in subta-

Fig. 15–25. Measurement of supination and pronation of the calcaneus (rearfoot inversion and eversion) (non–weight-bearing).

lar neutral and the forefoot locked (Fig. 15–26).
      i. In order to accomplish locking of the forefoot in the open-chain position the forefoot must be loaded against the neutral subtalar rearfoot. This is accomplished by applying a dorsiflectory force against the fourth and fifth metatarsal heads so that the forefoot is fully pronated on a neutral rearfoot. In order to fully lock the forefoot, also called loading the forefoot, at the midtarsal joint the dorsiflectory force should be applied only until resistance is appreciated. The relationship of the neutral subtalar position and a fully pronated forefoot against the rearfoot results in

Fig. 15–26. Measurement of forefoot valgus or varus (non–weight-bearing).

the neutral position of the foot in the open-chain position. It is not necessary to dorsiflex the foot to 90° or lift the leg from the supporting surface. Slightly adduct the forefoot to ensure complete midtarsal joint pronation.

ii. Place one arm of the goniometer along the posterior calcaneal bisection and the other arm along the plantar aspect of the heel. Align the latter arm with the plane of the forefoot (an imaginary line from the head of the fifth metatarsal to the head of the first) and read the degrees of forefoot deviation. Deviation from a normal perpendicular relationship with a line bisecting the calcaneus represents a

difference between alignment of forefoot to hindfoot.

iii. Forefoot valgus is commonly found in the varus foot. Forefoot varus may require increased pronation to adequately contact the surface while running or walking.[49,93]

iv. The calcaneal position, varus or valgus, can also be determined at this time.

d. Dorsiflexion

i. Position the patient prone with his foot over the edge of the table. Place a 4-inch roll underneath the distal anterior thigh to ensure full knee extension. Place the foot into subtalar neutral. While maintaining subtalar neutral, manually assist dorsiflexion of the foot on the leg while the patient actively dorsiflexes the foot to its end range.

  ii. Repeat with the knee flexed to 90°.

  iii. Dorsiflexion is measured to the nearest degree.

  Note: The subtalar must be maintained in a neutral position during these motions. Pressure applied to the first ray will help prevent pronation.[72]

C. *Resisted isometric movements.* Resisted isometrics are done in the supine or sitting position. Resisted isometric knee flexion should be included because of the triceps surae action on the knee. With the patient's foot placed in the anatomical position the movements tested are as follows.

  1. *Dorsiflexion.* Pain may be due to a tendinitis. Painless weakness associated with a footdrop may be due to a lesion of the lateral popliteal or the L5 nerve root. Painful resisted dorsiflexion and inversion occurs in tendinitis of the anterior tibialis.

  2. *Plantar flexion.* Test in weight-bearing. Pain may be due to a lesion of the Achilles tendon or a tear in the gastrocnemius. A painless weakness may be due to S1 nerve-root pressure.

  3. *Inversion.* A painful weakness of inversion is usually due to tenosynovitis or tendinitis of the posterior tibialis muscle. Painless weakness may be due to a tendon rupture or L4 nerve root compression.

  4. *Extension of the great toe.* A painful weakness occurs with tenosynovitis of the extensor hallucis longus muscle. Painless weakness may indicate an L5 nerve root compression.

  5. *Toe extension.* A painful weakness may indicate a tenosynovitis of the extensor digitorum longus; painless weakness occurs in an L5 nerve root lesion.

D. *Joint-play movements.* Assess for hypermobility or hypomobility and presence or absence of pain. (See Chapter 6, Peripheral Joint Mobilization Techniques.)

  1. Distal tibiofibular joint—anteroposterior glide

  2. Ankle mortise (talocrural) joint

    a. Distraction of talus

    b. Anterior and posterior glide of talus. Anterior glide is an important test for integrity of the anterior talofibular lig-

ament. The patient is supine. Place one hand over the dorsum of the distal tibia and cup the other hand around the back of the calcaneus. The talus by way of the calcaneus is pulled forward in the mortise, and the movement is compared with the movement on the opposite side.

      i. Hypermobility will be present in the case of a chronic anterior talofibular ligament rupture.

      ii. Pain will be reproduced from a talofibular ligament sprain or adhesion.

  3. Subtalar joint

    a. Distraction of calcaneus

    b. Dorsal rock of calcaneus, plantar rock of calcaneus

    c. Inversion–eversion tilts of calcaneus. The range of calcaneal inversion and eversion is assessed and the two feet are compared. Capsular restriction will result in a greater loss of inversion than eversion.

  4. Transverse tarsal joint—dorsal-plantar glides

  5. Naviculocuneiform joint—dorsal-plantar glides

  6. Cuneiform-metatarsal joints

    a. Dorsal-plantar glides

    b. Pronation–supination twists

  7. Cuboid–fifth metatarsal joint—dorsal-plantar glides

  8. Intermetatarsal articulations—dorsal-plantar glides

  9. Metatarsophalangeal and interphalangeal joints

    a. Dorsal-plantar glides

    b. Internal-external rotations

    c. Medial-lateral tilts

    d. Distraction

IV. Neuromuscular tests. There are few localized neurologic problems that affect the foot. If a disorder affecting a relevant nerve root (L4, L5, S1, or S2) is suspected, or if a problem affecting a peripheral nerve supplying the foot is suspected, the necessary sensory, motor, and reflex testing should be performed. The segmental and peripheral nerve innervations, as well as the related reflexes, are listed in Chapter 4, Assessment of Musculoskeletal Disorders.

V. Palpation

  A. *Skin*

    1. Moisture or dryness. Abnormal moisture, usually associated with pain and joint restriction, may accompany a reflex sympathetic dystrophy. Vascular disorders may also cause changes in the moisture or texture of the skin.

2. Texture
3. Mobility. Skin mobility may be restricted after prolonged immobilization, especially following a surgical procedure.
4. Temperature. Inflammatory lesions will often result in increased skin temperature over the site of the lesion. Fairly precise documentation of the degree of inflammation may be made by using a thermister probe. This often offers a convenient guide as to the effect of treatment procedures on the state of the lesion as well as a guide to the state of the inflammatory process in general. For example, a baseline reading can be documented and measurements taken before and after each treatment session (these must be taken over precisely the same point and at the same time of day). A slight elevation of, say, 1°C can be expected after any treatment that imposes some mechanical stress, such as mobilization, massage, or exercise. However, it is important that the elevation does not persist over more than a few hours. If so, the treatment program may be too vigorous. If some decline in temperature is noted, it may be a sign that resolution is taking place. Thermister readings, as with most tests, are significant when compared with a normal side.

B. *Soft tissue*
   1. Swelling
      a. Localized extra-articular swelling may accompany ankle sprains, usually involving the lateral aspect of the ankle below the lateral malleolus.
      b. Localized articular effusion of the ankle mortise joint manifests as a loss of definition over the malleolar regions. Subtle joint effusion can be detected by applying firm pressure with the thumb and index fingers over the regions below the medial and lateral malleoli simultaneously. This will force the fluid into the anterior capsular region and cause a fullness over the dorsum of the ankle.
      c. Generalized edema of the foot may follow major trauma, or it may accompany systemic, more generalized vascular or metabolic disorders.

2. Mobility
3. Consistency
4. Pulses
   a. The pulse of the dorsalis pedis artery may be palpated just lateral to the tendon of the extensor hallucis longus over the dorsum of the foot.
   b. The pulse of the posterior tibial artery is palpated behind the tendons of the flexor digitorum longus and flexor hallucis longus posterosuperior to the medial malleolus.
5. Other specific tendons, ligaments, and muscles should be palpated, as indicated by findings to this point in the examination. A guide to palpation of these structures is included in the section on surface anatomy in this chapter.

C. *Bony structures and tendon and ligament attachments*
   1. Palpate joint margins to assess structural alignment and to note any hypertrophic changes.
   2. Palpate tendon and ligament attachments as indicated in the section on surface anatomy.

COMMON LESIONS AND THEIR MANAGEMENT

The common disorders affecting the foot are in the majority of cases the result of some biomechanical disturbance. As indicated in the preceding section, such biomechanical disorders may be of local origin, or the primary problem may involve one of the other weight-bearing segments. For this reason, evaluation of chronic, subtle foot disorders requires that structural and functional assessments of the other weight-bearing joints be made. Similarly, evaluation of patients with problems in these other regions may necessitate examination of the foot. In understanding the rationale of the evaluative and treatment procedures related to foot disorders, it is essential that the practitioner have a basic knowledge of the biomechanics of the foot and how they relate to the biomechanics of the other weight-bearing joints.

Because the numerous joints of the foot contribute to make it a very mobile structure as a whole, it has the ability to attenuate the energy of forces applied to it. For this reason, traumatic lesions affecting the foot are relatively rare. On the other hand, the common lesions affecting the ankle are usually of traumatic origin.[13] While the individual joints making up the ankle are relatively trackbound or uniaxial, the ankle complex allows some movement in the sagittal, frontal, and transverse planes. However, transverse rotations are of limited range because they do not occur about a true vertical axis. Also, eversion is normally quite restricted because the fibular malleolus extends distally to create an abutment that limits this movement. Forces that move the ankle past its physiological limits of motion will tend to cause damage, usually to the osseus or ligamentous components of the ankle complex, or to both. Excessive forces to the ankle producing such damage are often the result of forces from the ground acting over the lever-arm provided by the foot, or by forces of the center of gravity of the body acting over the lever-arm of the lower extremity with the foot fixed. Because of these lever-arms over which forces acting on the ankle may be applied and because certain ankle motions are normally limited, the ankle is often the site of acute traumatic injuries such as sprains and fractures.

Except in situations in which there is malalignment of bony constituents, such as following healing of a fracture, or in situations in which there is marked restriction of movement of one of the ankle joints, such as following arthrodesis of the subtalar joints, degenerative joint disease affecting the ankle is rare. Rheumatoid arthritis often affects the foot, but less often the ankle.

Both the foot and ankle may be the site of fatigue disorders. Such disorders result from abnormally high stresses occurring over relatively short periods of time or from mildly abnormal stresses occurring over a long period of time. The former situation usually occurs in athletes or others who have undergone an abrupt increase in activity level. In such cases, the degree of microtrauma affecting certain tissues exceeds the rate at which the body is able to repair itself; the result is a fatigue yielding of the involved tissue. Examples are stress fractures, blisters, and many of the tendinitis conditions affecting this region. Milder stresses occurring over longer periods of time tend to result in tissue hypertrophy that may contribute to certain painful disorders. Typical examples are heel spurs and various callus formations.

ANKLE SPRAIN

The most common lesion affecting the ankle is a sprain or tear of one of the ligaments.[13,35] The anterior talofibular ligament is the most commonly sprained ligament at the ankle and is probably the most commonly sprained ligament in the body. The next most frequently sprained ligaments at the ankle

are the calcaneocuboid and the calcaneofibular ligaments. Portions of the deltoid ligament may also be sprained, but more often a forceful eversion stress will result in an avulsion of the tibial malleolus rather than damage to the ligament.[14,20]

I. History

  A. *Onset of pain.* The patient will invariably recall the traumatic incident. The common mechanism of injury for an anterior talofibular ligament sprain is a plantar flexion–inversion stress.[38,40,53,77] Typical examples include a jumper coming down on the lateral border of the plantarly flexed foot, a person wearing high-heeled shoes or walking on uneven ground who catches a toe on the lateral side of the foot, or a person stepping off a curb or step who rolls over the lateral side of the plantarly flexed foot. If the forefoot is forced into supination or adduction, the calcaneocuboid ligament may be injured instead or as well. The calcaneofibular ligament restricts inversion with the foot in a more neutral or dorsiflexed position. It may be injured along with the talofibular ligament if, at the time of injury, the person retains good contact of the foot with the ground but continues to force the foot into inversion.

   When torn, the deltoid ligament is usually injured because the foot is forced into external rotation and eversion with respect to the leg. As mentioned, it is more common for a portion of the tibial malleolus to avulse with the deltoid ligament attachment. The anterior tibiofibular ligament may be torn with a similar mechanism, since as the talus rotates within the mortise, it tends to wedge the tibia and fibula apart, producing a diastasis.[1,14,20] In order for the talus to rotate enough to produce a diastasis and to tear the anterior tibiofibular ligament, the deltoid ligament is torn or the tibial malleolus is avulsed as well.[1]

  B. *Site of pain.* This usually corresponds well with the approximate location of the injury. Some pain may be referred distally into the foot or proximally into the lower leg.

  C. *Nature of pain or disability.* Similar to ligamentous lesions at the knee, the degree of pain and disability immediately following an injury to an ankle ligament does not necessarily correlate well with the severity of the lesion.[48] A person sustaining a mild or moderate sprain may describe more pain and be more reluctant to continue a particular activity than one who completely ruptures a ligament. This is because in the event of a rupture there is complete loss of continuity of the structure and there are no longer intact fibers to be stressed and from which pain can be elicited.

Repeated episodes of anterior talofibular ligament sprains are not uncommon. Usually the initial injury results in somewhat more pain and disability than with subsequent occurrences. These patients typically describe intermittent giving way of the ankle, often during athletic activities, followed by pain and effusion lasting for a few days.[32,90]

II. Physical examination

  A. *Observation*. A patient seen soon after injury may hobble into the office walking with a characteristic "foot flat," short-stance gait; both heel-strike and push-off are lacking. If the pain is more severe, the patient may present walking with the aid of crutches or hopping in on one leg.

  B. *Inspection*. Localized swelling over the region of the involved ligament is usually present within several hours following the injury. Since the anterior talofibular ligament and the deep fibers of the deltoid ligament blend with the ankle mortise joint capsule, there may be some associated articular effusion. Within a day or so following most ankle sprains, there is diffuse ecchymosis in the region of the injury, which may extravasate distally into the foot.

  C. *Selective tissue tension tests*

    1. Active movements. In the acute stage there is likely to be considerable difficulty in heel and toe walking and other weight-bearing activities involving ankle movements. The examiner must exercise judgment in requesting the patient to perform these movements to avoid undue discomfort or stress to the part.

    2. Passive movements and joint-play movements (key objective tests)

      a. If the ankle mortise joint capsule has been stressed with subsequent articular effusion, the ankle movements will be limited in a capsular pattern; plantar flexion will be slightly more restricted than dorsiflexion.

      b. In the case of a mild or moderate ligamentous sprain, pain will be repro-

duced with movements that stress the involved ligament. There will usually be an associated muscle-spasm end feel. Painless hypermobility will be noted in the presence of chronic ruptures. Acute ruptures will also demonstrate hypermobility; however, a false-negative finding may be elicited because of protective muscle spasm. Take care to ensure maximal relaxation of the part when performing passive movements. The common ligaments injured and the passive movements used to test their integrity are as follows:

      i. Anterior talofibular ligament. Combined plantar flexion–inversion–adduction of the hindfoot and anterior glide of the talus on the tibia[13,60]

      ii. Calcaneocuboid ligament. Combined supination–adduction of the forefoot

      iii. Calcaneofibular ligament. Inversion of the hindfoot in a neutral position of plantar flexion–dorsiflexion

      iv. Deltoid ligament. Anterior fibers —combined plantar flexion–eversion–abduction of the hindfoot; middle fibers—eversion of the hindfoot

    3. Resisted movements. These should be strong and painless. Occasionally the peroneal tendons are strained in conjunction with an inversion ligamentous strain. In this case, isometric resistance to eversion will be strong and painful.

  D. *Neuromuscular tests*. Results are noncontributory.

  E. *Palpation*

    1 Tenderness will usually correspond to the site of the lesion in acute injuries. There is also likely to be diffuse tenderness in the presence of marked swelling from extravasation of blood into the tissues.

    2. Joint effusion from synovitis or extra-articular swelling will be palpable in the acute stages.

    3. Skin temperature will be elevated over the region of the involved structure in the acute stages.

III. Management

  A. *Acute sprains—immediate measures*. At this early stage, there is little that needs to be done to, or for, the patient that he cannot do on his own. Ice, elevation, compression, mobility exercises, and strengthening can be carried out easily at home by most patients. This does, however, require very clear and precise instruction by the therapist. Do not spare words or time in making sure that the patient understands exactly what he should or should not be doing with the ankle. A follow-up visit after 2 or 3 days should be scheduled so that a reassessment can be made and the program appropriately progressed. At this point, there should be evidence of reduction of the acute inflammatory process; pain, temperature, and swelling should be decreased. It is important, in the subacute stage, to carefully reassess joint-play movements, since at this stage the therapist can determine more easily whether there has been some loss of integrity of the involved structure. Often in the acute stage, muscle spasm precludes accurate determination of the extent of the damage.

1. Reduce stress to the ligament to allow healing without undue lengthening.
   a. Ankle strapping will help reduce movement in response to mild (non–weight-bearing) stresses. Swelling should have stabilized by the time of application. A felt or foam rubber "horseshoe" should be used to fill in the submalleolar depressions so as to obtain even compressions of the area with application of tape or an elastic bandage.
   b. Crutches should be used to relieve stress and pain during ambulation. A three-point, partial weight-bearing crutch gait should be instituted; non–weight-bearing is usually not necessary and should be avoided because of its nonfunctional nature.
2. Reduction of the acute inflammatory process to reduce pain and to prevent undue tissue damage from localized pressure and proteolytic cellular responses
   a. Ice—To decrease blood flow and reduce capillary hydrostatic pressure, thus reducing extravasation of blood fluids
   b. Compression—Increased external pressure to the area will minimize capillary leakage by effectively reducing the volume of the tissue spaces. This can be maintained by appropriate ap-

plication of an elastic bandage with a horseshoe pad below the malleolus.
   c. Elevation—Reduces capillary hydrostatic pressure to minimize fluid loss and assists the venous and lymphatic return.
3. Prevention of residual disability
   a. Institute motion of the part in planes that do not stress the healing ligament to minimize residual loss of movement and optimize circulation in the area.
   b. *Isometric exercises* to the muscles in the area should be started as early as pain allows, to maintain strength of the muscles of the lower leg and foot.

B. *Acute sprains—subsequent measures*
1. Mild sprains. In the case of a simple sprain, in which there is no hypermobility on the associated passive movement tests, gradual return to normal activities should be allowed as the inflammatory process resolves. Weight-bearing should be increased and the crutches discarded, usually by the fifth day. Range of motion, strength, and joint play should be restored to normal. Most patients may regain normal motion and strength with careful instruction in home exercises. Before discharging the patient from care, the therapist must ascertain that normal joint play has returned. If it has not, the restricted movements must be restored with passive joint mobilization techniques. Friction massage, initiated in the subacute stage, may promote healing of the ligament in a mobile state and prevent adherence to adjacent tissue.

   As the swelling subsides in the subacute stage, strapping should be substituted for the elastic bandage to provide support and to increase proprioceptive feedback as the patient resumes functional use of the part. Use of strapping should continue until good strength, range of motion, and joint play are restored. The athlete should continue to strap the ankle when participating in vigorous activities. Studies suggest that ankle strapping does play a role in preventing ankle sprains.[37] This is probably not due to actual mechanical support provided by the tape, since movement of the bones within the skin (to which the tape is adhered) is probably still sufficient to allow a ligament to be stretched. However, the added proprioceptive input provided by the tape may enhance protective reflexes (such as contraction of the peroneal muscles) in response to forces tending to stress the ankle ligaments.

Return to vigorous activity must be gradual. Clinical evidence of healing does not indicate that a ligament has regained normal strength. In fact, maturation of the new collagen laid down during healing may take weeks or months. The necessary stimulus for maturation and restoration of normal ligamentous strength is stress to the ligament produced by functional use of the part. This induces formation of the appropriate collagen crosslinks and realignment of the new collagen fibers along the normal lines of stress. However, the ligament must not be overstressed before normal strength is regained, since it is susceptible at this point to reinjury. The athlete should begin by jogging, then running, in straight lines. When normal muscle strength and joint motion have been regained, figure-of-eight patterns that impose some lateral stress to the part may be initiated. Gradually, the patient should progress to sharp cutting drills. When these can be performed well and without pain, competitive activity may be resumed.

Also during the later stages of rehabilitation, balance drills should be instituted to facilitate the restoration of normal protective reflexes.[31,33] Progression may proceed from challenging one-legged standing to one-legged standing on a rocking board to one-legged standing on a board supported on half a sphere (free to tilt in all planes).

2. Moderate sprains and complete ruptures. The related literature reflects some controversy regarding the management of ruptured ligaments at the ankle. Most authorities would agree that injuries involving extensive damage, with rupture of both the anterior talofibular and calcaneofibular ligaments, should be repaired surgically to restore passive stability to the ankle.[2,90] Good results are favored by early surgery, since the torn ends will tend to atrophy and retract with time, making apposition and suturing technically difficult or impossible. Similar considerations apply to rupture of the deltoid ligament.

There is more divergence of opinion, however, with respect to management of isolated ruptures, in which some hypermobility of anterior glide of the talus in the mortise is demonstrable. While some clinicians favor early surgical intervention to suture the torn ends and minimize residual and structural instability, others favor early return to function following some period of restricted activity and immobilization. There is evidence from studies by Freeman that suturing of the ligament does result in a more stable joint, but in the end, the functional status of those undergoing surgery is really no better than those treated "conservatively."[31-33] In fact, those patients treated conservatively returned to normal function significantly sooner than those undergoing surgery, if they were not immobilized in plaster for a prolonged period of time. Of those treated conservatively, there was very little difference in residual mechanical stability between those who were immobilized in plaster for 6 weeks and those treated with strapping and early mobilization. The incidence of residual pain and swelling several months following injury was highest in the surgical group. The only way to guarantee increased mechanical stability following rupture of the anterior talofibular ligament is to reappose the torn ends with sutures. However, it seems that the residual disability resulting from prolonged immobilization in those treated with surgery outweighs whatever advantage this form of management may have in producing a more stable ankle. Further studies by Freeman suggest that there is no correlation between mechanical instability, as determined by stress roentgenograms, and the incidence of residual disability resulting from chronic swelling and pain.[31-33]

Conservative (nonsurgical) management of patients in whom there is evidence of actual loss of integrity of the ligament should follow the same approach as management for less serious injuries; the primary difference should be that those ankles with more extensive damage will need to be protected, by crutches and strapping, somewhat longer, perhaps as long as 2 weeks. However, early motion and strengthening at pain-free intensities should be initiated as resolution of the acute inflammatory process ensues. Also, in cases of more extensive damage, return to normal and, especially, to vigorous activity levels should be more gradual. Again, it must be emphasized that although new collagen is laid down within the first 1 or 2 weeks following injury, it takes months for this new tissue to mature to normal strength. During the period of maturation, the ligament is weaker than normal and, therefore, more susceptible to reinjury.

C. *Chronic recurrent ankle sprains.* Following initial injury, especially to the anterior talofibular ligament, a certain number of patients will suffer recurrent giving way of the ankle, with subsequent pain and swelling. There are three possible causes of this to be considered and to which assessment should be directed

1. Healing of the ligament with adherence to adjacent tissues. In this situation, the healed ligament does not allow the joint play necessary for normal functioning of the part.[20] With repetitive stress to the tightened structure, pain and swelling will result from a fatigue phenomenon. With forceful stress to the structure, the adhesion will rupture, producing another sprain. This type of problem will present as a painful, minor restriction on passive plantar flexion–inversion of the hindfoot and on anterior glide of the talus. Treatment consists of deep, transverse friction massage to the ligament and specific joint mobilization in the directions of restriction. Normal mobility to the ligament is thus gradually restored.

2. Loss of protective reflex muscle stabilization. Normally, stress to some aspect of a joint capsule or to a joint ligament results in firing of specific receptors in the structure, through a reflex arc, to produce contraction of the muscles overlying the stressed structure. This "booster" mechanism of dynamic joint stabilization protects joint ligaments from injury under conditions of heavy loading. Thus, when the anterior talofibular ligament is stressed, the peroneus tertius is called to reduce the load to the ligament. Damage to a ligament with subsequent immobili-

zation may result in interference of this protective mechanism. Freeman has shown good results in management of such cases by instituting a program of balance training (as described above).[33] The therapist must also make sure that good muscle strength has been restored.

3. Gross mechanical instability of the joint. If both the anterior talofibular ligament and the calcaneofibular ligament are ruptured, or if there has been extensive capsular disruption with an anterior talofibular ligament rupture, the resultant mechanical instability of the joint may not allow certain functional weight-bearing activities to be performed without giving way. Such patients will present with obvious hypermobility on joint-play movement tests. If an aggressive muscle strengthening and balance training program is not sufficient to compensate for the instability, surgical reconstruction may be contemplated.

Thus, the therapist should direct assessment of the chronically unstable ankle toward determining if there is some residual increase or decrease in joint play, if good muscle strength has been regained, and whether the person is able to balance well during one-legged standing under various unstable conditions (*e.g.*, on a tilt board). It is important to realize that giving way of the joint is not necessarily the result of structural instability and that some degree of structural instability can be compensated for by muscle strengthening or balance training.

PROBLEMS RELATED TO ABNORMAL FOOT PRONATION

Pronation of the hindfoot with respect to the forefoot is a relatively common disorder that may or may not give rise to foot pain. Also, because of the biomechanical interplay between the foot and other weight-bearing segments, the pronated foot may result in dysfunction in other regions of the lower extremity, especially the knee. Similarly, a pronated foot may be caused by some local structural abnormality of the tarsal skeleton, or it may be caused by some structural deviation in segments either distal or proximal to the hindfoot.

Pain resulting from a pronated foot is usually of the fatigue type from prolonged increased stress on the affected tissues. In some patients, pain may arise with normal activity levels, while others may get along well until they engage in some activity, such as jogging, involving increased stress levels or frequency. Pain of local origin usually has its source in one of the plantar structures responsible for maintaining the twisted configuration of the foot—the plantar aponeurosis, the short plantar ligament, or the long plantar ligament. Pain may also arise from fatigue of the intrinsic muscles of the foot, in which activity may be increased in an attempt to prevent undue stress to the plantar aponeurosis and ligaments. In association with increased tensile stress to the plantar aponeurosis, a calcaneal periostitis may develop from the added pull to the proximal attachment of the aponeurosis on the plantar surface of the calcaneus. Excessive pulling on the periosteum in this region occasionally results in a bony outcropping (heel spur) that in itself may give rise to localized pressure to the overlying soft tissue. Periostitis and eventually osteophyte formation should be considered as resulting from increased stress to the plantar aponeurosis. It must be emphasized that spurring can develop in the absence of pain and that a cartilaginous spur may be present that is not visible in roentgenograms. Another source of local pain occurring in association with a pronated foot is pressure from the shoes against the talar head or the navicular, which becomes prominent medially when the foot untwists.

A pronated foot may be the cause of, or be associated with, pain in the forefoot, leg, or the knee. Pain from pressure over the first one or two metatarsal heads may result from increased weight bearing over the medial side of the forefoot. This occurs if the talar head and navicular drop downward and inward, shifting the center of gravity line medially. Since hallux valgus often accompanies pronation of the hindfoot, either as a cause or as a result, pressure over a prominent first metatarsophalangeal joint may also occur with increased pronation of the foot. Leg pain may result from increased tension on the anterior or posterior tibialis muscles, which are dynamic supporters of the arch of the foot. Chronic periostitis at the proximal attachment of these muscles may result and is often referred to as *shin splints*. The knee tends to assume a valgus position when the foot pronates. Such an angulation tends to increase the lateral pull on the patella during loaded quadriceps contraction. This may predispose to pain from patellar tracking dysfunction at the knee (see Chapter 14, The Knee).

As mentioned, pronation of the hindfoot may occur from some local structural disorder or from structural deviations elsewhere. The common local causes are capsuloligamentous laxity and bony abnormalities. Capsuloligamentous laxity may be a hereditary condition, or it may accompany some specific disease state, such as rheumatoid arthritis. The common *bony* anomaly resulting in flatfoot is tarsal coalition, in which the talus and calcaneus are fixed to one another in a pronated orientation through fibrous or osseous union.[27] The common malalignment problems affecting other regions that predispose to abnormal pronation of the hindfoot are femoral anteversion, internal tibial torsion, a shortened Achilles tendon, and adduction of the first metatarsal. The excessive internal rotation imposed by anteversion of the femur or internal tibial torsion during stance phase is at least partially absorbed by the subtalar joint, bringing the hindfoot into pronation. In the presence of a short Achilles tendon, the midtarsal joint attempts to compensate for lack of dorsiflexion at the ankle; in order to do so, the foot must untwist to unlock the midtarsal joints. Because of the oblique orientation of the first cuneiform–first metatarsal joint, adduction of the first metatarsal also involves a component of dorsiflexion. This effectively supinates the forefoot, which necessitates a compensatory pronation of the hindfoot in order to get the foot flat on the ground. Each of these possible causes must be considered when examining the patient with a pronated foot.

Finally, it must be remembered that abnormal foot pronation during gait is not always associated with a "pronated foot" seen on structural examination with the patient standing. The typical example is a person with increased tibial varum. The foot usually appears normal or even supinated during relaxed standing. However, when running or walking there is a tendency to heel-strike on the lateral border of the heel and the foot must undergo increased hindfoot pronation in order for the heel to become flat on the ground. So, even though the foot appears not to be pronated, it will be subject to increased pronatory stresses. Similar considerations apply to the patient with either femoral anteversion or external tibial torsion, in which case the cause of pronation is not localized to the foot itself.

I. History

A. *Onset of pain* is usually insidious, since the pathologic tissue conditions associated with biomechanical abnormalities such as a pronated foot are typically fatigue phenomena. Often the onset can be related to some increased activity level, such as long-distance running. Another common predisposing factor is a period of disuse, such as immobilization of the foot in a cast. In such cases, the muscles of the foot weaken, and when activity is resumed, they no longer contribute their share to stabilizing the arch of the foot. This results in increased stress to the capsuloligamentous structures. Occasionally, a change in footwear, for example, to lower heel height, can be related to the onset. Lowering the heel height increases the tension on the Achilles tendon, which may in turn result in increased pronation of the hindfoot in the same way as described for a shortened Achilles tendon. A lowered heel also results in reduced dorsiflexion of the toes during the stance, decreasing the windlass effect on the plantar aponeurosis and reducing the twisted configuration of the foot.

B. *Site of pain.* Foot pain associated with abnormal pronation usually is felt over the plantar aspect of the foot. Pain from calcaneal periostitis and heel spurs is fairly well localized over the bottom of the heel, often more medially; it may be referred anteriorly into the sole of the foot. Pain from fatigue stress to the plantar ligament or aponeurosis is felt over the sole of the foot, usually more medially. Keep in mind that the bony and soft-tissue pathologic processes referred to previously may occur concurrently.

Forefoot pain arising secondary to a pronated foot condition may be felt in the region of the medial metatarsal heads, if due to abnormal weight distribution, or it may be felt over the medial aspect of the first metatarsophalangeal joint, if caused by pressure over the joint resulting from a hallux valgus deformity.

Knee pain related to a pronated foot is typically from patellofemoral joint problems (see section on patellar tracking dysfunction in Chapter 14).

C. *Nature of pain.* Pain is from increased stress to the plantar ligaments, fascia, capsules, or calcaneal periosteum under conditions in which increased untwisting of the foot takes place. This typically occurs in a person whose foot undergoes an abnormal degree of pronation during stance phase or whose foot remains in a pronated position during prolonged standing. The muscles controlling the twist, or arch, of the foot will protect these structures for a certain period of time. However, once the muscles fatigue, more

stress is transmitted to the ligaments and fascia, which are responsible for the passive stabilization of the arched configuration of the foot. In some cases, this may occur with normal activity levels, such as after walking some distance or after standing for a long period of time. In others, increased activity, such as long-distance running, provides the added stress to bring on the pain. Once a low-grade inflammation develops, the pain is brought on with less stress and may be relatively continuous during weight-bearing. In these more severe cases, pain is typically pronounced on initial weight-bearing, subsiding somewhat as the muscles contract more to protect the painful structures, then increasing again as the muscles fatigue.

II. Physical Examination

A. *Observation and inspection of structural alignment.* Evidence of excessive pronation of the foot and associated biomechanical abnormalities may be noted when the patient walks or stands.

1. Flattening of the medial arch. The region of the navicular and the talar head may appear to be prominent medially and depressed inferiorly.
2. Abduction of the forefoot on the rearfoot.
3. Adduction of the first metatarsal, perhaps with a valgus deformity of the first metatarsophalangeal joint.
4. Valgus position of the heel maintained throughout stance phase.
5. Internal tibial torsion. The feet may be pointed inward while the patellae face straight forward.
6. Femoral anteversion. The patellae face inward when the feet are in normal alignment. This must be differentiated from external tibial torsion, which may present similarly. External tibial torsion is evidenced by an increased external rotation of the intermalleolar line with respect to the frontal plane (in excess of about 25°). Femoral anteversion is suggested when the total range of motion at the hip is about normal, but the range of internal rotation is increased and the range of external rotation is proportionally decreased.
7. Genu valgum. This often exists in conjunction with femoral anteversion.

B. *Inspection (supine)*
1. Structural alignment

a. Forefoot varus. This is the most common intrinsic deformity resulting from abnormal pronation.[21,82,95] Root and co-workers describe it as a frontal plane deformity that is compensated at the subtalar joint by eversion or a valgus position of the calcaneus in weight-bearing.[81]

b. Dorsiflexed and hypermobile first ray producing hallux valgus, which is subluxation of the metatarsophalangeal joint of the big toe in the sagittal and transverse plane.[81]

2. Skin. Inspect for signs of pressure over the navicular tubercle, first metatarsophalangeal joint, and medial metatarsal head. As a result of first ray insufficiency, callus or keratosis may develop under the head of the second metatarsal.[46]

3. Soft tissue. Inspect for muscle atrophy that may relate to loss of dynamic support of the arch of the foot.

4. Inspect the shoes (see page 387).

C. *Selective tissue tension tests*

1. Active movements. If inspection of structural alignment reveals a pronated position of the hindfoot, observe the effect of raising up on the toes and externally rotating the leg over the fixed foot. Both of these movements should decrease the pronation and cause an increased twisting and arching of the foot. If not, a rigid flatfoot, caused by some fixed structural abnormality such as tarsal coalition, probably exists.

2. Passive movements. Unless a rigid flatfoot exists (a relatively rare condition), a pronated foot is usually a hypermobile foot. Hypermobility, especially of the midtarsal joints, may be noted.

a. If a tight heel cord or restricted ankle mortise joint capsule is a contributing cause, dorsiflexion of the hindfoot will be restricted. One must lock the foot by supinating the calcaneus and pronating the forefoot when testing ankle dorsiflexion to avoid misinterpreting movement of the forefoot as being movement at the ankle. There should be about 10° to 20° of dorsiflexion. If dorsiflexion and plantar flexion are both restricted, the joint capsule is probably at fault. If dorsiflexion is restricted with the knee straight, but not

with the knee bent, the gastrocnemius is tight. If dorsiflexion is restricted regardless of the position of the knee, the soleus is probably at fault.

b. If anteversion of the hip is a contributing factor, hip range of motion will be relatively normal but skewed toward internal rotation with restriction of external rotation.

c. Joint play. Movements of the tarsal joints are likely to be hypermobile. Excessive arthrokinematic movements typically occur between four bones: calcaneus, talus, navicular, and cuboid.[21]

d. Pain from low-grade inflammation of the plantar fascia or ligaments, or from calcaneal periostitis, may be reproduced by passively everting the heel, supinating the foot, and dorsiflexing the toes.

3. Resisted movements. Results are usually noncontributory.

D. *Neuromuscular tests.* Determine whether weakness, either neurogenic or atrophic, of any of the muscles controlling movement and stability of the foot exists.

E. *Palpation.* Localized tender areas may exist that relate to areas of low-grade inflammation occurring in response to abnormal tissue stresses. As usual, the finding of localized tenderness to palpation, in itself, must not be taken to be diagnostic of any specific disorder because of the common phenomenon of referred tenderness associated with lesions of deep somatic tissue.

Typical areas of tenderness associated with abnormal foot pronation might include the calcaneal attachment of the plantar fascia and long plantar ligament, especially at the medial tubercle; the plantar fascia, usually over the medial aspect of the sole of the foot; the navicular tubercle; the spring ligament, between the sustentaculum tali and the navicular tubercle; the medial one or two metatarsal heads; and the medial aspect of the first metatarsophalangeal joint.

Areas of skin or subcutaneous tissue hypertrophy may be distinguished on palpations as localized indurated regions. Such calluses, associated with pronation, might be found over the medial one or two metatarsal heads or over the medial aspect of the first metatarsalphalangeal joint.

III. Management. Symptoms arising in association with abnormal foot pronation are the result of increased stress to some pain-sensitive tissue. Proper management, then, must involve selective reduction of abnormal stresses. The approach used must be in accordance with findings on evaluation, including information relating to the patient's activity level. In developing a program of management, it must be kept in mind that the tissue pathology resulting in the painful condition may be due to normal stresses occurring at too great a frequency, to abnormally high stresses occurring at normal frequencies, or to some combination thereof. Either situation may result in tissue fatigue in which the rate of tissue breakdown exceeds the rate at which the tissue is able to repair itself. However, the approach to management will differ, depending on which condition prevails. In general, management of conditions associated with pronation of the foot involves measures to reduce either the frequency or the magnitude of stresses, or both.

In the case of the pronated foot, forces are typically increased by structural malalignments that cause changes in the direction in which forces occur and changes in the degree of movement of skeletal parts during functional activities. The most common postural malalignment causing abnormal foot pronation is probably increased femoral anteversion, which is usually accompanied by increased genu valgum (knock knees). As mentioned earlier, the other common structural deviations predisposing to increased pronation of the foot are adduction of the first metatarsal and increased internal tibial torsion. Each of these conditions results in untwisting of the tarsal skeleton during ambulation, such that a greater tensile stress is imposed on the plantar ligaments, fascia, and joint capsules. Under such conditions, the foot loses the normal passive stability normally produced by becoming twisted during stance phase. To compensate, the intrinsic muscles of the foot must contract more to prepare the foot for push-off. Pain may arise from increased stress to the plantar capsuloligamentous structures, from fatigue of the abnormally contracting muscles, or both.

Persons with long-standing pronation from a congenital structural malalignment or from a malalignment acquired early in life are likely to have a permanent hypermobility of the joints of the foot. The ligaments and joint capsules will have been elongated from the chronic increased stresses applied to them throughout development. By the time they are adults, these persons are not likely to have pain arising from the already lengthened ligaments and fascia during normal activity levels. They are, however, likely to have feet that tire easily from increased activity of the intrinsics and other muscles supporting the arch during gait. They are also more predisposed to developing problems elsewhere, such as metatarsalgia, hallux valgus, and patellofemoral joint dysfunction.

Persons with more subtle structural deviations resulting in an increased tendency toward pronation are likely to have problems only with increased activity levels, such as long-distance running, that increase the magnitude and frequency of pronatory stresses. The mobility of the joints of the foot in these persons allowed by the capsules and ligaments is likely to be fairly normal. It is especially important in patients experiencing pain suggestive of increased pronation, but who have relatively normal structural alignment, to consider nonstructural causes. The most common of these would include a tight heel cord and inappropriate footwear. It is these patients, having subtle structural deviations or nonstructural causes of increased pronation, who are likely to experience pain and develop pathologic lesions associated with increased strain to specific tissues. The most common tissues involved are the supporting plantar structures of the foot, including the periosteum of the plantar aspect of the calcaneus, and the Achilles tendon.

A. *Techniques*

1. Instruction in appropriate activity levels. As in any common musculoskeletal disorder, appropriate instruction in exactly what the patient should and should not do, and to what degree, is an essential component of the treatment program too often overlooked. With respect to problems related to increased foot pronation, this is especially important in the person experiencing problems primarily with increased activity levels. Treatment of the long-distance runner experiencing pain from plantar fasciitis, Achilles tendinitis, or other pronation-related disorders simply involves advising the patient to not run so much. But this is not adequate management of the problem since, as with any disorder, the therapist must be concerned primarily with restoring opti-

mal function. From the patient's standpoint, optimal function may be running long distances! The role of the therapist should be first to decide whether the patient's functional expectations are realistic. The patient with considerably increased femoral anteversion, knock knees, and hypermobile flat feet probably should not be engaging in activities, such as long-distance running, that involve high-frequency, weight-bearing stresses. However, this condition should not prevent the person from engaging in other vigorous conditioning exercise, such as swimming and bicycling.

If there are no gross structural malalignments predisposing to pronation-type problems, the therapist must then determine what can be done to reduce the stresses to the involved tissues, to allow them to heal and to prevent further pathologic processes and pain. As far as healing is concerned, the most important step to be taken is to reduce the stresses that caused the problem. The most reliable method of doing this is to reduce the activity level. The long-distance runner experiencing chronic, persistent pain must be advised to markedly reduce or stop running for a period of 1 to 2 weeks to allow the tissue to heal. Complete immobilization, however, is seldom, if ever, indicated for fatigue disorders such as these. During this period of relative rest the therapist should determine what can be done to reduce stresses when the activity is resumed. Other procedures to help restore the involved tissue to its normal state may also be instituted.

2. Muscle strengthening and conditioning. Strengthening and endurance exercises for the intrinsic muscles of the foot as well as for the extrinsic muscles, such as the anterior and posterior tibialis that help maintain a twisted configuration of the foot, are important in the management of virtually all foot problems resulting from abnormal pronation. Improving the function of these muscles will allow the person with the hypermobile flat foot to stand or walk for longer periods of time before muscle fatigue sets in. It will also help relieve strain on the plantar fascia and ligaments in patients suffering from strain of

these structures by increasing the dynamic support of the arch, thus allowing the muscles to take a greater portion of the load.

3. Proprioceptive balance training
    a. Because the pedal intrinsic muscles appear to function similarly to the plantar fascia in stabilization of the foot, pedal intrinsic strengthening exercises should be prescribed.[66] Foot doming is a particularly beneficial exercise.[22,66]
    b. Dorsiflexors are often found to be weak. Before strengthening, according to Janda, it is better to stretch the tight structures (gastrocnemius–soleus). Both eccentric and concentric exercises should be included.[51]
    c. The tibialis posterior, flexor digitorum longus, and flexor hallucis longus exert a supinatory force at the subtalar joint. These muscles help control pronation by working eccentrically. Marshall prefers to strengthen the supinators eccentrically by using the BAPS balance board (Camp International, Inc., Jackson, Michigan).[66]
4. Strapping. Strong muscles are of little use unless they contract with sufficient force and at the appropriate time to perform the desired function. Abnormal foot pronation can be controlled to varying degree by contraction of the muscles that affect an increased twisted configuration of the foot. Most important among these are the anterior and posterior tibialis muscles and the peroneus longus. Theoretically, muscle function can be enhanced by providing additional input along the afferent limb of the reflex arcs that normally invoke muscle contraction during functional activities. One method of doing so is to strap the part in a manner that will cause increased tension to the straps, and therefore the skin, when movement occurs in the undesired direction. The added afferent input from the tension and pressure produced by the straps serves to enhance activity of muscles that normally check the undesired movement. This is apparently the means by which ankle strapping helps to "stabilize" the ankle against inversion sprains.[35] Although empirically there seems to be evidence for

the efficacy of such procedures, electromyographic studies have yet to be performed to substantiate the proposed mechanism.

For an excellent review of the literature, the reader is referred to the work of Metcalf and Denegar.[73] The low-dye taping technique that was designed by Ralph Dye in an attempt to provide functional mechanical support of the joints of the feet is recommended by Newell[76] and by others[3,4,25,44,54,85,97,98] to restrict abnormal foot pronation. The ability of low-dye taping to modify forces on the medial arch during weight-bearing has been clearly demonstrated by Scranton and colleagues.[85] It is meant to bring the ground up to the foot to eliminate the need for the foot to pronate to reach it.[97] It may be used to protect the passive stabilizing structures of the foot, such as the plantar fascia and associated structures, during the rehabilitation phase following injuries and to assess what effect more permanent stabilizing measures, such as a biomechanical functional foot orthosis or shoe modification, may have.

A number of variations have been developed (modified low-dye, cross X technique, Herzog taping) and have been used in rehabilitating posterior tibial syndrome, posterior tibial tendinitis, peripatellar compression pain, Achilles' tendon problems, and jumper's knee.[49,76,96,97] James and associates demonstrated effectiveness of this type of treatment for overuse injuries when combined with rehabilitation exercises.[49] These procedures pull the medial aspect of the foot toward the supportive surface and secure it in this position with tape (see Appendix B for one variation of this technique).

5. Ultrasound and friction massage. These may be important treatment measures in cases of plantar fasciitis, Achilles' tendinitis, and tibialis periostitis. The resultant increased blood flow may assist in the healing process. Transverse frictions will promote the development of a mobile structure and help prevent adhesions as healing ensues.

6. Achilles' tendon stretching. This is especially important when evaluation reveals a tight heel cord as a possible contributing cause of the patient's problem and in cases of Achilles' tendinitis.

McCluskey and co-workers were one of the first groups to report the beneficial effects of calf muscle stretching to reduce ankle injuries.[67] Ten degrees of dorsiflexion with the knee extended and the subtalar in neutral is the amount considered necessary for normal walking.[82] James suggests at least 15° talocrural joint dorsiflexion is required for running.[50] One must take care to ensure that the stretching force is applied to the hindfoot since using the forefoot as a lever to stretch the heel cord will result in dorsiflexion of the transverse tarsal joint in addition to dorsiflexion at the ankle mortise (talocrural) joint. This may result in hypermobility of the transverse tarsal joint, which may add further to a tendency toward pronation of the foot.

When stretching of the calf muscle is attempted, it is important that the subtalar joint is maintained in a neutral position. To ensure that this position is maintained, the patient should either stretch out in a biomechanical orthotic device or place a lift under the medial aspect of the barefoot to maintain a neutral position of the subtalar joint during stretch.

In the more acute stages of Achilles tendinitis, the therapist must not be overly vigorous in restoring mobility to the heel cord since the condition could be aggravated. However, since most cases of Achilles tendinitis are fatigue disorders, an acute stage never exists. Some gentle stretching may be initiated carefully from the outset since the slow, short-termed stress produced by such stretching procedures in no way approximates the high-frequency, high strain-rate stresses that produce this type of disorder. In fact, early stretching, performed judiciously, will help prevent the fibers from healing in a shortened state.

Increasing the load and speed of contraction with a emphasis on eccentric training has been found to be particularly helpful.[89] This can be carried out with the rear foot over the edge of a step to allow for greater range of dorsiflexion – plantar flexion and eccentric control. To ensure normal weight-bearing alignment, a tennis ball can be placed between the patient's medial malleoli and the patient instructed not to lose contact with the ball throughout the exercise, since this may invoke excessive supination or pronation.[74]

7. Shoe inserts and modifications. When abnormal foot pronation is due to some structural malalignment, whether marked or subtle, only surgery can remedy the true cause of the disorder. However, nonsurgical management is effective in the majority of cases. In order to optimize function, while at the same time preventing stresses sufficient to cause painful pathologic processes, the excessive untwisting of the foot must be reduced. This can be accomplished by altering the orientation of the segments of the foot as they contact the ground during stance phase, by producing direct support to the arched configuration of the foot, or by both.

If the joint capsules and ligaments of the foot are not elongated, as in the hypermobile flat foot accompanying gross malalignment, the twist in the foot during stance phase can be increased by increasing the pronatory orientation of the forefoot or by increasing the supinatory orientation of the hindfoot. This can be done by providing a lateral wedge for the forefoot or a medial wedge for the heel. A trial, temporary insert can be made by cutting such a wedge from a piece of 1/8-inch to 3/16-inch felt to fit inside the shoe. However, if it is to be used on a permanent basis, the wedge should be incorporated into the sole or heel of the shoe by one experienced in shoe modifications or should be incorporated into an orthosis.

If the tarsal joints of the foot are lax, then the twisted configuration cannot be restored by indirect means such as wedging, since these rely on taking up the slack in the joint capsules to effect a twisting of the tarsal skeleton. In the case of a hypermobile, pronated foot, some direct support must be provided to prevent the head of the talus and navicular from dropping downward and medially in a pronatory fashion. For the severely pronated foot, such an arch support may be used in conjunction with wedging of the sole or heel.

Such wedging may be built into the orthosis or into the shoe. Regardless of the type of shoe modification or insert used, in order for the support to be effective the calcaneus must be stabilized by a firm shoe counter or a calcaneal cup built into an orthosis. If the calcaneus is not held firmly, it will tend to compensate for attempts to increase the twist of the foot by rolling farther over into a valgus position (pronation). Thus, many orthoses now in use have a heel cup incorporated into the orthosis itself, obviating the need for an extra-firm shoe counter. Such an orthosis can be used, for example, in athletic shoes, which often do not have very stiff counters.

When chondromalacia of the knee occurs as a result of abnormal pronation of the foot, the use of arch supports or shoe modification may be a necessary component of the treatment program.

The progression of a hallux valgus deformity may also be retarded by use of orthoses or shoe modifications, if the adduction of the first metatarsal is a result of abnormal foot pronation.

In cases of metatarsalgia, if reducing the degree of pronation with appropriate orthotic devices or shoe modification does not adequately relieve the pressure over the metatarsal heads, a metatarsal insert may be used. This simply reduces the stress to the metatarsal heads by increasing the weight-bearing surface area behind the heads. Metatarsal pads are available "ready-made" with an adhesive backing, or a metatarsal support may be incorporated into an arch-supporting orthosis. To place the pad properly in the shoe, tape it to the patient's foot in place just behind the metatarsal heads with the widest dimension of the pad forward. Outline the bottom of the pad with lipstick or some substance that will leave a mark on the insole of the shoe when the patient steps down. The patient then puts on the shoes and walks about to make sure they are reasonably comfortable, realizing, of course, that they will at first feel somewhat peculiar. The shoes are then removed and the pad adhered to the insole of the shoe in the appropriate place as indicated by the marks left on the insole by the lipstick.

Several devices designed to modify forces in the foot have been reported to be helpful for the patient with plantar heel pain. Heel pads have been used to reduce the shock of weight-bearing and shift vertical forces forward and away from the heel.[4,6,36] Some authors have suggested the use of a heel cup to prevent calcaneal eversion and thus reduce tension on the plantar fascia.[11,26,52,85]

PROBLEMS RELATED TO ABNORMAL SUPINATION

Abnormal supination of the entire foot occurs when the subtalar functions in a supinated position.[82] There are three basic classifications for abnormal supination: pes equinovarus, pes cavus, and pes cavovarus.[63,93] A pes equinovarus foot demonstrates a fixed plantar flexed forefoot and an equinus forefoot. The rear foot in weight bearing is in neutral.[21] A pes cavovarus foot demonstrates a fixed medial column or first ray. In the weight-bearing position the calcaneus is in varus or inverted.[21]

Root and co-workers define forefoot valgus as eversion of the forefoot on the rear foot with the subtalar joint in neutral.[82] The compensation for a forefoot valgus is inversion of the calcaneus in the weight-bearing position.[79,93] Forefoot valgus and/or a fixed plantar-flexed first ray are the most common intrinsic deformities resulting in abnormal supination of the subtalar joint.

Functionally abnormal supination is a failure of the foot to pronate, resulting in a foot with inability to compensate normally. There is prolonged supination during the stance phase and a delayed pronation during the gait cycle. Stress fractures, metatarsalgia, plantar fasciitis, and Achilles' tendinitis are common in this type of foot.

In general, treatment consists of stretching, mobilization, exercises, and orthoses.[95] The flexible cavus foot responds well to conventional biomechanical orthotic foot control. The rigid cavus foot requires a special orthosis or a shoe with shock-absorbing materials such as Spenco Insoles (SpencoMedical Corp., Waco, Texas) and Sorbothne Inserts (Spectrum Sports, Twinsburg, Ohio) to lessen the strain on the lower extremities.

ORTHOSES

Ultimately, the patient exhibiting a true intrinsic biomechanical fault should be fitted with custom-made functional biomechanical orthosis to correctly balance the foot during weight-bearing activities. Orthotic devices are most often used to correct excessive pronation and thus may be effective in the

management of related shin splints, chondromalacia, and, occasionally, trochanteric bursitis.

The orthosis made from a positive mold of the foot in its neutral position is designed for restoration of normal alignment of the subtalar and midtarsal joint by controlling excessive pronation and supination and reducing the abnormal forces through the kinetic chain. In basic terms it is directed toward preventing the foot from compensating, allowing normal motion to take place in its proper sequence.

When the orthosis is in place, the foot should function near its neutral position. It is important to evaluate muscle imbalances extrinsic and intrinsic to the foot, in addition to evaluating forefoot and rear foot deformities. Softer flexible types of orthoses can be fabricated in the clinic as a temporary measure or may be made of flexible materials molded to a positive cast of the patient's foot. Most clinics are not equipped for fabrication of the rigid orthosis, which is custom fabricated (also from a positive model). There are a number of podiatry laboratories specializing in these types of orthotic appliances. Many excellent texts and articles are available describing orthotic fabrication and shoe modifications.*

Shoe styles and features are constantly changed by the manufacturers so that it is almost impossible for the clinician to keep abreast of current shoe models, particularly the athletic shoe. The basic functions of any quality shoes are to enhance shock absorption and foot control and to provide good traction and protection. Lasting or curve of the sole of the shoe should generally conform to the patient's own foot shape. In general, most patients will do well with a relatively straight last. Many manufacturers now provide information on shoes that have been selectively designed to limit common foot abnormalities such as overpronation or oversupination of the subtalar joint.

Since foot problems and related disorders are common and because alteration of footwear is often an important component of management of these problems, it is important that the therapist develop a close working relationship with an orthotist, podiatrist, or other professional possessing these skills.

* References 8,10,11,16–19,23,24,28,30,41,49,55,57,66,68,69,80, 92,96.

REFERENCES

1. Alldredge RH: Diastases of the distal tibiofibular joint and associated lesions. JAMA 115:2136–2140, 1940
2. Anderson KJ, LeCocq JF: Operative treatment of injuries to the fibular collateral ligament of the ankle. J Bone Joint Surg 36(A):825–832, 1954

3. Anderson JL, George F, Krakauer LJ, Separd RJ, Torg JS: Year Book of Sports Medicine. Chicago, Year Book Medical Publishers, 1982

4. Appenzeller O, Atkinson R: Sports Medicine: Fitness Training, Injuries. 2nd ed, pp 413–414. Baltimore, Urban & Schwarzenberg, 1983

5. Barnett CH, Napier JR: The axis of rotation at the ankle joint in man: Its influence upon the form of the mobility of the fibula. J Anat 86:1–9, 1952

6. Bateman JE: The adult heel. In Jahss MH (ed): Disorders of the Foot, vol 1, chap 27. Philadelphia, WB Saunders, 1982

7. Bates B: Running biomechanics. Presented at the American Orthopedic Foot Society Meeting, New Orleans, 1982

8. Bates BT, Osternig LR, James MS, James LS: Foot orthotic devices to modify selected aspects of lower extremity mechanics. Am J Sports Med 7:338–342, 1979

9. Boeing DD: Evaluation of a clinical method of gait analysis. Phys Ther 57:795–798, 1977

10. Brody DM: Running injuries. Clin Symp 32:2–36, 1980

11. Campbell JW, Inman VT: Treatment of plantar fasciitis and calcaneal spurs with the UC-BL shoe insert. Clin Orthop 103:57–62, 1974

12. Carson WG: Diagnosis of extensor mechanism disorders. Clin Sports Med 4:231–246, 1985

13. Cedell CA: Ankle lesions. Acta Orthop Scand 46:425–445, 1976

14. Cedell CA: Supination-outward rotation injuries of the ankle. Acta Orthop Scand (Suppl) 110:1–148, 1967

15. Close JR, Inman VT, Poor PM, Todd FN: The function of the subtalar joint. Clin Orthop 50:159–179, 1967

16. Colson JW, Berglund G: An effective orthotic design for controlling the unstable subtalar joint. Orthotics Prosthetics 33:39–49, 1979

17. Cook SD, Kester MA et al: Biomechanics of running shoe performance. Clin Sports Med 4:619–626, 1985

18. D'Ambrosia RD: Orthotic devices in running injuries. Clin Sports Med 4:611–618, 1985

19. D'Ambrosia RD, Drez D: Orthotics. In D'Ambrosia RD, Drez D (eds): Prevention and Treatment of Running Injuries. Thorofare, NJ, Charles B. Slack, 1982

20. De Souza Dias DL, Foerster TP: Traumatic lesions of the ankle joint: The supination external rotation mechanism. Clin Orthop 100:219–224, 1974

21. Donatelli R: Abnormal biomechanics of the foot and ankle. J Orthop Phys Sports Ther 9:11–16, 1987

22. Dowd I: In honor of the foot. Contact Q, Fall 1986, pp 33–39

23. Doxey GE: The semi-flexible foot orthotic: fabrication and guidelines for use. J Orthop Sports Phys Ther 5:526, 1983

24. Drez D: Running footwear. Am J Sports Med 8:140–141, 1980

25. Duggar GE: Plantar fasciitis and heel spurs. In McGlawry ED (ed): Reconstructive Surgery of the Foot and Leg. pp 67–73. New York, Intercontinental Medical Book Co, 1974

26. Du Vries HL: Surgery of the Foot, 4th ed, pp 287–291. St. Louis, CV Mosby, 1959

27. Dwyer FC: Causes, significance, and treatment of stiffness in the subtaloid joint. Proc R Soc Med 69:97–102, 1976

28. Eggold JF: Orthotics in the prevention of runner's overuse injuries. Phys Sports Med 9:125–131, 1981

29. Eltman H: The transverse tarsal joint and its control. Clin Orthop 16:41–46, 1960

30. Festa S, Schuster R: Ask the expert what the doctor says. Runner 9:61, 1986

31. Freeman M: The etiology and prevention of instability of the foot. J Bone Joint Surg 47(B):678–685, 1965

32. Freeman M: Instability of the foot after injuries to the lateral ligament of the ankle. J Bone Joint Surg 47(B):669–677, 1965

33. Freeman M: Treatment of ruptures of the lateral ligament of the ankle. J Bone Joint Surg 47(B):661–668, 1965

34. Fromherz WA: Examination. In Hunt GC (ed): Physical Therapy of the Foot and Ankle, pp 59–90. New York, Churchill Livingstone, 1988

35. Fulp MJ: Ankle joint injuries. J Am Podiatr Med Assoc 65:889–911, 1975

36. Furey JG: Plantar fasciitis: The painful heel syndrome. J Bone Joint Surg 57(A):672–673, 1975

37. Garrick JG, Requa RK: Role of external support in the prevention of ankle sprains. Med Sci Sports 5:200–203, 1973

38. Gerbert J: Ligament injuries of the ankle joint. J Am Podiatr Med Assoc 65:802–815, 1975

39. Gray GW: When the Feet Hit the Ground Everything Changes. Toledo, Ohio, American Physical Rehabilitation Network, 1984

40. Gross AE, MacIntosh DL: Injuries to the lateral ligaments of the ankle: A clinical study. Can J Surg 16:115–117, 1973

41. Henderson WH, Campbell JW: UC-BL shoe inserts: Casting and fabrication. Bull Prosthet Res 10:11:215–235, 1969

42. Hicks JH: The mechanics of the foot: I. The joints. J Anat 87:345–357, 1953

43. Hicks JH: The mechanics of the foot: II. The plantar aponeurosis and the arch. J Anat 88:25–30, 1954

44. Hlavac HF: The Foot Book. Mountain View, CA, World Publications, 1977

45. Hunt GC: Examination of lower extremity dysfunction. In Gould JA, Davies GJ (eds): Orthopaedic and Sports Physical Therapy. St. Louis, CV Mosby, 1985

46. Hutton WC, Dhanedran M: The mechanics of normal and hallux valgus feet: A quantitative study. Clin Orthop 157:7–13, 1981

47. Inman VT: The Joints of the Ankle. Baltimore, Williams & Wilkins, 1976

48. Jackson DW: Ankle sprains in young athletes: Relation of severity and disability. Clin Orthop 101:201–219, 1974

49. James SI: Bates BT, Ostery LR: Injuries to runners. Am J Sports Med 6:40–50, 1978

50. James SL: Chondromalacia of the patella in the adolescent. In Kennedy JC (ed): The Injured Adolescent Knee, pp 214–228. Baltimore, Williams & Wilkins, 1979

51. Janda V: Muscle Function Testing. Boston, Butterworths, 1983

52. Katoh Y, Chao EY, Morrey BF, Laughman RK: Objective technique for evaluating painful heel syndrome and its treatment. Foot Ankle 3:227–237, 1983

53. Kleiger B: Mechanisms of ankle injury. Orthop Clin North Am 5:153–176, 1974

54. Kosmahl EM, Koshmahl HE: Painful plantar heel, plantar fasciitis, and calcaneal spur: Etiology and treatment. J Orthop Sports Phys Ther 9:17–24, 1987

55. Kwong PK, Kay D, Voner RT, White MW: Plantar fasciitis, mechanics and pathomechanics of treatment. Clin Sports Med 7:119–126, 1985

56. Lamoreux L: Kinematic measurements in the study of human walking. Bull Pros Res 10-15:3–84, 1971

57. Langer S: Posting: Theory and practice. Larger Lab Biomech News Lett 1:3, 1973

58. Leonard MH: Injuries of the lateral ligaments of the ankle: A clinical and experimental study. J Bone Joint Surg 31(A):373–377, 1949

59. Level AS, Inman VT, Blosser JA: Transverse rotation of the segments of the lower extremity in locomotion. J Bone Joint Surg 30(A):859–872, 1948

60. Lindstrand A: New aspects in the diagnosis of lateral ankle sprains. Orthop Clin North Am 7:247–249, 1976

61. Lutter LD: The knee and running. Clin Sports Med 4:685–698, 1985

62. MacConnaill MA, Basmajian JV: Muscles and Movements: A Basis for Human Kinesiology, pp 74–84. Baltimore, Williams & Wilkins, 1969

63. Mann RA: Biomechanics of running. In Mack RP (ed): Symposium on the Foot and Leg in Running Sports, pp 1–29. St. Louis, CV Mosby, 1982

64. Mann RA, Hagy JL: Running, jogging and walking: A comparative electromyographic and biomechanical study. In Bateman JE, Trott AW (eds): The Foot and Ankle. New York, Brian C. Decker, 1980

65. Manter JT: Movements of the subtalar and transverse tarsal joints. Anat Rec 80:397–410, 1941

66. Marshall P: The rehabilitation of overuse foot injuries in athletes and dancers. Clin Sports Med 7:175–191, 1988

67. McCluskey GM, Blackburn TA, Lewis T: Treatment of ankle sprains. Am J Sports Med 4:158–161, 1976

68. McKenzie DC, Clements DB, Taunton JE: Running shoes, orthotics and injuries. Sports Med 2:334–347, 1985

69. McPoil TG, Brocato RS: The foot and ankle: Biomechanical evaluation and treatment. In Gould JA, Davies GJ: Orthopaedic and Sports Physical Therapy. St. Louis, CV Mosby, 1985

70. McPoil TG, Schuit D, Knecht HG: A comparison of three positions used to evaluate tibial varum. J Am Podiatr Med Assoc 78:22–28, 1988

71. McRae R: Clinical Orthopedics. New York, Churchill Livingstone, 1983

72. Melillo TV: Gastrocnemius equinus: Its diagnosis and treatment. Arch Podiatr Med Foot Surg 2:159–205, 1975

73. Metcalf GR, Denegar CR: A critical review of ankle taping. Athletic Training 187:121, 1983

74. Molnar ME: Rehabilitation of the injured ankle. Clin Sports Med 7:193–204, 1988

75. Murray MP, Draught AP, Kory RC: Walking patterns in normal men. J Bone Joint Surg 46(A):335–360, 1964

76. Newell SG, Nutler S: Conservative treatment of plantar fascial strain. Phys Sports Med 5:68–73, 1977

77. Nichols JA: Ankle injuries in athletes. Orthop Clin North Am 5:153–176, 1974

78. Peiyer E, Wright DW, Mason L: Human locomotion. Bull Pros Res 10–12:48–105, 1969

79. Ramig D, Shadle J, Watkins A, Cavolo D: The foot and sports medicine: Biomechanical foot faults as related to chondromalacia patellae. J Orthop Sports Phys Ther 2:48–50, 1980

80. Reed JK: Orthotic devices, shoes and modifications. In Hunt GC (ed): Physical Therapy of the Foot and Ankle. New York, Churchill Livingstone, 1988

81. Root ML, Orien WP, Weed JH: Biomechanical Examination of the Foot, Vol 1. Los Angeles, Clinical Biomechanics Corp, 1971

82. Root ML, Orien WP, Weed JN: Clinical Biomechanics, Vol II, Normal and Abnormal Function of the Foot. Los Angeles, Clinical Biomechanics Corp, 1977

83. Sammarco GJ, Burstein AH, Frankel VH: Biomechanics of the ankle: A kinematic study. Orthop Clin North Am 4:75–95, 1973

84. Saunders JB, Dec M, Inman VT, Eberhart HD: The major determinants in normal and pathological gait. J Bone Joint Surg 35(A):543–558, 1953

85. Scranton PE, Pedegana LR, Whitsel JP: Gait analysis alterations in support phase using supportive devices. Am J Sports Med 10:6–11, 1982

86. Sgarlato TE: A compendium of podiatric biomechanics. San Francisco, College of Podiatric Medicine Press, 1971

87. Shore M: Footprint analysis in gait documentation, an instructional sheet format. Phys Ther 60:1163–1167, 1980

88. Smith JW: The ligamentous structures in the canalis and sinus tarsi. J Anat 92:616–620, 1958

89. Standish WD, Curwin S, Rubinovich M: Tendinitis: The analysis and treatment for running. Clin Sports Med 4:593–609, 1985

90. Staples OS: Ruptures of the fibular collateral ligaments of the ankle: Result study of immediate surgical treatment. J Bone Joint Surg 57(A):101–107, 1975

91. Subotnick SI: Biomechanics of the subtalar and midtarsal joints. J Am Podiatr Med Assoc 65:756–764, 1975

92. Subotnick SI: Orthotic foot control and the overuse syndrome. Phys Sports Med 3:75, 1975

93. Subotnick SI, Newell SG: Podiatric sports medicine.

In Fielding MD (ed): Podiatric Medicine and Surgery. Mount Kisco, NY, Futura Publishing Co, 1975

94. Subotnick SI: The cavus foot. Phys Sports Med 8:53–55, 1980

95. Tax H: Flexible flatfoot in children. J Am Podiatr Med Assoc 67:616–619, 1977

96. Wallace L: Lower Quarter Pain: Mechanical Evaluation and Treatment. Cleveland, 1984

97. Wallace L: Foot pronation and knee pain. In Hunt GC (ed): Physical Therapy of the Foot and Ankle, pp 101–122. New York, Churchill Livingstone, 1988

98. Whitesel J, Newell SG: Modified low-dye strapping. Phys Sports Med 8:129–131, 1980

99. Wright DG, Desai SM, Henderson WH: Action of the subtalar and ankle complex during stance phase of walking. J Bone Joint Surg 469(A):361, 1964

16 The Temporomandibular Joint

Darlene Hertling

TEMPOROMANDIBULAR JOINT AND THE STOMATOGNATHIC SYSTEM

Disease and dysfunction of the temporomandibular joints and the adjacent structures affect a large number of persons. It is estimated that over 20% of the average population at one time or another has symptoms relating to the temporomandibular joint.[64] Practitioners of dentistry and medicine have long been aware that the temporomandibular joints are among the few joints in the body that, like the vertebral joints, function as a unit in a sliding–gliding action because of the mandible, which links the two condyles together. However, the many intricacies of the temporomandibular joint are just beginning to be appreciated.

In referring to the temporomandibular joints, the masticatory systems, its component structures, and all the tissues related to it, the term *stomatognathic system* is used. The designation includes a number of systematically related organs and tissues that function as a whole. The components of this system include the following:

— Bones of the skull, mandible, maxilla, hyoid, clavicle, and sternum
— Temporomandibular and dentoalveolar joints
— Muscles and soft tissues of the head and neck and the muscles of the cheeks, lips, and tongue
— Vascular, lymphatic, and nerve supply systems
— Teeth

The stomatognathic system functions almost continuously, not only in mastication and swallowing but also in respiration and speech. It also directs the intricate postural relationships of the head, neck, tongue, and hyoid bone, as well as movements of the mandible. It must be constantly kept in mind that the entire system governs the movements of the mandible. Impaired physiological function results in breakdown not only of an individual tissue but also of the interdependent structures and eventual function of the other parts, thus setting up a chain reaction.

The relationship of the head and neck must be considered. Postural maintenance must consider the shoulder girdle, clavicle, sternum, and scapulae as the fixed base of operation. The head may be said virtually to teeter on the atlanto-occipital joint. Since the center of gravity of the head lies in front of the occipital condyles, it follows that a balance force must be applied to hold the head erect. That force is provided by the large posterior muscles of the neck. Normal balance of the head and neck unit requires normal balance of the anterior and posterior muscles, mandible and cranial relationship, and occlusion of the teeth. If one element is off balance, the normal relationship is broken, leading to eventual dysfunction. Therefore, the entire system must be evaluated and treated.

A faulty relationship of the mandible and maxilla may result in faulty posture of the cranium on the first and second cervical vertebrae, or an imbalance between these vertebrae may result in symptoms referable to the mouth, ear, face, or even the thoracic cavity. Furthermore, faulty curvature of the cervical spine, along with the strains it produces, often is responsible for pain and dysfunction of the head, temporomandibular joints, shoulders, upper extremities, and chest.[4]

Management of the stomatognathic system is not limited to the discipline of any one particular field but encompasses in part nearly every specialty within dentistry and medicine. Treatment involves a team approach that may include physical, myofunctional, and speech therapists; the general dentist; oral-maxillofacial surgeon; orthodontist; otolaryngologist; psychologist; neurologist; allergist; and others.

FUNCTIONAL ANATOMY

OSTEOLOGY

The mandible, the largest and strongest bone of the face, articulates with the two temporal bones and

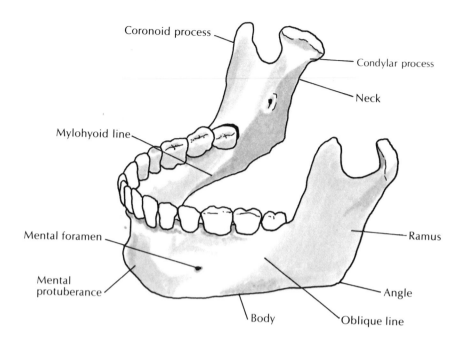

Fig. 16–1. Lateral and frontal aspects of the mandible.

accommodates the lower teeth. It is composed of a horizontal portion, the body, and two perpendicular portions, the rami, which unite with ends of the body nearly at right angles (Fig. 16–1).

The external surface of the body is marked by a midline, the mental protuberance, bilateral mental foramina (for passage of the mental artery and nerve), and the oblique line. Muscle attachments include the platysma, depressor anguli oris, depressor labii inferioris, mentalis, and buccinator. The internal surface is concave from side to side. The superior or alveolar border, wider posteriorly than anteriorly, consists of the dentoalveolar cavities for reception of the teeth. Extending upward and backward on either side of the internal surface is the mylohyoid line, to which the mylohyoid muscle attaches (see Fig. 16–1). Other muscle attachments include the digastric and medial pterygoid muscles.

The ramus, which is quadrilateral in shape, has two processes, the coronoid process and the condylar process. The coronoid process serves as an insertion for the temporalis and masseter muscles. The triangular eminence varies in shape and size; its anterior border is convex, and its posterior border is concave. The condylar process consists of two portions, the neck and the condyle. The condyle, which is convex in shape, articulates with the meniscus of the temporomandibular joint. The mandibular condyle is 15 to 20 mm long and 8 to 10 mm thick and resembles a little cylinder laid on its side. Its long axis is directed medially and slightly backward. An imaginary line drawn through the axis to the middle line would meet a line from the opposite condyle

near the anterior margin of the foramen magnum (Fig. 16–2).* The lateral pterygoid inserts into a depression on the anterior portion of the neck of the condyle.

THE JOINT PROPER AND ITS LIGAMENTOUS STRUCTURES

The temporomandibular joint is located between the temporal fossa (glenoid fossa) on the inferior surface of the temporal bone and the condylar process of the mandibular bone (Figs. 16–3 and 16–4). Just posterior to the joint is the external auditory meatus. The temporal portion consists of the temporal fossa, which is concave, and an anteriorly placed articular eminence, which is convex (see Fig. 16–4).

The temporal fossa is bounded in front by the articular eminence (tubercle) and posteriorly by the postglenoid process (spine) (see Figs. 16–3 and 16–4). The postglenoid process separates the articular surface of the temporal fossa from the anterior margin of the tympanic part of the temporal bone (see Fig. 16–3). The temporal fossa (squamous part of the temporal bone) is made up of thin compact bone). The articular surface, which is smooth, oval, and deeply concave, articulates with the articular disk or meniscus of the temporomandibular joint. After the mid 20s, there is no fibrocartilage in the posterior portion of the mandibular fossa.†

---

* This relationship is an important consideration in the application of mobilization techniques.

† Moffett BC: Personal communication, 1979

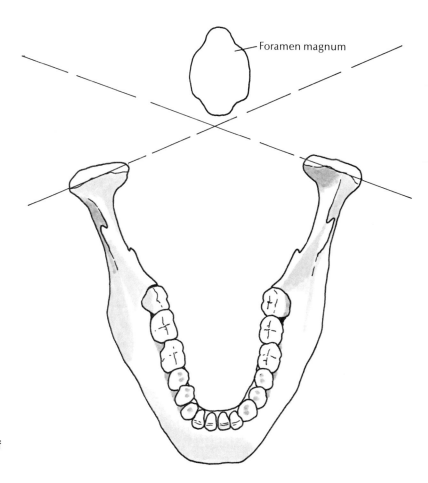

Fig. 16–2. Schematic representation illustrates how extensions of the long axis of the condyles meet near the anterior margin of the foramen magnum.

From a functional point of view, the concave fossa serves as a receptacle for the condyles when the jaws are approximated and as a functional component in lateral movements of the jaw. During opening, closing, protrusion, and retrusion, the convex surface of the condylar head must move across the convex surface of the articular eminence. The existence of the meniscus (inter-articular disk) compensates functionally for the incongruity of the two opposing convex bony surfaces. In addition, the meniscus divides the joint into two portions, sometimes referred to as the upper and lower joints. The meniscus is concavoconvex on its superior surface to accommodate the form of the mandibular fossa and the articular tubercle. The inferior surface is concave over the condyle. In function both the condylar head and articular eminence of the temporal bone are not in contact with each other but with the opposing surfaces of the meniscus. The upper cavity is the larger of the two. The outer edges of the meniscus are connected to the capsule. Synovial membranes line the two cavities above and below the meniscus (see Fig. 16–5). The superior portion of the joints acts as a

gliding joint that allows forward, backward, and lateral movements of the joint. During horizontal lateral jaw movements, the ipsilateral condyle rotates with a slight lateral shift (Bennett movement), with a corresponding forward translation and rotation of the other condylar head. On opening of the mouth, the meniscus rotates and translates forward under the articular eminence.

The meniscus follows the condyle closely in normal function, being pulled forward as the lateral pterygoid contracts to open the mouth and back by the elasticity of its posterior attachment. Arthrography has shown that the disk also changes shape during function as well as moving bodily.[41]

Rees has described the disk or meniscus as having three parts: (1) a thick anterior band (pes meniscus), (2) a thicker posterior band (pars posterior), and (3) a thin intermediate zone (pars gracilis) between the two bands (Fig. 16–6).[75] It is the intermediate band that is both avascular and aneural, with its fibrous tissue being most dense. The intermediate band is positioned between the pressure-bearing articulating surfaces to the temporal bone and the mandibu-

Fig. 16–3. Temporal bone, articular area: temporal fossa (1), articular eminence (2), postglenoid process (3), external auditory meatus (4), tympanic bone (4a), and zygomatic arch (5). (Alderman MM: Disorders of the temporomandibular joint and related structures. In Lynch MA [ed]: Burket's Oral Medicine, Diagnosis and Treatment, 7th ed. Philadelphia, JB Lippincott, 1977)

lar condyle. The anterior and posterior bands have both vascular and neural elements present.

The disk envelopes the condyle much as a cap envelopes the head of a jockey, with the anterior and posterior bands converging medially and laterally to be inserted rigidly onto the medial and lateral poles.[54] The two terms *meniscus* and *disk* usually given to this structure do not describe it adequately. It is not the shape of a meniscus (a crescent-shaped body) or a disk, suggesting a flat structure interposed between the bony surfaces.[45] The articular disk or meniscus has the following attachments[45,54,74]:

—**Anterior attachment** (see Fig. 16–6). Anteriorly,

Fig. 16–4. Temporomandibular joint, right view of bony relations. Note the mandibular condyle and the incongruity of the articular surfaces (1) and the lateral view of articular eminence of temporal bone (2). (Alderman MM: Disorders of the temporomandibular joint and related structures. In Lynch MA [ed]: Burket's Oral Medicine, Diagnosis and Treatment, 7th ed. Philadelphia, JB Lippincott, 1977)

the disk is attached to the capsule. Fibers from the upper head of the lateral pterygoid muscle attach through the capsule into the medial part of the anterior edge of the disk.

—**Medial and lateral attachments** (Fig. 16–7). Medially and laterally, the disk inserts into the corresponding poles of the mandibular condyle, via the medial and lateral collateral ligaments.

—**Posterior attachments** (see Figs. 16–6 and 16–7).[54,74] The posterior-superior disk attaches to the superior stratum, which then attaches to the postglenoid spine. The posterior-inferior disk attaches to the inferior stratum, which then attaches to the neck of the mandibular condyle. The disk also attaches to the posterior capsule. The superior and inferior (lower) strata or laminae enclose an area termed the *bilaminar zone*.[75] This bilaminar zone consists of loose neurovascular connective tissue referred to as the *retrodiskal pad*.[36] Since the retrodiskal pad consists of both vascularized and innervated tissue within the capsule it may be a source of nonarthritic intracapsular inflammation and arthralgia.

An excellent comprehensive study by Rees provides a more detailed analysis of the function and structure of the temporomandibular joint.[75]

Ligamentous Structures

The ligamentous structures around the temporomandibular joint include the following:

—Articular capsule (capsular ligament)
—Lateral ligament (temporomandibular ligament)
—Sphenomandibular ligament (internal lateral ligament)
—Stylomandibular ligament

The capsular ligament is attached to the circumference of the mandibular fossa and the articular tubercle superiorly and to the neck of the mandibular condyle inferiorly. It is a sleeve of thin, loose, fibrous connective tissue. The capsule is especially lax anteriorly in the superior cavity but very taut in the inferior cavity between the head and disk. Therefore, when the condyle moves forward, the disk follows (Fig. 16–8).

The temporomandibular ligament, a thickening of the joint capsule, is attached superiorly to the lateral surface of the zygomatic arch and articular eminence; inferiorly it attaches to the lateral surface and the posterior border of the neck of the mandible. The ligament prevents extensive forward, backward, and lateral movements and is the main suspensory liga-

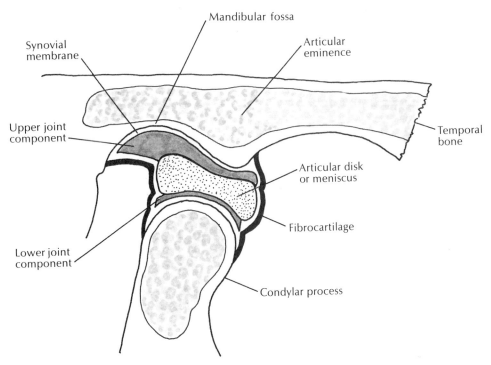

Fig. 16–5. Articular structures of the temporomandibular joint in the closed position.

ment of the mandible during moderate opening movements (see Fig. 16–8).

The sphenomandibular ligament, an accessory ligament, originates from the spine of the sphenoid and attaches to the lingula of the mandible at the mandibular foramen. It serves as a suspensory ligament of

the mandible during wide opening. Following moderate opening, the temporomandibular ligament relaxes and the sphenomandibular ligament becomes taut (Fig. 16–9). The medial pterygoid is associated with its medial surface.

The stylomandibular ligament is also considered

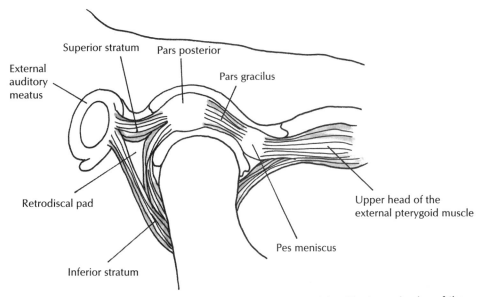

Fig. 16–6. Parasagittal section of the temporomandibular joint. The lower lamina of the bilaminar zone is inserted into the condylar neck and the upper lamina is inserted into the squamotympanic fissure.

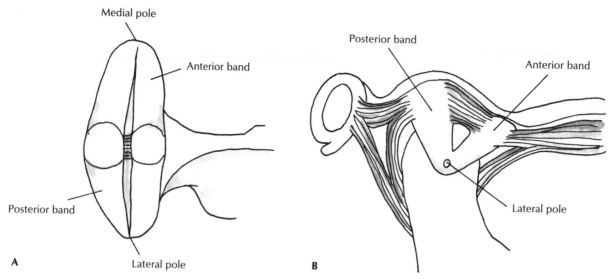

Fig. 16–7. Schematic drawing showing the normal meniscus (right side) seen from above *(A)*, and from the side *(B)*. The posterior and anterior bands are seen converging, to be inserted at the medial and lateral poles.

an accessory ligament. It runs from the styloid process of the temporal bone to the posterior portion of the ramus of the mandible and separates the masseter and medial pterygoid muscles. It acts as a stop for the mandible during extreme opening, preventing excessive anterior movement (see Fig. 16–9).

The mandibular-malleolar ligament has been demonstrated by Pinto and others.[70] This ligamentous structure was found connecting the neck and anterior process of the malleus to the medioposterior part of the joint capsule, the meniscus, and the sphenomandibular ligament. According to Ermshar this anatomical association of the joint and middle ear may well explain many of the middle ear complaints associated with temporomandibular dysfunction.[23]

MANDIBULAR MUSCULATURE

Function of all of the muscles of the upper quadrant need to be understood because of their impact on temporomandibular joint function and dysfunction. Movements of the mandible are a result of the action of the cervical and jaw muscles. The cervical muscles stabilize the head to increase the efficiency of the mandibular movements.

The three major closing muscles of the mandible are the temporalis, the masseter, and the medial pterygoid. The superior head of the lateral pterygoid is also actively involved in mandibular closure.[53,59]

The *temporalis* muscle, which is fan shaped, arises from the temporal fossa and deep surface of the temporal fascia. The anterior fibers of the muscle are vertical, and the middle are oblique, and the posterior are nearly horizontal. The fibers converge as they descend, becoming tendinous, and insert into the medial and anterior aspects of the coronoid process of the ramus. The temporalis muscle functions primarily as an elevator of the mandible, moving the jaw vertically and diagonally upward. The posterior fibers also retract the mandible and maintain the condyles posteriorly (Fig. 16–10).

The *masseter* is a thick quadrilateral muscle composed of two bellies, the deep and superficial. The superficial portion arises from the lower border of the zygomatic arch and maxillary process; it extends down and back and inserts into the angle and the inferior half of the lateral surface of the ramus. The muscle itself is formed by an intricate arrangement of tendinous and fleshy bundles that make it extremely powerful (Fig. 16–11*A*). The smaller, deeper portion is fused anteriorly to the superficial portion but is separated from it posteriorly. It arises from the entire length of the zygomatic arch and passes anteriorly and inferiorly, inserting in the lateral surface of the coronoid process and superior half of the ramus (Fig. 16–11*B*). The masseter functions primarily as an elevator of the mandible. The superficial fibers also protrude the jaw a little, and the deep portion acts as a retractor as well.

The *medial pterygoid* is located on the medial aspect of the ramus. Although less powerful than the

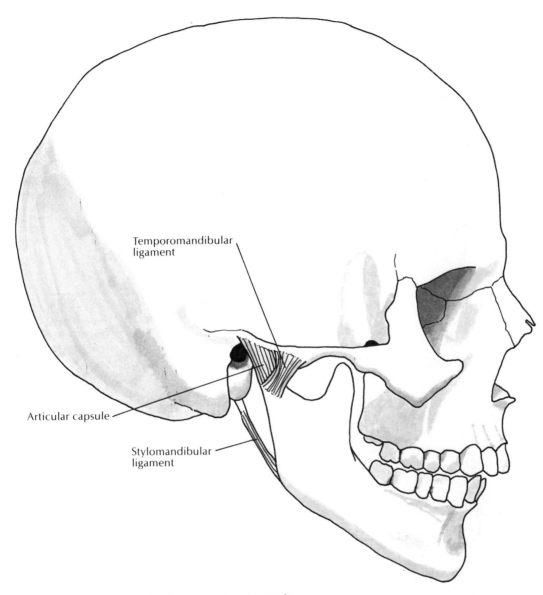

Temporomandibular
ligament

Articular capsule

Stylomandibular
ligament

Fig. 16 – 8. Temporomandibular ligament and capsule.

masseter, its construction is similar to the masseter in that it is characterized by an alternation of fleshy and tendinous parts. The medial pterygoid, which is quadrilateral in shape, arises from the medial surface of the lateral pterygoid plate and pyramidal process of the palatine bone. The fibers pass laterally, posteriorly, and inferiorly and insert onto the medial surface of the ramus and angle of mandible. Its primary function is closing and elevation of the mandible. It also protrudes and laterally deviates the jaw (Fig. 16 – 12).

The major muscles that depress the mandible are the lateral pterygoids and the anterior strap muscles, the suprahyoid and infrahyoid groups. The supra-

hyoid muscles are the digastric, stylohyoid, mylohyoid, and geniohyoid. They are all either opposed or assisted synergically by the infrahyoid muscles.

The *lateral pterygoid* is a thick conical muscle and consists of two bellies. The superior head arises from the infratemporal crest of the greater wing of the sphenoid bone. The inferior head arises from the lateral surface of the pterygoid plate. The two heads form a tendinous insertion in front of the temporomandibular joint. The lower fibers run horizontally and insert on the neck of the condyle, with some fibers attaching to the medial portion of the condyle as well. Fibers from the superior head are attached to the articular disk and capsule as well as to the condy-

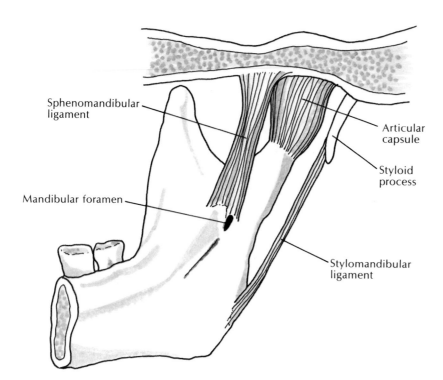

Fig. 16–9. Sphenomandibular and stylomandibular ligaments as viewed from medial aspect of mandible.

lar head (see Fig. 16–12).[59,71] The attachment of the lateral pterygoid to the condyle and disk is significant in stabilizing the temporomandibular joint during bilateral protrusion, retrusion, and closing of the mandible. Lateral movement of the mandible is achieved by the action of the lateral and medial pterygoid on one side and the contralateral temporalis muscle. The lateral pterygoid, especially its inferior head, is also the primary muscle used in opening the mouth, and in protrusion of the mandible. The superior head is believed to play an important role in stabilizing the condylar head and disk against the articular eminence during closing movement of the mandible.[59] This muscle is particularly important in cases of temporomandibular joint dysfunction and is the muscle most frequently involved.

The *digastric* muscle consists of an anterior and posterior belly connected by a strong round tendon. The anterior belly arises from the lower border of the mandible close to the symphysis. The posterior belly, which is considerably longer than the anterior one, arises from the mastoid process of the temporal bone. Both bellies descend toward the hyoid bone and are united by the intermediate tendon, which is connected to the hyoid bone by a loop of fibrous tissue (Fig. 16–13). The function of the digastric is to pull the mandible back and down. The digastric, assisted by the suprahyoids, plays a dominant role in forced opening of the mandible when the hyoid bone

is fixed by the infrahyoid muscle group. It also aids in retraction of the jaw and elevation of the hyoid bone.

The *stylohyoid* muscle arises from the styloid process of the temporal bone and inserts on the hyoid bone. Along with the geniohyoid it determines the length of the floor of the mouth. It also acts in initiating and assisting jaw opening and draws the hyoid bone upward and backward when the mandible is fixed (see Fig. 16–13).

The *geniohyoid* is a narrow muscle, wider posteriorly than anteriorly, that lies adjacent to the midline of the floor of the mouth and above the mylohyoid muscle. It arises from the symphysis of the mandible and inserts onto the anterior surface of the hyoid bone. Like the digastric, it acts to pull the mandible down and back when the hyoid bone is fixed and assists in elevation of the hyoid bone (Fig. 16–14).

The *mylohyoid* muscle arises from the whole length of the medial surface of the mandible, from the symphysis to the last molar teeth, and makes up the floor of the mouth. The fibers pass downward, with some meeting in the median raphe and some attaching directly to the hyoid bone. The mylohyoid elevates the floor of the mouth. It also assists in depression of the mandible when the hyoid is fixed and elevation of the hyoid bone when the mandible is fixed (see Fig. 16–14).

The *infrahyoid* muscles (sternohyoid, thyrohyoid,

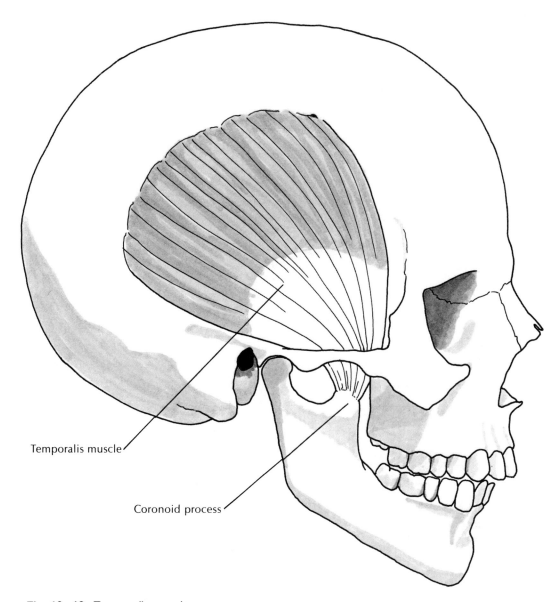

Temporalis muscle

Coronoid process

Fig. 16-10. Temporalis muscle.

and omohyoid) act together to steady the hyoid bone or depress it and therefore allow the suprahyoids to act on the mandible (see Fig. 16-13).

Other muscles that have a close neurophysiological relationship to the temporomandibular joint and that are innervated by the fifth cranial nerve include

Tensor tympani—Controls movement of the tympanic membrane. It is contained in the bony canal superior to the bony part of the auditory tube, from which it is separated by a thin bony septum.

Tensor veli palatini—Controls diameter of the eustachian tube. This thin triangular muscle lies lateral to the medial pterygoid plate, the auditory

tube, and the levator veli palatini. Its lateral surface is in contact with the upper and anterior part of the medial pterygoid.

Abnormal muscle contraction or spasms of any of the temporomandibular muscles, including clenching of the jaw, may affect the tensor veli palatini and tensor tympani muscles and, indirectly, the stapedius muscle of the ear.[11,43]

Muscle Group Action

Mandibular movements are complicated owing to the wide range of positions that the mandible can potentially assume. Briefly, group action might be summarized as follows:

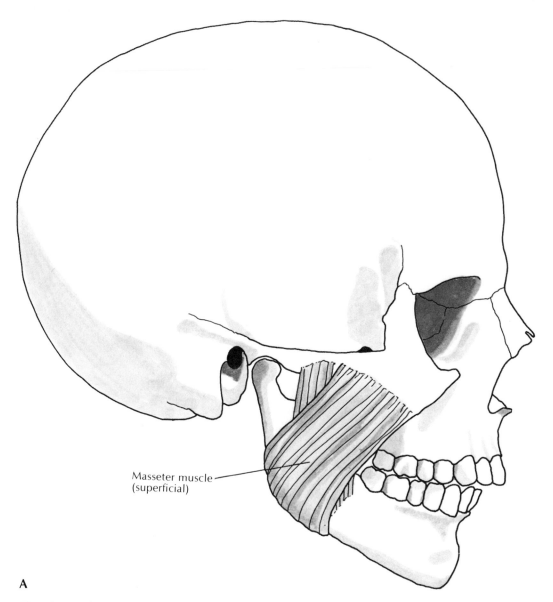

A

Fig. 16-11. Superficial *(A)* and deep *(B)* layers of masseter muscle.

Mandibular Elevators. The mandibular elevators include the coordinated action of the masseter, temporalis (for retrusion), superior head of the lateral pterygoid (for stabilization), and the medial pterygoid (for protrusion).

Mandibular Opening. The inferior head of the lateral pterygoid and the anterior head of the digastric are considered the primary muscles used in opening the mandible. The inferior head of the lateral pterygoid acts synergistically with the suprahyoid muscle group in the translation of the condylar head downward, inferiorly, and contralaterally during opening movements. Opening is assisted by the other suprahyoid muscles, which also act in initiating motion

when the hyoid bone is fixed by the infrahyoid muscles. The masseter and the medial pterygoid muscles also help draw the jaw slightly forward.

Retrusion of the Mandible. The posterior fibers of the temporalis draw the condyles backward during retrusion and are assisted by the digastric and suprahyoids.

Protrusion of the Mandible. Protrusion is performed by the masseter and medial and lateral pterygoids.

Lateral Movements. Action is achieved primarily by the lateral and medial pterygoids on one side and the temporalis muscle on the contralateral side. When the mandible moves to the right side, the left lateral

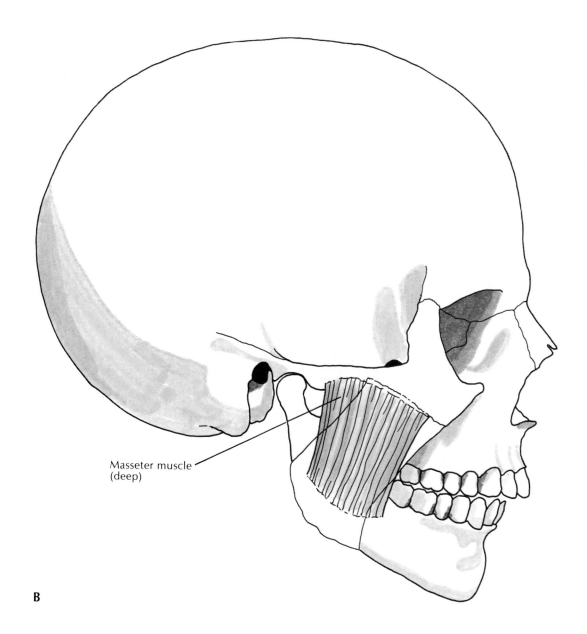

Masseter muscle
(deep)

B

pterygoid and medial pterygoid move the chin across the midline toward the right side. The digastric, geniohyoid, and mylohyoid also are actively involved.

DYNAMICS OF THE MANDIBLE AND TEMPOROMANDIBULAR JOINTS

Before evaluating the dynamics of the various mandibular movements, certain physiological positions of the jaw should be defined. These are the rest position, occlusal positions, hinge position, and centric position. The terminology of some of these positions is confusing and controversial. No basic termi-

nology has been universally adopted, and each investigator has had to establish his or her own.

The *rest position* of the mandible is considered the position the jaw assumes when there is minimal muscle-action potential. It usually implies that the head is also in its normal rest position when the person is in an upright posture. The mandibular rest position is considered to be an equilibrium between the tonus of the gravity, or jaw opening muscles and that of the antigravity, or jaw closing muscles. The residual tension of the muscles at rest is termed *resting tonus*. In this position there is no occlusal contact between the maxillary and mandibular teeth. The space between the upper and lower teeth is called the

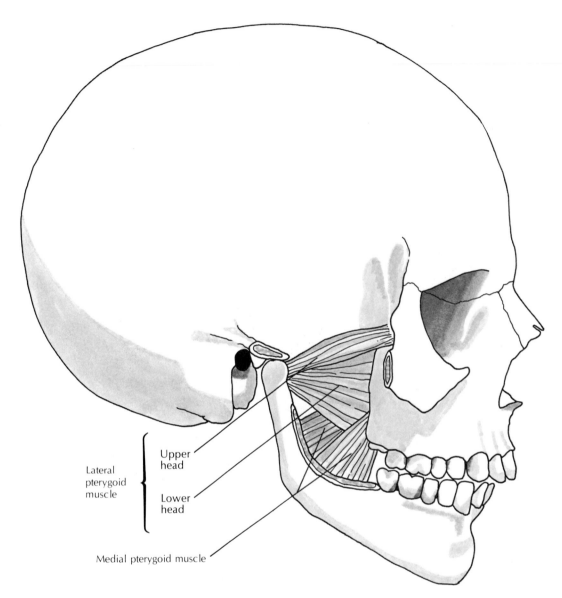

Fig. 16–12. Medial and lateral pterygoid muscles.

free-way space or *interocclusal clearance*. It normally measures from 2 to 5 mm between incisors.

The rest position of the tongue, often referred to as the *postural position*, is up against the palate of the mouth.[27] The most anterosuperior tip of the tongue lies in the area against the palate just posteriorly to the back side of the upper central incisors. The rest position of the tongue by way of neuroreflexors (jaw–tongue reflex) provides a foundation for the resting muscle tone of the elevator muscles of the mandible and for the resting activity of the tongue.[2]

The importance of the rest position lies in the fact that it permits the tissues of the stomatognathic system to rest and thus repair themselves. If the vertical dimension is abnormally decreased (eliminating the interocclusal space), the teeth will be in constant contact. This eliminates the rest position and creates constant muscular tension and stress on the supporting structures and teeth. Factors that influence muscle tonus and the rest position are function, sleep, pathologic conditions, and the normal aging process.

Occlusal positions are functional positions in which contact between some or all of the teeth occur. One occlusal position, termed *median occlusal position* by Sicher and DuBrul, is highly significant.[86] This is the position in which the jaws are closed so that all upper and lower teeth meet, result-

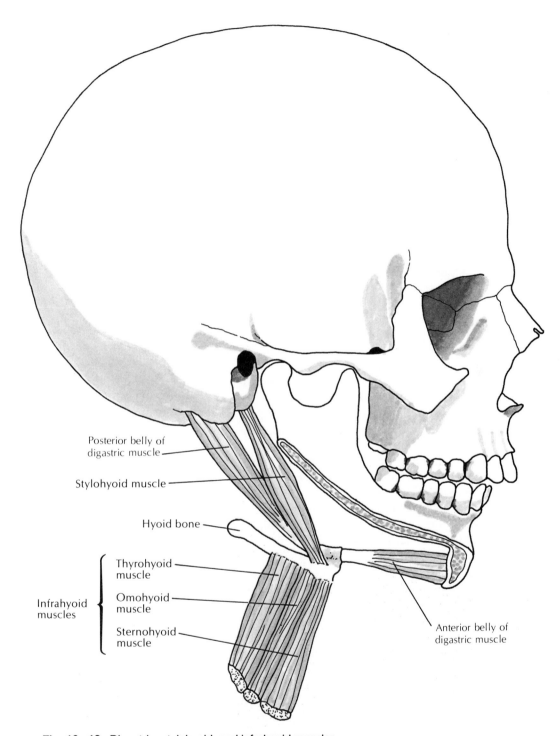

Fig. 16–13. Digastric, stylohyoid, and infrahyoid muscles.

ing in full occlusion with a balanced intercuspation of the upper and lower dental arches. From the median occlusal position, the mandible can move forward into protrusive occlusal positions, laterally, and backward to a limited extent in all normal jaws. Absent or abnormally positioned teeth can displace the mandible from the normal median occlusal posi-

tion, disturbing the complete balance between the teeth, temporomandibular joints, and the musculature.

The *hinge position* is the position of the mandible from which a pure hinge opening and closing of the jaw can be made.[86] In the hinge position, the condyles are in the most retruded position that the mus-

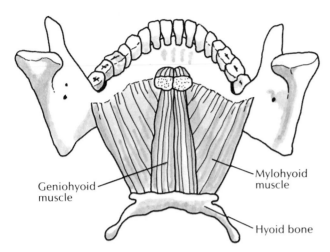

Fig. 16–14. Mylohyoid and geniohyoid muscles viewed from above and behind the floor of the mouth.

cles of the jaw can accomplish; it is determined by the length of the temporomandibular ligaments. The position is considered a retruded position or "strained relationship" that the mandible can assume actively or passively. Determination of this position is useful for some clinical procedures.

Centric position, or centric relation occlusion, denotes a concept of normal mandibular posture. Centric position implies the most retruded, unstrained position of the mandible from which lateral movements are possible and the components of the oral apparatus are in balance. Normal centric position is slightly forward of the most posterior position that the mandibular musculature can actually achieve. Ideally, median occlusal position should coincide with centric position.

Mandibular movements are complicated owing to the wide range of positions that the mandible can assume. Involved and integrated in mandibular movements are the shape of the fossae, the degree of tension of the associated ligaments, the menisci, the neuromuscular system, and the guiding incline of the teeth.

Kinematically, the mandible may be considered a free body that can rotate in any angular direction. It has, therefore, three degrees of freedom; each of these degrees of freedom of motion is associated with a separate axis of rotation.[92] The two basic movements required for functional motion are rotation and translation. The mandible is capable of affecting these movements in three planes—sagittal, horizontal, and frontal. The joint has three functional motions—opening and closing, protrusion and retrusion, and lateral motions. A considerable degree of rotation is also possible.

When the mouth is opened, the condyles first rotate around a horizontal axis. This motion is then combined with gliding of the condyles forward and downward with the lower surface of the meniscus at the same time as the meniscus slides forward and downward on the temporal bone. This movement results from the attachment of the meniscus to the medial and lateral poles of the head of the mandible and from the contraction of the lateral pterygoid, which carries the condyle with the meniscus onto the articular eminence. The forward sliding of the meniscus ceases when the fibroelastic tissue attaching to the temporal bone posteriorly has been stretched to the limits. Thereafter, there is some further hinging and gliding forward of the condyle until it articulates with the most anterior part of the meniscus and the mouth is fully opened. The condyles essentially rotate on an axis in the horizontal plane and translate against the posterior slope of the articular eminence in the sagittal plane.

Opening movements of the mandible are caused by the synergistic action of the lateral pterygoid muscles and the depressors of the mandible. Although the lateral pterygoid pulls the condylar head and meniscus forward, the digastric and geniohyoid muscles pull the mandible downward and backward, affecting rotation. This blending of muscle action makes possible the rotatory and translatory movements of jaw opening. This motion affects all the other muscles anchored to the mandible. The elevators of the mandible must lengthen to ensure smoothness of performance, and the muscles of the cranium and hyoid bone must act as holders to establish a fixed position (Fig. 16–15).

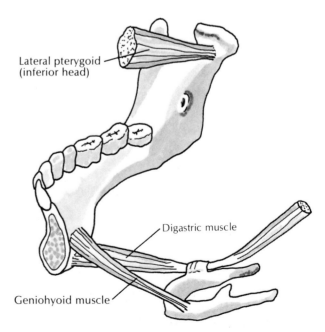

Fig. 16–15. Mandibular muscles involved in opening.

In mandibular closure, the movements are reversed. In the first phase of the movement, the condyles glide backward and then hinge on the menisci, which are held forward by the lateral pterygoids. The backward glide of the mandible results from interaction between the retracting portions of the masseter and temporal muscles and the retracting portions of the depressors. During the second phase, the inferior head of the lateral pterygoids relaxes while the upper head allows the menisci to glide backward and upward on the temporal bone along with the condyles.[53] The second phase begins with the contraction of the masseter, the medial pterygoid, and temporalis muscles; it ends with intercuspation of the teeth. The onset of superior head, or lateral pterygoid, function is usually concurrent with that of the elevator musculature.[59]

In protrusion, the teeth are retained throughout in the occlusal position, so far as possible, and the lower teeth are drawn forward over the upper teeth by both lateral pterygoids. In contrast to opening movements, the condyles and menisci move downward and forward along the articular eminences without rotation of the condyles around a transverse axis. To prevent the mandible from falling, the elevating muscles exhibit some degree of contraction. They must make the necessary adjustment with the balancing depressor–retractors as they lengthen to allow the mandible to slide forward just free of the interlocking dentition.

In retraction, the mandible is drawn backward by the deep portion of the masseter muscles and by the posterior fibers of the temporalis muscles to the rest position. At the same time, the geniohyoid and the digastric muscles and the elevators synergistically balance each other to maintain the mandible in the horizontal position.

In lateral movements of the mandible, asymmetrical muscular patterns develop on both sides. In this movement, one condyle and meniscus slides downward and forward in the sagittal plane and medially in the horizontal plane along the articular eminence. At the same time, the other condyle rotates laterally on a sagittal plane around a shifting vertical axis and translates medially in the horizontal plane while remaining in the fossa. The condylar translation in the horizontal plane is known as the Bennett movement.[86,93,94] If one views the mandible from above, it will be seen that the medial pole of the condyle juts far medially from the plane of the jaw, while the coronoid process leans laterally. The lateral pterygoid muscle, inserted on the medial pole of the condyle, pulls inward and forward in the horizontal plane, while the horizontal fibers of the temporalis muscle, inserted on the coronoid process, pull outward and backward (Fig. 16–16). These muscles, operating as a force-couple, contribute to the torque of rotating the condyle that is necessary to effect chewing on this side. The condyle is known as the working-side condyle. Therefore, in lateral deviation to the left,

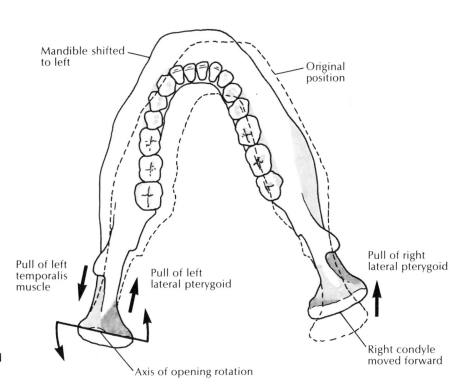

Fig. 16–16. Mandibular muscles involved in lateral movement of the mandible to the left. The suprahyoid muscles are not shown.

Mandible shifted to left

Original position

Pull of left temporalis muscle

Pull of left lateral pterygoid

Pull of right lateral pterygoid

Axis of opening rotation

Right condyle moved forward

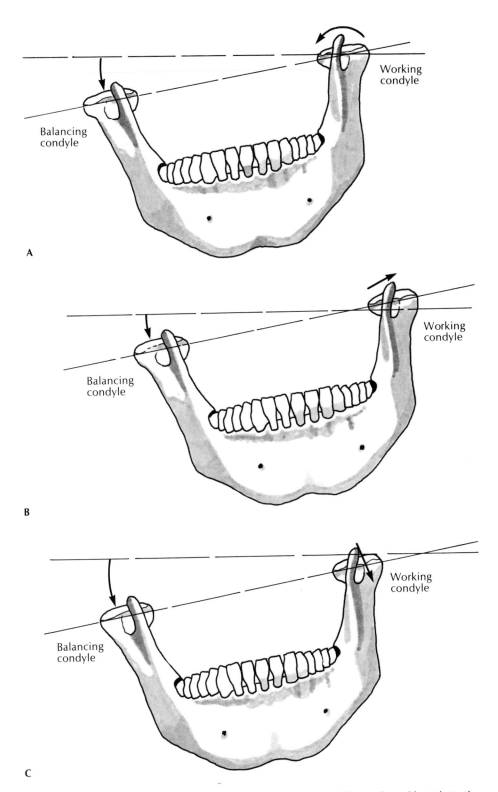

Fig. 16–17. The basic types of working condylar motions are *(A)* rotation with no lateral shift; *(B)* rotation with movement backward, upward, and/or laterally; *(C)* rotation with movement downward, forward, and laterally. *(Figure continues.)*

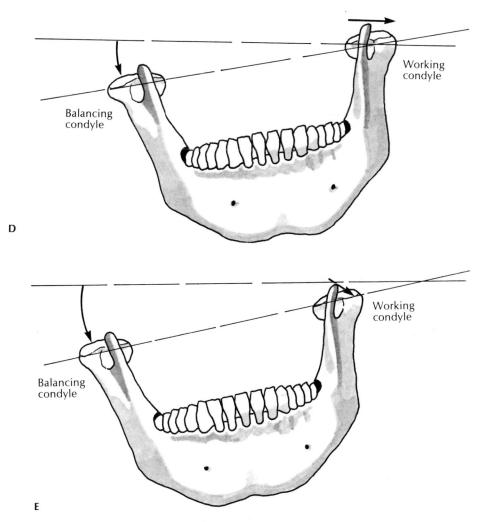

Fig. 16-17 *(continued). (D)* rotátion with a lateral shift; and *(E)* rotation with movement downward, backward, and laterally. (After Weinberg LA: An evaluation of basic articulators and their concepts: I. Basic concepts. J Prosthet Dent 13:622–644, 1963)

the lateral pterygoid on the right, together with the right and left anterior bellies of the digastric and geniohyoid, contract. This causes the right condyle to move downward, forward, and medially, while the actions of the left temporalis and the lateral pterygoid rotate the left condyle in the fossa and displace the mandible to the left. This is described as left lateral excursion with a Bennett shift to the left. The left condyle is called the *working side condyle* and the right condyle is the *nonworking condyle*, or balancing condyle. Basic types of working condylar motions include:[94]

—Rotation with no lateral shift (Fig. 16-17*A*)
—Rotation with movement backward, upward, and/or laterally (Fig. 16-17*B*)

—Rotation with movement downward, forward, and laterally (Fig. 16-17*C*)
—Rotation with a lateral shift (Fig. 16-17*D*)
—Rotation with movement downward, backward, and laterally (Fig. 16-17*E*)

It is apparent that the right lateral pterygoid has also entered into the force-couple system. In the closing stroke, the force-couple changes in direction and components. Thus, in the rotatory movements of grinding or chewing, these alternating movements swing the mandible from side to side.

Although masticatory movements are highly complex, they become automatic in each person as a result of the integration of the proprioceptive mechanism and muscular action. All of the muscles of mastication are involved in the act of chewing because it involves all four movements of the mandible—elevation, depression, protrusion, and retrusion.

RELATIONSHIP OF HEAD POSTURE AND REST POSITION OF THE MANDIBLE

Functionally the temporomandibular joint, the cervical spine, and the articulations between the teeth are intimately related. The neuromuscular influence of the cervical and masticatory region actively participate in the function of mandibular movement and cervical positioning.[40,69,88,99] Many factors influence the masticatory muscles and affect the rest position and path of mandibular closure.[50,60,62,72,73] A change in head position caused by cervical muscles changes the mandibular position.[13,18,33,62,76] This change affects occlusion and the masticatory muscles, and the masticatory muscles then affect the temporomandibular joint.[28,79] The balance between the flexors and extensors of the head and neck is affected by the muscles of mastication and the suprahyoid and infrahyoid muscles.[78] Dysfunction in either the muscles of mastication or the cervical muscles can easily disturb this normal balance.

Cervical posture change affects the mandibular path of closure,[72] the mandibular rest position,[13] masticatory muscle activity,[40,57,72] and, subsequently, the occlusal contact pattern. Neurologically the cervical apophyseal joints and increased gravitation forces on the head can directly alter muscular activity about the jaw. Electromyographic studies have indicated increased masticatory levels with cervical backward bending and cervical flexion: backward bending increases activity of the temporalis muscles and cervical flexion increases activity of the masseter and digastric.[8,9]

A common postural defect that increases the gravitational forces on the head and leads to hyperextension of the head on the neck is the forward head posture (anteriorly positioned head). When the head is held anteriorly, the line of vision will extend downward if the normal angle at which the head and neck meet is maintained. To correct for visual needs there is a tilting of the head backwards, flexion of the neck over the thorax, and posterior migration of the mandible.[79] The posterior cervical muscles are shortened isometrically and are forced to contract excessively to maintain the head in this position while the anterior submandibular muscles are stretched to cause retrusive forces on the mandible and an altered occlusal contact pattern. The mandible is forced posteriorly by the rebound effect of the stretched platysma and other anterior cervical muscles.[29] The contracted posterior cervical muscles may entrap the greater occipital nerve and refer pain to the head.[10] Excessive mandibular shuttling between opening and closing, necessary for functional activities such as eating, leads to joint hypermobility because the temporomandibular joint capsule is stretched.[28] Increased muscular activity in the cervical (longus colli) and hyoid muscles will in turn cause tightness in the throat and difficulty swallowing.[79]

NERVE SUPPLY

The innervation of the temporomandibular joint is supplied by three nerves that are part of the mandibular division of the fifth cranial nerve. The posterior deep temporal and masseteric nerves supply the medial and anterior regions of the joint. The auriculotemporal nerve supplies the posterior and lateral regions of the joint (see Fig. 18–11). The auriculotemporal nerve is the major nerve innervating the posterior lateral capsule, the retrodiscal pad, the temporomandibular ligaments, and the capsular blood vessels. The auriculotemporal nerve also sends a few branches to the tympanic membrane, the external auditory meatus, the superior one half of the auricle on its lateral aspect, and the skin of the temples and scalp.[19,35] The central part of the disk is not innervated.[74]

All four types of joint mechanoreceptors have been identified with respect to the joint structures of the temporomandibular joint. For a detailed understanding of their morphologic and functional characteristics see Chapter 2, Arthrology, and articles by Clark,[12] Klineberg,[48] and Wyke.[99] The general characteristics of type I, II, and III mechanoreceptors are postural and kinesthetic perception, reflexive influence on motor neuron pool activity, and inhibition of nociceptor-mechanoreceptor activity. The major contribution to position sense of the mandible is believed to come from these joint receptors, although the presence of spindles in the muscles of mastication and pain impulses from the periodontal membrane also contribute to afferent information. This mechanoreceptor system is polysynaptic and heavily influences (both inhibitory and facilitory) the reflex coordination of masticatory activity.

There is also an abundant supply of type IV, nonadapting, high-threshold pain receptors, which are nonactive under normal conditions. Abnormal activity of these receptors results when related tissue is subject to marked deformation or other noxious mechanical or chemical stimulation (i.e., intracapsular pressure changes, capsular tightness, and strained positions of the mandibular condyles).[47] As a result there will be altered perception of mandibular movement and positioning as well as altered muscle activity of those muscles innervated by the fifth cranial nerve.

APPLIED ANATOMY

Subluxation of the Jaw

The temporomandibular joint can subluxate itself through its own muscular dynamics. Subluxation occurs when the condyle translates onto the articular tubercle and then back to the articular eminence. Predisposing factors that allow the subluxation to occur more easily in some persons more than others is a decrease in the slope of the articular eminence or a flattened articular eminence (see Figs. 16–4 and 16–5) and stretching of the ligamentous attachments of the meniscus into the condylar pole.[44,45,100] Signs of subluxation include excessive mandibular opening (greater than 40 mm), movement of the lateral poles too far anteriorly (too much translation), and joint noise at the beginning of closing. If unilateral subluxation occurs, there will be a quick deviation from midline to the contralateral side at the end of opening.

Translation Occurring Too Soon in Opening

In this condition or dysfunction, translation occurs within the first 11 mm of opening. Such a movement is contrary to normal arthrokinematic movements of the jaw in which translation begins only after the first 11 mm of opening. Both translation occurring too soon and subluxations are conditions that are believed to involve muscle imbalances. There may be no actual temporomandibular joint dysfunction present with these two conditions, and they may occur separately or together in some patients. Their long range effect on the temporomandibular joint, however, can lead to temporomandibular joint dysfunction.

If either or both of these conditions are observed, it is important to control them to minimize the stress placed on the intracapsular tissues and prevent the perpetuation of temporomandibular joint dysfunction that is present and may be a hindering factor to the treatment.

Dislocation of the Jaw

Dislocation may result from actual trauma to the chin during opening of the mouth or may occur without actual trauma, for example, with a sudden muscular spasm during a yawn. This dislocation is always anterior and may be unilateral or bilateral, resulting in displacement of one or both condyles forward into the infratemporal fossa anterior to the articular eminences.[84] In bilateral dislocations, the chin is displaced forward so that the patient shows some degree of prognathism with an open bite. In unilateral dislocation the mandible is displaced toward the noninjured side.

Reduction is accomplished unilaterally by depressing the mandible with the thumb placed on the last molar teeth and at the same time elevating the chin. The downward pressure overcomes the spasm of the elevating muscles, and elevating the chin repositions the condyles backward behind the articular eminences. Reduction is usually followed by several days of rest.[82]

Habitual dislocation, subluxations, or self-reducing dislocations are not especially rare. According to Dufourmentel and Axhausen, there are two kinds of habitual subluxation that patients themselves may learn to adjust either by a special jaw movement or with the hand. These are luxation in the upper cavity (meniscotemporal) and luxation in the lower cavity (meniscocondylar).[3,21]

Derangement of the Meniscus

Trauma, overclosure of the mouth with backward displacement of the condyle, or malocclusion may cause derangement of the meniscus. Trauma to the meniscus can vary from an inflammatory condition to a complete or partial tearing of the meniscus from its capsular attachment. If the meniscus remains attached to the anterior capsule and the external pterygoid, an anterior dislocation of the meniscus occurs. It may be manifested by displacement of the mandible toward the affected side and possible blockage of mandibular opening and closing.[84] If the meniscus remains attached to the posterior capsule, a painful blockage in closing the mandible results.[84]

The most widely accepted view is that clicking is the result of derangement of the meniscus. However, many investigators have reported various other theories of its etiology in addition to derangement of the meniscus. Among these are incoordinate contraction of the two bodies of the lateral pterygoid, so that the meniscus snaps over the condyle rather than following the movement smoothly and coordinately when the mouth is open; deterioration of the meniscus and cartilaginous surfaces; and stretching of the joint ligaments by frequent subluxation.[85]

Clicking may occur as one or more clicks in one joint, or clicking may occur in both joints; it may or may not be associated with pain. Various types of clicking noises have been observed during sagittal opening, including an opening click, an intermediate click during the opening phase, and a full opening click. Each of these clicks appears to be associated with various pathologic occlusions.

An opening click is believed to be due to an anterior displacement of the meniscus, with the condyle displaced posteriorly and superiorly. As the mandible opens, the condyle must pass over the posterior surface of the meniscus.[85]

Clicking during various parts of the opening of the mandible is believed to result from incoordinate movements of the upper and lower heads of the external pterygoid, so that the condyle cannot remain in its normal relationship with the meniscus.[85] More likely causes are possible anteroposterior displacement of the disk and ruptures or rents of the disk.[98]

A final click occurring in the full opening phase may be caused by the condyle passing over the anterior portion of the meniscus, by the meniscus being pulled forward of the condyle, or by both the meniscus or condyle passing over the articular eminence.[85]

In addition to clicks produced during mandibular opening, clicks may be produced by eccentric movements. Again these may be largely due to structural changes in disks or incoordinate functioning of the parts of the joint.[85]

Crepitus has been associated with perforation in the disk. Moffett and co-workers demonstrated that perforation of the disk is usually followed by osteoarthritic change on the condylar surface, which is in turn followed by similar bony alterations on the opposing surface of the fossa.[61] The most common disk–condyle derangements that present clinically are anterior disk derangements in which there are anterior disk dislocations that reduce and those that do not reduce.[25]

The classic signs of the type of anterior disk dislocation that reduces are (1) a distinguished, sometimes loud click during mandibular opening, signifying that the disk has relocated itself with respect to the condyle, and (2) a more subtle click usually occurring during mandibular closing and signifying that the disk has displaced itself anterior to the mandibular condyle. The sign of an anterior disk dislocation that does not reduce is the absence of joint noises with a series of reproducible restrictions during mandibular movements. These restrictions are due to the disk blocking translatory glide.

COMMON LESIONS

TEMPOROMANDIBULAR JOINT DYSFUNCTION SYNDROME

A common temporomandibular joint disorder found clinically is temporomandibular joint dysfunction syndrome, also referred to as mandibular pain–dysfunction syndrome, arthrosis temporomandibularis,[85] temporomandibular joint arthrosis, and myofascial pain syndrome.

Temporomandibular joint dysfunction syndrome cannot be considered a disease of aging or senility, since it commonly occurs in patients between the ages of 20 and 40 years.[82] It is most frequently found among women. The early incoordination phase associated with clicking, subluxation, and recurrent dislocation is most commonly found among women in the third to fourth decade of life and in men during the third decade. The later limitation phase occurs most frequently in women in the fourth to fifth decades.[83]

Signs and symptoms of the early incoordination phase are usually unilateral but may be bilateral. They may include muscular tenderness, limited motion, and a dull aching pain in the periarticular area often radiating to the ear, face, head, neck, and shoulders and aggravated by function. Usually, the syndrome first manifests itself in the form of functional incoordination of the mandibular muscles with symptoms of clicking in the temporomandibular joint, which is otherwise asymptomatic, and subluxation or recurrent dislocation. Additionally, clinical examination often reveals hypermobility of the joints or a tendency to protrude the mandible or both during the initial opening movement.[87] These symptoms are followed in many cases by spasms of the masticatory muscles characterized by pain on movement of the joint, especially during mastication. Gradually, the pain becomes worse and is accompanied by decreased mobility. Pain and mobility tend to be worse in the morning. In unilateral conditions, the mandible deviates to the symptomatic side, resulting in compensation of the contralateral joint by hypermobility, subluxation, and irregular mandibular opening and closing movements. Mandibular "catching" or "locking" in certain positions may also occur on opening. Often pain may accompany movement of the hypermobile joint and may require treatment as well.

The temporomandibular joint dysfunction syndrome is usually reversible, but its perpetuation may and often does result in organic changes. When spontaneous recovery does not occur and when spasm is not relieved by treatment, such spasm may set up a sustaining cycle. If dysfunction is of a long duration, contracture of the masticatory muscles with limited painless mandibular movement may occur. This is referred to as the *limitation phase*. At this stage, pathologic changes are noted and are mainly degenerative. They are located in the fibrous covering of the articular eminence, in the condylar head, and in the fibrous articular meniscus. There is, however, little evidence to support the view that there is a relationship between degenerative changes within the joint and symptoms of temporomandibular joint dysfunction.[82] Marked changes are often seen without symptoms, and frequently marked symptoms are seen without radiographic evidence of changes in structure. When arthrosis of the temporomandibular joint shows extreme changes in the structure of the joint or joints, the disease is sometimes referred to as *arthrosis temporomandibularis deformans*.[85]

It is generally accepted that temporomandibular joint dysfunction–pain syndrome is a neuromuscular or joint dysfunction and that the etiology of pain is multicausal. The five major causes of pain may be (1) neurologic, (2) vascular, (3) the joint itself, (4) muscular, or (5) hysterical conversion.[97] Pain that originates from the joints themselves can be caused by infection, disk derangement, condylar displacement, microtrauma, and traumatic injury.[95] Many patients, particularly those with painful limited mandibular movements, complain of sudden onset of symptoms on awaking, after rapid or extensive mandibular opening (*e.g.*, yawning or following a long dental appointment), or when changes are made in occlusion (*e.g.*, through restoration, grinding, or the use of a dental appliance).

Many authors point out that many conditions called temporomandibular joint disorders are not in the strict sense of the word disorders of the joint at all but simply dysfunction of the masticatory muscles.[66] The presence of painful areas within the muscles and signs of mandibular dysfunction were Schwartz's most constant finding.[82] Such painful areas and accompanying dysfunction have been given various names such as *myalgia, myositis, fibrositis,* and *myofascial pain syndromes*. The precipitating factor is believed to be motion that stretches the muscle, setting off a self-sustaining cycle of pain, spasm, and pain. The muscles that are commonly involved are the masseters, medial and lateral pterygoids, temporalis, suprahyoids, infrahyoids, sternocleidomastoids, scaleni, and rhomboids. The muscles most frequently involved are the lateral pterygoids.

Emotional tension may also play a predominant role. With stress, the tension of the skeletal muscles increases, often with clenching of the teeth or bruxism resulting in local disharmony of the masticatory apparatus. When hypertonicity occurs in the masticatory muscles for a long period of time, pain–dysfunction syndrome, occlusal wear, and tooth mobility may be evident. Once the pattern is established, it appears to be self-perpetuating. Other habit manifestations seen in these patients that cause pathologic occlusal contact are numerous and include unilateral mastication, abnormal swallowing, and "tooth doodling" during the waking hours.[31,87] What the patient does to his occlusion in reaction to stress seems to be more important than any existing malocclusion. Certainly malocclusion, by mechanically increasing the amount of force or altering its direction, can make the chance of injury more likely. More important than the type of malocclusion, however, may be the amount and kind of muscular activity and the reaction of the person to such activity. In some persons, change in proprioception, no matter how slight, seems to be more important than a longstanding malocclusion, no matter how irregular.

Diagnostic procedures to establish the presence of temporomandibular joint dysfunction and a definitive diagnosis include

—An accurate history
—Determination of the patient's emotional state and daily habits
—Examination of mandibular movements
—Measurement of mandibular opening, lateral deviation, and protrusion
—Palpation of the temporomandibular joint and muscles of mastication
—Dental and oral examination
—Occlusal analysis
—Roentgenograms
—Electromyography
—Physical examination of related structures (cervical spine)
—Neurologic testing

The primary methods of therapy revolve around the correction of occlusal disharmonies and tension habits, as well as physical therapy to eliminate spasm and increase range of motion through therapeutic exercise and mobilization techniques.

DEGENERATIVE JOINT DISEASE–OSTEOARTHRITIS

Although osteoarthritis may occur at any age, it is considered primarily a disease of middle or old age.

It is estimated that it may be found in 80% to 90% of the population over 60 years of age.[38,64]

The etiology is generally believed to be the result of normal wear and tear associated with aging and function, as well as the result of repeated minor trauma. It is speculated that damage consists primarily of degeneration of the chondroitin–collagen–protein complex.[37] Roentgenographic examination may reveal narrowing of the temporomandibular joint space with condensation of bone in the region of the articular cortex, spur formation, and marginal lipping at the articular margins of the condylar head.[37] In some cases there is considerable thickening of the synovial membrane due to chronic synovitis. There may be perforation of the disk without bony changes. Erosion of the condylar head, articular eminence, and fossa may be noted.

Symptoms do not seem to be related to the extent of articular damage. Osteoarthritis may be asymptomatic even in the presence of extensive articular damage, while on the other hand, articular findings may be completely absent in patients with acute symptoms. The onset is generally insidious with mild symptoms. Pain, which is usually a dull aching in or around the joint, is usually not constant. Typically, painful stiffness of the jaw muscles is noted in the morning or following periods of rest. With use, the symptoms may disappear and then reappear with fatigue at the end of the day. Pain may be precipitated on opening or during mastication. Crepitation, crackling, or clicking may occur in one or both joints. Subluxation and locking of one or both joints during certain movements are common complaints. The patient may also complain of symptoms of the ear, impaired hearing, frequent headaches, and dizziness. At the onset, symptoms are usually short-lived, but as degeneration progresses they occur more frequently and last longer. Crepitation and limited motion are the most constant findings.

Diagnostic procedures to establish the presence of osteoarthritis can be difficult but again depend on an accurate history, the determination of the patient's emotional state, physical examination, and roentgenograms. Physical examination may or may not reveal discrete painful areas in the musculature; minimal emotional tension may be noted. Loss of movement is greatest in the upper joint compartment. There is limitation in a capsular pattern of restriction. In unilateral conditions, contralateral excursions and opening are most restricted; protrusion and retrusion are both restricted. There is an ipsilateral deviation of the mandible at the extreme range of opening. Accessory movements are limited and reproduce temporomandibular pain.

The primary method of therapy is directed at symptoms and may involve correcting the occlusion of the teeth or prosthesis, drug therapy, and physical therapy. During the painful phase, the application of hot packs may help to reduce muscle spasm and pain. Active range of motion exercises (often in conjunction with ultrasound), passive range of motion exercises, mobilization techniques (preceded by deep friction massage to the capsule[16]), and stretching may be used during the chronic phase. Graded exercises involving a few simple movements performed frequently during the day are often prescribed as a home treatment. Advanced bony changes within the joint may necessitate arthroplasty with joint debridement.

RHEUMATOID ARTHRITIS

There is little agreement regarding the incidence of patients with rheumatoid arthritis who also develop the disease in the temporomandibular joints; estimates vary from 20 to 51%.[37] Women are affected more often than men.

There are three groups of symptoms—transitory, acute, and chronic. Transitory symptoms include limitation of motion and referred pain. Acute symptoms consist of transitory symptoms plus joint pain, swelling, and warmth lasting 6 to 10 weeks. Chronic symptoms are characterized by severe pain and limitation of motion. The joint and muscle symptoms are most severe in the morning and diminish with the day's activity. Inflammatory changes are noted in the synovial membrane and periarticular structures by atrophy and rarefaction of bone. A serious sequela of ankylosis may restrict or even eliminate movement. If symptoms are not relieved by conservative management, surgical intervention may be indicated.

The primary method of therapy is directed at symptoms and may involve drug therapy, if indicated by specific signs and symptoms, and physical therapy. In the acute phase, immobilization is contraindicated but rest in the form of a soft or liquid diet is advocated. After inflammation has subsided, treatment is directed at reducing muscle spasm and restoring mandibular movements by corrective exercises.

Surgical procedures such as condylectomies and condylotomies frequently used in the past are now believed to be obsolete for the most part but are occasionally performed.[81] Following surgery, corrective exercises and exercises of mandibular excursions, using mouth props to ensure that range of motion is not compromised, should be performed several times a day.[55]

TRAUMA AND DISORDERS OF LIMITATION

One of the most frequent causes of temporomandibular joint dysfunction is a direct or indirect blow to the area, including resultant fracture in the region of the condyle. When there is no fracture, injuries may result in edema and possible soft-tissue damage, such as tearing of the capsular ligaments or meniscus and simple dislocations and subluxations. Other causes of limitation include postoperative trismus following tooth extraction and whiplash injuries.

There is adequate proof that whiplash injuries are responsible for many temporomandibular joint dysfunctions. Whiplash can be explained as a deceleration effect on the mandible and thus on the temporomandibular joint either through direct injury or through neurologic involvement. When the head is snapped back abruptly, the mouth flies open, evoking a stretch reflex of the masseter. The capsule, ligaments, and inter-articular meniscus act as a restraining ligament; tearing or stretching these tissues may result. Immediately following, the jaw snaps shut; this may strain the attachment of the meniscus if malocclusion is present. Cervical traction, commonly used in the management of the cervical spine, may also produce temporomandibular joint dysfunction, or the primary temporomandibular joint dysfunction may be aggravated.

Treatment and management of such injuries will depend on the structures involved, the extent of displacement, the effect on function, and the degree of pain. During the acute phase, soft and liquid diets, head bandages or intermaxillary immobilization, and splints may be used to rest the joint. Surgical procedures, open and closed reduction, and manipulations may be necessary.

Physical therapy may consist of heat and other methods to reduce pain and muscle spasm; early mobility exercises after surgery or following immobilization to ensure range of motion is not compromised; and muscle re-education and corrective exercises. Stretching and mobilization techniques may be necessary to treat contracture of the musculature or capsules. When cervical traction is considered necessary in the treatment of the neck and whiplash injuries, the temporomandibular joint should be protected with bite plates or soft splints and the proper use of traction.[97]

OTHER CONDITIONS

Other conditions that may cause temporomandibular joint dysfunction include a variety of neurologic and muscular disorders, bone disease, tumors, infections, psychogenic disorder, growth and developmental disorders, diseases causing disturbance of the occlusion of the teeth or supporting structures, faulty habits of the jaw, improper swallowing, orofacial imbalance, and others.

PHYSICAL THERAPY

Temporomandibular joint dysfunction, arthritic conditions, ankylosing diseases, traumatic injuries, and postsurgical entities may be a few of the causes that bring a patient to the physical therapist.

When degenerative disease, bony or fibrous ankylosis, fractures, occlusal disharmony, and other conditions necessitate surgery, follow-up physical therapy may become necessary to maintain or regain motion, as well as regain normal mandibular osteokinematics. In the majority of postsurgical cases, muscle tonus remains good, except after long-term ankylosis or degenerative joint disease. In these cases there is greater possibility that the muscles have atrophied, making rehabilitation more difficult and necessitating a more extensive program of therapeutic exercises to increase the physiological elasticity and strength of the muscles.

Following condylectomy, one must keep in mind that the lateral pterygoid's attachment to the condyle has been severed, and that the jaw will increasingly deviate ipsilaterally. Postoperative rehabilitation for the lost function should encourage the similarly functioning muscles of the masseter, temporalis, and suprahyoid muscles on the healthy side to perform with increased strength. At least partial use of the lateral pterygoid muscle should be stressed so that it is able to contribute to contralateral mandibular excursion and to prevent posterior drifting of the ramus in its tonic state.

Signs and symptoms of the temporomandibular joint syndrome vary but generally include a cluster of symptoms.

—Pain and tenderness of the masticatory muscles
—Limited or altered mandibular function (*i.e.*, hypermobility or a tendency to protrude the mandible in the initial opening phase)
—Crepitation or clicking
—Deviation of the mandible on opening
—Disturbed chewing patterns
—Locking of the jaw
—Vague, remote subjective complaints

The means of treatment of temporomandibular joint syndrome is basically like that for other myofascial pain syndromes—anesthetics, exercise, and physical and pharmacologic agents. There are, however, additional considerations. There are two traditional concepts of the etiology of temporomandibular joint dysfunction. Some clinicians stress malocclusion as the causal factor. They advocate treatment involving mainly mechanical methods, such as equilibration of the occlusion.[16,39] Others emphasize that psychological factors, especially response to stress, and harmful habits of the jaw may influence both the onset and course of symptoms. They advocate patient education, the elimination of habitual protrusion or other harmful habits, and muscular relaxation.

The effective management of temporomandibular joint disorders requires first of all a diagnosis based on a complete history, thorough physical examination, and when indicated, adjuncts such as a detailed study of the patient's occlusion, roentgenography, and electromyography.

TREATMENT OF LIMITATION DISORDERS

STRETCHING TECHNIQUES

For the purpose of increasing limited mandibular movements, a variety of exercises involving the muscles of mastication may be employed. They are used, on one hand, to help break up the muscle spasm, and on the other, to maintain and increase limited jaw movement to full physiological function.

Active Stretch

The patient actively opens his mouth as wide as possible several times following a series of warming up exercises.[83] By having the patient repeat a gentle, rhythmic, hingelike movement a number of times before active stretch, muscle spasm can be physiologically diminished or eliminated. With the patient in a comfortable, relaxed, reclining position or in a recliner chair, have him place his tongue in contact with the hard palate as posteriorly as possible, while keeping the mandible in a retruded position. In this position with the tongue on the hard palate, the patient's articular movements are mainly rotatory and early protrusion is avoided. It is helpful to have the patient palpate the condyles so that he can feel the movement. If glide occurs too early, with little or no rotatory motion, there is an early protrusion problem. Instruct the patient to open his mouth slowly and rhythmically within this limited range ten times

or so in succession. He then performs active stretch by opening his mouth as wide as possible within the pain-free limit, as slowly as he can two or three times. The opening position should be held for 5 seconds, followed by relaxation in the rest position for 5 seconds. In the case of a unilateral limitation, the tip of the tongue is positioned on the palatal surface behind the canine teeth on the contralateral side. The application of a vapocoolant spray or ultrasound may be an effective adjunct during active stretch.

During normal mandibular opening, translation begins beyond 11 mm.[50] Improving translation is therefore accomplished by having the patient place a finger (six or so tongue blades or a wooden pencil) horizontally between the teeth, which will open the mandible approximately 11 mm. The patient can then actively practice protrusive, retrusive, and lateral excursions of the mandible but avoid any jamming effects that might occur if translation is done within the first 11 mm of opening.

Yawning is recommended as a home program exercise. It is an active stretching movement that is accomplished by strong reflex inhibition of the mandibular elevators.

These active exercises should be repeated often during the day for brief periods. These procedures must be applied cautiously in the presence of roentgenographic evidence of temporomandibular joint arthropathy and if done soon after disk plication or graft.

RELAXATION—HOLD-RELAX

A variety of neuromuscular facilitation exercises may be used when range of motion is limited by shortening, contracture, or spasm.[48,82,98] One of the most frequently used methods is hold-relax to make stretching of the masticatory muscles more effective. This technique implies a contraction of the antagonist against maximal resistance followed by relaxation and then active or assistive stretch of the agonist. For example, to increase mandibular opening, the patient is asked to close his mouth tightly as resistance is applied gently and slowly to the mandible. This is followed by a relaxation and then by active or passive motion. Isometric contraction of the mouth elevator muscles facilitates their relaxation. The resultant stimulation of the jaw opening muscles permits increased active or passive stretch. The therapist might use the following commands:

1. "Just hold your jaw closed and don't let me move

it." Apply resistance gently and slowly to the mandible.

2. "Let go." Maintain gentle support of the mandible and wait for relaxation to occur.
3. "Open your mouth." Have the patient move the mandible actively with or without resistance.

Unresisted reversing movements may also be used as a follow-up procedure by either active or assistive stretch.

A variety of similar techniques, such as maximal resistance superimposed on an isotonic or isometric contraction, slow-reversal-hold, and contract-relax, may be used.[48,82,98] Such exercises may also be used for increasing range of protrusion, retrusion, and lateral deviation. The therapist provides resistance, or the patient may be asked to do so with his own hand.[82] By using resistance, the patient effects an increased relaxation of the antagonist muscles. This sets up a reflex mechanism called reciprocal inhibition.

PASSIVE AND ASSISTIVE STRETCH

Prolonged static stretch is often advantageous and may be accomplished by using a series of tongue blades built up, one on top of the other, between the anterior incisors for bilateral limitation or between the upper and lower teeth (far back on the involved side) in the case of unilateral limitation.[56] This places the capsule and tight elevator muscles on moderate stretch. The tongue blades are not meant to be used as a forced stretch but rather to take up the slack and maintain the mandible in a relaxed open position. The use of cold (ice or vapocoolant spray) or ultrasound may be administered while on passive stretch. As the jaw begins to relax, additional tongue blades may be added. Prolonged stretch is usually applied for 15 to 20 minutes. Following temporomandibular joint surgery, no more than 1 or 2 minutes of stretching is recommended.

Tongue blades can also be used for home treatment, both as a static stretch and for briefer periods of active and passive stretch. Tongue blades, however, must be used with caution since too vigorous application may cause injury. Shore recommended the use of a tapered cork.[85] The cork, which is approximately 15 mm at its narrow end and 30 mm at its widest end, is gradually inserted (small end first) into the patient's mouth until the jaws are separated. Once the jaw begins to relax, the cork can be placed farther into the mouth, thus progressively opening the jaw wider and wider. Shore recommends using

this technique as a home treatment for 30-second periods every 2 hours.

Direct Methods

With the patient sitting, the therapist stands behind and places both thumbs over the patient's lower teeth and his index fingers over the upper teeth. A sterile gauze or a cloth may be placed over the lower teeth. The patient is instructed to support the mandible with one hand under the chin. The mandible is then opened with gentle but maximal effort. If a less vigorous stretch is indicated, the therapist uses one hand, with the index finger and thumb in the same position, and supports the patient's mandible with the opposite hand.[82]

The patient may be taught to use this method as a form of self-treatment, using the thumb and index finger in a reverse position and supporting the mandible with one or both hands.[82]

All of these exercises should emphasize movement without pain or undue force. Stretching should be done slowly and can be done actively (with or without resistance to the mandible) or passively.

Reflex relaxation of the elevator muscles followed by active stretch, as used for the opening movement, as well as passive and assistive stretch may also be applied to lateral, protrusive, and retrusive movements. With instruction, the patient can carry out many of these exercises alone.

MOBILIZATION TECHNIQUES

Mobilization techniques in the treatment of temporomandibular joint disorders are aimed at restoring normal joint mechanics in order to allow full, pain-free osteokinematics of the mandible to occur. The techniques described are based on courses presented by Rocabado and the works of Kaltenborn.[46,77] They are restricted to a description of manual techniques, which are best learned and practiced under supervision in a postgraduate course or in physical therapy schools.

Temporomandibular Joint

1. *Caudal Traction*
   P—Lies supine on a semi-reclining table or in dental chair that supports the head and trunk.
   O—Stands at patient's side and faces left side of patient's head. Right hand and forearm are placed around patient's head, fixating head against the table. A stabilizing belt across the

Fig. 16–18. Caudal traction.

forehead may be used instead. Left hand holds with thumb in the mouth over the left inferior molars and with the fingers outside around the patient's jaw.

M—Ask patient to swallow. While maintaining the forearm in a straight line (hand and forearm act as a unit), apply traction caudally (Fig. 16–18). Reverse for the opposite side.

Comments: Caudal traction may be combined with ventral and dorsal glide (protraction and retraction). The mandible is first distracted caudally, and while traction is maintained the mandible is glided ventrally, then dorsally, followed by a gradual release of caudal traction.

2. *Protrusion*—ventral glide

P—Lies supine on a semi-reclining table or in dental chair that supports the head and trunk.

O—Stands at patient's side and faces left side of patient's head. Right hand and forearm are placed around the patient's head, fixating against the operator's body. Left hand holds onto the angle of the ramus with index and third finger. The rest of the hand contacts the patient's jaw.

M—Ask patient to swallow. While maintaining the forearm in a straight line, glide the mandible ventrally into protrusion (Fig. 16–19). Reverse for the opposite side.

Comments: An alternate handhold would be to place the thumb in the mouth on the right

Fig. 16–19. Protrusion (ventral glide).

inferior molars and the fingers outside around the right side of patient's jaw. This same handhold can be used for retrusion (dorsal glide).

Gliding movements ventrally may be combined with a little rotation. The right mandible is first glided forward, as described, and then rotated to the left by rotation of operator's body.

3. *Medial-Lateral Glide*

a. Rotation of the left joint and forward glide of the right joint

P—Lies supine on a semi-reclining table or dental chair that supports the head and trunk

O—Stands behind patient. Right hand holds around the patient's head, fixating head against table. Left hand is positioned so that the hypothenar eminence is placed just caudal to the left temporomandibular joint with the fingers wrapped around the patient's jaw.

M—Ask patient to swallow. The hypothenar eminence acts as a pivot point as the mandible is glided forward and medially to the left (Fig. 16–20). Reverse for opposite side.

b. Alternate technique

P—Lies supine on a semi-reclining table or in dental chair that supports the head and neck.

O—Stands at patient's side and faces left side of patient's head. Right hand is placed around patient's head, fixating head

Note: P—patient; O—operator; M—movement.

Fig. 16–20. Medial-lateral glide.

against table. Left hand holds with thumb in mouth on medial aspect of body of mandible near the right inferior molars, with the fingers (outside) wrapped around the jaw.

M—Ask patient to swallow. With the thumb acting as a pivot point, move the wrist ulnarly so that the right condyle moves outward, forward, and laterally as the mandible is moved medially to the left (Fig. 16–21). Reverse for opposite side.

Many of the semi-reclining techniques described above may be carried out in a sitting position. The patient's head may b stabilized against the opera-

Fig. 16–21. Medial-lateral glide (alternate technique).

tor's body and supported with the free hand. However, the semi-reclining or supine position is preferred since the head and mandible are in a better position for fixation. Furthermore, if a stabilizing belt is used, the operator's other hand is free to assist the mobilizing hand or to palpate the joint to determine if correct motion is obtained. Mobilization techniques using pressures against the head of the mandible, which have been developed by Maitland, are particularly useful (Fig. 16–22).[56,91] One of the greatest difficulties encountered when mobilizing the jaw is the patient's inability to relax the jaw completely. By mobilizing the condyle directly rather than through the mandible (which involves large movements), the patient is often able to relax more readily and treatment is often more successful. Also, overstretching of the upper joint compartment is avoided. Medial glide is particularly useful in restoring rotation (lower joint compartment).

TREATMENT OF DISK DERANGEMENT AND CONDYLAR DISPLACEMENT

Signs and symptoms of early temporomandibular joint dysfunction include primarily muscular hyperactivity and pain, disturbed chewing habits, clicking, "catching" or "locking" of the jaw (recurrent subluxations), and limited motion or hypermobility of the joints. Palliative therapy is directed at reducing muscle spasm (the pain–spasm–pain cycle) and relieving intrajoint symptoms caused by trauma, inflammation, condylar displacement, or disk derangement.[97] Treatment may include drug therapy, injections, application of various forms of heat or cold, disengagement of the occlusion by prostheses or voluntarily, and alterations in dietary and oral habits.

Causative therapy procedures may include manipulations and joint mobilization techniques to restore normal joint mechanics; correction of condylar displacements with the use of occlusal repositioning splints or occlusal equilibration; and correction of disk derangement by mandibular manipulations or repositioning appliances.[51,56,67,85,97] Occasionally, surgical correction may be necessary.

Adjunctive therapy may include the use of ultrasound, electrical stimulation, patient education, relaxation techniques, psychotherapy, biofeedback, and exercises. According to Somers, treatment directed toward patient education, the elimination of poor oral habits, and the acquisition of muscle relaxation are often all that is required to relieve the patient's symptoms.[87]

Fig. 16-22. Mobilization techniques (here a medial glide) may be applied directly to the condyle.

PATIENT EDUCATION

A most important step is to educate patients regarding the functioning of their joints, the reason for their symptoms, and the means of removing those symptoms. Advice should include reassurance, which is often simply gained by understanding the anatomy of the joint and the physiological mechanisms at work.

Use of a skull, the patient's roentgenograms, or simple diagrams will help the therapist to explain the structure and function of the temporomandibular joints and the rationale for the various procedures that must be undertaken. Instructions should emphasize diet and careful use of the jaw.[85] The harmful effects of wide opening, yawning, biting off large mouthfuls of hard food, habitual protrusion, diurnal clenching, or nocturnal bruxism should be explained. Because an emotional overlay is often present, counseling on how emotional conflicts are translated into muscle tension and pain is usually an important consideration. Point out that methods to achieve muscle relaxation and abolish well-established patterns of inappropriate muscular activity and methods to acquire new ones are important means of eliminating symptoms.

RELAXATION TRAINING

In addition to patient education, relaxation training for jaw and facial muscles is often considered, although it may be difficult to achieve. Muscle tension is one of the most frequent single contributing causes of muscular derangements of the temporomandibular joint, whether or not the derangement occurred through trauma. A report by Heiberg and colleagues indicates that of a group of patients with a diagnosis of temporomandibular joint syndrome almost all exhibited tense muscles in the neck and back as well, indicating that muscular tension is not confined to the masticatory muscles alone. Increased muscular tension, especially in the erector trunci, was present in 95% of these patients.[42] Typically these patients present with a tightly closed jaw, stiffened neck and back, elevated shoulders, and a forward head. Faulty respiration patterns are also a common finding.

Relaxation of the whole body or body regions is frequently indicated in the treatment of these overly tense patients. More often than not, general relaxation techniques will have to precede training for local relaxation. (See Chapter 9, Relaxation.) Relaxation exercises such as those modified from Jacobsen, autogenic training, and reflex relaxation exercises may all be used.

The therapist can show the patient the presence of unnecessary muscular contraction at the end of the initial physical examination or during the first treatment session. Most patients are unable to relax the jaw muscles so that the mandible can be moved freely by the therapist. They are unable to let the head loll back when the shoulders are supported since the neck muscles remain rigid. They cannot permit their elevated arm to fall limply to the treatment table when requested by the examiner.

Perhaps one of the hardest of all relaxation procedures to achieve is elimination of overcontraction of the jaw muscles. An example of a local technique using a modification of Jacobson's approach follows:

—Clench the jaw firmly and concentrate on feeling the sense of tightness in the temples as well as the jaw itself.
—Switch off and let the jaw fall open.
—Push the jaw open against the pressure of an assistant's hand.
—Relax completely.
—Move the jaw sideways to the left as far as possible with or without resistance and experience the sensation this gives to the jaw and temples before relaxing.
—Repeat the same exercise to the left.
—Complete the sequence by clenching the jaw firmly again, and let the jaw drop open loosely.

Somers suggests that total relaxation cannot be assumed until the assistant can take the patient's chin between the thumb and forefinger and tap the teeth together rapidly without any opposition from the jaw muscles.[87] It is often most helpful for the patient to adapt this method for use from time to time to assess the degree of tension and his progress in attempting to achieve relaxation. Autosuggestion techniques to guard against clenching and tooth contact are also helpful. He may be told to repeat the following after each meal: "Lips together, teeth apart." He should also be instructed to make frequent checks during the day for jaw clenching and to attempt to maintain the rest position of the mandible in which only the lips touch while the teeth are held apart. These methods of treatment are often considered the first line of defense against clenching and nocturnal bruxism.[85]

The use of biofeedback methods to guide the patient in controlling muscle activity and promoting relaxation has increased in recent years.[39,68,89,90]

Feedback from electromyography of the frontal, temporal, and masseter muscles has been popular.

In addition, the therapist must spend time instructing the patient in good body mechanics, postural control, and correct body positioning for maximum relaxation of the cervical spine and masticatory muscles. Cervical traction, exercises, and mobilization may also be indicated when associated cervical symptoms or pathologic processes coexist. Occlusal splints may be indicated to create relaxation of the elevator muscles and disorientation of an acquired noxious occlusal sensory input. Splints may also be used to disorient the sensory input in patients who clench by changing the quality of afferent touch information.[51,85] Occlusal analysis and equilibration, if indicated, are usually best deferred until relaxation has been achieved.

Many clinical manifestations of pain in the upper quarter have their source not in an isolated joint disorder but in chronic upper quarter dysfunction spanning several body segments. It is estimated that 70% of patients presenting with craniomandibular dysfunction (temporomandibular disorders) will also present with craniocervical dysfunction.[78] Based on clinical studies and experience of numerous practitioners, there are several findings that are common to a population of patients presenting with temporomandibular joint dysfunction. Some of the findings include the following:

—Abnormal forward or lateral head postures
—Compensatory abnormal shoulder girdle postures (protracted shoulders)
—Changes in the position of the mandible (condylar retrusion and diminished interocclusal distance)[22]
—Mouth and upper chest breathing
—Abnormal resting position of the tongue
—Deviant swallow

Postural or orthostatic evaluation and treatment of these patients is extremely important because an altered biomechanical relationship will always produce accommodations and even subsequent adaptations if the accommodations are maintained.[63,79]

A system of upper quarter re-education methods has been developed by Rocabado[79] and Kraus[50] that addresses these common imbalances. Methods of treatment encompass correcting abnormal head posture and craniocervical dysfunction, instructions in the normal sequence of swallowing and the proper resting position of the tongue and mandible, and techniques to enhance proper use of the diaphragm (nasodiaphragmatic breathing) and thoracic spine mobility.[22,50,77,79]

EXERCISE THERAPY

The use of retraining exercises to overcome spasm and incoordination of the mandibular musculature, to promote harmonious coordinated mechanism, to reduce momentary luxation of the disk, and to increase muscle strength have long been advocated; however, they are now considered controversial.[6,17,67,82,83]

Cyriax believed that clicking of the jaw due to momentary luxation of the intra-articular meniscus can usually be relieved by strengthening the muscles of mastication. Opening, protrusion, and lateral resistive movements are performed. It is usually not necessary, he believes, to develop the closing muscles since most patients usually maintain normal strength of these muscles by chewing.[16]

Schwartz and Bertoft recommend a training program of exercises against resistance to promote reflex relaxation of the antagonistic muscles. This stimulates the maximum number of motor units within the lateral pterygoids during opening and lateral mandibular movements.[6,82,83]

Paris advises that major derangements should be treated in the same manner as subluxations by mobilization techniques. Minor derangements, however, are best treated by isometrics to the lateral pterygoids (*i.e.*, protrusion and lateral movements).[67] Regardless of the type of exercises used, they should always be carried out without clicking and pain.

Such strengthening-resistive exercises, according to Weinberg, are not indicated in the temporomandibular joint pain–dysfunction syndrome because the neuromuscular mechanism involved is associated with overfunction rather than underfunction.[95,96] Such exercises do not seem to have a rational basis as an effective therapy. Strengthening and re-education exercises may be indicated when true muscle weakness is found (as in the limitation phase) or when habits such as deviant swallowing or habitual protrusion reverses normal muscle function and contributes to the temporomandibular joint pain–dysfunction syndrome.[87,97]

TREATMENT OF OROFACIAL IMBALANCES

Muscles of the entire stomatognathic system and the orofacial complex play a major role in proper balance and function of the temporomandibular joint. It should be kept in mind that the orofacial muscles are under stress 24 hours a day. Swallowing takes place 2000 times a day as a reflexive act. Forces during eating, drinking, speech, and the rest position of the tongue must be taken into consideration. If there is an imbalance of forces, there will be a tremendous amount of pressure against normal balance of forces of the temporomandibular joint that can cause malfunction of the joint apparatus.

Protrusion of the mandible resulting in an abnormal palatal swallow may be caused by ankylotic tongue, shortened frenulum, or abnormal use of facial muscles, particularly the mentalis.[30,34] Abnormal use or position of the tongue at rest, muscle imbalance of the masseter, decreased strength of the orbicularis oris, neuromuscular problems, post-traumatic and surgical conditions (*e.g.*, unilateral condylectomies), pain conditions of the head, face or cervical spine, and other pathologic processes can result in malfunction of the temporomandibular joint.

In many of these conditions, real or apparent reduction in muscle strength of one or more muscles may be disclosed during examination. This may point to lack of use (*e.g.*, in unilateral function), atrophy of muscle fibers, muscular fibrositis, and other pathologic conditions localized in or near the muscle and its tendon, causing pain on contraction. Although strengthening-resistive exercises are usually not indicated in muscles that are already refusing to relax, they do need to be considered in the proper balance and function of the temporomandibular joint complex when weakness exists, from whatever cause.

FACILITORY EXERCISES

There is a wide variety of well-known facilitory and strengthening-resistive exercises that are at the therapist's disposal.[24,30,49,80,82,83] Exercises employing postural reflexes, brushing, vibration, synergistic muscle action of the facial and cervical muscles, and activities of daily living may be used as facilitory techniques. Stimuli—consisting of stretch, maximal resistance, pressures, stroking, or tapping—may be given manually. Popping or clucking of the tongue on the hard palate may be used to strengthen the muscle of the tongue and encourage greater range of motion of the jaw. Gargling after each brushing helps facilitate mandibular depressors. Resistive tongue exercises may be used to facilitate the three major jaw muscles. Resisted neck motion may facilitate tongue motions as well as mandibular motions. In general, facial and mandibular motions that require depression or downward motions are facilitated by neck flexion; conversely, facial and mandibular motions that require elevation and upward motions are facilitated by neck extension. Neck rotation reinforces motion on the side of the face or the mandible toward which the head is turned.

Early protrusion of the mandible during opening that is due to an imbalance of the synergistic action of the suprahyoids and lateral pterygoids is often revealed during examination. A translatory rather than a rotatory movement is occurring; its abolition should be a major step in management. An excellent, initial exercise requires the patient to place his tongue as posteriorly as possible in contact with the hard palate, to effect retrusion. By assuming this position, protrusion of the lower jaw is eliminated, since the patient's articular movements are mainly rotatory and limited by the constraints of the internal pterygoids. By limiting the movement to the interocclusal clearance, any subsequent translatory movement is eliminated. Instruct the patient to open his mouth slowly and rhythmically within the pain limits several times in succession. He should practice this simple exercise frequently during the day.

The next step is to instruct the patient to repeat this exercise with the addition of one critical modification, voluntary resistance. The patient should grasp the chin firmly or position a closed fist under the mandible to resist the motion of pressing the jaw down and back.

Both of these exercises rely on synergistic action of the suprahyoids and lower bodies of the lateral pterygoids. In normal opening, all of these muscle pairs contract strongly. However, when the lateral pterygoids contract more strongly than the suprahyoids, the mandible will protrude. These exercises are believed to help train the suprahyoids to contract more forcefully than the lateral pterygoids.

Another useful exercise for the development of the suprahyoids, described by Shore, consists of teaching the patient to perform isometric contraction of these muscles in front of a mirror.[85] The patient is taught to contract these muscles with the mouth closed and the teeth in light contact. He then makes a conscious effort to retrude the jaw and depress the floor of the mouth without actually moving it. Once acute spasms have subsided, the patient repeats the exercise with the mouth slightly open. Each day he can gradually increase the extent of mouth opening until coordinated mandibular muscular action is achieved.

Once the patient has mastered rotation during limited opening without forward condylar movement, the range of opening is gradually increased. While the patient is looking in a mirror, he is asked to place his index finger over each condylar head or his palms over the sides of the face to monitor and correct any abnormal protrusion of the condylar head during opening and closing. He should also note any irregular movements such as one condylar head preceding movement of the other. Keeping the hands in place, the patient is instructed to carry out slow rhythmic full opening and closing within the pain-free range, avoiding any clicking, abnormal protrusion, or lateral deviation of the jaw. If abnormal deviation or protrusion does occur, he is taught to guide the motion with his thumb or forefinger positioned on his chin so that the mandible moves smoothly in a coordinated hingelike fashion without protrusion.[82] Initially, this exercise should be performed with the therapist, who assists by guiding the motion of the mandible as the patient actively opens and closes his mouth.

Of particular interest is the rehabilitation of unilateral condylar fractures following immobilization. Residual mandibular kinesiopathy often persists and is referred to as *postfracture condylar syndrome*. It consists of deviation of the mandible on depression and inadequate mandibular excursion toward the contralateral side. Begin management by first explaining to the patient the difference between a hinge joint and a gliding joint and how he must develop a gliding joint to masticate with the contralateral side. He is then given a lateral tongue exercise to facilitate using the mylohyoid muscle to assist the weakened lateral pterygoid muscle in accomplishing lateral mandibular excursion. To perform this exercise, described by Gerry, the patient works before a mirror, places the tip of his tongue on the palatal surface of the contralateral maxillary molars, and presses as hard as he can while elevating and depressing his mandible.[32] It is suggested that this exercise be performed for 5 minutes hourly. As lateral excursions develop, periarticular fibrosis of the injured joint resolves and normal lateral pterygoid function tends to return.

TEMPOROMANDIBULAR EVALUATION

I. **History.** The general format of the initial evaluation should follow the same lines of questioning as set out in Chapter 4. Information on when the problem started and how it occurred as well as previous management and the results obtained by them is helpful. If the problem was caused by injury or surgical procedure, the therapist will need to know what was done by the attending personnel and physicians. A most important aspect of taking the history is the attempt to clarify any emotional factors in the patient's background that may provoke habitual protrusion or muscular tension.

The history may be handwritten from answers to your verbal questions. Perhaps a more complete history can be obtained, however, by using a personal history form, which is completed by the patient. After reviewing the form, all pertinent facts may be reviewed in detail with the patient. The work of Day,[20] Shore,[85] and Morgan and Rosen[65] provides excellent detailed outlines and the rationale for obtaining such information as a means of compiling a complete history relating specifically to temporomandibular joint disorders. Such forms have been designed to include most of the information that will be found useful in treating temporomandibular joint disorders and related orofacial problems. Certainly no specific set of questions is adequate, and more detailed questioning will usually be necessary. It is also unlikely that the therapist will obtain all relevant information at the initial evaluation. A few pertinent questions that apply particularly to temporomandibular joint disorders include the following:

1. Does the joint grate, click, pop, snap, or lock?
2. Do you have difficulty opening and closing your mouth?
3. Do you have frequent headaches? What area of the head? How long do they last?
4. Have you ever had a severe blow to the head or a whiplash injury?
5. Are your jaws clenched or your teeth sore when you awaken from sleep?

Perhaps one of the most common complaints of head pain is what is generally termed *tension headache*. Berry had studied 100 patients with mandibular dysfunction pain and reports that over 50% of his patients had headaches and pain in the neck, back, and shoulders.[5] This condition may be the result of structural cervical disease, may be associated with vascular pain syndrome, or may occur as a separate entity.[4,20]

II. Physical Examination

A. *Observation.* Record significant findings. The physical examination in a sense occurs simultaneously when the clinician takes the history. The appearance, general posture, and characteristics of bodily movements are often revealing. Physically the typical patient with temporomandibular joint pain–dysfunction, with an emotional overlay, has a posture of elevated shoulders, forward head, stiff neck and back, and has shallow, restricted breathing.[42] Also observe facial expression and habits of the jaw (*i.e.,* clenching or grinding the teeth, biting the fingers, or twitching the masseter).

B. *Inspection of the head, face, and neck.* Record significant findings.

    1. *Skin.* Examine the face for blemishes, moles, pigmentations, scars, and texture.

    2. *Soft tissue.* Note any swelling. Swelling of the joint must be moderate or marked before it is apparent on inspection. If swelling is detectable, it appears as a rounded bulge just anterior to the external meatus. The face should be further examined for atrophies and hypertrophies. Asking the patient to clench his jaws together may help to disclose asymmetry.

    3. *Bony structure and alignment.* Record significant findings. The profile of the face in both the frontal and sagittal plane will reveal the relative development of the skull, face, and mandible. The size of the mandible should be compared with that of the skull and abnormal positions or asymmetry of the jaw noted. Asymmetry may be indicative of a growth or developmental problem or unusual muscular activity. Take particular note of the occlusal and rest positions of the jaw. An abnormal protrusive position may be associated with tongue thrust (deviant swallowing) or habitual protrusion. The evaluation described by Kraus to determine the presence of an acquired adult tongue thrust is helpful.[50] The patient is asked to swallow water several times, pausing between each swallow while the therapist palpates the hyoid bone and the suboccipital muscles. Normally a quick up and down movement of the hyoid should be felt with minimal contraction of the suboccipital muscles. With an acquired anterior adult tongue thrust, a slow up and down movement of the hyoid bone is felt along with significant suboccipital muscle contraction. Excessive forward movement of the entire head and neck and lip may be noted.

    The examiner should briefly inspect the upper spine, shoulder girdles, and arms for obvious muscle atrophy or deformities.

C. *Selective tissue tension tests.* Record significant findings. Before examining the temporomandibular joint movements, the resting position of the mandible and tongue is noted by the clinician by parting the patient's lips (or using a lip separator) to reveal the alignment of the incisors as well as any evidence of abnormal resting position of the tongue or a deviant swallow (see section on dynamics of the mandible and temporomandibular joint).

1. *Active movements* (with passive overpressure). Observe the general patterns of active movements (depression, elevation, lateral deviation, protraction, retraction) for freedom of movement, range, and symmetry. Ascertain if any pain accompanies active movements and in what part of the range it occurs and where. Pain may be felt in the area of the joint and about the ear, but often it is also felt diffusely through the face, teeth, jaws, and mouth. Masticatory pain is typically not well localized. (During the palpation portion of the examination, actual sites of tenderness can be established.)

   Abnormal movements such as "jumps" or "facet slips" should be noted. In particular the patient is asked to open his mouth to a limited extent (about 1 cm) while the examiner observes whether the mandible is making an initial rotation or translatory movement. Forward movement will be revealed by a reduction in incisal overjet and by excessive prominence of the condylar heads.

   The restriction of movement, deviations to one side, and asynchronous patterns of movement are recorded; the maximum opening the patient can achieve without pain is measured. Lateral movements to the left and right, using the bite position as the control as well as protrusion–retrusion, again using normal bite as control, should be recorded when restricted. Lateral motion may be lost earlier and to a greater degree than vertical motions.

   Note whether pain is provoked when the jaws are in firm occlusion and when the patient is asked to bite against a tongue blade on one side. Such tests help distinguish muscle spasms from diskitis and retrodiskitis.[4]

2. *Passive movements* (anatomical ranges). With passive movements, in addition to seeing how easily the jaw can be moved and making a comparison with active range of motion, note the type of end feel as well as the presence of pain and spasms. To determine the nature of the end feel, have the patient open his mouth and then apply additional pressure with the thumbs and index fingers on the edge of the upper and lower teeth, noting the type of end feel present. Passive movements should routinely include depression, elevation, protraction, retraction, and lateral movements.

3. *Resisted movement* (static tests). Determine the strength and presence of pain by applying resistance to mandibular opening, protrusion, and lateral deviations. Pain arising in the pterygoid muscles may be provoked by resisted deviation to the painful side as well as clenching the teeth. Weakness of the muscles that close the mouth is rather uncommon, since strength is usually maintained by mastication.

4. *Passive joint-play movements*. Routinely include accessory posteroanterior, transverse movements, and longitudinal movements (cephalad and caudal to the heads of the condyle) with and without compression.[56,90] Note stability, mobility, presence of pain, guarding, spasm, and behavior.

D. *Palpation*

1. *Skin*. Palpate for warmth, tenderness, temperature, moisture, and mobility.

2. *Muscles*. Palpate for consistency, mobility, continuity, tenderness, pain, and signs of spasm. Palpation of the muscles of mastication should routinely include the origin and insertion of the masseter, temporalis, internal pterygoid, and the insertion of the external pterygoid (see Fig. 18–28).[82]

   When indicated, all the muscles of the maxillofacial region should be palpated, including the facial muscles, sublingual and suprahyoids, and the cervical muscles, especially the sternocleidomastoid and trapezius. Various structural or functional cervical diseases may result in spasms of the masticatory muscles. A comprehensive thesis on the musculature and differential diagnosis of orofacial pain is described by Bell.[4]

3. *Temporomandibular joint*. First, palpate the condylar heads laterally with the mouth closed; then palpate the distal aspect with the jaw apart for tenderness. Determine if any such tenderness is definitely accentuated when the mandible is moved contralaterally. This maneuver brings the condyle more firmly under the

palpating finger. The posterior aspect can be palpated through the external auditory meatus with the palpating finger. Pain and tenderness on palpation suggests a capsulitis, particularly if tenderness is found posteriorly. Abnormal capsular thickening, warmth, and swelling should also be noted. Moderate degrees of swelling in the joint prevent the fingertip from entering the depressed area overlying the joint. Swelling of a marked degree may be palpable as a rounded, often fluctuant mass overlying the joint.

The range and dynamics of condylar motion can also be ascertained by means of palpation. From a position behind the patient, the examiner's forefingers are placed on the lateral aspects of the condylar heads as the patient actively opens his mouth. Inability to feel protrusion of the condylar head suggests a lack of forward movement.

The examiner can determine the presence and the amount of rotation by placing the fingertips in the ear. Palpation should be done bilaterally so that a comparison of both joints can be made and any asymmetrical movements ascertained. Palpable snapping, clicking, or jumps should also be noted.

Bony palpation should include palpation of the zygomatic arch, the hyoid bone, and the upper cervical spine.

4. *Auscultation.* Palpation of the temporomandibular movements often reveals the presence of clicking or crepitus. However, such sounds can be more accurately evaluated with the bell of a stethoscope placed over the condylar head as the patient actively opens his mouth. Note the type of sound associated with the movements and particular phase of movement in which it occurs. All movements—opening, closing, lateral deviation, protrusion, and retrusion—should be assessed.

E. *Selective loading of the temporomandibular joint can aid in determining intracapsular pathologic conditions.* Tests may include the following:

1. *Dynamic loading of one joint.* Have the patient bite forcefully on a cotton roll or tongue blade on one side. This procedure loads the contralateral temporomandibular joint and may elicit pain.

2. *Posterior loading (compression) of both temporomandibular joints.* Grasping the mandible with both hands. The thumbs are placed on the most distal molars or alveolar ridge with the fingers beneath the mandible. The mandible is then tipped down and back to compress the joints. The mandible may also be moved forward or backward to localize tenderness in the posterior or inferior parts of the joint.

3. *Distraction (unloading) or caudal traction.* Using the same handhold as above, distraction of both joints is performed at the same time or caudal traction of each joint separately (see Fig. 16–18) is performed.

Frequently the incisors are not aligned, with the mandible being deviated to one side. To assess the relevance of this deformity to the patient's symptoms, the examiner passively attempts to correct the deformity.[90] If the deviation is a protective deformity, then this test will increase the pain.

F. *Dental and oral examination.* Make a general survey of the oral cavity, since both facial pain as well as temporomandibular joint disorders may have their origin in dental or oral lesions.[58] The examination of the teeth and their supporting structures, other oral structures, and mucosa is important.

By having the patient open his mouth maximally, the examiner is able to observe the oropharynx, tonsillar areas, and surfaces of the palate and tongue. Any alteration in the color and texture of the lingual tissues is noted. Palpations are included.

Cavities and restored and missing teeth should be noted. Wear of biting edges and chewing surfaces that appears excessive for the patient's age often points to tensional oral habits such as bruxism. Also, the occlusion of the teeth, premature contact, overclosure of the vertical dimension, and the degree of overjet are noted.[14] Detailed occlusal analysis should always be deferred until muscle relaxation has been achieved.

G. *Sensory and motor response.* Masticatory and orofacial functioning and the neurologic system that integrates it are complex. Involvement of the muscles innervated by the 5th to 12th cranial nerve and at least the upper three cervical spinal nerves may be reflected in masticatory malfunctioning or pain.[5] Not only the chief masticatory and secondary muscles but also the muscles of the lips, cheeks, tongue, floor of the mouth, neck, palate, and pharynx may be involved. Sensory as well as motor function testing may be indicated.

H. *Other tests.* A cervical–upper extremity scan examination is frequently indicated in the evaluation of temporomandibular joint disorders (see Chapter 19, The Cervical-Upper Extremity Scan Examination). It should be noted that the upper cervical spinal nerves are more likely sources of pain that refer or spread to the masticatory region than are the lower cervical nerves. The upper cervical joints (occipitoatlantal, atlantoaxial) and sub-occipital muscles that are supplied by C1 to C3 nerves have been shown to refer pain into the frontal retro-orbital, temporal, and occipital areas of the head.[15,26,28,52] Passive movements (physiological) and passive joint-play movements of the upper cervical spine should be included (see Chapter 18, The Cervical Spine).[56,90]

Adjuncts, such as roentgenography and electromyography, may be indicated. Only electromyography can reveal how a muscle acts at any point during mandibular movements and postures; some researchers believe that electromyography is more reliable diagnostically than roentgenograms of the temporomandibular joints.[7,56,64]

Analgesic blocking of tender muscles of the joint proper may be needed to confirm the source of pain as well as to help identify secondary pain effects.[4]

Examination of the ear, nose and throat may be necessary to exclude a variety of diagnosable and treatable conditions that may be confused with temporomandibular joint pathology. In addition to the history and clinical examination, further procedures are often necessary to evaluate tinnitus, hearing loss, and vertigo to establish or rule out otologic or neurologic cause for these symptoms.

REFERENCES

1. Alderman MM: Disorders of the temporomandibular joint and related structures. In Lynch MA (ed): Burket's Oral Medicine: Diagnosis and Treatment, 7th ed. Philadelphia, JB Lippincott, 1977
2. Atwood DA: A critique of research of the rest position of the mandible: J Prosthet Dent 16:848–854, 1966
3. Axhausen G: Pathology and therapy of the temporomandibular joint. Fortschr Zahnaerz 6:101–215, 1932
4. Bell WE: Orofacial Pains: Classification, Diagnosis, Management, 3rd ed. Chicago, New Year Medical Publishers, 1985
5. Berry DC: Mandibular dysfunction pain and chronic minor illness. Br Dent J 127:170–175, 1969
6. Bertoft G: The effect of physical training on temporomandibular joint clicking. Odontol Revy 23:297–304, 1972
7. Bessette RW, Mohl ND, DiCosimo CJ: Comparison of results of electromyographic and radiographic examination in patients with myofascial pain-dysfunction syndrome. J Am Dent Assoc 89:1358–1364, 1974
8. Boyd CH: The effect of head position on electromyographic evaluations of representative mandibular positioning of muscle groups. J Craniomandib Pract 5:51–53, 1987
9. Bratzlavsky M, HanderEecken H: Postural reflexes in cranial muscles in man. Acta Neurol Belg 77:5–11, 1977
10. Cailliet R: Neck and Arm Pain, 2nd ed. Philadelphia, FA Davis, 1981
11. Campbell CD, Loft GH, David H, Hart DL: TMJ symptoms and referred pain patterns. J Prosthet Dent 47:430–433, 1982
12. Clark R, Wyke B: Contributions of temporomandibular articular mechanoreceptors to the control of mandibular posture: An experimental study. J Dent 2:121–129, 1974
13. Cohen S: A cephalometric study of rest position in edentulous persons: Influence of variations in head position. J Prosthet Dent 7:467–472, 1957
14. Curnutte DC: The role of occlusion in diagnosis and treatment. In Morgan DH, Hall WP, Vamvas SJ (eds): Disease of the Temporomandibular Apparatus: A Multidisciplinary Approach, 2nd ed. St. Louis, CV Mosby, 1982
15. Cyriax J: Rheumatic headache. Br Med J 2:1367–1368, 1982
16. Cyriax J: Textbook of Orthopaedic Medicine, Vol I, Diagnosis of Soft Tissue Lesions, 8th ed. London, Balliere Tindell, 1978
17. Dachi SF: Diagnosis and management of temporomandibular dysfunction syndrome. J Prosthet Dent 2:53–61, 1968
18. Darling DW, Kraus S, Glasheen-Wray MB: Relationship of head posture and the rest position of the mandible. J Prosthet Dent 52:111–115, 1984
19. Davis D: Gray's Anatomy Descriptive and Applied, 34th ed. London, Longmans Green, 1967
20. Day LD: History taking. In Morgan DH, Hall WP, Vamvas SJ (eds): Disease of the Temporomandibular Apparatus: A Multidisciplinary Approach. St. Louis, CV Mosby, 1977
21. Dufourmentel L: Chirugie de l'Articulation Temporomaxillaire. Paris, Masson, 1920

22. Ellis JJ, Makofsky HW: Balancing the upper quarter through awareness of RTTPB. Clin Man 7:20–23, 1987

23. Ermshar CB: Anatomy and neuroanatomy. In Morgan DH, Hall WP, Vamvas SV (eds): Disease of the Temporomandibular Apparatus: A Multidisciplinary Approach. St. Louis, CV Mosby, 1977

24. Farber SD: Sensorimotor Evaluation and Treatment Procedures, 2nd ed. Bloomington, IN, Indiana University Press, 1974

25. Farrar W, McCarty W Jr: Outline of Temporomandibular Joint Diagnosis and Treatment, 6th ed. Montgomery, AL, Normandy Study Group, 1980

26. Feinstein B, Lanton NJK, Jameson RM, Schiller F: Experiments on pain referred from deep somatic tissues. J Bone Joint Surg 36(A):981–997, 1954

27. Fish F: The functional anatomy of the rest position of the mandible. Dent Prac 11:178, 1961

28. Friedman MH, Weisberg J: Temporomandibular Joint Disorders: Diagnosis and Treatment. Chicago, Quintessence Publishing Co, 1985

29. Friedman MH, Weisberg J, Agus B: Diagnosis and treatment of inflammation of the temporomandibular joint. Semin Arthritis Rheum 12:44–51, 1982

30. Garliner D: Myofunctional Therapy. Philadelphia, WB Saunders, 1976

31. Gelb H: The craniomandibular syndrome. In Garliner D: Myofunctional Therapy. Philadelphia, WB Saunders, 1976

32. Gerry RG: Condylar fractures. In Schwartz L: Disorders of the Temporomandibular Joint. Philadelphia, WB Saunders, 1959

33. Goldstein DF, Kraus SL, Williams WB, Glasheen-Wray M: Influence of cervical posture on mandibular movement. J Prosthet Dent 52:421–426, 1984

34. Greene BJ: Myofunctional therapy. In Morgan DH, Hall WB, Vamvas SJ (eds): Disease of the Temporomandibular Apparatus: A Multidisciplinary Approach 2nd ed. St. Louis, CV Mosby, 1982

35. Greenfield B, Wyke B: Reflex innervation of the temporomandibular joint. Nature 211:940–941, 1966

36. Griffen C: A neuro-myo-arterial glomus in the temporomandibular meniscus. Med J Aust 48:113–116, 1961

37. Grokoest A: Osteoarthritis. In Schwartz L: Disorders of the Temporomandibular Joint. Philadelphia, WB Saunders, 1959

38. Grokoest A, Chayes CM: Rheumatic disease. In Schwartz L, Chayes CM: Facial Pain and Mandibular Dysfunction. Philadelphia, WB Saunders, 1968

39. Grossan M: Biofeedback. In Morgan DH, Hall WP, Vamvas SJ (eds): Disease of the Temporomandibular Apparatus: A Multidisciplinary Approach, 2nd ed. St. Louis, CV Mosby, 1982

40. Halbert R: Electromyographic study of head position. J Can Dent Assoc 23:11–23, 1958

41. Hargreaves A: Dysfunction of the temporomandibular joints. Physiotherapy 72:209–212, 1986

42. Heiberg AN, Heloe B, Krogstad BS: The myofascial pain dysfunction: Dental symptoms and psychological and muscular function: An overview. Psychother Psychosom 30:81–97, 1978

43. Jonck LM: Ear symptoms in temporomandibular joint disturbances. South Afr Med J 54:782–786, 1978

44. Juniper RD: Temporomandibular joint dysfunction: A theory based upon electromyographic studies of the lateral pterygoid. Br J Oral Maxillofac Surg 22:1–8, 1984

45. Juniper RD: The pathogenesis and investigation of TMJ dysfunction: Br J Oral Maxillofac Surg 25:105–112, 1987

46. Kaltenborn F: Manual Therapy for the Extremity Joints. Oslo, Olaf Norlis Bokhandel, 1974

47. Kawamura Y, Majina T, Kato I: Physiologic role of deep mechanoreceptors in temporomandibular joint capsule. J Osaka Univ Dent School 7:63–76, 1967

48. Klineberg I: Structure and function of temporomandibular joint innervation. Ann R Coll Surg 49:268–288, 1971

49. Knott M, Voss DE: Proprioceptive Neuromuscular Facilitation. New York, Harper & Row, 1962

50. Kraus SL: Physical therapy management of TMJ dysfunction. In Kraus SL (ed): TMJ Disorders, Management of Craniomandibular Complex. New York, Churchill Livingstone, 1988

51. Krogh-Poulsen WG: Management of the occlusion of the teeth. In Schwartz L, Chayes CM: Facial Pain and Mandibular Dysfunction. Philadelphia, WB Saunders, 1968

52. Lazorthes G, Gaubert J: L'innervation des articulations interapophysaires vertebrales. In: Comptes Rendus de l'Association des Anatomistes, 1956, pp 488–494

53. Luschei ES, Goodwin GM: Patterns of mandibular movement and muscle activity during mastication in the monkey. J Neurophysiol 35:954–966, 1974

54. Mahan P: Temporomandibular problems: Biologic diagnosis and treatment. In Solberg WK, Clark GT (eds): Temporomandibular Joint Problems. Chicago, Quintessence Publishing Co, 1980

55. Mahan P, Kreutziger KL: Diagnosis and management of temporomandibular joint pain. In Alling C, Mahan P (eds): Facial Pain. Philadelphia, Lea & Febiger, 1977

56. Maitland GDP: Peripheral Manipulations, 2nd ed. Boston, Butterworths, 1977

57. McLean LF, Brenman HS, Friedman MGF: Effects of changing body position on dental occlusion. J Dent Res 52:1041–1050, 1973

58. McNamara DC: Examination, diagnosis and treatment of occlusion pain-dysfunction. Aust Dent J 23:50–55, 1978

59. McNamara JA: The independent function of the two heads of the lateral pterygoid muscle. Am J Anat 138:197–205, 1973

60. Mintz VW: The orthopedic influence. In Morgan DH, Hall WP, Vamvas SJ (eds): Diseases of the Temporomandibular Apparatus: A Multidisciplinary Approach, 2nd ed. St. Louis, CV Mosby, 1982

61. Moffett BC, Johnson LC, McCabe JB, Askew HC: Ar-

ticular remodeling in the adult human temporomandibular joint. Am J Anat 115:10–130, 1964

62. Mohl ND: Head posture and its role in occlusion. NY State Dent J 42:17–23, 1976

63. Mohl ND: The role of head posture in mandibular function. In Solberg W, Clark G (eds): Abnormal Jaw Mechanics: Diagnosis and Treatment. Chicago, Quintessence Publishing Co, 1984

64. Morgan DH, Hall WP, Vamvas SJ (eds): Disease of the Temporomandibular Apparatus: A Multidisciplinary Approach, 2nd ed. St. Louis, CV Mosby, 1982

65. Morgan DH, Rosen LM: Interpretation of radiograph. In Morgan DH, Hall WP, Vamvas SJ (eds): Disease of the Temporomandibular Apparatus: A Multidisciplinary Approach, 2nd ed. St. Louis, CV Mosby, 1982

66. Munro RR: Electromyography of the masseter and anterior temporalis muscles in the open-close-clench cycle in temporomandibular joint dysfunction. Monogr Oral Sci 4:117–125, 1975

67. Paris SV: The Spinal Lesion. Christchurch, New Zealand, Pegasus Press, 1965

68. Peck C, Kraft G: Electromyographic biofeedback for pain related to muscle tension: A study of tension headache, back, and jaw pain. Arch Surg 112:889–895, 1977

69. Perry C: Neuromuscular control of mandibular movements. J Prosthet Dent 30:714–720, 1973

70. Pinto OF: A new structure related to the temporomandibular joint and the middle ear. J Prosthet Dent 12:95–103, 1962

71. Porter MR: The attachment of the lateral pterygoid muscle of the meniscus. J Prosthet Dent 24:555–562, 1970

72. Prieskel HW: Some observations on the postural position of the mandible. J Prosthet Dent 15:625–633, 1965

73. Ramfjord SP: Dysfunctional temporomandibular joint and muscle pain. J Prosthet Dent 11:353–374, 1961

74. Rayne J: Functional anatomy of the temporomandibular joint. Br J Oral Maxillofac Surg 25:92–99, 1987

75. Rees LA: The structure and function of the temporomandibular joint. Br Dent J 96:125–133, 1954

76. Robinson MJ: The influence of head position on TMJ dysfunction. J Prosthet Dent 16:169–172, 1966

77. Rocabado M: Management of the temporomandibular joint. Presented at a course on physical therapy in dentistry. Vail, Colorado, January 1978

78. Rocabado M: Advanced Upper Quarter Manual. Tacoma, Washington, Rocabado Institute, 1981

79. Rocabado M: Diagnosis and treatment of abnormal craniomandibular mechanics. In Solberg W, Clark G (eds): Abnormal Jaw Mechanics: Diagnosis and Treatment. Chicago, Quintessence Publishing Co, 1984

80. Rood M: Neurophysiological reactions as a basis for physical therapy. Phys Ther 34:444–449, 1954

81. Scherman P: Surgery of the temporomandibular articulation. In Gelb H (ed): Clinical Management of Head, Neck and TMJ Pain and Dysfunction: A Multidisciplinary Approach to Diagnosis and Treatment. Philadelphia, WB Saunders, 1977

82. Schwartz L (ed): Disorders of the Temporomandibular Joint. Philadelphia, WB Saunders, 1959

83. Schwartz L, Chayes CM (eds): Facial Pain and Mandibular Dysfunction. Philadelphia, WB Saunders, 1968

84. Shira RB, Alling CC: Traumatic injuries involving the temporomandibular joint articulation. In Schwartz L, Chayes CM (eds): Facial Pain and Muscular Dysfunction. Philadelphia, WB Saunders, 1968

85. Shore MA: Temporomandibular Joint Dysfunction and Occlusal Equilibration. Philadelphia, JB Lippincott, 1976

86. Sicher H, Du Brul EL: Oral Anatomy, 8th ed. St. Louis, CV Mosby, 1988

87. Somers N: An approach to the management of temporomandibular joint dysfunction. Aust Dent J 23:37–41, 1978

88. Thompson JR, Brodie AG: Factors in the position of the mandible. J Am Dent Assoc 29:925–941, 1942

89. Trott PH, Goss AN: Physiotherapy in diagnosis and treatment of the myofascial dysfunction syndrome. Int J Oral Surg 7:360–365, 1978

90. Trott PH: Passive movements and allied techniques in the management of dental patients. In Greives GP (ed): Modern Manual Therapy of the Vertebral Column. New York, Churchill Livingstone, 1986

91. Trott PH: Examination of the temporomandibular joint. In Grieves GP (ed): Modern Manual Therapy of the Vertebral Column. New York, Churchill Livingstone, 1986

92. Viener AE: Oral surgery. In Garliner D (ed): Myofunctional Therapy. Philadelphia, WB Saunders, 1976

93. Weinberg LA: An evaluation of basic articulators and their concepts: I. Basic concepts. J Prosthet Dent 13:622–644, 1963

94. Weinberg LA: The etiology, diagnosis, and treatment of TMJ dysfunction-pain syndrome: I. Etiology. J Prosthet Dent 42:654–664, 1979

95. Weinberg LA: The etiology, diagnosis and treatment of TMJ dysfunction-pain syndrome: II. Differential diagnosis. J Prosthet Dent 43:50–70, 1980

96. Weinberg LA: The etiology and treatment of TMJ dysfunction-pain syndrome: III. Treatment. J Prosthet Dent 43:186–196, 1980

97. Wetzler G: Physical therapy. In Morgan DH, Hall WP, Vamvas SV (eds): Disease of the Temporomandibular Apparatus: A Multidisciplinary Approach, 2nd ed. St. Louis, CV Mosby, 1982

98. Whinery JG: Examination of patients with facial pain. In Alling C, Mahan P (eds): Facial Pain. Philadelphia, Lea & Febiger, 1977

99. Wyke BD: Neuromuscular mechanisms influencing mandibular posture: A neurologist's review of current concepts. J Dent 2:111–120, 1972

100. Yale S, Allison B, Hauptfuehrer J: An epidemiological assessment of mandibular condyle morphology. Oral Surg 21:169–177, 1966

Part Three
CLINICAL APPLICATIONS — THE SPINE

17 *The Spine—General Structure and Biomechanical Considerations*

Darlene Hertling

General Structure

The spine is divided into five regions: cervical, thoracic (or dorsal) lumbar, sacral, and coccygeal (the "tail" or coccyx). The spine usually has 33 segments —seven cervical, 12 thoracic, five lumbar, five sacral, and four coccygeal (Fig. 17–1). The sacral vertebrae are fused together and serve as an attachment to the pelvic girdle. The "presacral" vertebrae, with which we are most concerned clinically, most often total 24. However, occasionally there are supernumerary thoracic or lumbar vertebrae, or perhaps an unfused sacral vertebra, rather than an actual additional segment. It is questionable whether the above-stated variations hold much clinical significance, although a spine in which a lumbar vertebra is sacralized is felt to gain stability at the expense of mobility, and a spine in which a sacral vertebra is not fused tends to be mobile but less stable.[4,24,44] Unilateral sacralization or lumbarization, in which only one side of the vertebra is involved, is often thought to be of more significance, presumably leading to asymmetry in mobility and stability. However, this may not always be the case, because osseous fusion on one side is often accompanied by fibrous fusion (not evident on roentgenograms) on the opposite side. Another not uncommon finding is fusion of two upper cervical vertebrae, which again may have little clinical significance.[21,40,47]

The spine is a flexible, multicurved column. When viewed in the sagittal plane, the cervical and lumbar regions are in lordosis (lordotic curve); the thoracic, sacral, and coccygeal regions are in kyphosis (kyphotic curve) (see Fig. 17–1C). These normal anatomical curves give the spinal column increased flexibility and augmented shock-absorbing capacity, while at the same time maintaining adequate stiffness and stability at the intervertebral joints.[2,155] In humans, the thoracic spine is partially splinted by the rib cage. The thoracic curve is structural and is secondary to less vertical height at the anterior thoracic vertebral border, as opposed to the posterior border. This is also true of the sacral curve. Although the sacrum is rigid, slight motions occur *in vivo* in the sacroiliac joint, decreasing with age (see Fig. 17–1)[28,39,118,121,189] The coccyx, which is not well developed in humans, has no functional role (see Fig. 17–1A,C).

In contrast, the cervical spine and lumbar spine are quite flexible, yet still are able to support heavy loads. The demanding functional role they play is felt to be a major reason why these regions of the spine are the most likely to become symptomatic. Curvature of the cervical and lumbar regions is largely due to the wedge-shaped intervertebral disks.[194] These disks are entirely responsible for the existence of a normal cervical lordosis, because the cervical vertebral bodies are actually shorter in height anteriorly than posteriorly (see Fig. 17–1C). They are largely responsible for the lumbar lordosis in the upper lumbar spine, but less so in the lower lumbar spine, where the vertebral bodies are wedge-shaped so as to form the lordosis. Thus, in both the cervical and lumbar regions the disks are of greater height anteriorly than posteriorly. In the thoracic spine the kyphosis is almost entirely caused by the shape of the vertebral bodies—the disks being of equal height anteriorly and posteriorly.

The spine has at least four biomechanical functions: 1) housing and protection, 2) support, 3) mobility, and 4) control.[155,194] Its most important function is to protect the delicate spinal cord from potentially damaging forces or motions. From a support standpoint, it transfers the weight and bending movements of the head and trunk to the pelvis. Facilitated by the ribs, it functions as a framework for attachment of the internal organs.

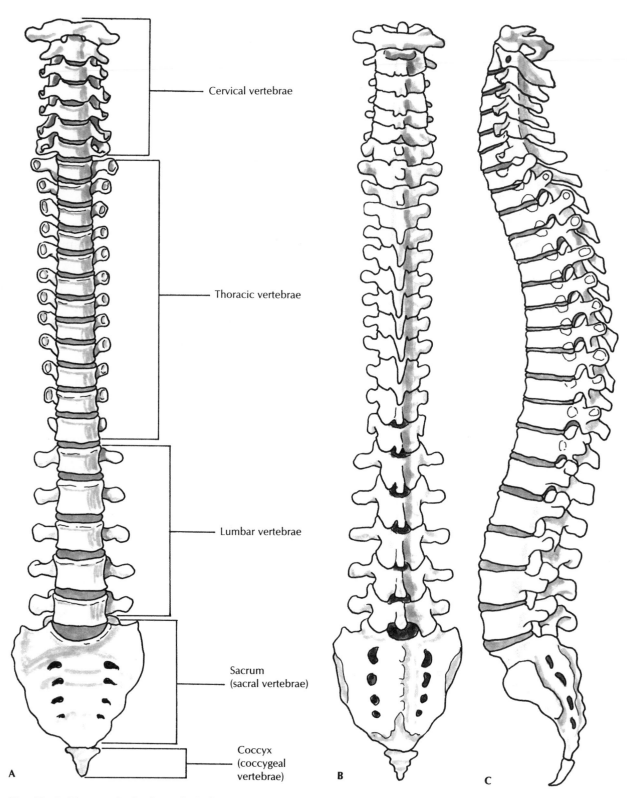

Cervical vertebrae

Thoracic vertebrae

Lumbar vertebrae

Sacrum
(sacral vertebrae)

Coccyx
(coccygeal
vertebrae)

A

B

C

Fig. 17–1. The vertebral column, including sacrum and coccyx, as seen on *(A)* anterior,
(B) posterior, and *(C)* left sagittal views.

The human neck has been described as a cylindrical conduit that supports the head and renders it mobile.[105] It provides avenues of passage for essential connections in the respiratory, gastrointestinal, nervous, and vascular systems and serves as a locus for vital ductless glands and for the organs of phonation, vocalization, and ventilation. As such, it is a compact aggregate of numerous critical structures related to the cervical spine, which serves as the major architectural member. The cervical spine is a highly mobile structure that functions principally to position the head in space, permitting effective adaptation of the organism to the environment. Motions of the neck are therefore inseparably linked with motions of the head, and this linkage is a critical concept in both normal and pathologic states.[105]

Mobility allows for physiological motion to occur between the parts of the spine. Thus, instead of a single rigid column, the spine is a flexible stack of rigid blocks with flexible soft tissue in between. The basic functional unit of the spine is the *spinal motion segment*, which may be defined as comprising the adjacent halves of two vertebrae, the interposed disk and articular facet joints, as well as the supporting structures (*i.e.*, ligaments, blood vessels, nerves, and muscles).[40,149,155,170] It should be noted that in the cervical spine there are no disks between the atlas and the occiput and the atlas and the axis. The disks permit intervertebral movement, while the posterior articulations control the amplitude and direction of the movement. This concept leads to a more functional than anatomical approach to pathology.

REVIEW OF FUNCTIONAL ANATOMY

Although a detailed description of the anatomy of the spine is beyond the scope of this chapter, the reader is referred to several other, comprehensive sources.[44,51,91,128,166,167,194] Briefly, the following constituents of the spinal segment and how they respond to motion and load are reviewed:

1. Support system—vertebral bodies, posterior elements, articular facet (apophyseal) joints, intervertebral disks, and vertebral foramen
2. Control system—both contractile (muscles) and noncontractile (ligaments, fascia, capsules, and vertebral innervations) elements
3. Other support systems—intra-abdominal and thoracic pressures

THE SUPPORT SYSTEM: INDIVIDUAL STRUCTURES

Vertebrae

The special anatomical features of the vertebrae are probably best described in relation to their biomechanical functions. Probably the earliest biomechanical study of the human spine with respect to strength measurements of the vertebrae was conducted by Messerer more than 100 years ago.[120]

Each vertebra consists of two major parts—the anterior vertebral body, which is the major weight-bearing structure of the vertebra, and the posterior vertebral arch (Fig. 17–2). The vertebral arch is composed of the pedicle, which joins the arch to the body and to which the superior articular process is attached. This superior process articulates with the inferior process by means of the articular facet (apophyseal) joint and the transverse and spinous processes.

The basic design of the vertebrae in the various regions of the spine is the same. The size and mass of the vertebral bodies increase all the way from the first cervical to the last lumbar vertebra (see Fig. 17–1A). This is a mechanical adaptation to the progressively increasing loads to which the vertebrae are subjected.[194] There are individual differences in the various regions of the spine. Unique to the typical cervical vertebra (C2–C7) are lateral prominences called *uncinate processes;* the transverse processes contain *foramina* (foramen transversarii) through which the vertebral artery passes (Fig. 17–3B,C). The thoracic vertebrae have articular facets for the ribs (Fig. 17–4A,C) and the lumbar spine has *mammary processes* (roughened raised areas on each articular pillar that serve for muscle attachment for the multifidi) (Fig. 17–5A,C). Of course the sacral spine, being fused, is unique.

Anterior Portion of the Motion Segment

Although the articular facets carry some compressive load, it is the vertebral bodies that are primarily designed to sustain these loads. A compressive load is transmitted from the superior end-plate of a vertebra to the inferior end-plate by way of two paths, the *cortical shell* and the *cancellous core*. The body consists of spongy bone covered with a thin, dense bony cortex, whereas the neural arch and its processes are thinner and have proportionally more cortical bone. The cortical bone of the upper and lower surfaces of the bodies (vertebral plateaus) reflects the structure of the overlying cartilaginous end-plate, with a somewhat concave center and a more dense ringed epiphyseal plate peripherally. As the superimposed weight of the upper body increases, the vertebral bodies become larger. The bodies in the lumbar spine have a greater height and cross-sectional area than those in the thoracic and cervical spine; their increased size allows them to sustain the greater loads to which this part of the spine is subjected.[108]

The vertebral bodies are about six times stiffer and three times thicker than the disks. Thus the vertebral bodies deform about half as much as the disks under compression. Because the vertebrae are filled with blood, it is possible that they behave like hydraulically strengthened shock absorbers.[93,94]

Vertical and oblique trabecular systems that correspond to the stresses placed on the bodies are found within the spongy bone (Fig. 17–6).[55,91] Verti-

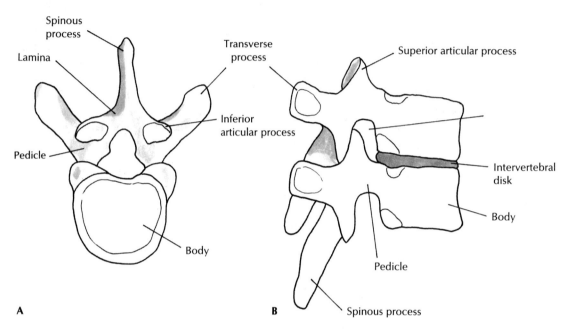

Fig. 17–2. Parts of a vertebra, viewed from *(A)* inferiorly and *(B)* sagittally.

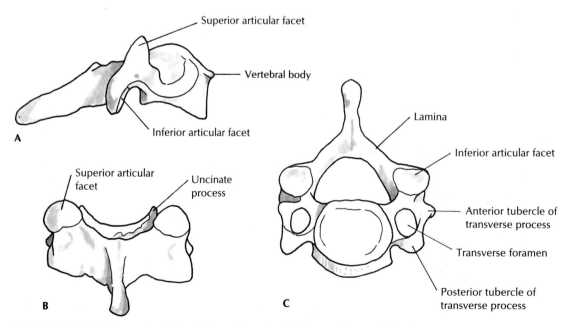

Fig. 17–3. Typical lower cervical vertebra: *(A)* sagittal, *(B)* posterior, and *(C)* inferior views.

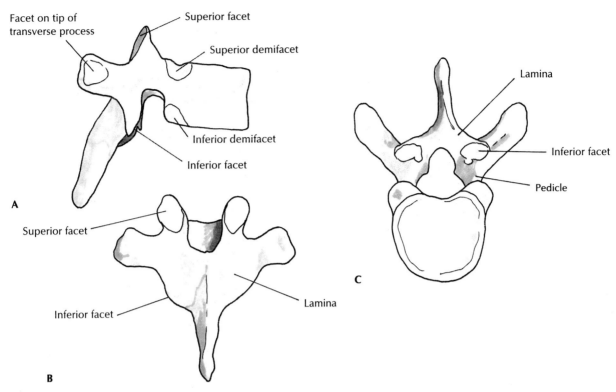

Fig. 17-4. Typical thoracic vertebra: *(A)* lateral, *(B)* posterior, and *(C)* inferior views.

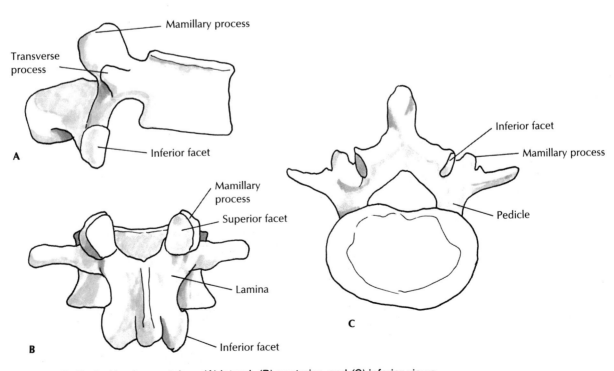

Fig. 17-5. Typical lumbar vertebra: *(A)* lateral, *(B)* posterior, and *(C)* inferior views.

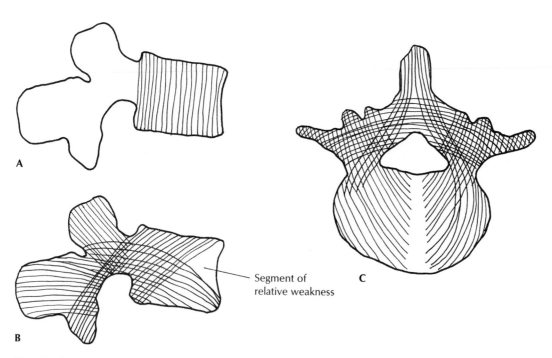

Fig. 17–6. Trabecular arrangement of vertebrae. *(A)* Vertical trabeculae, *(B)* inferior and superior oblique patterns (note segment of relative weakness), and *(C)* oblique patterns viewed from above.

cally directed trabeculae mainly support the body and the compressive forces and help to sustain (see Fig. 17–6A) the body weight. The other trabecular systems help to resist shearing forces. At both the lower and upper surfaces of the body there are oblique trabeculae, which aid in compressive load-bearing function and also serve to resist the bending and tensile forces that occur at the pedicles and spinous processes (see Fig. 17–6B,C). In osteoporosis there is a greater loss of horizontal trabeculae in comparison to the vertical trabeculae of cancellous bone; the effect on the strength of the vertebrae is considerable. In pathologic processes of the spine, the type of failure may be related to whether the spine was loaded in flexion or extension, with flexion tending to cause anterior collapse where trabeculae are weakest.[155] This also explains the wedge-shaped compression fracture of the vertebrae that occur.[91]

Krenz and Troup found that the pressure was higher in the center of the end-plate than in the periphery during compressive loading.[103] This is a common site for failure in which the nucleus apparently ruptures the end-plate. Again, this may be a significant problem for those who have diminished bone strength, as in osteoporosis. Central fractures of the end-plate typically occur in nondegenerated disks, whereas peripheral fractures are found to be related to degenerated disks.[151,152,165]

Regionally, the lumbar vertebral bodies alter in shape from the first lumbar vertebra (more squared) to the fifth lumbar vertebra (more rectangular), giving the articular end-plate a broader surface area (see Fig. 17–5C). The bodies of the middle thoracic vertebrae are almost heart-shaped because of the pressure of the descending aorta (see Fig. 17–4C). The thoracic vertebral bodies are proportionally higher than the lumbar vertebrae and more squared in the transverse plane. Unique to the cervical spine (C2–C7) are lateral uncinate processes on the superior surface of each vertebral body, which articulate with the beveled edge of the inferior surface of the vertebral body (see Fig. 17–3B). At this junction there is usually a synovial joint called the *joint of Luschka*.[69,186]

The atypical cervical vertebrae (C1 and C2) are characterized by the absence of a vertebral body at C1 (the *atlas*) and by the embryological fusion of the C1 body with C2 (the *axis*), forming a prominent pillar on the surface of C2 known as the *odontoid process* or *dens* (Fig. 17–7A,B,D).[186]

Each vertebral body has its primary nutrient foramen located in the center of the posterior aspect and *in situ* is covered by the *posterior longitudinal ligament* (Fig. 17–8A,B).[166,167] In general the upper and lower surfaces of the vertebral bodies are slightly concave.

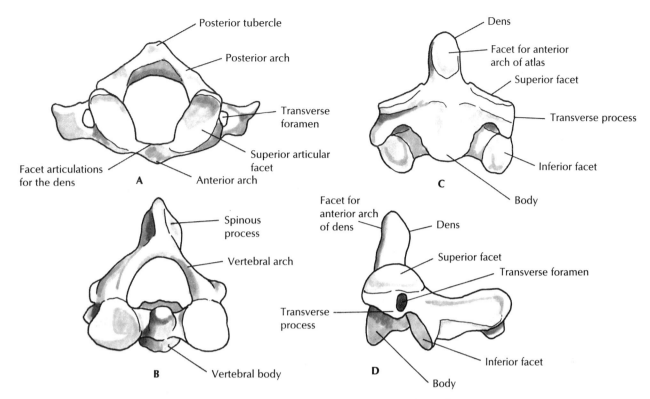

Fig. 17–7. First and second cervical vertebrae. *(A)* The atlas (C1), as viewed from above; *(B)* the axis (C2), as viewed from above; *(C)* anterior view of axis; and *(D)* sagittal view of axis.

Posterior Elements and Facet Joints

The vertebral arch is more complex than the body, because it has many projections, including four articulating facet (apophyseal) joints and three processes (see Fig. 17–2). The processes, two transverse and one spinous, provide for the attachment of ligaments and muscles. The arch is divided into a short anterior portion and a long posterior portion by the articulating projections and transverse processes. The anterior half of the arch consists of the pedicles, which attach the arch anteriorly to the upper posterior wall of the vertebral body (see Fig. 17–2). The laminae join to form the peak of the arch and continue to form the spinous process. At the site where the lamina takes origin from the pedicle, the lamina is narrowed, an area referred to as the *pars interarticularis* or *isthmus* (see Fig. 17–5*B*). Whereas pedicles rarely fracture, the pars is a frequent site of a distinctive fracture, apparently secondary to fatigue of bone rather than a sudden or acute fracture; this defect is commonly found in athletes.[2] Because the pars interarticularis is actually part of the neural arch forming a part of the posterolateral boundary of the arch, these lesions are often referred to as *neural arch defects*.[62] These defects are known as either *spondylolysis*, which consists of a single fracture of the pars, or as *spondylolisthesis*, which consists of a bilateral fracture often accompanied by some degree of forward slippage of the vertebral body (see Chapter 20, The Lumbar Spine).

The trabecular systems of the vertebral arch extend into the vertebral body (see Fig. 17–6). The area where the transverse process and articular facets arise is reinforced by many crossing trabeculae. The alignment of the trabeculae in the vertebral body and posterior element indicates that the facet articulations must function to some extent as a fulcrum between the anterior vertebral body and the laminae and spinous processes; although the compression forces seen by the posterior elements in direct axial compression are markedly relieved by the compression strength of the body and disk system and by the potential for tensile elongation of the ligaments and muscles posteriorly.[91]

The articular facet joints are extensions of the laminae and are covered with hyaline cartilage on their articulating surfaces (Fig. 17–9*A*). The articular facets are particularly important in resisting torsion and shear, but also play a role in compression. They may carry large compressive loads (25% to 33%), depending on the body posture, and they also

Fig. 17–8. The ligaments of the vertebral column include *(A)* the posterior longitudinal ligament (posterior view); *(B)* the ligamentum flavum and anterior longitudinal ligament (anterior view); *(C)* the supraspinous and interspinous ligaments (sagittal view); and *(D)* and intertransverse ligaments (superior view).

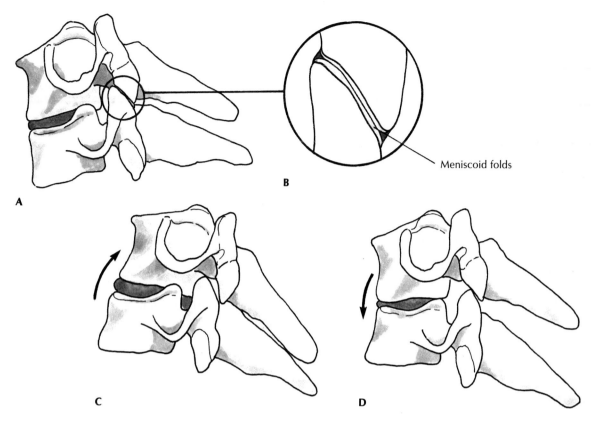

Fig. 17–9. Sagittal section of an articular facet joint *(A)*, with an enlarged view *(B)* showing the meniscoid folds. The articular surfaces tend to approximate during extension *(C)* and separate during flexion *(D)*.

provide (in equal proportion to the disk) 45% of the torsional strength of a motion segment.[44,81,95,110]

The amount of load-bearing by the articular facet joints is related to whether the motion segment is loaded in flexion or extension. Differences in interdiskal loading between erect sitting and standing can be explained in part by load-bearing of the articular facet joints while in extension or lordosis. Theoretically, the disk would be protected from both torsional and compressive loads when the motion segment is in extension. However, excessive loading of the spine in extension may cause failure of this secondary load-bearing mechanism; that is, loads transmitted through the articular facet joints may produce high strains in the pars interarticularis, leading to spondylolysis.

The apophyseal or articular facet joints are usually described as *plane diarthrodial synovial joints* (except for the joints between the first two cervical vertebrae), although there is a "meniscus" (fatty synovial mass) in most of the joints (see Fig. 17–9A).[96] The superior processes (prezygapophyseal) always bear an articulating facet whose surface is directed dorsally to some degree (see Figs. 17–3A,B; 17–4A,B; and 17–5A,B); the inferior articulating processes (postzygapophyseal) direct their articulating surfaces ventrally (see Figs. 17–3A, 17–4A, and 17–5A).[166,167] The joint consists of a cartilaginous articular surface, a fluid-filled capsule, and numerous ligaments surrounding and reinforcing the capsule. In degeneration the synovium is redundant, and the capsule frequently is redundant or torn and may contribute to malfunction as trapped menisci do in other joints.[97,149]

Generally motion between two vertebrae is extremely limited and consists of a small amount of gliding or sliding. The net effect of small amounts of gliding at a series of vertebrae produces a considerably large range of motion for the spinal column as a whole. The motions available to the column may be likened to that of a joint with three planes of motion: flexion and extension, lateral flexion (sidebending), and rotation.[142] In addition, a small amount of vertical compression and distraction is possible. The type and amount of motion that are available differ from region to region and depend on the orientation of the facets and the fluidity, elasticity, and thickness of the intervertebral joint. Although the degree of movement at the spinal segment is largely determined by the disks, the patterns of movement of the spine depend on the shape and orientation of the articulating processes of the articular facet joint surfaces. If the superior and inferior articular facets of the three adjacent vertebrae lie in the sagittal plane, the motions of flexion and extension are facilitated. Conversely, if the articular facets are placed in the frontal plane, the predominant motion is that of lateral flexion or sidebending.

Regionally (except for C1 and C2, whose articular facets are oriented in the transverse plane), the articular facets of the intervertebral joints of the cervical spine are oriented at 45° to the transverse plane and parallel to the frontal plane (see Fig. 17–3A). This alignment of the intervertebral joints allows flexion, extension, sidebending, and rotation. The angle increases at descending levels, approaching vertical at C7 in the frontal plane. The superior articular facet surface is convex, and the inferior facet surface is concave. The articular facet joint surfaces tend to separate during forward bending and approximate during backward bending (see Fig. 17–9C,D). Sidebending and rotation occur together to the same side. This is because the articular facet joint surfaces are positioned approximately halfway between the frontal and transverse planes. As one articular facet joint slides forward and upward, its mate slides backward and downward, translating to a sidebending component in the frontal plane and a rotatory component in the transverse plane. In this way, sidebending and rotation from C2–C3 to about T1 involve essentially an identical movement between articular facet joint surfaces. The only difference between sidebending and rotation of the cervical spine results from differences in movement at the upper cervical spine. The unique joint configuration found in the alantoaxial complex is discussed in Chapter 18, The Cervical Spine. According to Kapandji, combined movement of flexion and extension for these segments is approximately 100° to 110°.[91] When combined with movement of the atlantoaxial complex, the total range of motion is 130°.

In the erect spine, sidebending and rotation in the thoracic and lumbar regions tend to occur to opposite sides. The reasons may be more complex than at the cervical spine, but again seem to be largely the result of the orientation of the articular facet planes (Figs. 17–4A, 17–5A). In the thoracic spine, all 12 thoracic vertebrae support ribs and show facets for the articulation of these structures. Unlike the spinous processes in the lumbar and cervical areas,

where the tip of the spinous process is found directly posterior to the body of the vertebra, the tip of the spinous process lies posteriorly and inferiorly to the body (see Fig. 17–4A,B). The spinous processes are long and triangular in section. Those of the upper and lower four thoracic vertebrae are more bladelike and are directed downward at an angle of 60° so that their spines completely overlap the next lower segment (see Fig. 17–1C).[166,167] This elongation limits the amount of extension possible at each segment. The thoracic pedicles are longer than in the cervical and lumbar areas, giving the vertebral canal an oval appearance and diminishing the possibility of stenosis of the canal (see Fig. 17–4A,C). The transverse processes are characterized by having a concave facet that receives the tuberculum of the rib and being angled backward; this encourages rotation movements by the attached muscles.

The articular facets of the thoracic vertebrae are oriented 60° to the transverse plane and 20° to the frontal plane (see Fig. 17–4A,C),[98,108,114] allowing sidebending, rotation, and some flexion and extension. Because of the articular facet alignment and stabilization of the vertebral bodies laterally, rotation is the most accessible movement. Gregerson and Lucas concluded from a study on rotation of the trunk that approximately 74° of rotation occurred between the first and twelfth thoracic vertebrae. (The average cumulative rotation from the sacrum to the first thoracic vertebrae was 102°.)[63] The superior articular facets form a stout, shelflike projection. The ovoid surfaces of the superior articular facets are slightly convex, whereas the inferior articular facets are slightly concave (similar to the articular facet joint surfaces in the cervical spine), which is opposite to the articular facets in the lumbar spine.[59]

The majority of thoracic vertebrae adhere to the basic structural design of all vertebrae, except for some minor variations. The C7–T3 segments are a transitional zone between the cervical lordosis and thoracic kyphosis, with all ranges being diminished although flexion and extension are freer than in the lower thoracic spine. The first thoracic vertebra is considered the transitional vertebra, whereas the second thoracic vertebra, which can be distinguished by an enlarged pedicle, is thought to be developed to carry that portion of the weight borne by the articular facets into a more forward position, so that at levels below the second thoracic vertebra the weight is carried principally by the vertebral bodies and disks.[149] The physiological movement combinations are the same as for the typical cervical regions (*i.e.*, sidebending accompanied by rotation).[66] At the T3–T10 segments, both sidebending and rotation are limited by the bony thorax. Amplitudes of movement, especially in the sagittal range, increase progressively as the restriction offered by the ribs begins to decrease. The T11–L1 segments are a transitional zone between the thoracic kyphosis and lumbar lordosis. While the articular facet joints remain vertically oriented, they begin to change from the frontal to the sagittal plane. The last thoracic vertebrae (T12), acting as a bridge between the thoracic and lumbar regions, has its inferior articular facets in the sagittal plane to match those of L1.[91]

Rib Cage Articulations

According to Maigne, involvement of the rib cage in pathologic processes is often neglected. Yet costal sprain is very frequent and is expressed by thoracic or upper lumbar pain.[114] It follows either a contusion, an unusual effort, or a faulty movement (generally in rotation). The ribs are thus mechanically significant articulations of the thoracic spine. The 12 pairs of thin arc shaped bones form a protective cavity for the heart, lungs, and great vessels.[31] They also provide attachment for muscles necessary for respiration, posture, and arm function. The rib cage has several important biomechanical functions related to the spine. It acts as a protective barrier for any traumatic impact directed from the sides or anterior aspect, and it stiffens and strengthens the thoracic spine. The moment of inertia provided by the rib cage is its most important biomechanical aspect, according to White and Panjabi.[194] The increased moment of inertia stiffens the spine when it is subjected to any kind of rotatory forces, such as bending movements and torques.

The transverse dimensions of the thoracic spine are increased manifold by the inclusion of the sternum and ribs. Cartilaginous junctions fix the ribs to the sternum. Characterized as *true ribs*, the first seven attach to the sternum by individual cartilages (Fig. 17–10A). The eighth, ninth, and tenth ribs have a common junction with the sternum and are called *false ribs.*

The ends of the true ribs join this costal cartilage by means of the costochondral joint. The first rib is joined firmly to the manubrium by a cartilaginous joint, while the second rib articulates with demifacets on both the manubrium and the body of the sternum by way of synovial joints (see Fig. 17–10A). The cartilages of the third to seventh ribs have small synovial joints which attach to the body of the sternum.[194] Later in life these joints become ankylosed or obliterated.[66]

The ribs and vertebrae are united at two locations.

The radiate ligament anchors each rib head to two adjacent vertebral bodies and the disk between them (see Fig. 17–10B,C).[153] This occurs at the superior and inferior costal demifacets located at the junction of the vertebral body and posterior arch, and forming the costovertebral joint (a synovial joint) (see Fig. 17–10B). Costotransverse ligaments join the rib tubercle and corresponding vertebral transverse process (see Fig. 17–10B,C). To accommodate this articulation, each long transverse process is capped by a costal facet. The costotransverse joint is also a synovial joint surrounded by a capsule but it is primarily strengthened by three costotransverse ligaments.[91]

Each rib is a curved lever which has its fulcrum immediately lateral to the costotransverse joint, and each has its own range and direction of movement differing slightly from the others. Although it is fair to surmise that each rib has its own pattern of movement, certain generalizations can be made. The first ribs form a firm horseshoe-shaped arch, which moves upward and forward as a unit (Fig. 17–11A,B). This movement occurs at the heads of these ribs and is a simple elevation of the manubrium upward and forward.[113] The false ribs combine the elevation of their anterior ends with a caliper-like opening (Fig. 17–11C).[113] Following direct trauma or secondary to some attempts at trunk rotation, the false ribs induce pain somewhat analogous to that of lumbago. The pain is typically located in the lumbar fossa, radiating toward the groin, and is acutely intensified by certain movements.[114]

The final two (eleventh and twelfth) ribs are free floating (termed *floating ribs*) and simply end in the trunk musculature of the abdominal wall. Their loose attachment at their heads and lack of union with the transverse processes leaves them subject to push and pull in any direction, hinging on the head.[113] The twelfth rib is the shortest and may be so short that it fails to project beyond the lateral border of the back muscles that cover it.[79]

With respect to spinal motion, both sidebending and rotation of the thoracic spine are limited by the rib cage. When a thoracic vertebra rotates, the motion is accompanied by distortion of the associated rib pair. The ribs on the side to which the body rotates become convex posteriorly, while the ribs on the contralateral side become flattened posteriorly.[142] The amount of rotation that is possible depends on the ability of the ribs to undergo distortion and the amount of motion available in the costovertebral, costotransverse, and costochondral joints.

Because the rib cage actually encloses the thoracic spine, any external stabilizing force must be indi-

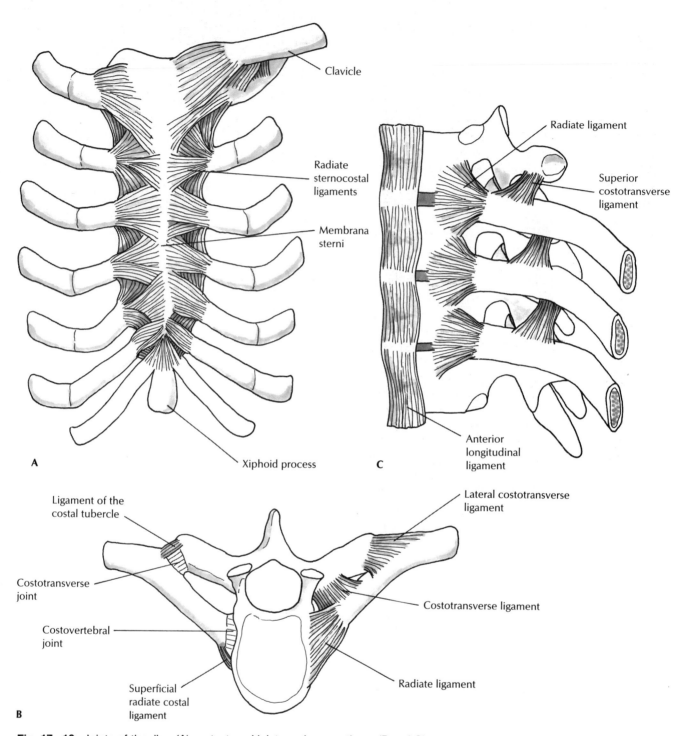

Fig. 17-10. Joints of the ribs: *(A)* costosternal joints and connections; *(B and C)* costovertebral joints, on superior and sagittal views.

rectly applied through the ribs. Because of their size and configuration, the ribs are more plastic than the vertebral bodies.[163] As such they readily yield to applied forces, and their shape will be altered before any corrective effect is noted on a rigid spine.[31]

Most rib lesions are accompanied, if not caused, by spasm of the intercostal muscles. A sneeze or cough with a violent contraction of the musculature of the thoracic cage may leave a persistent contraction of one intercostal muscle, leading to approximation of two adjacent ribs which may persist. The net effect of sustained contraction in one intercostal muscle is to

Fig. 17-11. Movements of the ribs: *(A)* the first rib and manubrium with upward and forward movement; *(B)* the typical vertebrosternal ribs with bucket-handle movement; and *(C)* the caliper-like movements of the lower ribs.

A

B

C

elevate the lower rib (an inspiration-type lesion). Expiratory-type lesions in which the lower rib is held downward can only occur in the lower ribs, mainly the eleventh and twelfth, because of the attachment of the quadratus lumborum.

Lumbar Articulations

The average plane of inclination of the lumbar articular facets is almost 90° to the transverse plane and 45° to the frontal plane (see Fig. 17–5A,B). The articular facets face in almost a lateromedial direction are therefore aligned in the sagittal plane, whereas the articular facets of the fifth lumbar vertebra face obliquely forward and laterally toward the frontal plane.[166,167,194] This alignment allows flexion, extension, and sidebending, but almost no rotation. Sidebending is limited to a range of approximately 5° between each successive vertebra, whereas rotation is limited to approximately 3°.[2]

The lumbosacral intervertebral joints differ from the other intervertebral joints in the lumbar spine. The orientation and shape of the facets at this level allow more rotation.[111] Most L4–L5 articular facet joints are angled about 43° from the coronal or frontal plane, while most L5–S1 articular facets are angled about 52°. Unlike the more superior lumbar joints, the articular facets of the inferior articulating process of L5 vertebra faces forward and slightly downward to engage the reciprocally corresponding articular processes of the sacrum. The most essential function of the lumbosacral articulations involves their role as buttresses against the forward and downward displacement of L5 vertebra relative to the sacrum.[166,167] Because the sacrovertebral angle produces the most abrupt change of direction in the column, and the center of gravity which passes through L5 segment falls anterior to the sacrum, there is a marked tendency for the thick, "edge-shaped" fifth lumbar disk to give way to the shearing vector that the lumbosacral angularity produces. The resulting condition, spondylolisthesis, most frequently reveals a deficiency in the laminae that fails to anchor L5 to the sacrum and allows it to displace forward.

All of the articular pillars of the lumbar vertebrae have convex surfaces on the inferior articular process, forming in most cases one third or one half of a sphere with a greater curvature in the transverse than in the longitudinal section. The superior articular process carries a corresponding concave surface so that the joints have two principal movements— translation (slide) and distraction (gapping). Unlike the intervertebral disks, which allow motion in all

planes, the articular facet joints restrict the motion segment, assisted by the ligaments. The capsules of the lumbar articular facets are quite fibrous and extend upward and medially onto the laminae above, which enables them to restrict forward bending.[34,149]

According to White and Panjabi, "mechanical load-sharing" between the facets and disks is rather complex.[194] Other authors have made quantitative estimates of the biomechanics, including Nachemson who found that 18% of the compressive load is borne by the articular facet;[131] King, who reported that 0% to 33% of the axial load was borne by the facet, depending on the position or posture of the joint;[95] and Farfan, who attributed 45% of torsional stiffness to the articular facets and capsules.[44] The articular facet joints make a major contribution to the rotational stiffness of the lumbar spine; this is important because *in vitro* testing of loaded motion segments in rotation alone and rotation with either flexion or sidebending can produce the types of disk lesions seen clinically. The importance of asymmetrical articular facet orientation for pathologic processes of the intervertebral disk has been well documented by Farfan and Sullivan, who established a highly significant correlation between asymmetry of the articular facet joints and the level of disk involvement and between the side of the more oblique articular facet orientation and side of sciatica.[46] Most articular facet planes have a difference in angle of less than 10°, but "gross" asymmetry is seen in about 25% of an essentially random population by conventional roentgenography.[44] This may be associated with asymmetrical vertebral bodies or with unilateral laminar hypertrophy and is clearly associated with early disk degeneration at the level of the asymmetry. When such asymmetry is present, it is the side with the most oblique articular facet that acquires early posterolateral annular damage.

Intervertebral Disks

The spine, which is composed of alternating rigid and elastic elements, possesses a considerable degree of flexibility that is primarily attributable to the intervertebral disks. The amount of flexibility depends on the material characteristics, the size and shape of the disk, and the amount of restraint offered by the invertebral ligaments. Normally the disks may be considered to act as universal joints, permitting motion in four directions between vertebral bodies: (1) translational motion in the long axis of the spine, occurring because of compressibility of the disk; (2) rotary motion about a vertical axis; (3) anteroposterior bending; and (4) lateral bending.[128]

Each successive vertebral body is linked by an intervertebral disk, which acts as a symphysis between the vertebrae. There are no disks between the occiput and atlas nor between the atlas and axis. The disk "spaces" in the young adult contribute to as much as 20% to 33% of total vertebral column height. The ratio between the height of the disk and the corresponding vertebral bodies in part determines the amount of motion that may occur in a particular region. It has been shown that the flexibility varies directly with the square of the vertical height of the disk and indirectly with the square of the horizontal diameter of the body.[130] Because of the proportionally greater height in the lumbar region, the range of intervertebral motion is greater in the lumbar region; but because of the greater horizontal diameter, the flexibility is less than in the thoracic region.[128] Motion is greatest in the cervical spine. The unique composition of the intervertebral disks allows for a more even distribution of weight transmitted to the adjacent vertebral bodies during movement.

It is often mentioned that the disks act as shock absorbers during vertical compressive loading. While this may be true to some extent, shock absorption on vertical loading is largely related to the fact that the spine is a curved, "spring-loaded," flexible column, rather than a rigid rodlike structure.

The cervical disks are largely responsible for the existence of a normal cervical lordosis in the upper spine; the lumbar disks are somewhat less responsible for the normal lumbar lordosis, which is mostly caused by the wedged-shaped vertebral bodies. In the thoracic spine the normal kyphosis is almost entirely caused by the shape of the vertebral bodies.

The disk is composed of several structures, including the nucleus pulposus, which is the central fluid-filled portion of the disk; and the annulus fibrosus, the series of elastic fibers that surround the nucleus (Fig. 17–12). The disk is bounded above and below by cartilaginous end-plates, to which the annular fibers are firmly anchored. These end-plates are then attached to the body surface of the vertebral bodies. The inner fluid nucleus (a remnant of the embryonic notochordal tissue) is surrounded by a zone of irregular connective tissue bands that are also rich in fluid and are in turn surrounded by the lamellae of the annulus fibrosus.[149] The overall shape of the nucleus mimics that of the body, and takes up about 25% of the disk area.[44] The fluid mass of the nucleus pulposus is composed of a colloidal gel rich in water-binding glucosaminoglycans with a few collagen fibers randomly embedded within. It is centrally located in the disk, except in the lower lumbar segments where it is located more posteriorly. Both the relative size of the nucleus and its capacity to take on water and swell are greatest in the cervical and lumbar spine. It is well suited for its essential function to resist and redistribute compressive forces within the spine. Because of its high water content and plastic nature, its functions follow closely the laws of hydrodynamics. Typically, the nucleus pulposus occupies an eccentric position within the confines of the annulus, usually close to the posterior margin of the disk (Fig. 17–12*B*). Being avascular, the nucleus depends on its exchange of fluid across the cartilaginous end-plate with the vascularized vertebral body for its nutrition. The tendency of imbibition of fluid by the nucleus is greatest when weight-bearing is reduced through the disk. As a result, a young person tends to be taller (¼ to ¾ inch) in the morning than at the end of the day. During the day the disk fluid is expressed from the disk to complete the nutrient cycle. In addition to being expressed, the disk fluid can be relocated by the assumption of specific postures.[100] Examples of this include the loss of normal lordosis after assuming a flexed position when gardening, or a lateral shift associated with low back injury.[149] The mucopolysaccharide gel changes in its biochemical characteristics with damage and age. These biochemical changes decrease the water-binding capability of the nucleus. Hendry demonstrated that a disk will give up water more readily if it is degenerated because of damage or age.[75] Normally, the nucleus contains between 70% and 88% water, which makes it nearly incompressible, and thus it acts as a distributor of force at the vertebral level. As the disk becomes dryer and its elasticity decreases, it loses its ability to store energy and to distribute stresses and is therefore less capable of resisting loads.

The annulus fibrosus consists of fibroid cartilage with bundles of collagen fibers, arranged in a crisscross pattern which allows them to withstand high bending and torsional loads (see Fig. 17–12*A*). These fibers run obliquely between vertebral bodies such that the fibers in one layer run in the opposite direction to the fibers in adjacent layers. The outer layer of fibers blends with the posterior longitudinal ligament posteriorly and with the anterior longitudinal ligament anteriorly. These outer fibers attach superiorly and inferiorly to the margins of the vertebral bodies by Sharpey's fibers. The fibers of the outermost ring of the annulus extend beyond the confines of the disk and blend with the vertebral periosteum and longitudinal ligaments. The inner fibers attach superiorly and inferiorly to the cartilaginous end-plates. The cartilaginous end-plate is composed of hyaline cartilage that separates the outer two components of the disk from the vertebral body (see Fig.

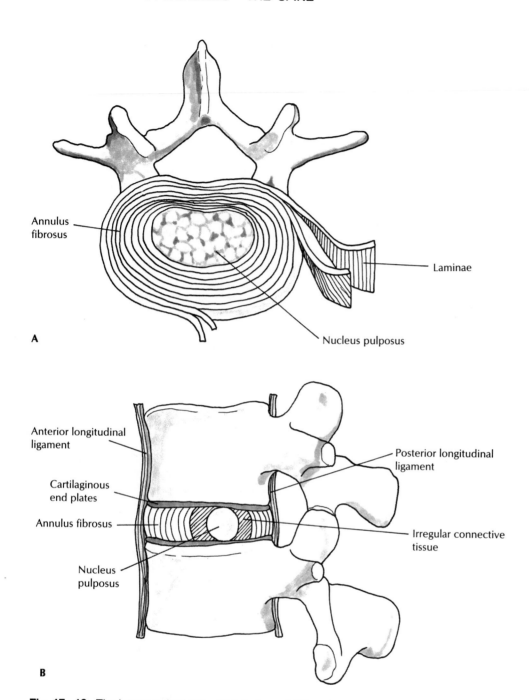

Fig. 17–12. The intervertebral disk: (A) inferior and (B) sagittal views.

17–12B). In addition to absorbing forces, the annulus contains the nucleus pulposus, which acts as
the fulcrum of movement for the three planes of motion available at each vertebral level.[91] One of the
major functions of the annulus is to withstand tension, whether the tensile forces are from the horizontal extension of the compressed nucleus, from torsional stress of the column, or from the separation of
the vertebral bodies on the convex side of spinal flex-

ion.[166,167] The entire unit is then ensheathed by the
periosteum, which extends over the vertebrae and in
effect the intervertebral disks, displaying a thickening both anteriorly (anterior longitudinal ligament)
and posteriorly (posterior longitudinal ligament).[174]
According to Paris, the location where this sheath
covers the disk has been found to be both innervated
and vascularized and possesses, in effect, a neurovascular capsule.[149] Innervation from the sinuvertebral

nerve has been substantiated by findings of Cloward and others. It is proposed that the diseased disk, in which parts of the annulus have been torn and repaired, contains a richer innervation from the ingrowth of nerve tissue with granulation.[27] This may be of some importance clinically in patients with spinal pain. Surgically removed disk tissue has been reported to contain some complex as well as free nerve endings.

In the young, healthy disk a positive pressure is present within the nucleus pulposus at rest and increases as loads are applied to the spine. This pressure approximates 1.5 times the mean applied pressure over the entire area of the end-plate.[139] Knowledge of these pressures is of importance therapeutically when designing activity and exercise programs for patients with disk problems. Disk pressures have been extensively studied in various postures and seating configurations. A more detailed description can be found in other sources and will not be covered here.[3,5–13,64,66,67,70,71,126,127,129,131,133–137,139] The "preloaded" spinal column in the healthy nucleus maintains a continuous pressure to separate the adjacent vertebrae. This preloaded condition and the incompressibility of the nucleus serve to form a self-righting system in which, with a compressive force or angular movement in any direction, the resultant intradiskal pressure changes are such that the disk favors movement back to the "neutral" position. Note, however, that this self-righting system also depends on the tensile strength and the elasticity of the annulus. Tensile strength or stiffness must be provided in the horizontal direction in order to withstand the intermittent stresses applied to it from the nucleus. Elasticity of the annulus, and/or movement between adjacent planes of annular fibers, is necessary in a vertical direction to allow angular movement between adjacent vertebral bodies. Loss of a balance between this extensibility and stability of the annular fibers is probably a contributing factor in disk disorders.

In axial compression, the increased intradiskal pressure is counteracted by annular fiber tension and disk bulge, rather analogous to inflating a tire (Fig. 17–13A).[155] Some disk-space narrowing also occurs. Because of the incompressibility of the fluid-like nucleus, forces acting on the nucleus will act to move it, change its shape, or both. In flexion, extension, and lateral bending, the same process occurs. Because the annular fibers are somewhat elastic and because the annulus allows vertical and tangential movements between vertebral bodies, in the healthy disk the nucleus may either change in shape or move within the limits allowed by the annulus.[172] Its vol-

ume, however, must remain the same. Displacement of the nucleus within the disk has been disputed more recently.[66,99] Because the nucleus is roughly spherical, some have considered it as a ball that allows one vertebra to rotate over its neighbor. The nucleus is said to move backward during flexion and forward during extension. However, others have not confirmed this observation, and Krag and associates found little motion of the nucleus.[99]

In the consideration, then, of an angular movement forward (flexion) of one vertebral body on another in a weight-bearing situation, the forward shift of weight will result in an increased compressive force on the anterior aspect of the disk. This causes the anterior annular fibers to bulge backward and causes the nucleus to shift backward, transferring the vertical compressive force to a horizontally directed force backward against the posterior annulus (Fig. 17–13B). Because the healthy nucleus is fluid-like, an even distribution of pressure results across the inner annular layers. The posterior annular fibers, which are normally bulged somewhat backward in the neutral position, tend to straighten because of the increase in distance between the posterior vertebral bodies. However, because of the pressure against the posterior annulus from the nucleus, there is also a tendency to maintain this posterior bulge and thus bring the vertebrae back to a neutral relationship—the self-righting mechanism discussed earlier. Looking at it from another perspective, the straightening of the annular fibers tends to increase the counterpressure against the posteriorly bulging nucleus, which effects a counter force against the original vertical compressive force. In this way an equilibrium must be reached between the transformation of the vertical loading to a horizontal pressure against the annulus and the tendency for the annulus to reconvert this pressure, in a self-righting manner, to counter the compressive loading. In extension and lateral bending, the same process occurs (Fig. 17–13C, D). Of clinical significance is the fact that changes in this equilibrium favor pathologic changes in the related tissues, while, conversely, pathologic tissue changes result in a change in the equilibrium; the resultant cycle of events should be obvious. For example, a weakening of the annular fibers results in less tendency to resist the horizontal forces exerted by the nucleus, which will result in further weakening of the annulus. Osteoporosis of the vertebral bodies results in a decreased ability to withstand reactive vertical forces with erosion of disk material into the vertebral bodies; the so-called vacuum phenomenon.

In axial rotation, a compressive force causes an

Fig. 17–13. Nucleus pulposus: *(A)* during axial compression, *(B)* in spine flexion, *(C)* in spine extension, *(D)* in lateral bending, and *(E)* during axial rotation.

increase in intradiskal pressure and tends to narrow the joint space (Fig. 17–13E). When rotation occurs, the annular fibers—which are oriented in the direction of rotary movement—become taut, while the fibers oriented in the opposite direction tend to slacken. Mathematical models based on the geometry of the disk demonstrate that torsion produces stress concentration of the region of the posterior lateral annulus, which is a common site of disk herniation.[101,178] Torsional loading of spinal segments *in vitro* produces fissures in the annulus in the same posterolateral location and is thought to be one of the common early causes of acute low back pain.[156] During daily activities the disk is loaded in a complex manner, usually by a combination of compression, bending, and torsion. Flexion, extension, and lateral flexion of the spine produce mainly tensile and compressive stresses in the disk, whereas rotation produces shear stress. The tensile stress in the posterior part of the annulus fibrosus in the lumbar spine has been estimated to be four to five times the applied axial load.[54,131] The thoracic annuli fibrosi are subjected to less tensile stress than the lumbar annuli fibrosi because of their geometric difference. The ratio of disk diameter to height is higher in the thoracic disk than the lumbar disk.[104]

The entire intervertebral disk in the adult is avascular. Up to the time of skeletal maturity, blood vessels do enter the disk from the vertebral bodies through the cartilaginous end-plates. These vessels are gradually obliterated, leaving scars in the end-plate where they penetrated.

Intervertebral Foramina

The intervertebral foramen is the aperture that gives exit to the segmental spinal nerves and entrance to the vessel and nerve branches that supply the bone and soft tissues of the vertebral canal. This aperture or canal is superiorly and inferiorly bounded by the respective pedicles of the adjacent vertebrae (see Fig. 17–2). Its ventral and dorsal relations involve the two major intervertebral articulations. Ventrally it is bounded by the dorsum of the intervertebral disk, covered by the posterior longitudinal ligament, and dorsally by the capsule of the articular facet and ligamentum flavum (see Fig. 17–8A,C). Spur formation within the foramen can decrease the available space and create compression forces on the spinal nerves exiting through the foramen or on the structures that reenter the foramen, such as the sinuvertebral nerve, which innervates the posterior longitudinal ligament (see Vertebral Innervation, page 474).

Nerve-root entrapment may also result from clo-sure or narrowing of the vertebral foramen, through any of the following mechanisms: (1) approximation of the pedicles resulting from narrowing of the intervertebral disk; (2) hypertrophic degenerative arthritic changes of the articular facet joints; and (3) thickening of the ligamentum flavum. The existence of additional ligamentous elements in relation to the intervertebral foramen (*e.g.*, the transforaminal ligaments, found frequently in the lumbar region) could be critical.[24,166,167] The transforaminal ligaments are strong, unyielding cords of collagenous tissue that pass anteriorly from various parts of the neural arch to the body of the same or adjacent vertebra.

THE CONTROL SYSTEM: NONCONTRACTILE SOFT TISSUES

Ligaments

The ligaments are vital for the structural stability of the spinal system. Their principle role is to prevent excessive motion. The ligaments are also the principal tensile load-bearing elements and, along with the apophyseal capsules, provide the central nervous system with information in regard to posture and movement.[199] Unlike muscles, ligaments are passive structures so that their tension depends on their length. Ligaments are viscoelastic in nature, with their deformation and type of failure being dependent on the rate of loading. Like all materials, ligaments fatigue and can fail with repetitive loading.[155,190] They readily resist tensile forces but buckle when subject to compression.

The ligaments that connect the anterior elements of the spine are the broad *anterior longitudinal ligament*, which extends from the basiocciput to the sacrum, and the *posterior longitudinal ligament*, which also extends from the basiocciput to the sacrum on the anterior aspect of the neural canal, behind the vertebral bodies. These ligaments are interlinked at each level by the disk which adds support to the disk and vertebral body network (see Fig. 17–8). The annulus fibrosus of the intervertebral disk may be considered a part of the ligamentous structure. These ligaments deform with separation of the vertebrae and bulging of the disk.[194] Richly supported by nerve fibers, they respond to painful stimuli. The remaining ligaments of the spine support and link the posterior elements.

The anterior longitudinal ligament is one ligamentous structure placed anterior to the center of rotation of the intervertebral joint. It thus acts to prevent hyperextension, along with the capsular ligament of the articular facet joint (see Fig. 17–8). It begins as a rather narrow band from the basiocciput and broadens as it descends from C3 to the sacrum. It consists of long fibers along its length and short, arched fibers coursing between individual vertebrae and inserting into the anterior aspect of the intervertebral disk (see Fig. 17–18B).[91] Considered perhaps the strongest ligament in the body (with a tensile strength of nearly 3000 pounds per square inch), the anterior longitudinal ligament, along with the muscles about the spine, keeps a preload beam condition in the spine that helps to strengthen the spine during lifting.[43] In the lumbar spine it also resists the weight of the spine in its tendency to slip into the pelvic cavity.[149] Because of its breadth and tensile strength, this ligament provides strong support and reinforcement to the anterior disk during lifting, and Harrington and others have used the strength of the anterior ligament combined with Harrington rods to apply traction to fracture dislocations of the low back.[194]

The posterior longitudinal ligament extends from the basiocciput to the sacrum on the anterior aspect of the neural canal behind the vertebral bodies (see Fig. 17–8A,B,D). It is densely attached to the posterior annulus fibrosus at each level, with both vertical and transverse fibers that spread across the posterior annulus; however, as the posterior longitudinal ligament passes the vertebral bodies, it narrows and is not attached to them except at their margins.[166,167] This allows for the passage of the entrant arteries, veins, and lymphatics into and out of the posterior portion of the vertebral bodies. In flexion the posterior longitudinal ligament becomes taut and serves as a valve on these vessels, which do not have a valve mechanism of their own. It, like the anterior longitudinal ligament, is thickest in the thoracic (dorsal) spine. It is often reduced to a cordshaped filament in the lumbar spine. The lateral expansions over the disks are thin, whereas the central portions are much thicker. This is presumably why most posterior protrusions of the disk soon move laterally to become posterolateral protrusions. Although the posterior longitudinal ligament is not as massive as the anterior longitudinal ligament in terms of cross-sectional area, the tensile strength per unit area seems to be the same for both structures.[183] Functionally, the ligament limits forward bending and gives support to the disks, except in the lumbar region. Of interest is that in the midline the ligament does have a small amount of elastic tissue.[149] In the cervical spine the ligament is a broad band on the entire posterior aspect of the bodies, but because it is attached only in the region of the disk, with disk degeneration it produces folds that can press into the spinal canal on backward bending; this movement is therefore to be avoided in such conditions.

The segmental ligaments of the spine include the *ligamentum flavum*, the *interspinous* and *intertransverse ligaments*, and the *anterior and posterior capsular ligaments of the articular facet joints*. The biomechanical significance of these structures depends on their strength, stiffness, and distance from the axis of rotation of the joints they span.[194]

The ligamentum flavum extends from the anteroinferior border of the laminae above to the posterior border of the laminae below (see Fig. 17–8B,C,D). It connects the laminae from C2 to S1. The medial edges fuse with the contralateral ligament in midline and completely close the vertebral canal (a slight septum is provided for the passage of arteries and veins). At its lateral border, the ligamentum flavum blends with the capsules of the articular facets, particularly in the lumbar region (see Fig. 17–8B,C).[78] Histologically, the ligamentum flavum has the highest percentage of elastic fibers of any tissue in the body.[23,138] It checks the movement of the articular facet joints by exerting a constant pull on the capsule and thus assists in preventing the synovial lining and intra-articular menisci from being painfully nipped between the articular joint surfaces.[149] It owes much of this function to its yellow elastic fibers (hence, *flavum*).

During forward bending the ligamentum flavum permits considerable range and assists in return to neutral or the rest position of the spinal segments without the development of folds. It thus serves to protect the spinal canal from encroachment by soft tissues on flexion and extension. Nachemson and Evans found that in neutral the ligamentum flavum is prestrained by about 15% and that full physiological flexion can stretch it an additional 30% to 35%, while it retains a 5% stretch in full physiological extension.[138] This elasticity is lost to some extent in normal aging, but if the instant axis of rotation for flexion is in the region of the posterior annulus, the flexion–extension torque resistance in the ligamentum flavum is significant. There is appreciable strain of the ligamentum flavum on sidebending or lateral flexion.[147] The ligamentum flavum also provides some preloading of the disk (leading to disk nucleus pressures greater than atmospheric), even when there is no external load on the spine, which may reduce slack in the motion segment. In patients with severe spine degeneration, the ligamentum flavum may be thickened and less elastic and may produce narrowing of the spinal canal in extension. This narrowing occurs because of the buckling of the ligament. Thus, at the time of surgery for spinal stenosis, its excision may be necessary.

The intertransverse ligaments are well developed in the thoracic spine and are intimately connected with the deep muscles of the back.[194] They pass between the transverse processes and are characterized as rounded cords. These ligaments are barely mentioned in many texts on functional anatomy, particularly with respect to the lumbar spine, as being significant. Functionally, they tend to limit side-bending and rotation.

The interspinous ligaments, which connect the spinous processes, are important for the stability of the spinal column. They are reinforced, especially at the level of the thoracic and lumbar spine, by the supraspinous ligaments (see Fig. 17–8C,D). Their attachments extend from the root to the apex of each spinous process, proceeding in an upward and backward direction, *not* an upward and foreword direction, as often illustrated.[149] This upward and backward orientation permits increased range of motion during flexion while still resisting excessive range. Panjabi and associates found high strain in both the interspinous and supraspinous ligaments with flexion while these where relatively unstrained in rotation.[147] The interspinous ligaments are narrow and elongated in the thoracic region, only slightly developed in the cervical spine, and thicker in the lumbar spine.[194] In 90% of cadavers aged more than 40 years, Rissanen noted that the interspinous ligament between L4 and L5 had degenerated or was completely ruptured.[162]

The supraspinous ligament is a strong fibrous cord which connects the apices of the spines from the C7 to L4, and occasionally to L5 (see Fig. 17–8C, D).[149] At this level it is replaced by the interlocking fibers of the somewhat stronger erector spinae tendons of insertion. The supraspinous ligament is thicker and broader in the lumbar region than the thoracic, and it is intimately blended in both areas with the neighboring fascia. Between the spine of C7 and the external occipital protuberance, it is much expanded and called the *ligamentum nuchae* (see Fig. 18–4).[186] In the cervical region the spinous processes are buried deeply between the heavy muscles on the back of the neck so that the supraspinous ligament is represented by a thin septum between the musculature of the two sides. In quadrupeds with heavy heads, the ligamentum nuchae is a strong, thick band of elastic tissue and aids the muscles in holding up the head.[79] In humans, however, the supraspinous and interspinous ligaments and the ligamentum nuchae are largely collagenous tissue, relatively inelastic and of little strength; in the cervical and lumbar regions, where they should be most important in limiting segmental flexion, the interspinous ligaments are frequently defective or lacking in one or several interspaces.[79] Because the supraspinous ligament is the most superficial of the spinal ligaments and farthest from the axis of flexion it has a greater potential for sprains.[91]

Fascial Anatomy

Thoracolumbar Region. Although not technically a ligament, the thoracolumbar (lumbodorsal) fascia has a tensile strength of nearly 2000 pounds per square inch and serves as one of the most important noncontractile structures in the lumbar spine (see Fig. 17–14A).[44] In the lower thoracic and lumbar regions this fascia is much thicker than the rest of the spinal area, for it represents not only fascial tissue but the fused aponeuroses of several muscles.[79] It functions in many respects as a ligament, as it invests epaxial muscles that course along the spinous processes and is reinforced by the aponeurotic origin of the latissimus dorsi cranially and by the attachment of the erector spinae (epaxial paravertebral) muscle mass caudally into the sacrum and sacral ligaments. It spans the area from the iliac crest and sacrum up to the thoracic cage. The posterior layer is reinforced by the latissimus dorsi superficially and by the attachment of the sacrospinalis to its deep surface. The fascial aponeurotic sheet encloses the erector spinae muscle mass between the thoracic spines and the interspinous ligaments medially, and the laminae and ligamentum flavum anteriorly. Because the thorocolumbar fascia encloses a space on each side of the spine, contraction of the erector spinae muscle mass (with a consequent increase in the transverse muscle area) tends to greatly tighten the thoracolumbar fascia, so that it functions as part of an active mechanism for pulling the vertebrae posteriorly and controlling shear and flexion during lifting. On full flexion, as the muscles become electrically silent, the thoracolumbar fascia becomes the major force against further flexion.[113] On extension from a fully flexed position the gluteus maximus and hamstrings act in concert with the thoracolumbar fascia to initiate extension.[59] With increased activity of these muscles the fascia serves to increase their efficiency.[61] It also serves as a protective ligament against excessive flexion and as the muscle mass contracts, the increased diameter of the muscle exerts a wedging effect on the aponeurosis, which may relieve some of the shear load on the articular facet joints and disks in flexion–extension movements of the spine.[44] It has been further demonstrated on the basis of dissections and histological observations that the muscles of the abdomen have the potential to stabilize the vertebral column through the action of the thoracolumbar fascia. This

A

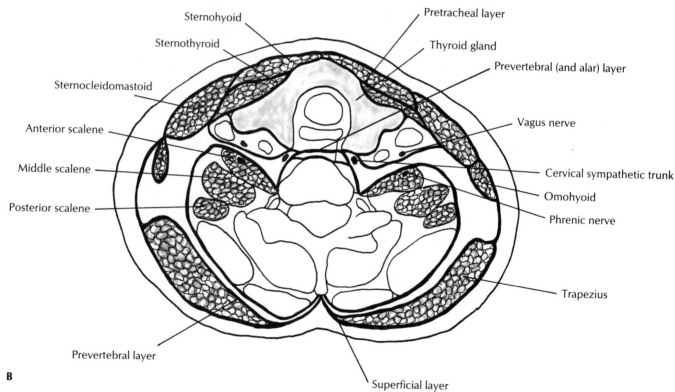

B

Fig. 17–14. *(A)* The thoracolumbar fascia, *(B)* a cross section of the neck, and *(C)* a longitudinal section of the fascial layers of the neck.

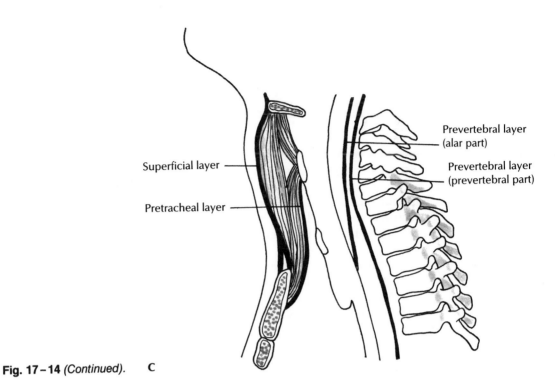

Fig. 17–14 *(Continued).* **C**

can be brought about, according to Tesh and associates, by (1) the intrinsic nature of the fascia without direct involvement of the vertebral ligaments; (2) muscle contraction modifying longitudinal ligament tension by the thoracolumbar fascia; or (3) a combination of both mechanisms.[182]

Cervical Region. The cervical spine, with its investing musculature, is housed within the vertebral compartment, situated centrally and posteriorly. The contents of this compartment provide points of anchorage and suspension for fascial layers defining all remaining compartments (see Fig. 17–14B).[105] Though these fascial layers provide stabilization to their contents, they are normally sufficiently lax to permit motion of the neck as a unit, as well as motion of one compartment relative to one another.

Prevertebral Fascia. The prevertebral fascia (see Fig. 17–14B,C) is a firm membrane lying anteriorly to the prevertebral muscles (longus colli, longus capitis, anterior, middle and posterior scalenes, and rectus capitis). It is attached to the base of the skull just anterior to the capitis muscles and descends downward and laterally to ultimately blend with the fascia of the trapezius muscles. In its course it covers the scalene muscles and also binds down the subclavian artery and the three trunks of the brachial plexus. The prevertebral fascia crosses medially to the transverse processes of the cervical vertebrae and covers all the cervical nerve roots. The fascia does not ensheath the subclavian or axillary veins, and therefore does not cause venous congestion. The fascia is firmly adherent to the anterior aspects of the cervical vertebrae. In the posture causing scapulocostal syndrome symptoms, the depressed scapula places strain on the fascia as well as the scapular musculature.[24] Obliteration of the radial pulse, as observed in Adson's maneuver, can be attributed to the tension of the cervical fascia on rotation of the head and neck. Traction on the lower trunk of the brachial plexus may well cause pain and numbness in the ulnar distribution of the hand, which is common in this syndrome.[185]

Capsules

The joint capsule of the spinal articular facet joints is composed of two layers, an outer layer known as the *stratum fibrosum* and an inner layer called the *stratum synovium.* The outer layer is attached to the periosteum of the component bone by Sharpey's fibers and is reinforced by musculotendinous and ligamentous structures that cross the joint. The outer layer is poorly vascularized but richly innervated. The nerve endings that are located in and around the joint capsule are sensitive to the rate and direction of motion tension and to compression and vibration.[68]

In contrast to the outer layer, the inner layer of the capsule is highly vascularized but poorly innervated.[76] The stratum synovium is insensitive to pain but undergoes vasodilatation and vasoconstriction in response to heat and cold. It produces the hyaluronic acid component of the synovial fluid and serves as an entry point for nutrients and an exit point for waste material.[76] The capsules of the articular facet joints possess two noteworthy recesses, one superior and one inferior, through which the synovium may distend during effusion or backward bending.[38,115] The superior recess is the weaker, and effusion here may protrude sufficiently to press on the mixed spinal nerve as it enters the intervertebral foramen.[38]

Capsules encompass all the articular facet joints in the spine including the articulation of the head with the atlas.[127] The capsules include separate thickenings which have different functional roles. The capsules and their ligaments guide and restrict the motion segments. Because they are far from the disks and therefore act on long moment arms, these ligaments have an important functional role in resisting spinal flexion.[155] In full flexion of the lumbar spine, the capsules support 40% of the body weight.[59] These fibers are generally oriented in a direction perpendicular to the plane of the articular facet joints. They are broader and more taut in the cervical region than the rest of the spine.[147] The capsules of the lumbar spine, which are often illustrated as being short and bunchy, in fact have a considerable medial extent and are quite fibrous, possessing an upward and medial direction that ideally suits them to restricting forward bending.[149] The capsular ligaments, along with the anterior longitudinal ligament, also act to prevent hyperextension of the spine.[44] Capsules are an important consideration with respect to the loose- and close-packed positions of the articular facet joints of the spine.[33,59] The concept of loose- and close-packed positions is useful in understanding when a joint may be less stable and more vulnerable. Loose-packed positions are those positions in a joint's range of motion in which the ligaments and capsules are slack; the area in contact with the articular surfaces are generally low and the joints are more vulnerable and less able to resist an external force. Close-packed positions, on the other hand, are those in which there is maximum contact between articular surfaces and maximum tautness of the ligaments.[14] The close-packed position of the articular facet joints from C3 to L5 is extension, whereas the close-packed position for the atlas and axis is full flexion.[59] The close-packed position is often lost following a pathologic process, trauma, or prolonged periods of poor posture. Inability to assume a full close-packed position results in the potential for increased dysfunction and, as a result, a more unstable, loose-packed position is maintained.

Vertebral Innervation

Because of the high frequency of patients presenting clinically with complaints of spinal pain or pain appearing to be of spinal origin, it is necessary for the clinician to have a thorough knowledge of spinal innervation. More specifically, the clinician must be aware of what structures appear to lack innervation totally. This information must be combined with an understanding of common pathologic processes and their clinical manifestations. In this way a more reliable judgment may be made as to the nature and extent of various disorders, and perhaps a better understanding of the often bizarre symptoms and signs that result.

Information relating to spinal innervation and pain-sensitive spinal tissues has come from two types of investigations: (1) actual experiments with human subjects in which attempts are made to isolate noxious stimuli to a particular tissue; and (2) laboratory tissue studies in which sensory endings are identified and attempts are made to trace the afferent pathways from these endings to central connections. For obvious reasons, those studies belonging to the first category of investigation are relatively few and results have at times been inconsistent or highly criticized. There have been numerous studies of the second type, however, and the results, for the most part, seem to be consistent. One must realize, though, that there is a limit as to how much can be inferred from tissue studies with respect to clinical significance. This is especially true when considering pain-sensitive tissue, because there is no direct correlation between the type of ending found within a particular tissue and the capacity for the tissue, when stimulated, to send signals to higher centers which result in the perception of pain (see Chapter 3, Pain). Presented here will be a summary of what seem to be reasonably well-accepted findings relating to spinal neurology. Spinal structures receive innervation largely from two sources, the sinuvertebral (recurrent meningeal) nerves and the medial branches of the posterior primary divisions of the segmental spinal nerves (Fig. 17–15A, B). Endings found in the dura mater and blood vessels are primarily of the free nerve plexus type (see Chapter 2, Arthrology). Endings found in the posterior longitudinal ligament and periosteum include free nerve endings and plexuses as well as encapsulated and nonencapsulated

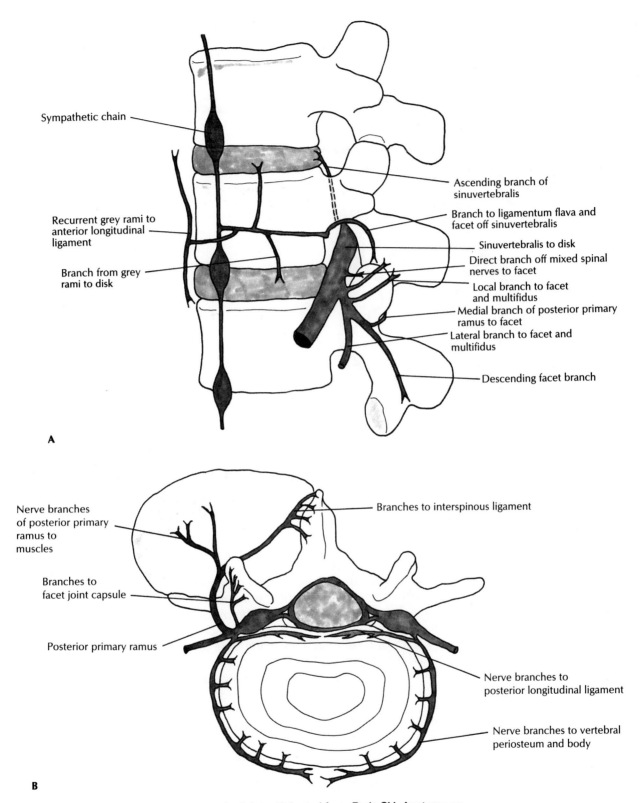

Sympathetic chain

Recurrent grey rami to anterior longitudinal ligament

Branch from grey rami to disk

Ascending branch of sinuvertebralis

Branch to ligamentum flava and facet off sinuvertebralis

Sinuvertebralis to disk

Direct branch off mixed spinal nerves to facet

Local branch to facet and multifidus

Medial branch of posterior primary ramus to facet

Lateral branch to facet and multifidus

Descending facet branch

A

Nerve branches of posterior primary ramus to muscles

Branches to facet joint capsule

Posterior primary ramus

Branches to interspinous ligament

Nerve branches to posterior longitudinal ligament

Nerve branches to vertebral periosteum and body

B

Fig. 17–15. *(A)* Innervation of the posterior joints. (Adapted from Paris SV: Anatomy as related to function and pain. Orthop Clin North Am 14:476, 486, 1983.) *(B)* Innervation of the spinal structures.

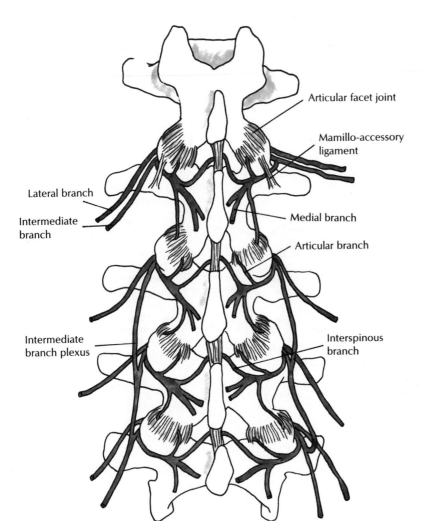

Articular facet joint

Mamillo-accessory ligament

Lateral branch

Intermediate branch

Medial branch

Articular branch

Intermediate branch plexus

Interspinous branch

Fig. 17–16. Posterior view of the branches of the lumbar posterior rami. The mamillo-accessory ligament has been left *in situ* covering the L2 medial branch.

nerve endings. It is assumed that the larger encapsulated nerve endings act primarily as mechanoreceptors. It is important to realize that each sinuvertebral nerve tends to innervate the tissues at its own level as well as sending ascending and descending branches to levels above and below (Fig. 17–15A). It follows that stimulation of endings supplied by a particular sinuvertebral nerve may result in the perception of pain or in reflex changes in muscle tone at levels of the spine other than the level at which the lesion lies. Also, because it is well documented that stimulation of deep somatic tissues often results in segmentally referred pain, we might assume that pain may be referred into a segment not corresponding to the vertebral segment (level) at which the lesion lies.

The posterior division of the spinal nerve divides into lateral, intermediate, and medial branches (see Fig. 17–16). The lateral branch innervates the skin and deep muscles of the back segmentally, while the medial branch innervates the articular facet joint

capsules, the posterior aspect of the ligamentum flavum, the interspinous ligaments, the supraspinous ligaments, and the blood vessels supplying the vertebrae. The medial branches of the posterior division also send ascending and descending branches to (usually) one level above and one level below, with the same clinical implications as discussed for the overlapping sinuvertebral nerves. Receptors found in the facet joint capsules, sending signals along the medial branch of the posterior division, include all four of the receptors discussed in the section on joint neurology (see Chapter 2, Arthrology).

Afferent fibers from both the sinuvertebral nerve and the medial branch of the posterior primary division approach the spinal cord through the dorsal roots. In the dorsal roots the small unmyelinated fibers, thought to be largely responsible for transmission of noxious stimuli, aggregate toward the anterior aspect of the dorsal root. These enter the spinal cord, sending branches to Lissauer's tract in which they may ascend or descend for a few segments before sending fibers to the substantia gelatinosa at the tip of the dorsal horn (see Chapter 3, Pain). Other fibers may pass directly to the base of the dorsal horn of the grey matter. From here they may ascend along the spinoreticulothalamic tract, or through internuncial neurons, and synapse with alpha motor neurons of segmentally related muscles (see Fig. 17–15A). In this way, noxious stimulation of sensitive spinal tissues may result in reflex muscle spasm (or perhaps inhibition) of segmentally related muscles. Thus muscle spasms, which are often a part of this clinical syndrome, may result from this proposed pathway or by yet undetermined sensory or motor-reflex pathways.[53] Note again that because of the overlapping distribution of sensory fibers, muscles of more than one segment are likely to be affected. The previously mentioned ascending tract tends to cross within a few segments before ascending, with only a few ascending ipsilaterally. Signals traveling along this tract are thought to contribute to the conscious awareness of pain.

The larger-diameter afferent fibers reach the spinal cord through the posterior rami of the dorsal roots. These contribute to the dorsal columns of the spinal cord, which supply information to higher centers, including proprioceptive and "fast-pain" input. Other large fibers synapse at the tip of the dorsal horn of the gray matter, the substantia gelatinosa, to contribute to modulation of afferent input to higher centers, as discussed in Chapter 3, Pain. Recall, however, that ultimate perception of pain is, in part, determined by the relative balance of large-fiber and small-fiber input to the substantia gelatinosa, and that an imbalance in favor of small-fiber input tends to facilitate pain perception.

Selective stimulation of spinal structures has been carried out in a number of investigations. These studies include distention of normal and pathologic disks, needling of various aspects of intervertebral disks, injection of hypertonic saline into interspinous ligaments, injections of facet joints, and mechanical stimulation of nerve roots and other structures during surgery carried out under local anesthesia. Back pain can be reproduced by injecting hypertonic saline into the supraspinatus, interspinous, and longitudinal ligaments; the ligamentum flavum; and facet capsules.[77,107,117] These structures and the peripheral third of the annulus fibrosus are innervated by nociceptive nerve fibers, which are afferent branches of the posterior primary rami.[19,200] The studies in which the intervertebral disks were distended by injection of dye during diskography suggests that, indeed, pain can result from

distention of the disk. It is noted that in most cases distention of a pathological degenerated or protruded disk resulted in much more severe pain than injection of a normal disk. In most cases pain was referred into the shoulder or hip girdles with cervical and lumbar injections, respectively, and often into the limbs. It was usually described as a deep, aching, poorly localized pain, whereas direct stimulation of a nerve root tends to result in a sharp, lancinating pain well localized to the related dermatome. On the basis of such findings, Rothman and Simeone distinguish between scleratogenous pain of spinal origin and neurogenic pain.[166,167] The former usually results from stimulation of the sinuvertebral nerve from a nuclear protrusion, putting abnormal mechanical pressure on the outer annular layers and/or the posterior longitudinal ligament. This results in a deep, aching, somewhat diffuse pain which may be referred to any part, or all, of the relevant sclerotome(s). Neurogenic pain is that of sharp, well-localized pain felt in a dermatomal distribution, resulting from actual nerve-root pressure.

Studies also show the spinal joints to be sensitive to pain.[199] Because the fibrous capsule is a primary pain-sensitive structure of the spinal joints, as it is in the peripheral joints, conditions that stretch, pinch, or otherwise stimulate the articular facet joint capsule may potentially cause pain. Pain elicited from joint stimulation also tends to be diffuse and poorly localized and may be referred into the related segment(s), keeping in mind the overlapping distribution of the medial branches of the posterior primary divisions.

THE CONTROL SYSTEM: CONTRACTILE TISSUES

Contractile Tissue Common to Most Areas of the Spine

The spinal column is the vertical supporting structure of the body and the only rigid link between the upper and lower parts of the body. However, this structure is in itself unstable and so is supported by the major trunk muscles, which act as guidewires to prevent excessive movement in a direction of inbalance. Gregerson and Lucas showed how an excised spine, with the ligaments intact but without muscles, buckles under even very small compressive forces whereas a muscled spine can, with abdominal support, carry the weight of the trunk, head, and upper extremities in addition to hundreds of added pounds.[63] These muscles also contract to produce motion of the trunk against the forces of gravity and may play a role in protecting the spine during trauma, if there is time for voluntary control, and possibly in the post-injury phase.[194] From a preventive and therapeutic standpoint, the muscles are very important structures of the spine. Under voluntary control they position the spine and stabilize it during awkward postures and provide the power necessary for lifting and carrying. Chaffin has demonstrated that workers with inadequate lifting strength working in relatively stressful lifting tasks have higher low-back injury rates than workers with equally stressful lifting tasks but better strength.[25] Apparently when lifting near the strength limit of these muscles, excessive strain may be transmitted to the other soft tissues, such as ligaments and disks.

The proper functioning of the mobile segment demands perfect synergy of the different muscles. A movement that is not anticipated or is poorly estimated can bring about a harmful distribution of forces on the intervertebral joints. Certain elements of the joints may be submitted to traction or compression forces beyond their capacity for resistance. Spasms of these muscles undoubtedly constitute a major factor in the genesis of the painful spine, susceptible to treatment by manual therapy.

The motor elements of the mobile segment comprise short and long paraspinal muscles. The former exert their action directly, whereas the latter act indirectly by affecting distal segments. These muscles are innervated by the posterior branches of the spinal nerves, which thus play a very important part in invertebral mechanical pathologic processes. Only a brief description of the musculature is appropriate here.

The posterior (epaxial) muscles in humans are organized in three planes with the shortest (myomeric) muscles being the deepest (see Chapter 1, Embryology of the Musculoskeletal System). The semispinalis, multifidi, and rotatores, although they have different sources, are often called the *tranversospinalis muscles* (Fig. 17–17). There are clearly fibers that course from spinous process to adjacent transverse process (interspinous); from transverse process to adjacent transverse process (intertransversalis); from transverse process to spinous process (multifidus), from transverse processes below to laminae above (musculi rotatores), and, in the thoracic region, from transverse processes to ribs (musculi levatores costrum).

The intermediate layer of the posterior musculature is masssive and courses from transverse process to spinous processes two to four segments above (multifidi) or multisegmentally (see Fig. 17–17). According to their regions, they are the multifidus (lumbosacral), thoracis, semispinalis cervicis, and semispinalis capitis (cervical). The deep and intermediate layers are of most interest to the motion segment. Of particular interest in the lumbosacral region is the complex multifidus. The multifidus is bipennate in both origin and insertion and is functionally significant with respect to its posterior insertion to the capsule of the articular facet joint.[149] Overlying the multifidi are the longer and more lateral muscles that arise from the sacrum and adjacent connections to insert on the lower six or seven ribs (iliocostalis) and the longest and most medial muscles that share the same origin but insert into the medial portions of the nine or ten lowest ribs and the transverse processes of the lower thoracic vertebrae (longissimus) (Fig. 17–18). These superficial and posterior muscles are collectively called the *erector spinae*. The active function of these muscles working together is to extend and stabilize the spine, while in groups they can rotate or sidebend it, often working with muscles in other groups.

The rotator muscles, although present at other levels, are most prominent in the thoracic region.[70] These muscles bring about rotation of the vertebrae in the direction opposite the side of the muscle and have a sensory role in monitoring rotation. Morris and colleagues found the longissimus thoracis and rotatores spinae to be continuously active during standing.[129] The trapezius and latissimus dorsi are common to most areas of the spine (Fig. 17–19, and see Fig. 18–6). Combined, the origin of the trapezius and latissimus dorsi span the entire spine from occiput to sacrum. The trapezius spans from the occiput to T12 and the latissimus overlaps the six segments from T6 to the sacrum. The trapezius then inserts on the stable portion of the shoulder complex (the scapula), whereas the latissimus dorsi inserts onto the mobile humerus. Together they act to position the shoulder and retract it during lifting, spreading the load of the upper extremity across the entire span rather than concentrating the force in the upper thoracic region.[59] The latissimus dorsi also produces extension of the lumbar spine, along with the serratus posterior. In addition, it acts in concert with the transverse abdominus, internal oblique, and gluteus maximus muscles as a dynamic stabilizer of the low back, by way of their attachments to the lumbodorsal fasciae or aponeuroses (see page 471). The trapezius also serves as one of the suspensor motors of the shoulder girdle, along with the rhomboids and the levator scapulae (see Fig. 18–6). These muscles, taking origin from the cervical and thoracic spine, suspend and mobilize the scapula and thereby link cervical and thoracic spine motions with upper limb motions.[105]

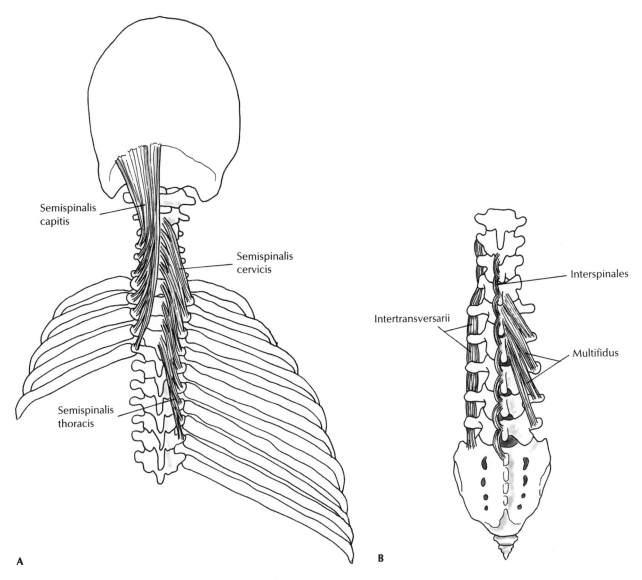

Fig. 17–17. Deep muscles of the back. The medial group (the transversospinalis, interspinalis, and intertransversarii) includes *(A)* the semispinalis (head, neck, and thoracic sections), and *(B)* the intertransversarii, interspinales, and multifidus. (*Note:* These muscles are only partially illustrated in each section so their relation to the bony structures of the spine can be seen.)

Muscles of the Thoracolumbar Spine

The lateral muscles of the trunk originate from the hypaxial portion of the lateral mesoderm, the quadratus lumborum, and psoas. The quadratus is the more posterior and is complex, filling the space between the iliac crest and the twelfth rib, while also attaching to the transverse processes of the lumbar vertebrae. It is a primary lateral bender of the lumbar vertebrae assisted by the psoas muscle. It is also described as a "hip hiker" that is active on gait, during the swing phase, to hold the pelvis in a neutral position.[82] If painfully restricted, it can limit chest or rib cage expansion and can contribute to a leg-length discrepancy.

The psoas is more ventral and is considered, by some, primarily a limb muscle,[79] but as Michele has stated, it is also a potential extensor of the spine and a flexor of the lumbar spine on the pelvis depending on the relative positions of the spine, pelvis, and femur.[122] The psoas major arises from the anterolateral aspect of the lumbar vertebral bodies and transverse processes, then crosses the hip before inserting with the iliacus on the lesser trochanter. The psoas minor (not always present) lies ventral to the psoas major and courses from the vertebrae of the thora-

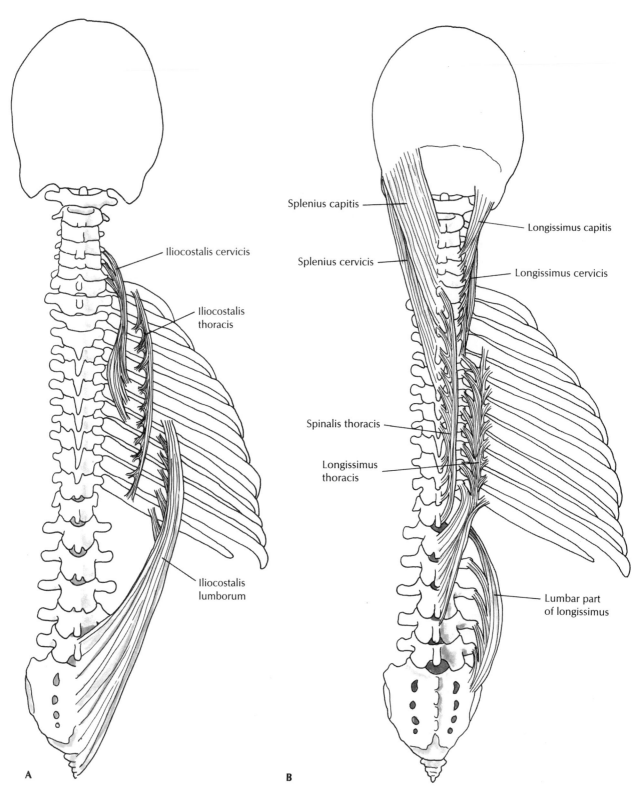

Iliocostalis cervicis

Iliocostalis thoracis

Iliocostalis lumborum

Splenius capitis

Splenius cervicis

Longissimus capitis

Longissimus cervicis

Spinalis thoracis

Longissimus thoracis

Lumbar part of longissimus

A

B

Fig. 17-18. Deep muscles of the back. The lateral group (erector spinae and the splenius) includes *(A)* the iliocostalis (cervical, thoracic, and lumbar sections) and *(B)* the longissimus (head and neck sections), splenius (head and neck sections), and the spinalis thoracis. *(Note:* These muscles are only partially illustrated in each section so their relation to the bony structures of the spine and ribs can be seen.)

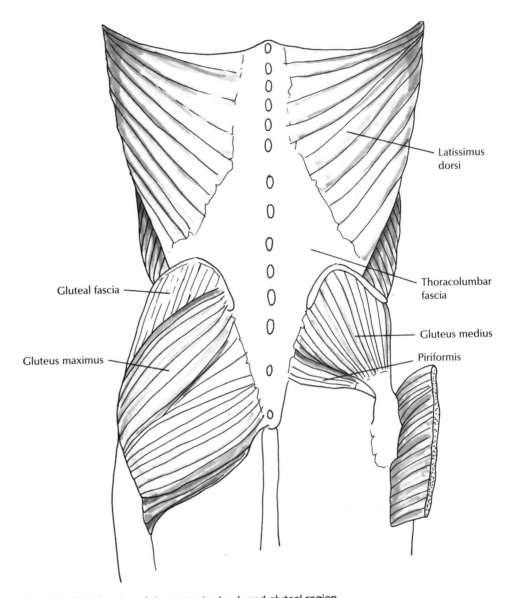

Fig. 17–19. Muscles of the posterior back and gluteal region.

columbar junction to insert on the superior pubis ramus, which allows it to work with the abdominal muscles in upward tilting of the pelvis.

The extensive fascial attachment of the gluteus maximus muscle, both at its origin and insertion, is well known (see Fig. 17–19). The crescent-shaped origin has widespread bony aponeurotic and ligamentous attachments. Approximately two thirds of the gluteus maximus muscle ends in a thick tendinous lamina, which inserts into the iliotibial band of the fascia lata. This offers strong control of the lower extremity during stressful activity. A comparison of the magnitude of action potentials elicited in the gluteus maximus muscle during a variety of exercises and activities demonstrates that the greatest

electrical activity occurs during muscle-setting contractions; these include exercises of hyperextension of the thigh accompanied by resistance, external rotation or abduction, and vigorous hyperextension of the trunk from the erect position.[48] The muscle seems to lack a major postural function in symmetrical upright positions at rest. Rotation of the trunk in a standing position activates the gluteus maximus contralateral to the direction of rotation, which is the corresponding function as an outward rotator of the leg when the trunk is flexed. Anteflexion of the trunk in the hip joint is attended by gluteus maximus activity, whose function probably is to fix the pelvis in its anteverted attitude.[92] Extension of the flexed thigh is performed primarily by action of the hamstrings, while extension beyond the relaxed standing position is associated with strong contraction of the gluteus maximus. EMG studies recorded during lifting activities indicate that hamstrings are activated earlier and to a greater extent during straight-knee lifts than during flexed-knee lifts. In contrast, the gluteus maximus and adductor magnus are more activated initially in the flexed-knee lift than the straight-leg lift.[48,140,141,150]

The human abdominal wall is developed from the body wall portion of the hyaxial mass of the lateral embryonic mesoderm. The two paired rectus muscles run alongside the midline from the sternum and costal cartilages to the pubis and, although they flex the spine powerfully, they do not increase interabdominal pressure. The transverse abdominus is the deepest of the lateral abdominal muscles, and runs from the lumbar vertebrae forward around the abdominal wall to merge with the contralateral transverse abdominus. In the lower abdomen the lower fibers of the transverse abdominus and those of the internal oblique muscle form the conjoint tendon. The transversus has a major role in developing intra-abdominal pressure and is an important tie between the muscle–fascia column formed anteriorly by the rectus abdominus and posteriorly by the sacrospinalis muscles and the thoracolumbar fascia.[70] The internal oblique muscle is the intermediate layer and has its fibers from the iliac crest to the lower ribs and the lateral margin of the rectus sheath oriented to flex the trunk and turn the upper body to the contracting side. The external oblique muscle is the most superficial abdominal muscle layer, and its fibers also run from the lower ribs to the rectus, the pubis, and the iliac crest. However, these fibers flex and rotate the trunk away from the side that is contracting. When the oblique muscles contract bilaterally and symmetrically, they also raise the intra-abdominal pressure[155] (see Other Support Structures, p. 483).

There is a fair concurrence of opinion about muscular activity in human posture based on EMG studies by many investigators.[44,79,132,194] Briefly, the activity of the lumbar spine muscles is low in relaxed standing and alternates with low levels of activity during body sway. There seems to be somewhat more constant activity in the paralumbar portion of the psoas major, both in standing and sitting, which provides additional preload to the spine and helps to maintain normal lumbar lordosis. Roentgenographic studies have shown that the line of gravity in most adults is 1 cm ventral to the center of L4, and that gravity would tend to straighten the lumbar spine without psoas activity. There is a small increase in activity of the lumbar spine muscles in sitting compared with standing. In the unsupported sitting posture, the muscle activity in the lumbar region was found to be about the same as that in the standing posture. In the thoracic region, Anderson and Örtengren found higher activity of the back muscles compared with that found in the standing posture.[5,7] These low levels of muscle activity imply that posture is maintained partly by active muscle contraction and partly by ligamentous and noncontractile support.

The lack of significant activity in the pelvic portion of the psoas major means that truncal equilibrium over the pelvis is fairly stable and is maintained by the strong ligaments anterior to this joint, as is also the case at the knee and sacroiliac joints. The line of force clearly falls behind the hip and in front of the knee, and there is no activity in the glutei at rest either.

During flexion from standing to sitting the glutei and erectors are active until full flexion is reached, at which time they are again quiet. They are active while initiating extension, and again at full extension. As the erector spinae muscles grade the rate of flexion, so do the abdominal muscles grade the rate of extension. During rotation, the longer erector muscles on the ipsilateral side, the short rotators and multifidi on the contralateral side, and the glutei on both sides are active, as is the tensor fascia lata on the ipsilateral side. Although the internal oblique muscles could assist with this motion, there is little abdominal activity in active rotation without resistance. Return to neutral is accomplished without significant muscular activity, evidently recovering some of the deforming force stored in the soft tissue. Sidebending is accomplished with ipsilateral activity of the back muscles unless the person is very tall and limber or is supporting external weight, in which case the contralateral muscles become active as soon as the equilibrium position is overcome by ipsilateral contraction.

A number of studies have scrutinized muscular function in control of the spine.* Several of the more recent studies have also reported results in patients with back disorders.† Most would concede the importance of muscular function both during posture and functional activities. Whether or not injury to these muscles is a common cause of spinal pain is still controversial.

---

* See references 3, 5–13, 15, 22, 49, 58, 83–89, 129, 130, 143–145, 147, 150, 158, 176, 187, 197, 198.
† See references 18, 29, 32, 49, 58, 60, 80, 102, 119, 155, 159, 173, 176, 177, 198.

Muscles of the Cervical Spine

In the cervical area special attention must be paid to a balance of the length and strength of posterior, anterior, and lateral musculature that control head-on-neck and neck-on-thorax movements.[91] The muscles of the cervical spine may be categorized into four groups: (1) cervicocapital motors; (2) visceral motors; (3) suspensor motors of the first ribs; and (4) suspensor motors of the shoulder girdle.[105] The cervicocapital motors consist of three groups, all of which move the cervical spine and skull. The first of these groups lies extrinsically to the spine, passing from the shoulder girdle to the skull in peripheral regions of the neck, producing primary motion of the head on the neck. The major members of this group are the sternocleidomastoid muscles (see Fig. 18–8). The sternocleidomastoid is especially important with respect to the position of the head and, when restricted, facilitates a forward head position and limits rotation toward the side of the tight muscle. The remaining two groups of cervicocapitals have origins directly from the spine and insertions onto either the spine or skull, and thus are intrinsic to the spine. They occur in right and left pairs and act to rotate and tilt the head and neck. One of these groups is located entirely anteriorly and includes the longus muscles (thoracis, cervicis, and capitis). When its members contract in concert, flexion occurs. The longus capitis and the longus colli (see Fig. 18–10) lie deep to the esophagus and are positioned in such a way that head and neck flexion and extension, rotation, and sidebending are resisted or assisted by the oblique or vertical fibers that make up these muscles.[91] The cervicocapital muscles are located entirely posteriorly, comprising the erector spinae and splenius muscles, which produce head and neck extension, often acting in concert (see Figs. 17–18, 18–6).

These long cervicocapital motors are supplemented by smaller muscles in the atlantoaxial region, which produce discrete motion (or fine tuning) of the structures in this special region (see Fig. 18–7). The four muscles that comprise the suboccipitals are the rectus major and minor and the obliquus superior and inferior. The rectus minor and the obliquus superior originate on the atlas and insert on the occiput. This places them in a good position to monitor and move the head into extension. The rectus major and the obliquus inferior act to move the head and C1 in rotation and are important in small neck movements (see Chapter 18, The Cervical Spine).

The visceral motors of the neck include those muscles associated with the pharynx, larynx, trachea, hyoid bone, thyroid bone, and thyroid gland. The suspensor motors of the first ribs are the scalene muscles, which pass from the spine to cover the domes of the thoracic cavities, thus they have an intimate relationship with vessels emerging to supply the head and upper limbs (see Fig. 18–8). The brachial plexus gains access to the thoracic outlet region by separating the muscle bundles of the scaleni. The scalene muscles, if unable to maintain their proper length, have a constrictive effect on the subclavian artery and veins as well as on the brachial plexus, all of which exit from the thoracic cavity and neck to the upper extremity.[70]

The suspensor motors of the shoulder girdle include the trapezius, rhomboids, and levator scapulae (see Fig. 18–6). These muscles, originating from the cervical and thoracic spine, suspend and mobilize the scapulae and thereby link neck motions with upper limb motions. The levator scapulae is clinically important in two ways. First, its origin allows the muscle to move the C1 to C2 area, especially when the shoulder is fixed. Second, it has a propensity for transferring symptoms from the upper cervical area to the superior angle of the scapula.[65] Pain in the upper cervical area creates an increased tension in the levator, which acts to elevate, migrate forward, and rotate downward the scapulae, resulting in rounded shoulders.

The muscles that serve the function of ventilation, mastication, vocalization, and phonation are collectively known as the *suprahyoids* and *infrahyoids* (see Figs. 16–13, 16–14 and 16–15, and Figs. 18–8 and 18–9).

OTHER SUPPORT STRUCTURES

The intra-abdominal pressure has been regarded as important for stabilization and relief of the spine when exposed to heavy loads, as when lifting. Both the abdominal and thoracic cavities have been shown to become pressurized during strenuous activity. The abdominal cavity can be pressurized by mechanical contraction of the muscles of the abdominal wall together with the diaphragm. Associated closing of the glottis (Valsalva maneuver) results in further pressurization.[35,36] This increased pressure tends to force the pelvic wall (floor of abdominal cavity) and the lung's diaphragm (roof of abdominal cavity) apart. This intra-abdominal pressure has been regarded as important for the stabilization and relief of the lumbar spine when carrying out heavy tasks (*e.g.*, lifting) by extending the spine and thus reducing the contraction force required in the extensor muscles. Bartelink showed that the rectus was not active but the transverse and oblique muscles were.[17] He maintained that strengthening of the rectus may have a positive effect on posture, but does little or nothing to brace the spine during lifting. Farfan has suggested that the thoracolumbar fascia can change the length of the dorsal ligament by means of a laterally directed force from the oblique musculature. This is said to shorten these ligaments.[44] He postulated that this is the mechanism by which intra-abdominal pressure creates an extension moment about the spine, and that this assists in compressive load-bearing. Other investigators have also shown that strengthening of the abdominal muscles does not generally effect intra-abdominal pressure during lifting.[72,106]

Recently, Hemborg and co-workers have conducted a number of studies with respect to intra-abdominal pressure and trunk muscle activity during lifting in both healthy subjects and low-back patients.[72-74] Various breathing techniques were assessed in order to elucidate the causal factors of increased intra-abdominal pressure during lifting and the effects of respiration. The intra-abdominal and intrathoracic pressures and the EMG activity of the oblique abdominals, the erector spinae, and at times, the puborectalis muscles were recorded. The trans-diaphragmatic pressure was calculated both during lifting and during the Müller maneuver.[56,168] The intra-abdominal pressure increase during lifting seems to be correlated to coordination between the muscles surrounding the abdominal cavity. Of these the diaphragm seems to be most important for the level of pressure. Closure of the glottis seems to be less important during lifting. Stillwell feels that the hydropneumatic effect of the abdominal support is facilitated by the bifolate shape of the diaphragm and by the change in shape of the abdominal wall that accompanies a deep breath taken before lifting.[179]

The general concept of spinal support from the abdomen has lead to a rationale for flexion exercises and protection of the spine by wearing a corset.[155] Davis has used this concept in determination of safe loads to be used in industry.[37] In lifting there is a linear relationship between the amount of weight lifted and the intra-abdominal pressure that can be measured in the stomach or rectum.[10,64] However, in a position of spinal flexion or axial rotation with altered mechanics, Gilbertson and associates have shown that an increase in intra-abdominal pressure may not decrease the activity of the dorsal musculature and therefore may not reduce the net axial loading of the disk.[57]

It is accurate to say that lifting is associated with high abdominal and thoracic pressures and that these pressures may reduce spinal compressive loads. However, it should be pointed out that lifting is only one type of loading that leads to spinal injury. Manning and co-workers have shown that slipping on wet or slippery floors is one of the most common events leading to a significant back injury; it is hard to see how strong abdominals and a deep breath can be used to prevent such an unexpected turn of events.[116] Other factors that protect the back in lifting include:

1. Stabilization of the vertebral column through the action of the thoracolumbar fascia (see Fascial Anatomy, p. 510)
2. The lever action of the thoracolumbar fascia, erector spinae muscles, and supraspinous ligaments. These structures pass some distance posteriorly to the spinous processes (and far posterior to the anterior column of the spine); however, they are firmly attached to them, and thus passive stretch of these structures can reduce the tendency toward flexion and forward shear of the lumbar vertebrae that would otherwise occur during lifting because of the orientation of the spinal elements. A shear resistance is created by the curve of the back, which imparts a posteriorly directed vector to the pull of the erector spinae muscles and the posterior ligaments of the lumbar vertebrae. Although this mechanical feature is lost in the upper lumbar spine with flexion, it is preserved in the lower lumbar spine.[1,44]
3. According to Adams and Hutton, the flexion position may strengthen the spine and obviate the need for a great deal of relief from increased abdominal pressure.[1] It is thought that the posture adopted by experienced weight-lifters (i.e., flexed lower lumbar spine, extended thoracic spine, and weight as close to the body as possible to reduce the bending moment) is the most efficient one biomechanically. The authors do not feel their studies negate the importance of abdominal pressure in increasing the margin of safety; rather, they state that the role of abdominal pressure is better defined as increasing the margin of safety, not making the lift possible in the first place, as others have implied.[1]
4. The lumbosacral rhythm, in which the spine does not perform its segmental motions in the most disadvantageous position of full trunk flexion, but only after the hip extensors have brought the trunk to approximately 45° and reduced the lever arm.
5. Action of the external and internal oblique muscles when asymmetrical loads are encountered.

Although the line of action of these muscles is anterior to the axis or rotation for flexion, these muscles are critical in preventing buckling and overrotation with asymmetrical loading.

SACROILIAC JOINT AND BONY PELVIS

The base of support for spinal movement is the pelvis, to which many of the back muscles attach and through which the muscles of the thigh exert their influence on posture. The pelvis supports the abdomen and links the vertebral column to the lower limbs. It is a closed osteoarticular ring made up of three bony parts and three joints. The three bony parts are the two iliac bones and the sacrum, a solid piece of bone resulting from fusion of the five sacral vertebrae. The three joints consist of the two sacroiliac joints and the pubic symphysis, which links the iliac bones anteriorly (Fig. 17–20).[91,186]

The major forces through the sacroiliac joints are borne by ligaments that tend to bind the sacrum into the ilia and lock the unusually shaped articular surfaces (narrow, curving in an earlike shape in their plane, and deeply modified by depressions and elevations) together. The pelvis is usually described as a ring or arch with the innominate bone as lateral pillars and the sacrum as the keystone. This analogy only holds if it is appreciated that the sacroiliac ligaments hold the arch together; in usual engineering practice it is the superimposed and lateral masses that hold an arch together and there is usually no tension member. The pelvis is an extremely stable system of joints maintained by some of the strongest ligaments in the body.

Movement of the sacroiliac joints has been described by many authors, with considerable effort being expended to try to precisely measure these movements by roentgenographic and physical means (e.g., pins placed in bones).[26,28,39,111] It is quite clear from this latter type of study that some motion does occur, but is of small amplitude, while at least one roentgenographic study indicated the potential for "significant" deflection of bones of the pelvis during various static manipulations.[52,196] Even if the motions of the joint are of small amplitude, the joint is located and constructed to serve as a shock absorber and thus there is little reason that it should fuse. In fact, careful anatomical studies indicate that although the joint undergoes severe degenerative changes, fusion is relatively unusual, except in ankylosing spondylitis.[20] With respect to degenerative changes it is interesting that the iliac articular surface is fibrocartilaginous throughout life, whereas the sacral surface is hyaline cartilage. In general, the sacral cartilage is also about three times thicker in early adult life than the iliac cartilage. Resnick and associates found that early degenerative changes occurred on the iliac surface rather than on both surfaces of the joint simultaneously.[161] Mitchell, in describing normal motion in the sacroiliac joints and in gait, suggests that the ilium rotates in a posterior direction at heel-strike and gradually moves from a posterior to an anterior direction as the person proceeds through the stance phase.[124] Elaborate descriptions of the possible axes and degree of motion have been described. These include a transverse axis through the pubic symphysis with rotation of the pubis to allow ilial motion in walking; a superior transverse axis, in the appropriate line of the second sacral segment, where some gross flexion occurs; a middle transverse axis, where additional gross flexion occurs; an inferior transverse axis, held to be the site of reciprocal motions of the joint during ambulation; and a set of oblique axes from the upper portion of one side of the sacrum to the lower portion of the contralateral joint.[124,191] Work by Weisl and others are not in total agreement about the amount and planes of motion.[28,188,196]

Kapandji describes the movements of nutation and counter-nutation (flexion and extension) of the sacrum within the ilia about a transverse axis posterior to the joint at the sacral tuberosity where the sacroiliac ligaments insert.[91] During nutation (flexion), movement of the sacral promontory is anterior and inferior, while the apex of the sacrum moves posteriorly. The iliac bones approximate and the ischial tuberosities move apart. Conversely, during counter-nutation (extension), the sacral promontory moves superiorly and posteriorly and the apex of the sacrum moves anteriorly. The iliac bones move apart while the ischial tuberosities approximate each other. These movements occur normally during the gait cycle and during activities such as forward and backward bending.

Understanding the position of the sacrum and ilia during gait and various body positions will help give the clinician an appreciation of the sacroiliac joint pain that may occur with locomotion. Despite differences of opinion regarding the movement center, most researchers agree that nutation and counter-nutation of the sacrum correspond to movements of the spine.[52,189] Therefore, in forward bending there is initially a backward bending (counter-nutation) of the sacrum, and as the spine completely extends there is a resultant forward bending (nutation) of the sacrum. Whereas the position of the sacrum is determined by a force that reaches it from above, the ilium

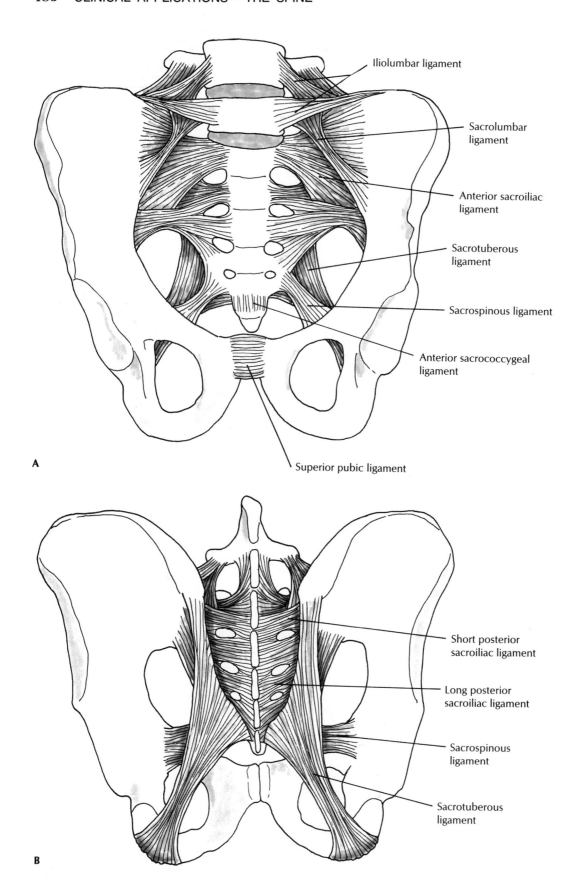

Fig. 17–20. Pelvic joints and ligaments. *(A)* Anterior aspect, *(B)* posterior aspect.

is controlled by movement of the femur. In standing, the base of the sacrum moves anteriorly. At heelstrike, the ipsilateral ilium is in a posteriorly rotated position. During the initial stance phase, sacral torsion occurs to that side. At midstance, increased tension of the iliopsoas encourages the ilium to move toward anterior rotation.[125]

Movement of the stable pelvic structure is made possible by the pelvic joints, consisting of the paired L5–S1 articular facet joints, the two sacroiliac joints, and the pubic symphysis. The two synovial sacroiliac joints are L-shaped when viewed from the side. The shorter and disposed cephalic limb of the sacral articulation is borne by the first sacral segment, while the longer and horizontally directed caudal limb is borne by the second and third sacral segments. Weisl has extensively studied these joints and has shown that a central depression can often be found at the junction of the two segments.[188,189] It has been noted that the cephalic limb of the sacral articular surface is more angled or wedged and is essentially vertical until it flares again inferiorly, as if to prevent it from sliding upward against the ilia.[177] The horizontal section of the sacrum has been described by Solonen as wedged dorsally in the upper portion of the joint and ventrally in the lower portion, whereas the ilial surface is convex superiorly and concave inferiorly.[177] The articular capsule is attached close to the margin of the articular surfaces of the sacrum and ilium.

The ligaments of the sacrum are a network of fibrous bands that fuse and intermingle to give added strength to the wedge of the pelvis. There are three main intrinsic and three main extrinsic ligaments. The three main *intrinsic ligaments* are the *anterior sacroiliac, short posterior sacroiliac,* and *long posterior sacroiliac ligaments* (see Fig. 17–20A,B).

The anterior sacroilac ligaments represent a thickening of the anterior and inferior parts of the fibrous capsule. They are particularly well developed at the level of the articular line but are thin elsewhere.[186] They stretch and tear easily upon slight pubic separation and allow the sacroiliac joints to gap during pregnancy.[169]

The short posterior sacroiliac ligaments pass from the first and second transverse tubercle on the dorsum of the sacrum to the posterior ilium. They prevent anterior (flexion) motion of the sacrum (see Fig. 17–20B).

The long posterior sacroiliac ligaments attach from the third transverse tubercle of the dorsum of the sacrum and the posterosuperior iliac spine, where they merge with the superior part of the sacrotuberous ligament and counteract the motion of downward slipping of the sacrum into the pelvis (see Fig. 17–20B).

The three main *extrinsic ligaments* are the *sacrospinous, sacrotuberous,* and *iliolumbar ligaments* (see Fig. 17–20A,B). The sacrospinous ligaments, which attach to the ischial spine and cross over to the anterior sacrum, and the sacrotuberous ligaments, which attach at the ischial tuberosity and traverse to the inferior sacrum, strongly stabilize the pelvis and anterior motion of the sacrum.

The iliolumbar ligament attaches from the iliac crest to the transverse processes of L4 and L5. It resists posterior rotation of the ilium and forward gliding of L5 on the sacrum (see Fig. 17–20A). According to Kapandji, the function of the superior band of the iliolumbar ligament is to check forward flexion of the vertebrae while the inferior or second band checks extension of the vertebral bodies.[91] Both bands of the iliolumbar ligament are also thought to be involved in lateral flexion (sidebending) of the lumbar spine and rotation.[157]

The pubic symphysis can be affected by excess motion in the sacroiliac joints and can be a source of symptoms (see Fig. 17–20A). It is a secondary cartilaginous joint of minimal mobility (if any at all), except in pregnancy.[91] Many forces act on this joint, especially those exerted by the muscles of the lower extremity.

While the strongest muscles of the body surround the sacroiliac joint, none are intrinsic to it and so do not play a major part in directly moving the sacrum between the ilia. According to Mitchell, sacral movement is a result of forces carried to it through the pull of ligaments and gravitational forces or both.[124] The muscles will indirectly affect the sacrum by their pull on the ilia and maintenance of poor sacral position after it has occurred. Conversely, these muscles have a direct effect on innominate movement. They can instigate or cause progression of iliosacral lesions.

Not unlike the shoulder girdle, the pelvic girdle serves as the fixed base of support of operation of the lumbar and thoracic spine. Static and dynamic disorders which alter this fixed base of support, such as differences in leg length (real or apparent) or malpositions of the pelvic bones, may often elicit symptoms over time and result in degenerative changes of the lumbar spine, hip, and sacroiliac joints. One should bear in mind that the sacroiliac joint is a common site for referred pain and tenderness derived from segmental diskogenic backache.

KINEMATICS

Motion in the spine is produced by the coordinated action of nerves and muscles. Agonistic muscles initiate and carry out motion, whereas antagonistic muscles often control and modify it. While the degree of movement at spinal segments is largely determined by the disk–vertebral height ratio, the types of movement that may occur depend on the orientation of the articular facets of the intervertebral joints at each level. The motion between two vertebrae is small and does not occur independently. Obviously, the degree and combination of the individual types of motion vary considerably in the different vertebral regions.

Skeletal structures that influence motion of the spine are the rib cage, which limits thoracic motion, and the pelvis, whose tilting increases trunk motion.

RANGES OF SEGMENTAL MOTION

In three-dimensional space, the spine has six planes of freedom. A vertebra may rotate about or translate along a transverse, a sagittal, or a longitudinal axis or move in various combination of these motions.[66,195]

Although the range of motion in an individual segment of the spine has been found to vary in different studies using autopsy material or roentgenographic *in vivo* measurements, there is agreement on the relative amount of motion at different levels of the spine. The phenomenon of *coupling*, in which two or more individual motions occur at the same time, has been well documented experimentally.[16,45,63,109,164,171,180,184] Frequently three motions will simultaneously take place during normal physiological spinal movement or function. The coupling effect occurs in the thoracic spine,[146,192,193] but is

more common in the cervical[112] and lumbar spine.[98,148]

Pure movement in any of the three principle planes very seldom occurs, because orientation of facet joint surfaces does not exactly coincide with the plane of motion and therefore modifies it to a greater or lesser extent.[66] For example, when the lumbar motion segment is rotated axially, it simultaneously bends in the sagittal plane and rotates axially.[194] Spinal movement is complex, and the intricacies of changing relationships observed on cineradiographic and other studies are sometimes difficult to explain.[66]

The occipitoatlantoaxial joints are the most complex joints of the axial skeleton, both anatomically and kinematically. Although there have been some thorough investigations of this region, there is considerable controversy about some of the basic biomechanical characteristics. In Chapter 18, The Cervical Spine, the best available information is analyzed with some discussion of representative values of range of segmental motion.

Representative values of other parts of the spine are presented here to allow a comparison of motion at various levels of the lower cervical (C2–C7), thoracic, and lumbar spine.[194] A representative value for flexion–extension is 8° at C2–C3, 13° at C3–C4, and 17° at C5–C6. A representative value for flexion–extension is 4° at T1–T4, 6° at T5–T10, and 12° at T11–T12. The range of flexion–extension progressively increases in the lumbar motion segments, reaching a maximum of 20° at the lumbosacral level (Fig. 17–21).

Fig. 17–21. Average ranges of segmental movement of the spinal joints. (From White AA, III, Panjabi MM: The basic kinematics of the human spine: A review of past and current knowledge. Spine 3:16, 1978)

Lateral flexion shows the greatest range in the C3–C4 and C4–C5 segments, which reach 11°. The greatest range in the thoracic spine is in the lower segments, where 8° to 9° is possible. In the lumbar spine, 6° of lateral flexion is common, except for the lumbosacral segments, where only 3° of lateral flexion occurs (see Fig. 17–21).[194]

Axial rotation is greatest in the midcervical spine, where 10° to 12° of motion is found. In the thoracic spine, axial rotation is greatest in the upper segments, where 9° is possible. The range of motion progressively decreases caudally, reaching 2° in the lower segments of the lumbar spine, but again increases in the lumbosacral segment to 5° (see Fig. 17–21).[194]

Segmental motion cannot be measured clinically and motion of the spine is a combined action of several segments. The degree of movement has clinical meaning in the spinal segment in relationship to its immediate neighbor and in general terms of the patient's body type.

Regional movement characteristics should also be appreciated. In general it can be said that in all sagittal starting positions of the cervical spine and in the flexed thoracic (below T3) and lumbar spines, sidebending is unavoidably accompanied by rotation to the same side; in the neutral or extended thoracic (below T3) and lumbar spines, sidebending is accompanied by rotation to the opposite side.[66]

In the upper thoracic spine there appears to be less consistency. According to White, the direction of coupled axial rotation is probably dominated by the middle sections of the thoracic spine, but sometimes the reverse is true.[192]

FUNCTIONAL MOTIONS OF THE THORACOLUMBAR SPINE

Normal values of functional range of motion of the spine do not exist because there are great variations among individuals. In fact, the range of motion in each of the three planes shows a Gaussian distribution, according to Lindl.[108] The range of motion also differs between the sexes and is strongly age dependent, decreasing by about 50% in old age.[126]

Flexion–Extension

Flexion is the most pronounced movement of the vertebral column as a whole. It requires an anterior compression of the intervertebral disks and a gliding separation of the articular facets in which the inferior set of an individual vertebra tends to move upward and forward over the opposing superior set of the adjacent inferior vertebra. The movement is checked mainly by the posterior ligaments and epaxial muscles. With respect to the thoracolumbar spine, the first 50° to 60° of spinal flexion occurs in the lumbar spine, mainly in the lower motion segments.[45] Forward tilting of the pelvis allows further flexion. There is an interconnection of movement between the spine and pelvis, particularly in total forward bending. Normally there is a synchronous movement in rhythmic ratio of the lumbar spine to that of pelvic rotation about the hips. As forward bending progresses, the lumbar curve reverses itself from concave to flat to convex. The sacrum is also moving within the ilia during forward bending. Initially, the sacrum flexes. As the pelvis is rotating anteriorly over the hips, the sacrum begins to counter-extend within the ilia. The thoracic spine contributes little to flexion of the total spine because of the orientation of the facets, the almost-vertical orientation of the spinous processes, and the restriction of the rib cage. Flexion is initiated by the abdominal muscles and the vertebral portion of the psoas. The weight of the upper body then produces further flexion, which is controlled by the gradually increasing activity of the erector muscles as the movement force increases.

Extension tends to be a more limited motion, producing posterior compression of the disk with the inferior articular process gliding posteriorly and downward over the superior set below. It is checked by the anterior longitudinal ligament and all the ventral muscles that directly or indirectly flex the spine. The laminae and spinous processes may also limit extension.[166,167] A reverse sequence of flexion is observed as the trunk returns from full flexion to the upright position. The lumbar spine becomes concave and the pelvis derotates and shifts forward as the spine extends. In some studies the concentric work performed by the muscles involved in raising the trunk has been shown to be greater than the eccentric work performed by the muscles during flexion.[52,90] When the trunk is extended from the upright position, the back muscles are active during the initial phase of motion. Activity decreases during further extension, and the abdominal muscles become active to control and modify motion.[108]

This arc of movement in forward and backward bending should normally be smooth and rhythmical, with a balance between lumbar reversal and pelvic rotation.[24]

Lateral Flexion

Lateral flexion is accompanied by some degree of rotation. It involves a rocking of the vertebral bodies upon their disks, with a sliding separation of the articular facets on the convex side and overriding of the articular facets related to the concavity.[166,167] Lateral flexion is limited by the intertransverse ligaments and the extension of the ribs. During lateral flexion, rotation may predominate in the thoracic or lumbar spine. In the lumbar spine the wedge-shaped spaces of the intervertebral joints show variation during motion.[160] The spinotransversal and transversospinal systems of the erector spinae are active in lateral flexion of the spine. The motion is initiated by ipsilateral contraction of these muscles and modified by the contralateral side.[108]

Rotation

Rotation is consistently combined with lateral flexion. The entire vertebral column rotates approximately 90° to either side of the sagittal plane, but most of this transversion is accomplished in the cervical and thoracic spine. With respect to the thoracic spine, the combined motion is most marked in the upper segments. The vertebral body rotates toward the concavity of the lateral curve of the spine.[192] A combined pattern of rotation and lateral flexion also exists in the lumbar spine.[123] In this region the vertebral body rotates toward the convexity of the curve. Lumbar rotation is extremely limited at the lumbosacral level because of the orientation of the facets. Pelvic motion is essential to increase the range of trunk rotation. During rotation, back and abdominal muscles are active on both sides of the spine as both ipsilateral and contralateral muscles cooperate.[108]

Measurements obtained during walking indicate that the pelvis and lumbar spine rotate as a functional unit.[63] In the lower thoracic spine, rotation diminishes gradually up to T7. This vertebra represents the area of transition from vertebral rotation in the direction of the pelvis to rotation in the opposite direction—that of the shoulder girdle.

REFERENCES

1. Adams M, Hutton WC: Prolapsed intervertebral disc: A hyperflexion injury. Spine 7:184–191, 1982
2. Alexander MJL: Biomechanical aspects of lumbar spine injuries in athletes: A review. Can J Appl Sports Sci 10:1–20, 1985
3. Andersson GBJ: Interdiscal pressure, intraabdominal pressure and myoelectric back muscle activity related to posture and loading. Clin Orthop 129:156–164, 1977
4. Andersson GBJ: Epidemiology of low back pain. In Bueger AA, Greenman PE (eds): Empirical Approach to the Validation of Spinal Manipulation. Springfield, IL, Charles C Thomas, 1985
5. Andersson GBJ, Jonsson B, Örtengren R: Myoelectric activity in individual lumbar erector spinae muscles in sitting: I. A study with surface and wire electrodes. Scand J Rehab Med (Suppl) 3:91–108, 1974
6. Andersson GBJ, Örtengren R: Lumbar disc pressure and myoelectric back muscle activity during sitting: II. Studies on an office chair. Scand J Rehab Med 6(3):115–121, 1974
7. Andersson GBJ, Örtengren R: Myoelectric back muscle activity during sitting. Scand J Rehab Med (Suppl) 3:73–101, 1974
8. Andersson GBJ, Örtengren R: Lumbar disc pressure and myoelectric back muscle activity during sitting: III Studies on a wheelchair. Scand J Rehab Med 6(3):128–133, 1974
9. Andersson GBJ, Örtengren R, Herberts P: Quantitative electromyographic studies of back muscle activity related to posture and loading. Orthop Clin North Am 8:85–96, 1977
10. Andersson GBJ, Örtengren R, Nachemson A: Intradiskal pressure and myoelectric back muscle activity related to posture and loading. Clin Orthop 129:156–164, 1977
11. Andersson GBJ, Örtengren R, Nachemson A: Quantitative studies of the load on the back in different working postures. Scand J Rehab Med 6:173–178, 1978
12. Andersson GBJ, Örtengren R, Nachemson A, et al: Lumbar disc pressure and myoelectric back muscle activity during sitting. Studies on an experimental chair. Parts I–III. Scand J Rehab Med. 6:104–127, 1974
13. Andersson GBJ, Örtengren R, Nachemson A, et al: Lumbar disc pressure and myoelectric back muscle activity during sitting: II. Studies on a car driver's seat. Scand J Rehab Med 6(3):128–133, 1974
14. Akeson WH, Amiel D, Woo SL: Immobility effect on synovial joints: The pathomechanics of joint contracture. Biorheology 17:95–110, 1980
15. Allen CEL: Muscle action potentials used in the study of dynamic anatomy. Br J Phys Med 11:66–73, 1948
16. Arkin AM: The mechanism of rotation in combination with lateral deviation in the normal spine. J Bone Joint Surg 32(A):180–188, 1950
17. Bartelink DL: The role of abdominal pressure in relieving the pressure on the lumbar intervertebral discs. J Bone Joint Surg 39(B):718–725, 1975
18. Basmajian JV: Electromyography of iliopsoas. Anat Rec 132:127–132, 1958
19. Bogduk N: The innervation of the lumbar spine. Spine 8:286–293, 1983
20. Bowen V, Cassidy JD: Macroscopic and microscopic anatomy of the sacroiliac joint from embryonic life until the eighth decade. Spine 6:620–628, 1980
21. Brain WR, Northfield D, Wilkinson M: The neurological manifestations of cervical spondylosis. Brain 75:187–225, 1952
22. Brasseur K, Melvin J: Myoelectric activity in deep muscles of the back: A review. Arch Phys Med Rehabil 59:546, 1978

23. Buckwalter JA, Cooper RR, Maynard JA: Elastic fiber in human intervertebral discs. J Bone Joint Surg 58(A):73–76, 1976
24. Cailliet R: Low Back Pain Syndrome, 3rd ed. Philadelphia, FA Davis, 1981
25. Chaffin JB, Park KS: A longitudinal study of low back pain as associated with occupational lifting factors. J Am Ind Hyg Assoc 34:513–525, 1973
26. Chamberlain WE: The symphysis pubis in the roentgen examination of the sacroiliac joint. J Bone Joint Surg 24:621–623, 1930
27. Cloward RB: Cervical diskography. Ann Surg 150:1052–1064, 1959
28. Colachis S, Worden R, Bechtol C, et al: Movement of the sacroiliac joint in the adult male: A preliminary report. Arch Phys Med Rehabil 44:490–498, 1963
29. Collins G, Cohen M, Naliboff B, et al: Comparative analysis of paraspinal and frontal EMG, heart rate and skin conductance in chronic low back pain patients and normals to various postures and stress. Scand J Rehab Med 14:39–46, 1982
30. Collis DK, Ponseti IV: Long term follow-up of patients with idiopathic scoliosis not treated surgically. J Bone Joint Surg 51(A):425–455, 1969
31. Cotch MT: Biomechanics of the thoracic spine. In Atlas of Orthotics: Biomechanical Principles and Applications. American Academy of Orthopaedic Surgeons. St Louis, CV Mosby, 1975
32. Cram J, Steeger J: EMG scanning in the diagnosis of chronic pain. Biofeedback Self Regul 8:229–241, 1983
33. Cyriax J: Textbook of Orthopedic Medicine, 8th ed, Vol 1, Diagnosis of Soft Tissue Lesions. London, Bailliere Tindal, 1982
34. Cyron BM, Hutton WC: The tensile strength of the capsular ligament of the apophyseal joints. Anatomy 132:145–150, 1981
35. Davis PR: Posture of the trunk during lifting of weights. Br Med J 11:87–89, 1959
36. Davis PR: The causation of herniae by weight lifting. Lancet 2:155–157, 1959
37. Davis PR: The use of intraabdominal pressure in evaluating stresses on the lumbar spine. Spine 6:90–92, 1981
38. Dory MA: Arthrography of the lumbar facet joints. Radiology 140:23–27, 1981
39. Egund N, Olsson TH, Schmid H, et al: Movement of the sacroiliac joint demonstrated with roentgen stereophotogrammetry. Acta Radiol 19:833–846, 1978
40. Ehni G: Cervical Arthrosis: Disease of the Cervical Motion Segments. Chicago, Year Book Medical Publishers, 1984
41. Eie N: Load capacity of the low back. J Oslo City Hosp 16:73–78, 1966
42. Eie N, Wehn P: Measurement of the intraabdominal pressure in relation to weight bearing of the lumbosacral spine. J Oslo City Hosp 12:205–217, 1962
43. Epstein BS: The Spine. Philadelphia: Lea & Febiger, 1962
44. Farfan HF: Mechanical Disorders of the Low Back. Philadelphia, Lea & Febiger, 1973
45. Farfan HF: Muscular mechanism of the lumbar spine and the position of power and efficiency. Orthop Clin North Am 6:135–144, 1975
46. Farfan HF, Sullivan JD: The relation of the facet orientation to intervertebral disc failure. Can J Surg 10:179, 1967
47. Fielding JW: Normal and selected abnormal motion of the cervical spine from the second cervical vertebra to the seventh cervical vertebra based on cineroentgenography. J Bone Joint Surg 46(A):1779–1781, 1964
48. Fischer FJ, Houtz SJ: Evaluation of the function of the gluteus maximus muscle: An electromyographic study. Am J Phys Med 47:182–191, 1968
49. Floyd WF: The function of the erector spinae muscles in certain movements and postures in man. J Physiol 129:184–203, 1955
50. Floyd WF, Silver PHS: Function of the erector spinae in flexion of the trunk. Lancet 1:133–134, 1951
51. Frankel V, Nordin M: Basic Biomechanics of the Skeletal System. Philadelphia, Lea & Febiger, 1980
52. Frigerio N, Stow R, Howe J: Movement of sacroiliac joint. Clin Orthop 100:370–371, 1974
53. Frymoyer JW: Back pain and sciatica. N Engl J Med 318:291–300, 1988
54. Galante JO: Tensile properties of the human lumbar annulus fibrosis. Acta Orthop Scand (Suppl) 100:9–96, 1967
55. Gallois J, Japoit T: Architecture interieuredes vertebre du point de vue statique et physiologique. Rev Chir (Paris) 63:689, 1925 (Cited in Steindler A [ed]: Kinesiology of the Human Body. Springfield, IL, Charles C Thomas, 1958)
56. Gibson GJ, Clark E, Pride NB: Static transdiaphragmatic pressures in normal subjects and in patients with chronic hyperinflation. Am Rev Respir Dis 124:685–689, 1981
57. Gilbertson LG, Krag MH, Pope MH: Investigation of the effect of intra-abdominal pressure on load bearing of the spine (abstr). Orthop Trans 7:313, 1983
58. Golding JSR: Electromyography of the erector spinae in low back pain. Postgrad Med J 28:401–440, 1952
59. Gould JA: The spine. In Gould JA, Davies GJ (eds): Orthopedics and Sports Physical Therapy. St. Louis, CV Mosby, 1985
60. Grabel J: Electromyographic study of low back muscle tension in subjects with and without chronic low back pain. Doctoral thesis, United States International University, 1973. Dissertation Abstracts International 34:292–293, 1974
61. Gracovetsky S, Farfan HF, Lamy C: The mechanism of lumbar spine. Spine 6:249–262, 1981
62. Grant JCB: Grant's Atlas of Anatomy. Baltimore, Williams & Wilkins, 1972
63. Gregersen GG, Lucas DB: An in vivo study of the axial rotation of the human thoracolumbar spine. J Bone Joint Surg 49(A):247–262, 1967

64. Grew ND: Intra-abdominal pressure response to load applied to the torso in normal subjects. Spine 5:149–155, 1980

65. Grieve GP: Manipulation therapy for neck pain. Physiotherapy 65:136–146, 1979

66. Grieve GP: Common Vertebral Joint Problems. New York, Churchill Livingstone, 1981

67. Grieve GP: Diagnosis. Physiotherapy Practice 4:73–77, 1988

68. Guyton AC: Basic Human Physiology: Normal Function and Mechanisms of Disease, 2nd ed, Philadelphia, WB Saunders, 1977

69. Hall MC: The Locomotor System: Functional Anatomy. Springfield, IL, Charles C Thomas, 1965

70. Hamilton WJ (ed): Textbook of Human Anatomy, 2nd ed. St Louis, CV Mosby, 1976

71. Hemborg B, Moritz V: Intra-abdominal pressure and trunk muscle activity during lifting: II. Chronic low-back patients. Scand J Rehab Med 17:5–13, 1985

72. Hemborg B, Moritz V, Hamberg J, et al: Intra-abdominal pressure and trunk muscle activity during lifting: Effect of abdominal muscle training in healthy subjects. Scand J Rehab Med 15:183–196, 1983

73. Hemborg B, Moritz V, Hamberg J, et al: Intra-abdominal pressure and trunk muscle activity during lifting: III. Effect of abdominal muscle training in chronic low back patients. Scand J Rehab Med 17:15–24, 1985

74. Hemborg B, Moritz V, Lowing H: Intra-abdominal pressure and trunk muscle activity during lifting: IV. The causal factors of intra-abdominal pressure rise. Scand J Rehab Med 17:25–38, 1985

75. Hendry NG: The hydration of the nucleus pulposus and its relation to intervertebral disc derangement. J Bone Joint Surg 40(B):132–144, 1958

76. Hettinga DL: Normal joint structures and their reaction to injury. J Orthop Sports Phys Ther 1:10, 1979

77. Hirsch C, Ingelmark BE, Miller M: The anatomical basis for low back pain: Studies on the presence of sensory nerve endings in ligamentous, capsular and intervertebral disc structures in the human lumbar spine. Acta Orthop Scand 33:1–17, 1963

78. Hollinshead WH: Anatomy for Surgeons, 2nd ed. New York, Harper & Row, 1969

79. Hollinshead WH, Jenkins DB: Functional Anatomy of the Limbs and Back. Philadelphia, WB Saunders, 1981

80. Hoyt W, Hunt H, De Pauw M, et al: Electromyographic assessment of chronic low back pain syndrome. J Am Osteopath Assoc 80:728–730, 1981

81. Hutton WC, Stott JRR, Cyron BM: Is spondylolysis a fatigue fracture? Spine 2:202–209, 1977

82. Inman VT, Ralston HJ, Todd F: Human Walking. Baltimore, Williams & Wilkins, 1981

83. Iwasaki T, Ito H, Yamada M, et al: Electromyographic study of lifting weights. J Jpn Phys Ther Assn 4:52–61, 1978

84. Jonsson B: The Lumbar Part of the Erector Spinae Muscle: A Technique for Electromyographic Studies of the Function of its Individual Muscles. Goteborg, Sweden, University of Goteborg, 1970

85. Jonsson B: Topography of the lumbar part of the erector spinae muscle: An analysis of the morphologic conditions present for insertion of EMG electrodes into individual muscles of the lumbar part of the erector spinae muscle. Z Anat Entwickl Gesch 130:177–191, 1970

86. Jonsson B: The function of individual muscles in the lumbar part of the spinae muscle. Electromyography 10:5–21, 1970

87. Jonsson B: Electromyography of the lumbar part of the erector spinae muscle. Medicine and Sport, Vol 6: In: Komi PV (ed): Biomechanics II, pp 185–188. Basel, S Karger, 1971

88. Jonsson B: Electromyography of the erector spinae muscle. Medicine and Sport, Vol 8: In Komi PV (ed): Biomechanics III, pp 294–300. Basel, S Karger, 1973

89. Jonsson B, Synnerstad B: Electromyographic studies of muscle function in standing. A methodological study. Acta Morphol Neerl Scand 6:361–370, 1966

90. Joseph J: Man's Posture: Electromyographic Studies. Springfield, IL, Charles C Thomas, 1960

91. Kapandji IA: The Physiology of the Joints, Vol 3: The Trunk and Vertebral Column. New York, Churchill Livingstone, 1974

92. Karlsson E, Jonsson B: Function of the gluteus maximus muscle: An electromyographic study. Acta Morphol Neerl Scand 6:161–169, 1965

93. Kazarian L: Dynamic response characteristic of the human vertebral column: An experimental study of human autopsy specimens. Acta Orthop Scand (Suppl) 146:1–186, 1972

94. Kazarian L: Creep characteristics of the human spinal column. Orthop Clin North Am 6:3–18, 1975

95. King AI, Prasad P, Ewing CL: Mechanism of spinal injury due to caudocephalad acceleration. Orthop Clin North Am 6:19–31, 1975

96. Kos J, Wolf J: Intervertebral menisci and their possible role in intervertebral blockage. Burkart SL (trans): Special Edition, Bull Orthop Sports Med Sect APTA 1:8, 1976

97. Kraft GL, Levinthal DH: Facet synovial impingement. Surg Gynecol Obstet 93:439–443, 1951

98. Krag MH: Three dimensional flexibility measurements of preload human vertebral motion segments, Ph.D. dissertation Yale University School of Medicine, 1975

99. Krag MH, Wilder DG, Pope MH: Internal strain and nuclear movements of the intervertebral disc. Proceedings of the International Society for Study of the Lumbar Spine, Cambridge, England, April 15, 1983

100. Krammer J: Treatment of the Lumbar Syndrome in Intervertebral Disk Disease. Chicago, Year Book Medical Publishers, 1981

101. Kraus H: Stress analysis. In Farfan HF (ed): Mechanical Disorders of the Low Back, pp 112–133. Philadelphia, Lea & Febiger, 1973

102. Kravitz E, Moore M, Glaros A: Paralumbar muscle

activity in chronic low back pain. Arch Phys Med Rehabil 62:172–176, 1981

103. Krenz J, Troup JDG: The structure of the pars interarticularis of the lower lumbar vertebrae and its relation to the etiology of spondylolysis with a report of healing fracture in the neural arch of a fourth lumbar vertebra. J Bone Joint Surg 55(B):735–741, 1973

104. Kuluk RF, Belytshko TB, Schultz AB, et al: Non-linear behavior of the human intervertebral disc under axial load. J Biomech 9:377–386, 1976

105. LaRocca H: Biomechanics of the cervical spine. In Atlas of Orthotics: Biomechanical Principles and Application. American Academy of Orthopedic Surgeons, St. Louis, CV Mosby, 1975

106. Legg SL: The effect of abdominal muscle fatigue training on the intra-abdominal pressure developed during lifting. Ergonomics 24:191–195, 1981

107. Lewis T, Kellgren JH: Observation relating to referred pain, visceromotor reflexes and other associated phenomena. Clin Sci 4:47–71, 1939

108. Lindl M: Biomechanics of the lumbar spine. In Frankel V, Nordin M (eds): Basic Biomechanics of the Skeletal System. Philadelphia, Lea & Febiger, 1980

109. Loebl WY: Regional rotation of the spine. Rheum Rehabil 12:223, 1973

110. Lorenz M, Patwardhan A, Vanderby R: Load-bearing characteristics of lumbar facets in normal and surgically altered spinal segments. Spine 8:122–130, 1983

111. Lumsden RM, Morris JM: An in vivo study of axial rotation and immobilization at the lumbosacral joint. J Bone Joint Surg 50: (A):1591–1602, 1968

112. Lysell E: Motion in the cervical spine. Acta Orthop Scand (Suppl) 123:1–61, 1969

113. MacConaill MA, Basmajian JV: Muscles and Movements. Baltimore, Williams & Wilkins, 1969

114. Maigne R: Orthopaedic Medicine. Springfield, IL, Charles C Thomas, 1976

115. Maldague B, Mathurin P, Malghem J: Facet joint arthrography in lumbar spondylosis. Radiology 140:29–36, 1981

116. Manning DP, Shannon HS: Slipping accidents causing low-back pain in a gearbox factory. Spine 6:70–72, 1981

117. McCall IW, Park WM, O'Brien JP: Induced pain referral from posterior lumbar elements in normal subjects. Spine 4:441–446, 1979

118. McGregor M, Cassidy JD: Post-operative sacroiliac syndrome. J Manipulative Physiol Ther 6:1–11, 1983

119. McNeill T, Warwick D, Andersson G, et al: Trunk strength in attempted flexion, extension and lateral bending in healthy subjects and patients with low-back disorders. Spine 5:527–538, 1980

120. Messerer O: Uber Elasticitat and Festigkeit der Meuschlichen Knochen. Stuttgart, JG Cottaschen Buchhandling, 1880

121. Meyer GH: Der mechanismus der symphysis sacroiliaca. Archiv fur Anatomie und Physiologie 1:1–16, 1978

122. Michele AA: Iliopsoas. Springfield, IL, Charles C Thomas, 1962

123. Miles M, Sullivan WE: Lateral bending at the lumbar and lumbosacral joints. Anat Rec 139:387–398, 1961

124. Mitchell FL: Structural Pelvic Function. Academy of Applied Osteopathy, Vol 2, Chicago Year Book Medical Publishers, 1965

125. Mitchell FL: An Evaluation and Treatment Manual of Osteopathic Muscle Energy Procedures. Valley Park, MO, Mitchell, Moran and Pruzzzo, 1979

126. Moll JMH, Wright V: Normal range of spinal mobility: An objective clinical study. Ann Rheum Dis 3:381–386, 1971

127. Mooney V, Robertson J: The facet syndrome. Clin Orthop 115:149–156, 1976

128. Morris JM: Biomechanics of the spine. Arch Surg 107:418–423, 1973

129. Morris JM, Benner G, Lucas DB: An electromyographic study of intrinsic muscles of the back in man. J Anat 96:509–520, 1962

130. Morris JM, Lucus DB, Bresler B: Role of the trunk in stability of the spine. J Bone Joint Surg 43(A):327–351, 1961

131. Nachemson AL: Lumbar interdiscal pressure. Acta Orthop Scand (Suppl) 43:9–104, 1960

132. Nachemson AL: The load on lumbar disc in different positions of the body. Clin Orthop 45:107–122, 1966

133. Nachemson A: Electromyographic studies on the vertebral portion of the psoas muscle with special reference to its stabilizing function of the lumbar spine. Acta Orthop Scand 37:177–190, 1966

134. Nachemson AL: The lumbar spine: An orthopaedic challenge. Spine 1:59–71, 1976

135. Nachemson A: Disc pressure measurements. Spine 6:93–97, 1981

136. Nachemson A: Low back pain including biomechanics of the intervertebral joint complex. In Straub LR, Wilson PD (eds): Clinical Trends in Orthopaedics. New York, Theime–Stratton, 1982

137. Nachemson A, Elfstrom G: Intravital dynamics pressure measurements in lumbar discs: A study of common movements, maneuvers and exercises. Scand J Rehabil Med 2 (Suppl 1):1–40, 1970

138. Nachemson AL, Evans J: Some mechanical properties of the third lumbar inter-laminar ligament (ligamentum flavum) J Biomech 1:211–219, 1968

139. Nachemson AL, Morris JM: In vivo measurements of intradiscal pressure: Discometry, a method for the determination of pressure in the lower discs. J Bone Joint Surg 46(A):1077–1092, 1964

140. Nemeth G: On hip and lumbar biomechanics: A study of joint load and muscular activity. Scand J Rehabil Med (Suppl) 10:1–35, 1984

141. Nemeth G, Ekholm J, Arborelius UP: Hip load moments and muscular activity during lifting. Scand J Rehabil Med 16:103–111, 1984

142. Norkin CC, Levengie DK: Joint Structure and Function: A Comprehensive Analysis. Philadelphia, FA Davis, 1983

143. Okada M: Electromyographic assessment of the muscular load in forward bending postures. Journal of the Faculty of Science, University of Tokyo 3:311–336, 1970

144. Okada M: An electromyographic examination of the relative muscular load in different human postures. J Hum Ergol 1:75–93, 1972

145. Örtengren R, Andersson GBJ: Electromyographic studies of trunk muscles with special reference to the functional anatomy of the lumbar spine. Spine 2:44–52, 1977

146. Panjabi MM, Brand RA, White AA: Mechanical properties of the human thoracic spine as shown by three-dimensional load-displacement curves. J Bone Joint Surg 58(A):642–652, 1976

147. Panjabi MM, Goel VK, Takata K: Physiologic strains in the lumbar ligaments: An in vitro biomechanical study. Spine 7:192–203, 1983

148. Panjabi MM, Krag MM, White AA, et al: Effect of preload on load displacement curves of the lumbar spine. Orthop Clin North Am 88:181–192, 1977

149. Paris SV: Anatomy as related to function and pain. Orthop Clin North Am 14:475–487, 1983

150. Pauly JE: An electromyographic study of certain movements and exercises: I. Some deep muscles of the back. Anat Rec 155:223–234, 1966

151. Perry O: Fracture of the vertebral end-plate in the lumbar spine. Acta Orthop Scand (Suppl) 25:3–101, 1957

152. Perry O: Resistance and compression of the lumbar vertebrae. In Ranninger K (ed): Encyclopedia of Medical Radiology. New York, Springer–Verlag, 1974

153. Platzer W: Color Atlas and Textbook of Human Anatomy, Vol 1, Locomotion System. Chicago, Year Book Medical Publishers, 1978

154. Poland JL, Hobart DJ, Payton OD: The Musculoskeletal System. New York, Medical Examination Publishing, 1977

155. Pope MH, Lehmann TR, Frymoyer JW: Structure and function of the lumbar spine. In Pope MH, Frymoyer JW, Andersson G (eds): Occupational Low Back Pain, New York, Praeger, 1984

156. Pope MH, Rosen JD, Wider DG, et al: The relation between biomechanical and psychological factors in patients with low back pain. Spine 5:173–178, 1983

157. Porterfield JA: The sacroiliac joint. In Gould JA, Davies GJ (eds): Orthopedics and Sports Physical Therapy. St Louis, CV Mosby, 1985

158. Portnoy H, Morin F: Electromyographic study of postural muscles in various positions and movements. Am J Physiol 186:122–126, 1956

159. Poulsen E, Jorgensen K: Back muscle strength, lifting and stooped working postures. Appl Ergon 2:133–137, 1971

160. Reichmann S: Motion of the lumbar articular processes in flexion–extension and lateral flexion of the spine. Acta Morphol Neerl Scand 8:261–272, 1970–1971

161. Resnick D, Niwayama G, Goergen TG: Degenerative disease of the sacroiliac joint. Invest Radiol 10:608–621, 1975

162. Rissanen PM: Comparisons of pathological changes in the intervertebral discs and interspinous ligaments of the lower part of the lumbar spine. Acta Orthop Scand 34:54–65, 1964

163. Roberts S, Chen PH: Global characteristics of typical human ribs. J Biomech 5:191–201, 1972

164. Rolander SD: Motion of the lumbar spine with special reference to the stabilising effect of posterior fusion. Acta Orthop Scand (Suppl) 90:1–144, 1966

165. Rolander SD, Blair WE: Deformation and fracture of the lumbar vertebral end-plate. Orthop Clinic North Am 6:75–81, 1975

166. Rothman RH, Simeone FA: The Spine, 2nd ed, Vol 1. Philadelphia, WB Saunders, 1982

167. Rothman RH, Simeone FA: The Spine, 2nd ed, Vol 2. Philadelphia, WB Saunders, 1982

168. Roussos CS, Macklem PT: Diaphragmatic fatigue in man. J Appl Physiol 43:189–197, 1977

169. Sashin D: A critical analysis of the anatomy and pathological changes of the sacro-iliac joints. J Bone Joint Surg 12:891–910, 1930

170. Schmorl G: Die pathologische anatomie der wirbel saule. Vern Dtsch Orthop Ges 21:3, 1927

171. Schultz A, Andersson G, Ortengren R, et al: J Bone Joint Surg 64(A):713–720, 1982

172. Shah JS, Hampson WGJ, Jayson MIV: The distribution of surface strain in the cadaveric lumbar spine. J Bone Joint Surg 60(B):246–251, 1978

173. Sherman RA: Relationships between strength of low back muscle contraction and reported intensity of low back pain. Am J Phys Med 64:190–200, 1985

174. Shore LR: On osteoarthritis in the dorsal intervertebral joint. Brit J Surg 22:833–849, 1935

175. Smidt GL, Amundsen LR, Dostal WF: Muscle strength of the trunk. J Orthop Sports Phys Ther 1:165–170, 1980

176. Soderberg GL, Barr Jo: Muscular function in chronic low-back dysfunction. Spine 8:79–85, 1983

177. Solonen KA: The sacro-iliac joint in the light of anatomical roentgenological and clinical studies. Acta Orthop Scand (Suppl) 26:9–127, 1957

178. Spilker RL: Mechanical behavior of a simple model of an intervertebral disk under compressive loading. J Biomech 13:895–901, 1980

179. Stillwell GK: The law of Laplace: Some clinical applications. Mayo Clin Proc 48:863–868, 1973

180. Stoddard A: Manual of Osteopathic Technique. London, Hutchinson, 1962

181. Tauber J: An unorthodox look at backaches. J Occup Med 12:128–130, 1970

182. Tesh JH, Evans J, Shawdunn J, et al: The mechanical interaction between the thoracolumbar fascia and the connective tissue of the posterior spine. In Bueger AA, Greenman PE (eds): Empirical Approach to the Validation of Spinal Manipulation. Springfield, IL, Charles C Thomas, 1985

183. Tkaczuk H: Tensile properties of human lumbar longitudinal ligament. Acta Orthop Scand (Suppl) 115:9–69, 1968
184. Troup JDG, Hood CA, Chapman AE: Measurements of the sagittal mobility of lumbar spine and hips. Ann Phys Med 9:308–321, 1976
185. Urschel HC, Razzuk MA, Wood RE, et al: Objective diagnosis (ulnar nerve conduction velocity) and current therapy of the thoracic outlet syndrome. Ann Thorac Surg 12:608–620, 1971
186. Warwick R, Williams P: Gray's Anatomy 35th ed, Philadelphia, JB Lippincott, 1978
187. Watanabe K: A study on the posture: The function of the man erector spinae. Jpn J Phys Educ 21:69–76, 1976
188. Weisl H: The articular surfaces of the sacro-iliac joint and their relation to the movement of the sacrum. Acta Anat 22:1–14, 1954
189. Weisl H: The movements of the sacro-iliac joint. Acta Anat 23:80–91, 1955
190. Weisman G, Pope MH, Johnson RJ: Cyclic loading in knee ligament injuries. Am J Sports Med 8:24–30, 1980
191. Weismantel A: Evaluation and treatment of sacroiliac joint problems. Bull Orthop Sports Med Sect APTA 3:5–9, 1982
192. White AA: Analysis of the mechanics of the thoracic spine in man. Acta Orthop Scand (Suppl) 127:8–105, 1969
193. White AA, Hirch C: The significance of the vertebral posterior elements in the mechanics of the thoracic spine. Clin Orthop 81:2–20, 1971
194. White AA, Panjabi MM: Clinical Biomechanics of the Spine. Philadelphia, JB Lippincott, 1978
195. White AA, Southwick WO, Panjabi MM, et al: Practical biomechanics of the spine for orthopedic surgeons. Instr Course Lect 23:62–78, 1974
196. Wilder DG, Msme, Pope MH, et al: The functional topography of the sacroiliac joint. Spine 5:575–579, 1980
197. Wolf SL, Basmajian JV: Assessment of paraspinal electromyographic activity in normal subjects and in chronic back pain patients using muscle biofeedback device. In Asmussen E, Gorgensen J (eds): International Series in Biomechanics, pp 319–323. Baltimore, University Park Press, 1977
198. Wolf SL, Basmajian JV, Russe CTC, et al: Normative data on low back mobility and activity levels. Am J Phys Med 58:217–229, 1979
199. Wyke BD: The neurology of joints. Ann Roy Coll Surg Engl 41:25–50, 1967
200. Wyke B: Receptor systems in lumbosacral tissues in relation to the production of low back pain. In White AA, Gordon SL (eds): American Academy of Orthopaedic Surgeons Symposium on Idiopathic Low Back Pain (Miami, FL, December 1980). St. Louis, CV Mosby, 1980

18 *The Cervical Spine*

Mitchell G. Blakney

REVIEW OF FUNCTIONAL ANATOMY

OSSEOUS STRUCTURES

The seven vertebrae of the cervical spine can be divided into two groups, according to structure and function. The vertebrae of the lower cervical spine (C2–C7) are similar in structure to the vertebrae of the thoracic and lumbar spine with clearly defined vertebral bodies and spinous processes (Fig. 18–1).[9] The transverse processes are abbreviated to allow better mobility, and there is a foramen to allow passage of the vertebral artery. The lateral portions of the vertebral bodies form the joints of Luschka, which also facilitate mobility of the lower cervical spine.[9] The facet joints of the lower cervical spine are in the sagittal plane and incline forward at approximately 45°. This forward inclination allows the facet joints to bear weight and guides the motion of the segment.

The bony structure of the upper cervical spine is specialized to allow a great deal of mobility and to protect the medulla oblongata (Fig. 18–2A,B). The inferior facet of C2 has the same form and function as the facets of the lower cervical spine. The joint surfaces of the superior facet of C2 are aligned in the horizontal plane to allow approximately 90° rotation. The dens portion of C2 is a vertical pin of bone that acts as a pivot around which the atlas rotates (Fig. 18–2C,D).[9] The atlas is a wide, thin ring of bone with a well-developed transverse process but no spinous process. There is no intervertebral disk between the C1 and C2 because the atlas, with concave joint surfaces above and below, serves the function of the disk. The anterior portion of the transverse ligament of the atlas forms a socket for the dens. The atlanto-occipital joint is the one true convex-on-concave joint in the spine. The superior facet surfaces of the atlas are oval, concave, and toed-in slightly. The convex condyles of the occiput are slightly larger than the joint surfaces of the atlas, making maximal congruence possible on only one side at a time, when

the occiput is laterally bent on the atlas. The anterior placement of the center of rotation of the atlas causes a lateral movement to the opposite side whenever the atlas is rotated (Fig. 18–3). This can be palpated as the transverse process becoming more prominent on the side opposite rotation. When viewed from the side, the superior facet joint of C2 is rounded as the atlas rotates. It rolls down the shoulder of the side of rotation and climbs up the shoulder of the side opposite rotation. This can be palpated as the transverse process of the atlas becoming higher and farther forward on the side opposite rotation and lower and more posterior on the side of rotation.[16]

The atlanto-occipital, atlantoaxial, and, arguably, the Luschka joint surfaces are lined with articular cartilage, have synovial membranes, and like other synovial joints, have rich proprioceptive and nociceptive innervation.[19]

JOINTS AND LIGAMENTS

The anterior and posterior longitudinal ligaments and the ligamentum flavum are present in the cervical spine from C2 through C7 and perform the same functions as in the thoracic and lumbar spine. The interspinous and supraspinous ligaments blend with the nuchal ligament of the cervical spine (Fig. 18–4). The nuchal ligament has its origins on the spinous processes of the cervical spine and its insertion on the occiput. Its function in quadruped animals is to support the head. Its function in humans is to prevent overflexion of the neck. The nuchal ligament tightens at the extreme of neck flexion. It also becomes tight, flattening out the cervical lordosis, with approximately 15° of nodding of the upper cervical spine.[16]

The posterior longitudinal ligament ends at C2. The tectorial membrane, which is thin and diaphanous through the rest of the spine, thickens into the tectorial ligament arising from C2, bypasses the atlas, and inserts on the occiput (Fig. 18–5). The tectorial ligament becomes tight with flexion of the head. Deep to the tectorial ligament is the cruciform ligament, which has both vertical and transverse portions (see Fig. 18–5). The vertical portion of the cruciform ligament has its origin on C2 and has the same insertion and function as the tectorial liga-

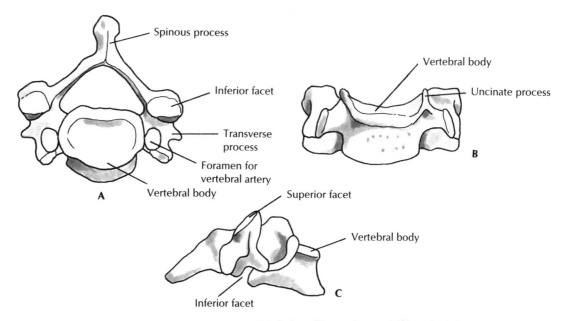

Fig. 18-1. A typical lower cervical vertebra. *(A)* Inferior, *(B)* anterior, and *(C)* sagittal views.

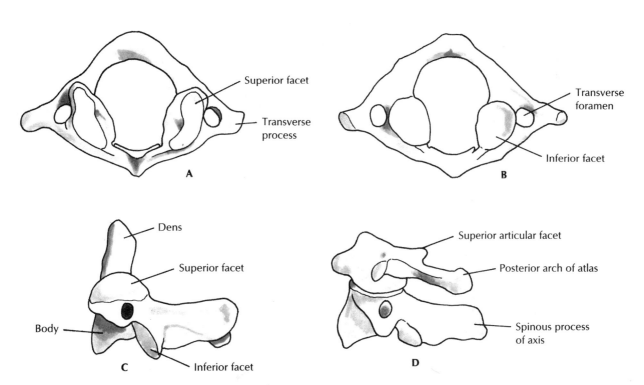

Fig. 18-2. The upper cervical spine. *(A)* Superior view of atlas, *(B)* inferior view of atlas, *(C)* lateral view of axis, and *(D)* lateral view of atlantoaxial articulation.

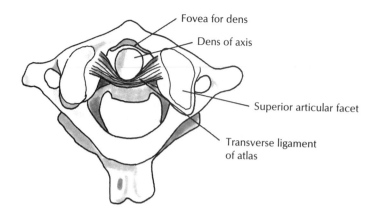

Fovea for dens

Dens of axis

Superior articular facet

Transverse ligament
of atlas

Fig. 18–3. The atlantoaxial joint from a superior view, showing the dens and the transverse ligament of the atlas.

ment. It also bypasses C1. The horizontal portion of the cruciform ligament has its origin and insertion on the interior surface of the anterior ring of the atlas. It encircles the dens to reinforce the transverse ligament of the atlas (see Fig. 18–3). The transverse ligament of the atlas has its origin and insertion on the interior surface of the anterior ring of the atlas. It encloses the dens and is lined with a synovial membrane and articular cartilage to provide lubrication

as the atlas rotates around the dens. If the transverse ligament of the atlas and the horizontal portion of the cruciform ligament are weakened by systemic inflammatory disease or injured in an accident, there is danger of damage to the medulla oblongata by dislocation of the dens. If this is suspected, traction or mobilization of the cervical spine should be considered gravely dangerous.

The alar ligament is a winglike structure that has

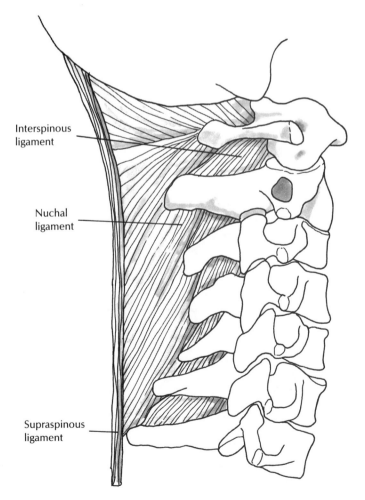

Interspinous
ligament

Nuchal
ligament

Supraspinous
ligament

Fig. 18–4. A lateral view of the cervical spine, showing the interspinous, supraspinous, and nuchal ligaments.

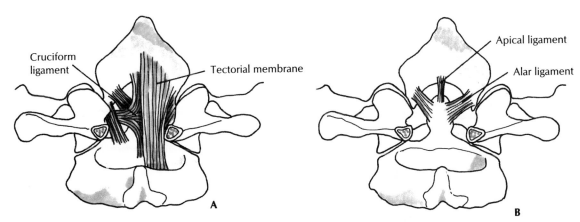

Fig. 18-5. A posterior view of the ligaments of the upper cervical spine. The more superficial tectorial and cruciform ligaments *(A)*, and the deeper alar and apical ligaments *(B)*. (*Note:* The cruciform ligament is not shown so that the deeper ligaments can be seen).

its origin on the lateral borders of the dens and its insertion on the occiput (see Fig. 18-5). It is a major portion of the stabilization system of the upper cervical spine. The configuration of the atlanto-occipital joints could allow considerable lateral flexion, which would damage the medulla oblongata. This lateral flexion is checked by the alar ligament. If the alar ligament is congenitally absent or damaged or if the dens is fractured or congenitally absent, mobilization or traction to the cervical spine should be considered gravely hazardous. The apical ligament has its origin on the tip of the dens and inserts on the occiput. It becomes taut when traction is applied to the head. The joint capsule of the atlanto-occipital joint is reinforced with ligaments. The lateral placement of the atlanto-occipital joint capsules and ligaments severely limits rotation of the occiput on the atlas.

Clinical Considerations

1. The ligaments of the upper cervical spine may be damaged in high-velocity accidents, weakened by rheumatoid arthritis or other types of systemic inflammatory diseases, or may be congenitally absent or malformed. Before any kind of mechanical treatment is begun, the integrity of the upper cervical ligament should be tested.
2. In order to distract by traction the atlanto-occipital or atlantoaxial joint, the head must be in a neutral or slightly extended position to slacken the nuchal and posterior longitudinal ligaments.
3. The upper cervical spine can be thought of as an upper joint which flexes and extends, has some sidebending but no rotation, and as an inferior joint that allows approximately 90° rotation, no sidebending, and limited flexion-extension;

therefore, if the lower cervical spine is locked in full flexion or sidebending, movements of the atlanto-occipital joint are tested by lateral flexion and movements of the atlantoaxial joint are tested by rotation.[9]

MUSCLE GROUPS

The muscles of the cervical spine can be considered in four functional groups: superficial posterior, deep posterior, superficial anterior, and deep anterior. Normal function of the cervical spine depends on proper flexibility and balance of these muscle groups.

The trapezius muscle is the largest, strongest, and most prominent of the posterior neck muscles (Fig. 18-6). It is very well developed in quadruped animals and serves to hold the head up against gravity. It inserts into the nuchal ligament and occipital ridge and extends the head and neck. In its function of maintaining the head in an erect position against the pull of gravity, the trapezius muscle works most efficiently when the head and neck are in their optimal position; that is, with the deepest part of the cervical lordosis no more than 4 to 6 cm from the apex of the thoracic kyphosis. The levator scapulae, splenius capitis, and splenius cervicis are other large superficial muscle groups that assist in extending the head and neck and holding the head up against gravity.

The multifidi and suboccipital muscles make up the deep posterior muscle group (Fig. 18-7). The multifidi have their origins on the transverse processes and insertions on the spinous process of the vertebra one to two segments above. When contracted together they extend the cervical spine; when contracted unilaterally they rotate the cervical spine to the opposite side and sidebend to the same side.

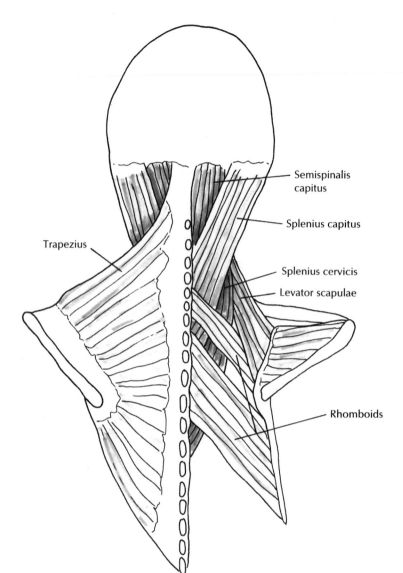

Semispinalis
capitus

Splenius capitus

Trapezius

Splenius cervicis

Levator scapulae

Rhomboids

Fig. 18–6. The superficial muscles of the head, neck, and shoulders. This posterior view shows the trapezius, levator scapulae, splenius capitis, splenius cervicis, and rhomboid muscles.

The sternocleidomastoid muscle is the largest and strongest of the anterior neck muscles (Fig. 18–8). From its dual origins on the sternum and clavicle, it inserts on the mastoid process, posterior to the center of gravity of the head. When both heads of the sternocleidomastoid are contracted together they are flexors of the neck but extensors of the head. When only one side is contracted, the head and neck are laterally flexed and are rotated to the opposite side. The sternocleidomastoid muscles are very strong, and when injured or in spasm, they hold the neck and head in the head-forward, chin-out posture.

The other major neck flexors are the scalenus muscles, having their origins on the first and second ribs and their insertions on the lateral tubercles of C2 to C7 (see Fig. 18–8). The scalenus anticus and scalenus medius are the anterior and posterior walls of the thoracic outlet. The first rib forms the bottom of the box, and the clavicle forms the top.[8] If the scalenus muscles are hypertrophied or in spasm, they may impinge on the lower roots of the brachial plexus or the subclavian artery as it passes through the thoracic outlet. Flexion of the head is accomplished by stabilization of the mandible by the muscles of mastication and a downward pull on the mandible by the strap (suprahyoid and infrahyoid) muscles (Fig. 18–9).[9]

The deep anterior neck muscles are the longus colli and longus cervicis (Fig. 18–10). They are small muscles with origins and insertions on the bodies of the cervical vertebrae. In spite of their size, they are very strong and have very good leverage. Their function is to prevent anterior collapse of the cervical lordosis to resist the compressive force of the long

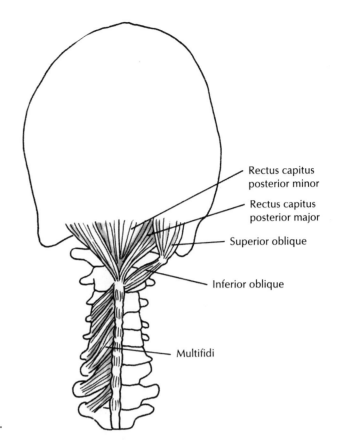

Rectus capitus
posterior minor

Rectus capitus
posterior major

Superior oblique

Inferior oblique

Multifidi

Fig. 18–7. A posterior view of the deep posterior neck muscles, showing the multifidi and suboccipital muscles.

cervical muscles. When these muscles are injured or in spasm, they exert a constant force that gradually flattens out the curve in the cervical spine.[9]

INNERVATION

Sensory and sympathetic innervation of the head and neck is a complex overlapping of cervical plexus and cranial nerves, making evaluation of pain complaints difficult. Sensory and sympathetic innervation of the face come from the facial and trigeminal nerves, both of which have sensory ganglia in the medulla oblongata and have anastomoses with sensory nerves of the cervical plexus (Fig. 18–11). The posterior portion of the head and upper cervical spine is primarily innervated by the greater and lesser occipital nerves, which arise from the cervical plexus, but also have twigs from the trigeminal nerve. The joint and ligamentous structures and the segmental spinal muscles of the cervical spine are innervated by the recurrent fibers of the segmental spinal nerves. The brachial plexus arises from the roots of the fifth through eighth cervical nerves and provides the sensory and motor innervation to the scapula and upper extremity.[7]

Clinical Considerations

1. Mechanical irritation of deep somatic structures in the cervical spine may refer pain to the face, head, upper extremity, or interscapular area.[4]
2. Neuritis and neuralgia of the cranial nerves, particularly V, VII, IX, and XI and also the greater and lesser occipital nerves, are common and may be mistaken for musculoskeletal pain.[1]
3. Peripheral entrapment of the brachial plexus is possible at the thoracic outlet, the shoulder, the elbow, and the carpal tunnel; this can produce symptoms that may be mistaken for shoulder tendinitis, elbow tendinitis, nerve root pain, or musculoskeletal pain of the neck or shoulder.
4. The nerve roots may be irritated by pressure from the bulging nucleus pulposus or by stenosis of the intervertebral foramen.

BLOOD SUPPLY

The blood vessels in the cervical region of particular interest to physical therapists are the subclavian arteries, which pass between the scalenus anticus and scalenus medius and may be compressed (see Tho-

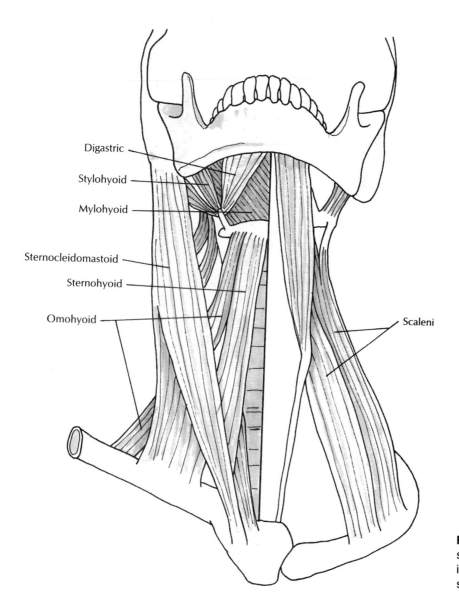

Digastric

Stylohyoid

Mylohyoid

Sternocleidomastoid

Sternohyoid

Omohyoid

Scaleni

Fig. 18–8. A frontal view of the superficial anterior neck muscles, showing the sternocleidomastoid, scaleni, suprahyoid, and infrahyoid muscles.

racic Outlet Syndrome on p. 511), and the vertebral artery. The vertebral artery passes upward through the lateral foramen of the cervical vertebrae. There is a redundant portion that allows full rotation of the atlas in both directions (Fig. 18–12). The vertebral arteries enter the cranium at the foramen magnum and come together to form the basilar artery.[10] The normal blood supply for the brain is through the carotid arteries if the circle of Willis is complete. If the circle of Willis is incomplete or if there is interruption of blood supply through the carotid arteries, the vertebral arteries may form a major portion of the blood supply for the brain, particularly the brain stem and cerebellum. The vertebral arteries are at least partially occluded by extension and rotation of the cervical spine; maximum occlusion occurs with the combination of extension and rotation. Brief occlusion of the vertebral artery is not a problem in a

patient who has normal carotid arteries and a normal circle of Willis; however, if there is interruption of the normal blood supply to the brain, occlusion of the vertebral artery may cause a reduction of blood flow to the brain stem and cerebellum, the symptoms of which are dizziness, nystagmus, slurring of speech, and loss of consciousness.[12]

There are many well-documented cases of coma and death secondary to vasospasm or thrombosis of the vertebral arteries caused by manipulation of the upper cervical spine.[3,10,13] The most common history of this type of catastrophe involves an attempt to rotate the atlas and usually involves an exceptionally forceful manuever. In many cases the patient felt violently ill, dizzy, briefly lost consciousness after manipulation, was manipulated again, and died several hours later. Because death may occur several hours after manipulation, it is possible that the num-

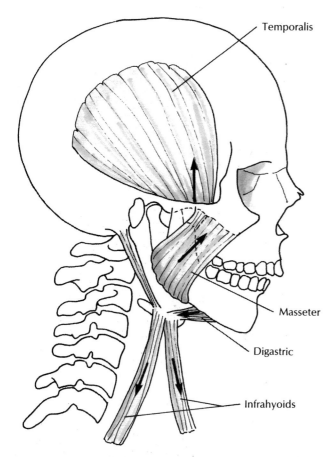

Fig. 18-9. A lateral view of the head, neck, and mandible showing the muscular forces that flex the head. The infrahyoid muscles pulling downward on the hyoid bone, the suprahyoids pulling down on the mandible, and the muscles of mastication stabilizing the jaw.

Fig. 18-10. The deep anterior neck muscles include the longus colli.

ber of catastrophic responses to upper cervical manipulation is actually underreported.

Blood vessels in the cervical spine have no nociceptive innervation, *per se,* but when overdilated, intense headaches (migraines) are perceived. Migraine headaches may be accompanied by blurring of vision from pressure of the distended cranial blood vessel on the optic nerves. They may also be accompanied by nausea and muscle spasm in the neck. The migraine headache may be distinguished from the musculoskeletal headache in that the pain is generally throbbing rather than constant, and the pattern of the headache is generally irregular and not related to trauma or activity.[1]

Clinical Considerations

1. Before using traction or mobilization techniques on the upper cervical spine, the vertebral arteries should be carefully tested one at a time by placing the neck in full rotation, extension, and lateral flexion to each side and holding for approximately 1 minute. The clinician should observe the patient for nystagmus, slurring of speech, blurring of vision, dizziness, or unconsciousness. Dizziness as a result of vertebral artery testing is fairly common and should be a warning sign to the practitioner to proceed very cautiously. Nystagmus, slurring of speech, or loss of consciousness should be considered contraindications to traction and mobilization of the neck, and the practitioner should take care when treating the patient to make sure that the neck is not positioned in extension or the extremes of rotation.[15]

2. If a patient has a history of throbbing headaches or headaches accompanied by blurring of vision and nausea, or if the history of headaches is irregular and not related to activity, the possibility of mi-

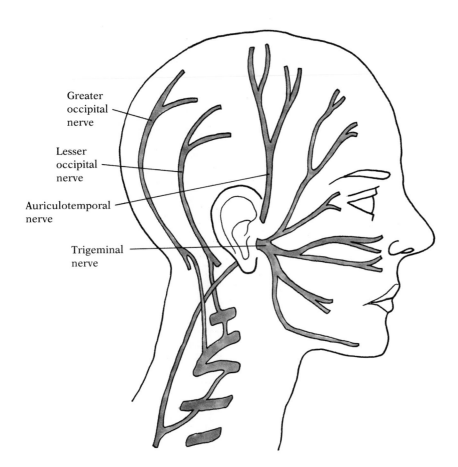

Greater
occipital
nerve

Lesser
occipital
nerve

Auriculotemporal
nerve

Trigeminal
nerve

Fig. 18-11. A lateral view of the neck, head, and face showing the cervical plexus, trigeminal, and occipital nerves.

Fig. 18-12. A posterior view of the upper cervical spine, showing the vertebral artery emerging from C2 with a redundant loop that allows mobility of the atlas.

graine headaches should be investigated before investing in a long course of physical therapy treatment.

JOINT MECHANICS

LOWER CERVICAL SPINE (C2-T1)

The facet joints of the lower cervical spine are planar; at the single-joint level the only motions possible are superior and inferior glide. In inferior glide or extension the joint surfaces are maximally congruent, and the facet and joint capsules are maximally taut. Extension is the close-packed position and the position of maximal stability of the cervical spine. In full flexion the ligaments of the joint capsule are also taut, but the surfaces of the joint are barely engaged, making flexion the position of instability.[16]

Clinical Considerations

1. When the cervical spine is positioned in slight lordosis, there is good passive stability from the facet joints and supporting ligaments. When the

cervical lordosis is lost or the cervical curve is reversed, passive stability is lost, and the segmental muscles must go into constant contraction to stabilize the spine.

2. When there is slight lordosis in the cervical spine, the facet joints are able to bear approximately one third each of the compressive forces on the spine.

When the cervical lordosis is lost, the entire compressive force is borne by the disk, causing excessive pressure and flattening.

Motion of a lower cervical segment involves movement of the vertebral bodies, using the disk as a pivot, as well as movement of the joints of Luschka and the facet joints. Flexion of a cervical segment is superior glide of both facet joints. Extension of the cervical spine is inferior glide of both facet joints. Rotation and sidebending of the lower cervical spine are the same movements. There is inferior glide of the facet joint on the side to which the spine is rotated or sidebent, and superior glide of the facet on the side opposite rotation. Because of the 45° slope of the facet joints, the lateral tubercle on the same side moves downward and backward while that on the opposite side moves upward and forward. With either rotation or lateral flexion, there is always slight extension of the segment as well.[9]

When the ring of the atlas lifts up posteriorly, there is approximately 20° of flexion–extension of the atlanto-occipital joint and approximately 15° of flexion of the atlantoaxial joint. When the atlanto-occipital joint is in extension, the ring of the atlas gets closer to the occiput and may compress the neurovascular structures in the suboccipital area. When the atlanto-occipital joint is flexed by nodding the head, the space between the atlas and occiput is maximally opened (Fig. 18–13). This can be seen clearly on mobility roentgenograms. Sidebending of the atlanto-occipital joint is always accompanied by a small conjunct rotation to the opposite side, which allows the condyle of the occiput on the side of lateral flexion to become congruent with the superior joint surface of the axis below. Lateral flexion is checked by the alar ligament, which because of its insertion on the dens, causes rotation of the axis toward the side of lateral flexion. This can be palpated as the spinous process of the axis swinging to the side opposite lateral flexion. Palpating for motion of the spinous process of the axis with sidebending of the atlanto-occipital joint is a test for integrity of the alar ligament. Rotation of the atlas around the axis always involves a swing to the side opposite rotation and an elevation of the transverse process opposite rotation as the atlas slides up the shoulder of the

Fig. 18–13. Mobility of the upper cervical spine. *(A)* Flexion, *(B)* extension. (Note: In flexion, the space between the occiput and C1 increases and decreases with extension.)

Fig. 18-14. An oblique view of the cervical spine showing full rotation: external rotation and lateral flexion of the lower cervical segments, rotation of alantoaxial joint, and flexion of the atlanto-occipital joint.

axis. This is accompanied by a tilting of the atlas toward the side of rotation, which may be palpated as the transverse process of the atlas moving posteriorly and inferiorly, and the transverse process on the side opposite rotation moving anteriorly and superiorly. Because the atlas has considerable mobility with relatively little ligamentous stability, it is possible for the atlas to be jammed or locked in a rotated position.

The combined movement of flexion of the head and neck involves full flexion of the atlanto-occipital joint, flexion of the atlas on the dens, and full flexion of the lower cervical segments. The combined movement of extension of the head and neck consists of extension of the atlanto-occipital joint, extension of the atlas on the axis, and extension of the lower cervical segments. As mentioned above, in the lower cervical spine there is no difference between rotation and sidebending. In the upper cervical spine,

rotation of the head and neck is rotation of the atlantoaxial joint to the same side and sidebending of the atlanto-occipital joint to the opposite side. Sidebending actually involves lateral flexion of only the atlanto-occipital joint, but rotation of the atlantoaxial joint to the opposite side. Both rotation and sidebending involve slight flexion of the atlanto-occipital joint to compensate for extension of the lower cervical spine (Fig. 18-14).[9]

Example. In left rotation of the head and neck, each segment of the lower cervical spine is in the combined movement of left lateral flexion and rotation, and each segment is slightly extended. The atlantoaxial joint is in full left rotation. The atlanto-occipital joint is in sidebending to the right and is slightly flexed.

In left lateral flexion of the neck and cervical spine, each segment of the lower cervical spine is as in left rotation, with lateral flexion, rotation, and slight extension. The atlantoaxial joint is fully rotated to the right. The atlanto-occipital joint is in sidebending to the left and in slight flexion.

The only difference between left lateral flexion of the head and neck and left rotation of the head and neck is what happens in the upper cervical spine.

Fig. 18-15. Clinical appearance of a boy with a rotated atlas.

HEAD-RIGHTING MECHANISM

The posture and righting mechanism seen in infants and lower animals are present in adult human beings as well. There is a strong tendency for the eyes to face forward and level in the horizontal plane. This means that any lateral or rotational deviation from normal posture must be compensated for in the upper cervical spine. This also means that if there is a rotational or sidebending fault in the upper cervical spine, it will impart scoliosis to the rest of the spine. For example, in an atlanto-occipital joint locked in left lateral flexion, the cervical spine will move into right sidebending to bring the eyes level, thus producing an S-shaped scoliosis in the rest of the spine. Another example would be a left leg-length discrepancy that imparts a long C-shaped scoliosis; this is compensated for by left lateral flexion at the atlanto-occipital joint to bring the eyes level (Fig. 18–15).[16]

EXAMINATION

I. **History** — In addition to the general musculo-skeletal history (see Chapter 4, Assessment of Musculoskeletal Disorders), the following factors should be considered:
   A. *Rule out migraines by determining if headache symptoms are:*
      1. Of an intermittent irregular pattern unrelated to activity or trauma
      2. Accompanied by nausea or blurring of vision
      3. Throbbing like a pulse rather than steady
      4. Relieved by beta blockers, ergotamine, or related compounds
   B. *Determine if pain is caused by neuritis or neuralgia:*[1]
      1. It is unrelated to activity or trauma.
      2. It is superficial, stimulating in quality, or electric.
      3. It follows the pattern of innervation of a cranial or peripheral nerve.
   C. *Evaluate upper extremity pain* — If the patient is complaining of upper extremity pain, is it in the pattern of a nerve root or peripheral entrapment?

II. **Observation**
   A. *Posture* — Observe in sitting and standing
      1. General alignment
      2. Does the head deviate from the optimal posture (4–8 cm from the apex of the thoracic kyphosis to the deepest point in the cervical lordosis)? (Fig. 18–16).[16]
      3. When the sternocleidomastoid muscle is in its normal rest position, it angles backward slightly. If the sternocleidomastoid muscle is vertical, this indicates forward head posture and/or tightness of the sternocleidomastoid muscle.
      4. Function — How willing is the patient to turn the neck when dressing, undressing, or filling out paperwork?

III. **Inspection**
   A. *Structure*
      1. Observe the angle of the head on the

Fig. 18–16. Measurement of head posture.

Fig. 18–17. Observation view of the head, neck, and shoulder girdle.

neck and the angle of the neck on the trunk (Fig. 18–17)

2. Are clavicles angled or horizontal?
3. Do the scapulae lie flat against the thoracic wall or are they winged?

B. *Soft tissue signs*
1. Muscle spasm or parafunctional activity of the muscles of mastication, the facial muscles, or muscles of the cervical spine
2. Segmental guarding or hypertrophy of muscle
3. Atrophy of the muscles of the neck, upper extremity, or scapula

C. *Skin*—neck, shoulder girdle, and upper extremity regions
1. Color
2. Moisture
3. Redness or swelling
4. Scars or blemishes

IV. Selective Tissue Tension
A. *Active range of motion*—test in sitting
1. Flexion–extension (see Fig. 18–18A,B)
2. Rotation (see Fig. 18–18C)
3. Sidebending (see Fig. 18–18D). (If side-

bending is severely limited, suspect capsular tightness of the lower cervical spine).
4. Lock lower cervical spine in full lateral flexion or full flexion. Test movement of the atlanto-occipital joint by testing lateral flexion. Test movement of the atlantoaxial joint by testing rotation (see Fig. 18–18E).

B. *Passive range of motion*—test supine. Repeat tests for active motion, noting the range of motion, end feel, muscle spasm, and pain.

C. *Isometrically resisted motions*
1. Gently test rotation, lateral flexion, and flexion of the cervical spine (see p. 535).
2. Test rotator cuff muscles, noting pain and/or weakness (see Ch. 10, The Shoulder).

D. *Joint play*
1. Atlanto-occipital joint
   a. Distraction (Fig. 18–19A)
   b. Lateral glide (Fig. 18–19B)
2. Atlantoaxial joint

Fig. 18-18. Active movements of the cervical spine. *(A)* Flexion, *(B)* extension, *(C)* rotation, *(D)* sidebending, and *(E)* atlantoaxial rotation.

A

B

Fig. 18–19. Joint-play movements of the atlanto-occipital joint. *(A)* Distraction, *(B)* lateral glide.

    a. Distraction
    b. Rotation (see Fig. 18–20).
  3. Lower cervical facets—Test glide by placing the web space of the thumb over the joint and gently gliding laterally (Fig. 18–21).
V. Neurological Testing
  A. *Neurological involvement suspected:*
    1. For neurological function in various sites, test the levels noted:
      a. Abduction—C5
      b. Biceps—C6

      c. Triceps—C7
      d. Pronator teres—C7
      e. Wrist extension—C6
      f. Wrist flexion—C7
      g. Finger abduction—C8
      h. Finger adduction—T1
    2. Reflex testing
      a. Biceps—C6 (Fig. 18–22*A*)
      b. Triceps—C7 (Fig. 18–22*B*)
      c. Wrist extensor—C6 (Fig. 18–22*C*)
  B. *Sensation*—Test sensation, particularly around the hand (Fig. 18–23) (see Chapter

Fig. 18–20. Joint-play movements of the atlantoaxial joint rotation.

19, The Cervical–Upper Extremity Scan Examination).
C. *Spurling test* (foramen compression)
  1. Place the neck in extension, lateral flexion, and rotation to one side. Watch for referred pain or neurological signs in the extremity (Fig. 18–24*A*).
  2. Apply traction to the neck and watch for improvement of referred pain and neurological symptoms (Fig. 18–24*B*).

D. *Carpal tunnel test* (see Chapter 12, The Wrist and Hand Complex) (Fig. 18–25)
E. *Tests for scalenus anticus and thoracic outlet* (Fig. 18–26) (see Chapter 19, The Cervical–Upper Extremity Scan Examination)
  1. Scalenus anticus (Fig. 18–26*A*)—Apply firm pressure over the lower bellies of the scalenus muscles near their origins on the first and second ribs. Maintain pressure for at least 30 seconds. The scalenus muscles, if involved, may refer pain to the anterior chest, neck, or interscapular area, even if there is no neurovascular compression.
  2. Test for neurovascular compression (Fig. 18–26*B*)
    a. Patient—in a sitting position
    b. Operator—standing behind and to one side
    c. Movement—Operator guides the motion of the patient's head to the extreme of rotation and into slight extension, holding this position for at least 30 seconds, palpating for pulse at the wrist, and watching for reproduction of radiating symptoms in the hand or arm.
  3. Neurovascular test with depression of the scapula (Fig. 18–26*B*). The patient and operator are in the same position as above (neurovascular compression test).

Fig. 18–21. Lateral glide movements of the lower cervical facets.

A

B

C

Fig. 18–22. Test of upper limb reflexes. (A) Biceps, (B) triceps, and (C) wrist extension.

In addition to rotating and extending the neck, the operator presses down on the shoulder, depressing the clavicle and closing down the thoracic outlet. Hold for 30 seconds and watch for the same signs and symptoms as above.

4. Neurovascular test with clavicle depressed and ribs elevated. Repeat the procedure in the previous test, and ask the patient to take a deep breath and hold for 30 seconds.

5. Overhead test (Fig. 18–26C). With the patient in the same position as above, place a 2- or 3-pound weight in the patient's hand, flex the shoulder, and repeatedly flex and extend the elbow (actively). If there is compression of the subclavian artery, the muscles of the elbow will fatigue very rapidly, and the symptoms may be reproduced.

VI. **Palpation**—The following structures should be carefully palpated for guarding, spasm, and particularly to see if deep palpation reproduces pain referred to another area.

A. **Trapezius**—Palpate inferior, middle, and superior portions (Fig. 18–27A).

Fig. 18–23. Sensory testing of the dermatomes of the hand. *(A)* C5, *(B)* C6, *(C)* C7, and *(D)* C8 sensory areas.

B. Levator scapula—Palpate particularly close to the origin.

C. Multifidi—Should be palpated segmentally from C2–C7, particularly noting segmental guarding at the C4, C5, or C6 segments (Fig. 18–27B).

D. Lesser occipital nerve (Fig. 18–28A)

E. Greater occipital nerve and suboccipital musculature (Fig. 18–28B)

F. Belly of the temporalis muscle (Fig. 18–28C)

G. Masseter muscle—Palpate bimanually with the thumb inside the mouth and fingers over the cheeks (Fig. 18–28D) and outside the mouth (Fig. 18–28E).

H. Inferior head of the lateral pterygoid muscle (Fig. 18–28F)

I. Medial pterygoid—Palpate at its insertion under the angle of the mandible.

J. The sternocleidomastoid muscle (Fig. 18–28G)

K. The thyroid cartilage and longus colli muscle (Fig. 18–28H)

L. The suprasternal notch and sternoclavicular joint (Fig. 18–28I)

M. The acromioclavicular joint (Fig. 18–28J)

A

B

Fig. 18–24. Spurling test.

N. The sternocleidomastoid in supine (Fig. 18–29)—Simultaneous palpation.

VII. Roentgenographic Analysis

    A. Cervical curve: normal or abnormal curvature.

        1. There should be a slight lordotic curve in the cervical spine.

        2. Note a straight or kyphotic spine suggesting spasms of the longus colli or over development of the anterior neck musculature.

        3. Ankylosis or instability on mobility films.

    B. Lipping or spurring of the vertebral bodies or unicate processes indicating abnormal weight bearing or degeneration of the disk. Also note disk height.

    C. Intervertebral foramina: Look for opening on an oblique film. Note any narrowing or encroachment.

    D. A 9–12 mm space between the ring of the atlas and the occiput. There should be a minimum of 9–12 mm of space on the x-ray between the occipital bone and the post arch of the atlas. Less than 9 mm of space

Fig. 18–25. Carpal tunnel test.

A

B

C

Fig. 18–26. Thoracic outlet tests. *(A)* Scalenus anticus test. *(B)* Neurovascular compression test with depression of the scapula. *(C)* Overhead test.

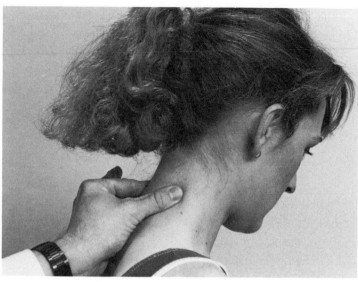

A   B

Fig. 18–27. Palpation of the *(A)* trapezius, and the *(B)* multifidi muscles (segmentally).

indicates extension of the upper cervical spine and possible compression of the neurovascular structures in the suboccipital area.

E. Through the mouth view for the relationship of the odontoid process to the adjacent bones.

COMMON DISORDERS

ACCELERATION INJURY

The mechanism of acceleration injury (or whiplash) is acceleration of the head and neck relative to the body. It usually results from the collision of two automobiles but also can result from contact sports such as football or high-velocity sports such as skiing. The most common mechanism of injury is an automobile at rest struck from behind. At the moment of impact, the trunk of the body, which is supported by the car seat, moves rapidly forward. The moment of inertia of the head creates a relative backward acceleration of the head and neck.[17] Acceleration injuries are not as dangerous as flexion injuries of the neck, in which the head is stabilized and the momentum of the body weight forces the neck into flexion, but they can be very persistent and difficult to treat. Because there is often a question of insurance compensation, and because roentgenographic reports, even in the most severe cases, are usually negative, the question arises as to whether there actually is an injury, and if so, which structures

are injured. As with low back injuries, there is a natural history to acceleration injuries; 80% of patients reporting symptoms following a motor vehicle accident will be better within 3 to 4 weeks.[5,6,14] If this is so, are there any factors that would allow us to predict from the physical examination who the 20% will be who will not improve spontaneously? These questions have been partially answered by experimental animal research and longitudinal studies of patients injured in automobile accidents.

In a study of 525 patients injured in automobile accidents, the direction of the initial impact was found to be an important predictor of prognosis. In this group, the 100 patients who were in cars involved in head-on collisions had no prolonged symptoms. The 200 cases where initial impact was from the side had lingering symptoms for a short period of time but no symptoms lasting more than a few months. Of the 250 patients in cars that were hit from the rear, 50% were still having symptoms 1 year after the accident.[11] The possibility of insurance compensation did not seem to be a factor in prognosis. Presumably, when the initial impact is from the front, the chin hits the chest before the cervical spine reaches its anatomical limit of motion. When the initial impact is from the side, the head hits the shoulder before the anatomical limit of range of motion is reached. When the impact is from behind, however, unless the back of the car seat is high enough, there is no anatomical stop to prevent hyperextension.

Acceleration injuries were simulated in monkeys

by strapping them to car seats and dropping them backward from various heights. The animals were sacrificed and dissected at intervals afterwards. The most common injuries found were complete and partial tears of the sternocleidomastoid muscle followed by complete and partial tears of the longus colli, complete and partial tears of the anterior longitudinal ligament, and finally, separation of the disks from the vertebral bodies.[11] Five patients who had persistent symptoms from rear-end impact were found at surgery to have disks torn away from the vertebral body.[11] Following anterior fusion, their symptoms were resolved, even though most of them had long since settled their insurance claims.

The two other predictors of a poor prognosis are: (1) roentgenographic evidence of degenerative joint disease and (2) neurological signs soon after the accident.[14]

Clinical Considerations

1. Patients with injuries from initial impact from the rear should be followed more closely and should be considered to be at higher risk for having prolonged symptoms. Patients who have roentgenographic evidence of degenerative joint disease or neurological signs soon after the accident must also be considered at higher risk and followed more closely.
2. Muscle injury to the anterior neck must not be overlooked, particularly the sternocleidomastoid and deep anterior neck musculature.
3. Acceleration injuries should be considered legitimate trauma with potential anatomical damage sufficient to cause the symptoms that most patients complain of.

   Acceleration injury should be considered in three phases: acute, subacute, and chronic. The injury should be classified according to the findings from examination, rather than the length of time since the accident.

Acute Phase

The acute phase begins at the moment of the accident and may last as long as 2 to 3 weeks. The most severe injury is from a rear impact. As the head hyperextends on the trunk, the sternocleidomastoid muscle becomes tight, and it is pulled or torn. With higher velocity impacts, the longus colli may be pulled or torn, the anterior longitudinal ligament may be pulled or torn, and the annulus of the disk may tear away from the vertebral body. The facet joints are hyperextended, and their capsules may be strained or torn. There is generally little pain and fairly free range of motion immediately after the accident with painful stiffness gradually developing over 24 to 48 hours. There is a possibility of fracture, traction injury to the nerve roots, contusion to the spinal cord, head injury, or tearing of the supporting ligaments of the upper cervical spine. These conditions cannot be ruled out definitively without a roentgenographic evaluation. Consultation with a physician prior to mechanical treatment is wise.

Evaluation. The patient will generally feel very little pain or stiffness immediately after the accident. As the large muscles swell and develop spasm, the patient will note onset of muscle soreness, stiffness, and swelling. The therapist may observe spasm of the sternocleidomastoid muscle, and the head will often be pulled into the head-forward posture. The skin may be red, and the muscles will be warm, rubbery, and tender to touch. Active range of motion will be quite limited with muscle spasm end feel. Passive range of motion will be greater than active. Joint play will be very difficult to assess because of muscle spasm. The sternocleidomastoid muscle will generally be warm, swollen, and in spasm. There may be palpable tears, particularly in the proximal third. There may be clearly delineated segmental spasm of the multifidi at the C4–C5 or C5–C6 level.

Treatment. The goal of treatment in the acute phase is to allow the cervical musculature to rest without becoming stiff and to progress to the subacute phase as rapidly as possible. Very little treatment is needed in the acute phase. The patient should be instructed in the use of heat or ice at home and in the use of a soft cervical collar. The patient should also be instructed in active rotation of the cervical spine within limits of pain to maintain joint range of motion. The patient should be given an explanation of the mechanics of the acceleration injury, including the information that most cases are completely healed in 4 to 5 weeks. The patient should be encouraged to be as active as possible and should be rechecked at approximately 1-week intervals.

Subacute Phase

In the subacute phase, which usually lasts 2 to 10 weeks, the larger muscles have healed and are no longer swollen or tender. General muscle guarding will be reduced, and a more detailed evaluation of the cervical spine will be possible.

Evaluation. The patient will report that the muscle pain originally experienced has gone away but has been replaced by deep, aching pain that may be referred to the head, the interscapular area, or the

(Text continued on p. 520.)

A

B

C

D

E

Fig. 18–28. Palpation of the occipital region, muscles of mastication, and the anterior neck muscles. *(A)* The lesser occipital nerve, *(B)* the greater occipital nerve and suboccipital musculature, *(C)* belly of the temporalis muscle, *(D)* the masseter muscle (inside the mouth), *(E)* masseter muscle (superficial fibers), *(F)* the inferior head of the lateral pterygoid, *(G)* the sternocleidomastoid muscle, *(H)* the thyroid cartilage and longus colli muscle, *(I)* the suprasternal notch and sternoclavicular joint, and *(J)* the acromioclavicular joint.

F

G

H

I

J

Fig. 18–29. Palpation of the sternocleidomastoid from its origin to its base. (Both sternocleidomastoids should be palpated simultaneously).

upper extremity. The large cervical muscles will no longer feel warm, rubbery, and swollen. There will be focal areas of intense tenderness in the sternocleidomastoid, suboccipital, multifidi, and deep anterior neck muscles. These areas of tenderness may refer pain to the head, shoulder, or upper extremity when palpated. Active range of motion will have increased considerably. The end feel will be capsular muscle guarding. If the facet joints have been injured, there will be capsular restriction of the neck with limitation of joint play when tested. The patient should be given a complete neurological screening, which in most cases will be negative. The major muscle groups of the neck should be carefully palpated noting tenderness, guarding, spasm, or anatomical shortening. The longus colli should be carefully palpated. As the patient progresses through the subacute phase, the longus colli should become progressively less tender. Roentgenograms may show flattening of the cervical spine from spasm of the longus colli.

Treatment. The treatment goal in the subacute phase is to restore flexibility to the cervical muscle groups and facet joints, if they are involved. Mechanical treatment is most effective in the subacute phase because muscle guarding has subsided, and stretching and mobilization will be fairly comfortable, but adhesions between muscle and joint fibers will not have solidified into scars.

Physical therapists have many effective techniques for dealing with tight, painful muscles. The following principles will make treatment of the muscles of the cervical spine more effective:

1. The most likely muscle to be injured in an acceleration injury is the sternocleidomastoid muscle. In order to stretch the sternocleidomastoid, the head and neck must be put into an extreme of rotation and lateral flexion, which can be uncomfortable and can also be damaging to joints and smaller muscles. The sternocleidomastoid muscle can be easily treated by massage.

2. The sternocleidomastoid muscles will be overshortened and very strong. Any strengthening program that increases the strength of the sternocleidomastoid or anterior neck musculature will contribute to muscle imbalance.

3. The most effective treatment for the longus colli and multifidi is to restore normal resting length (slight lordosis).[16]

4. Lordosis is a dynamic position and cannot be restored passively. Strengthening of the multifidus is the best way to restore cervical lordosis and to stabilize the midcervical spine. Multifidus strengthening through isometric exercise should be started as early as possible (see Treatment Techniques, p. 526).

5. The large posterior neck musculature should be strengthened but not stretched. These muscles need to be strong to counteract the anterior pull of the sternocleidomastoid muscle. All of the muscles of the cervical spine are accessory muscles of respiration. They can be aerobically strengthened by any activity that increases heart rate above the target level. Aerobic training of muscle is very helpful in reducing lactic acid to carbon dioxide. Blood flow to muscle can be increased by a factor

of one or two by massage, but with aerobic exercise, blood flow to muscle increases by a factor of six.

In addition to muscle therapy, attention must also be directed toward the facet joints. The cervical facet joints are approximately the same size as the distal interphalangeal joint of the little finger. The capsule and ligaments are delicate, and the mechanical forces that the facet joints undergo in an acceleration injury are severe. Because the facet joints are so deep, swelling, warmth, and redness are not apparent; however, the facet joints do go through the same stages that any acutely injured joint does. Mobilization or stretching that causes an increase in swelling will be harmful to the joint, because the presence of edema contributes to scarring. It is possible that overstretching or mobilization of swollen joints may lead to ankylosis or degenerative joint disease. Based on the information that we have about peripheral joint injuries, immobilization of injured joints also contributes to scarring.

The following guidelines are useful in treating the facet joints during the subacute phase:

1. During the acute phase, the patient should be instructed in active rotation within limits of pain to be done every hour.
2. Joint mobilization in the subacute phase should not be painful to the patient or cause lingering discomfort after treatment.
3. Hypermobile areas should be identified and mobilization avoided.
4. Gross passive stretching of the head and neck should be avoided because of the possibility of overstretching hypermobile segments. Range of motion should be restored by segmental joint mobilization (see Treatment Techniques, p. 528).

Chronic Phase

The chronic phase of an acceleration injury begins when the acute healing process is over. The large muscle groups will have completely healed, but they may be shortened and fibrotic. The longus colli remains in chronic spasm and will be acutely tender to palpation. The longus colli exerts a force that gradually flattens the cervical spine and may lead eventually to cervical instability. The multifidus at the C5 or C6 segment will be in constant contraction and may feel rubbery and inflamed as a result of overwork, attempting to stabilize the lower cervical spine.
Evaluation.   The patient will complain of symptoms which are consistent with irritation of the deep somatic structures. The pain will be deep, aching, vague, and often referred to the head, shoulders, interscapular area, or upper extremity. It is very common to have a headache in the suboccipital area, which begins in the morning and gets gradually worse with the day's activity. The patient will have hypertrophy of the sternocleidomastoid muscles and may have parafunctional hyperactivity of the anterior neck muscles and muscles of mastication. The patient will have a forward-head posture with protraction of the scapula and superior angulation of the clavicles. Active range of motion of the neck may be limited by as much as 50%. Active and passive ranges of motion will be approximately the same. When tested segmentally, the upper and midcervical spine will be limited in a capsular pattern with hypermobility of the C4, C5, or C6 segments. Neurological testing will generally be negative, but there is the possibility of nerve-root irritation or thoracic outlet syndrome from shortening and hypertrophy of the scalenus muscles. On palpation there will generally be segmental guarding of the multifidus muscle at the C5 or C6 segment. There may be tenderness and spasm of the suboccipital muscles from overcontracting in a shortened position from the forward-head posture. There may be tenderness of the greater or lesser occipital nerve from mechanical compression. The muscles of mastication should be carefully palpated if tenderness is present. A temporomandibular joint evaluation should be performed (see Chapter 16, The Temporomandibular Joint). The sternocleidomastoid muscle will be hypertrophied and may have palpable fibrous nodes. The longus colli will be acutely tender, particularly at the C4 through C7 segments.

Roentgenograms may begin to show flattening or kyphosis of the cervical spine. If retropharyngeal swelling is present, it may be seen along the anterior border of the cervical spine on the lateral roentgenogram. The intervertebral foramen will be open. There may be less than 8 mm of space noted on the lateral film between the occiput and atlas, indicating chronic extension of the upper cervical spine secondary to forward-head posture. If mobility films are taken, they may show hypermobility of C4, C5, or C6.
Treatment.   The treatment approach in the chronic phase must be gradual. Rapid increases in range of motion should not be expected because fibrosis of joints and muscles will respond well to gentle repetitive stretching, but attempts to overstretch will result in increased swelling and scarring. The emphasis of treatment must be to gradually restore cervical lordosis by mobilization into extension and specific segmental strengthening of the multifidus at the hypermobile segment. Normal muscle balance should

Fig. 18-30. The chin-tuck exercise.

also be restored by stretching the large anterior neck musculature and strengthening the posterior neck musculature.

Treatment of the acceleration injury in the chronic phase must be undertaken carefully and gradually, with a view not only to short-term symptoms but also to long-range outcome. A few precautions should be noted:

1. Stretching of the posterior neck musculature, particularly by pulling the head into flexion, may give temporary reduction of muscular symptoms, but in the long run will contribute to cervical instability.
2. The "chin-tuck" exercise (Fig. 18-30) may be helpful in stretching the suboccipital muscles, but it also completely flattens the curve in the cervical spine. When instructing a patient in this exercise, always give the precaution that it should be continued for no longer than 6 weeks.
3. Strengthening exercises should be light, as the multifidi are very small muscles. Care should be taken in the exercise instruction to avoid strengthening of the sternocleidomastoid or anterior neck muscles.

4. Vigorous rotatory mobilization or passive stretching may overstretch segments that are already hypermobile, contributing to cervical instability.
5. The patient should be encouraged to remain as active as possible, and 20 minutes of aerobic activity should be a component of every treatment program.

CERVICAL INSTABILITY

Passive stability of the cervical spine comes from the tripod configuration of the two posterior facet joints and the anterior disk. When the cervical spine is in its normal rest position of slight lordosis, the facet joints are engaged and bear approximately one third of the vertical compressive force. Very little muscle contraction is needed to maintain stability in this position. Passive stability may be lost as a result of an injury (see Acceleration Injury, earlier) or may develop after years of poor posture or activities that involve flexion of the neck. If cervical lordosis is lost, the facet joints disengage and are no longer capable of stabilizing rotational forces. The vertical compressive forces are shifted forward onto the disk, which gradually begins to lose height. Over time the annulus of the disk stretches out and weakens, and the vertebral bodies may show lipping and traction spurs as an attempt to compensate for increased vertical compressive forces (see Degenerative Joint Disease, p. 523). The multifidus muscle must be in constant contraction to prevent overrotation or overflexion. The segmental muscle will progress from constant guarding to spasm and inflammation. The annulus of the disk is weakened, and there may be acute episodes of bulging of nuclear material, either anteriorly or posteriorly. Patients with cervical instability may have chronic headaches, chronic neck pain, and chronic shoulder or interscapular pain. They also may have asymptomatic periods and acute episodes of disk bulging that happen suddenly for no apparent reason.

Evaluation. The patient may have a history of acceleration injury or an occupation that involves flexion of the neck such as office or laboratory work. The patient may have a forward-head posture but observation alone should not be relied on to determine cervical lordosis or compression of the upper cervical spine. There will generally be hypertrophy of the anterior neck and anterior chest and protraction of the scapula with elevation of the clavicles. Active and passive ranges of motion will be limited. When tested segmentally, the upper cervical spine will be restricted. There will be hypermobility of C4 or C5, usually accompanied by ankylosis of the segment below. The patient should be given a careful neurological examination. Neurological tests will generally be negative. There may be nerve irritation from peripheral entrapment or a bulging disk, but rarely from bony compression. The multifidi will be in segmental guarding or spasm and may feel rubbery or acutely inflamed. The sternocleidomastoid muscles are hypertrophied and may have localized areas of fibrosis that are acutely tender. The deep anterior neck musculature, particularly the longus colli, will be in spasm and may be acutely inflamed.

Treatment. The only effective conservative treatment for cervical instability is to restore the normal lordosis to the cervical spine. This should be accomplished by mobilizing the upper and midcervical spine to restore range of motion, segmental strengthening of the multifidus to hold the lordosis, followed by restoration of the muscular balance of the cervical spine. As with chronic acceleration injuries, care must be taken when working with the neck to avoid strengthening the sternocleidomastoid or anterior neck musculature and to avoid stretching segments that are already hypermobile.

ACUTE DISK BULGE

If the annulus of the disk is weakened, acute bulging of the disk, either anteriorly or posteriorly, may occur. If the disk bulges anteriorly, it presses on the anterior longitudinal ligament and may cause spasm of the longus colli. The patient may have difficulty swallowing or have the sensation of a sore throat. If the disk bulges posteriorly, it may press on the posterior longitudinal ligament, the spinal cord, or the nerve root.

Evaluation. Sudden onset of acute neck pain, usually noticed early in the morning, is probably from bulging of the disk. It has also been described as acute dislocation of a facet joint or entrapment of the synovial villi. The pain begins with clearly delineated, sharp neck pain and progresses during the day to generalized muscle spasm and inability to rotate the neck in one direction. The patient may present with the neck rotated and bent to one side and may be in acute distress. Active range of motion will be limited in rotation and lateral flexion to one side and fairly free to the opposite side. Active and passive range of motion will be limited by pain and muscle spasm, and passive range of motion will usually be considerably greater than active. A position of comfort is usually a combination of extension and lateral flexion to the opposite side, and traction often makes the condition immediately more comfortable.

Treatment. These conditions generally resolve in a few days if left untreated, but there is an excellent treatment method described by Cyriax (Part II, p. 76) that will provide greatly increased comfort and range of motion for the first few days.[2] This consists of placing the neck in as much extension as possible under fairly strong manual traction. Range of motion under traction is begun first to the pain-free side. When full range of motion of the pain-free side is achieved, range of motion under traction to the painful side is begun.[2]

The patient should be instructed to avoid flexion of the neck. A soft collar will be helpful for the first few days. The patient should be reassured and encouraged to be as active as possible. When the acute symptoms subside, treatment for cervical instability should begin.

DEGENERATIVE JOINT DISEASE

Degenerative joint disease begins as capsular restriction of the facet joints without bony changes on roentgenograms and gradually progresses over months or years to the characteristic flattening, lipping, and spurring of the vertebral bodies and facet joints that become clearly visible on roentgenographic studies. Degenerative joint disease must be considered a normal aging process (most older people have at least some evidence of it) but it should be considered abnormal in younger people. Degenerative joint disease may be accelerated by injury. Bony stenosis of the intervertebral foramen is possible and may cause symptoms of neck pain, shoulder pain, radiating pain in the arm, numbness in the extremity, or muscle weakness.

One of the paradoxes of degenerative joint disease is that the patient may have foraminal stenosis for many years without symptoms and then suddenly begin to have neurological signs and symptoms. After treatment with traction or passage of time, these signs or symptoms may resolve. Clearly the bony changes have not improved, so what accounts for the sudden appearance and disappearance of symptoms? Pain from compression of nerve roots is complex. In an experimental study, ligatures were placed around nerve roots at the time of surgery so that pressure could be applied after the surgical incision had healed. When pressure was applied to the healthy nerve roots, there were no symptoms of pain or paresthesia. When pressure was applied to injured nerve roots, there was a gradual onset of anesthesia, diminished reflex, and eventually motor weakness. If, however, the nerve root was ischemic, very light pressure by the ligature produced immediate pain and paresthesia in the arm.[18] A model of nerve-root

Fig. 18–31. Positional traction of the cervical spine.

irritation then might be that some unusual activity, probably involving extension or sidebending of the neck, causes the nerve root to swell. There is impingement of the blood supply to the nerve root, and it becomes extremely sensitive. When pressure is removed by traction or proper positioning, swelling of the nerve root diminishes, and the symptoms disappear. This would also seem to explain some of the complexities of peripheral entrapments. If the nerve root has slight compression and is ischemic, the nerve would be considerably more sensitive to pressure at the shoulder, wrist, or carpal tunnel.

Evaluation. The patient will generally give a history of gradual or sudden onset of neck pain, shoulder pain, and paresthesia in the upper extremity. (It is also possible to have motor weakness, muscle atrophy, and loss of reflex without symptoms of pain). The patient will generally have a forward-head posture, and the lower cervical spine will be kyphotic to palpation. Active rotation and lateral flexion toward the painful side will be limited by pain, as will extension. There will be capsular restriction of the lower cervical spine with possible ankylosis. The mobility of the upper cervical spine is generally quite good. The Spurling test will reproduce paresthesia in the upper extremity. There may be diminished reflex, motor weakness, anesthesia, or muscle atrophy. Roentgenograms may reveal generalized degenerative joint disease, stenosis of the intervertebral foramen, or both.

Treatment. The prognosis for treatment is much better if the symptoms are of a recent and sudden onset. Large-fiber nerves are more susceptible to pressure than small-fiber nerves, so as the pressure

increases, the signs and symptoms will progress from paresthesia to reflex loss, then to motor weakness and anesthesia. A patient who has a recent, sudden onset of only paresthesia has a very good prognosis compared with a patient who has a gradual, silent onset of muscle atrophy and weakness; the latter has a relatively poor prognosis.

Many patients will respond well to a combination of cervical traction and instruction to position the head in flexion and sidebending away from the painful side (positional traction) (Fig. 18–31), with reduction of symptoms being the best indicator of proper position. Mobilization of adjacent segments may reduce some of the mechanical forces on the involved segment. The patient should also be given instruction in activities of daily living to avoid extension. These may include thoracic extension exercises to improve back bending at the C6 and C7 segments, switching from bifocal glasses (which require extension of the neck to read) to reading glasses, and general avoidance of working above the head.

TREATMENT TECHNIQUES

I. Manual Techniques—Muscles

A. *Bimanual massage and manual stretching of the sternocleidomastoid muscle* (see Fig. 18–29).

P—Supine.

Note: For the sake of simplicity, the operator will be referred to as the male, and the patient as the female. All of the techniques described apply to the patient's left extremities, except where indicated. (P—patient; O—operator; M—movement)

Fig. 18–32. Stretching of the suboccipital muscles.

O—Seated at head of treatment table.
M—*Bimanual massage.* The sternocleido-mastoid muscle can be grasped between the thumb and fingers and rolled and massaged between them. Begin at the insertion behind the mastoid process and cover both the sternal and clavicular heads. (*Note:* Patient may be instructed to do this as a home program.) *Manual stretching.* Grasp the belly of the muscle between the thumb and fingers, holding the head and neck in slight lateral flexion to the opposite side. Glide the hand toward the table, stretching the belly of the sternocleidomastoid muscle.

B. *Stretching of the suboccipital muscle* (Fig. 18–32)
P—Supine.
O—Seated at head of treatment table. The thumb, forefinger, and web space of the right hand should be along the nuchal line. The left hand should be placed lightly on the patient's forehead to make the grip firmer.
M—3 to 4 lbs traction should be applied to the occiput. The patient's head should be in the chin-tuck position.

C. *Scalenus stretching* (Fig. 18–33)
P—Supine, with the neck in slight extension.
O—Seated at end of treatment table. If the scalenus muscles on the left are to be

stretched, the operator's right hand should be cupped underneath the neck. The heel of the left hand should be on the first and second ribs to stabilize them while the muscle is stretched. (Hand position is reversed if the right scalenus is to be stretched.)
M—The neck is rotated toward the side to be stretched and laterally flexed away from the side to be stretched. Vapor coolant spray may be helpful but is not necessary.

Fig. 18–33. Stretching of the scaleni muscles.

Fig. 18–34. Isometric strengthening of the multifidi.

D. *Isometric strengthening of the multifidus muscle*—This may be performed by the therapist or taught as a home program (Fig. 18–34).

  P—In a sitting position.

  O—Standing behind and to one side. A hand is cupped behind the neck, forming a slight backward curve. Light pressure is applied to the back of the head. The patient is asked to hold. (*Note:* The pressure should be applied with one finger only to avoid the possibility of overworking the multifidus muscle.)

Fig. 18–35. Segmental strengthening of the multifidus.

E. *Specific segmental strengthening of the multifidus muscle*—This may be done as a manual technique or taught as a home program (Fig. 18–35).[16]

  P—In a sitting position.

  O—Standing behind and to one side. Two fingers are placed at the level to be strengthened. The patient is asked to extend and sidebend the neck over the fingers. The patient is asked to hold while the force is applied in the direction of flexion and sidebending to the opposite side. As progress is made, this exercise may be modified by having the operator give the command to "push" and allowing 10° or so of motion.

F. *Antigravity strengthening of the multifidus* (Fig. 18–36)

  P—Prone, with head off the table. The top of the patient's head should be resting in the therapist's hand.

  O—Seated at the head of the table with the patient's head resting in a hand, which is supported by the knee. The operator lifts the patient's head until a slight backward curve can be palpated. The operator gives the command to "hold" and allows the multifidi muscles to take some of the weight. As progress is made, the therapist should allow the patient to accept more weight as long as the patient is strong enough to maintain a curve in the neck. (*Precaution:* If the patient's multifidus muscle is not

A

B

Fig. 18–36. Antigravity strengthening of the multifidi. *(A)* Lifting the head until a slight backward curve can be palpated, and *(B)* allowing the multifidi muscles to take some of the weight.

strong enough to support the weight of the head, this exercise should not be done.)

II. Manual Techniques — Joints

   A. *Manual traction to the upper cervical spine* (Fig. 18–37)

     P—Supine, with the upper cervical spine in slight extension with slackening of the suboccipital muscles and the nuchal ligament.

     O—Seated at the head of the table with the thumb, web space, and index finger of the right hand along the nuchal line.

The left hand is placed lightly on the patient's forehead to improve grip.

     M—The operator applies 3 to 5 lbs of traction by leaning backward, holding the arms rigid. (*Note:* Because motion has isolated the upper cervical spine, strong traction is not necessary. Traction may be sustained or oscillated, depending on patient response.)

   B. *Manual traction to the lower cervical spine* (Fig. 18–38)

     P—Supine, with the neck supported in flexion by a pillow. The upper cervical

Fig. 18–37. Manual traction to the upper cervical spine.

spine is flexed, drawing the nuchal ligament tight and transferring the force to the lower cervical spine.

O — Same position as for manual traction of the upper cervical spine.

M — The operator leans backward, applying 3 to 5 lbs of traction. Traction may be localized to a single segment by placing the web space of the hand at the desired level and laterally flexing the neck over the web space of the hand.

C. *Vertical oscillation extension* (Fig. 18–39)

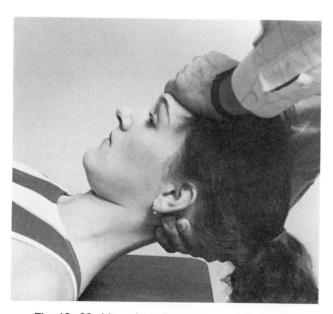

Fig. 18–38. Manual traction to lower cervical spine.

P — Prone, with two pillows under the chest and a small pillow under the forehead.

O — Standing next to the table, with thumb reinforced by a middle finger on the lamina of the joint to be mobilized.

M — For the atlantoaxial and atlanto-occipital joints, oscillatory motion from Grades I to IV (see Chapter 7, Peripheral Joint Mobilization Techniques) should be applied in a direction perpendicular to the table (see Fig. 18–39A). (The atlantoaxial, atlanto-occipital, and facet joints are all oriented in the horizontal plane.) For C2 to C7, the oscillation should be applied downward and forward at a 45° angle. (The lower cervical facet joints are aligned at 45° off the sagittal plane.) (Fig. 18–39B)

D. *Rotational oscillation* (Fig. 18–40)

P — Prone, with two pillows under the chest, forehead supported with a small block.

O — Standing beside table, with thumb on the lateral side of the spinous process of the segment to be mobilized.

M — The operator makes graded oscillating movements from Grades I to IV in a direction to induce rotation of the segment.

E. *Lateral glide* (Fig. 18–41)

P — Supine.

O — Seated at the head of the table, with the patient's head cupped in one hand and the web space of the other hand cup-

Fig. 18-39. Vertical oscillations to the joints of *(A)* the atlantoaxial, atlanto-occipital, and *(B)* C2–C7 segments.

Fig. 18-40. Rotational oscillations.

Fig. 18–41. Lateral glide.

ping the facet joint of the segment to be moved.

M—The operator takes up the slack by sidebending the neck over the web space of the hand and applies oscillations into sidebending Grades I to IV.

III. Positional Traction (Fig. 18–42)

A. *Positional traction*—This is a method of opening the intervertebral foramen by carefully positioning the head and neck.[15] Cervical traction may be applied in the positional traction position to further open the intervertebral foramen.

P—Supine.

O—Palpates the interspinous ligament at the segment to be distracted. The patient's head is elevated using small blocks or pillows until the interspinous ligament at the desired segment becomes taut, indicating the segment has flexed. The operator then places a hand on the lateral portion of the desired segment and, taking care to keep the head flexed at the same level, laterally flexes the neck over the finger. The patient can rest indefinitely in this position.

Fig. 18–42. Positional traction.

REFERENCES

1. Bell W: Temporomandibular Disorders: Classification, Diagnosis, Management. Chicago, Year Book Medical Publishers, 1986
2. Cyriax J: Textbook of Orthopedic Medicine, 11th ed, Vol 2: Treatment by Manipulation, Massage, and Injection. London, Balliere Tindall, 1984
3. Davidson KC, Welford EC, Dixon GD: Traumatic vertebral artery pseudoaneurysm following chiropractic manipulation. Radiology 115:651–652, 1975
4. Feinstein B: Referred pain from paravertebral structures. In Buerger AA, Tobis JF (eds): Approaches to Validation of Manipulation Therapy. Springfield, IL, Charles C Thomas, 1977
5. Gotten N: Survey of one hunderd cases of whiplash injury after settlement of litigation. JAMA 162:865–867, 1956
6. Hohl M: Soft tissue injuries of the neck in automobile accidents. J Bone Joint Surg 56(A):1675–1682, 1974
7. Hollinshead WH: Functional Anatomy of the Limbs and Back, 5th ed. Philadelphia, WB Saunders, 1981
8. Hoppenfeld S: Physical Examination of the Spine and Extremities. New York, Appleton–Century–Crofts, 1976
9. Kapandji IA: Physiology of the Joints. Vol 3: The Trunk and Vertebral Column. New York, Churchill Livingstone, 1974
10. Krueger BR, Okazak H: Vertebrobasilar distribution infraction following chiropractic cervical manipulation. Mayo Clin Proc 55:322–332, 1980
11. Macnab I: Acceleration injuries of the cervical spine. J Bone Joint Surg 46(A):1797–1799, 1964
12. McKenzie JS, Williams JF: The dynamic behavior of the head and cervical spine during whiplash. J Biomech 4:477–490, 1971
13. Miller RG, Burton R: Stroke following chiropractic manipulation of the spine. JAMA 229:189–190, 1974
14. Norris SH, Watt I: The prognosis of neck injuries resulting from rear-end vehicle collisions. J Bone Joint Surg 65(B):608–611, 1983
15. Paris S: Introduction to Spinal Evaluation and Manipulation. Continuing education course, May 19. Institute of Graduate Health Sciences, Los Angeles, California, 1978
16. Rocabado M: Advanced Upper Quarter, Continuing education course, Dec 10. Rocabado Institute, San Francisco, California, 1984
17. Severy DM, Mattewson JH, Bechtol CO: Controlled automobile rear-end collisions: An investigation of related engineering and medical phenomena. Can Serv Med J 11:727–759, 1955
18. Wyke B: Cervical articular contributions to posture and gait: Their relation to senile disequilibrium. Age Ageing 8:251–258, 1979
19. Wyke B: Neurology of the cervical spine joints. Physiotherapy 65:72–76, 1979

19 The Cervical–Upper Extremity Scan Examination

Randolph M. Kessler and Darlene Hertling

The extremities are derived from spinal segments: the myotomes, dermatomes, and sclerotomes corresponding to C4 through T1 extend into the arms, whereas those from L2 through S2 extend into the legs. The clinical significance of this is that symptoms and signs related to pathologic spinal processes are often referred into the extremities, and, conversely, symptoms from common extremity lesions are often referred to the spine (or other parts of the involved extremity). In the case of deep somatic lesions, referred symptoms and signs are the rule rather than the exception. This is most significant with respect to pain, since pain is the most frequent clinical manifestation of deep somatic disorders. Thus, the patient with a cervical problem is very likely to experience scapular, shoulder, or arm pain, perhaps even more so than cervical pain. In addition, paresthesias, weakness, or sensory changes may affect the related segment in the arm or hand. Similarly, it is not unusual for patients with common extremity disorders to experience pain that is referred in a retrograde direction to the proximal aspect of the extremity or the related spinal region. Indeed, patients with carpal tunnel syndrome often experience pain up the forearm and arm into the scapular region and neck.

The clinical problem encountered when dealing with the common phenomenon of referred symptoms is that information elicited from the history does not always reliably narrow the source of the problem to a particular region. When this is the case, the clinician may have trouble knowing in which area to direct the physical, or objective, examination. The situation may be compounded by the fact that many patients present with symptoms that occur as the result of summation of afferent input from two separate disorders affecting tissues innervated by the same segment. This is especially true for middle-aged and older people, since degenerative joint changes in the cervical spine are common by middle age and may cause "hyperexcitability" of the involved segments.

The purpose of performing a spinal-extremity scan examination is to help identify the major area of involvement so that the physical examination can be directed accordingly. It is most useful in cases in which the history or the referring diagnosis does not provide adequate information to indicate the area to be examined. It should be used with most middle-aged or older patients presenting with chronic musculoskeletal complaints because it will often reveal disorders, other than those identified by the referral or by the history, that are the primary cause. For example, a scan examination often reveals that the patient who describes symptoms suggestive of a C6 radiculopathy actually has carpal tunnel syndrome, that the patient with carpal tunnel syndrome may have symptoms that are enhanced by lower cervical facet-joint tightness, that a person with some lower cervical problem is also developing a frozen shoulder, or that someone who describes what sounds like pain referred distally into the C7 segment from the neck actually has pain referred proximally from a tennis elbow condition. Such situations are surprisingly common and can be a frequent source of error in evaluation and treatment planning unless recognized.

The tests that make up the scan examination include those that can be considered *key tests* for the common musculoskeletal lesions affecting the cervical spine and upper exremity, or the lumbar spine and lower extremity. Listed below are the key tests and positive findings for the common disorders for which the scan examination is intended to be sensitive.

COMMON DISORDERS OF THE CERVICAL SPINE AND UPPER EXTREMITY

A. *Localized cervical facet joint restriction*
  1. Typical subjective complaints include
     a. Aching in the scapular region, perhaps into the arm, usually unilaterally; occasional headaches
     b. Gradual onset with perhaps a history of cervical trauma or intermittent acute episodes of neck pain
     c. Worse at the end of the day and during periods of prolonged muscular tension such as during emotional stress and long periods of holding the head against gravity (*e.g.*, typing or reading)
     d. The patient is usually 25 to 50 years old.
  2. Key objective findings
     a. Active cervical movements with passive overpressure
        i. Pain at the extremes of sidebending and rotation to the involved side
        ii. Possible pain on extension
     b. Quadrant test (passive rotation, sidebending, and extension to one side). Pain when performed toward the side of involvement
B. *Generalized cervical degenerative changes.* Bilateral, multisegmental facet-joint capsular tightness is present
  1. Typical subjective complaints include the following:
     a. Gradual onset of neck stiffness with associated pain into shoulder girdles and perhaps the arms. Pain and stiffness may be bilateral, although they are usually worse on one side. Frequent headaches originate from the occiput and radiate to the frontal region.
     b. History of intermittent cervical problems over many years
     c. Stiffness and headaches noted in the morning, easing somewhat during midday, with increased neck and shoulder pain by evening
     d. The patient is usually 50 years old or older.
  2. Key objective findings. Active cervical movements with passive overpressure.
     a. Marked restriction of extension, moderate restriction of sidebending, mild to moderate restriction of rotations and flexion
     b. Pain at the extremes of some movements
C. *Cervical nerve root impingements* (see Ch. 18, The Cervical Spine)

  1. Typical subjective complaints include the following:
     a. Gradual or sudden onset of unilateral neck, scapular, or arm pain. Often paresthesias into fingers are described. Arm pain may be sharp or aching.
     b. Pain may be intense, relieved somewhat with recumbency, and worse with weight-bearing.
     c. The patient is usually 35 to 60 years old.
  2. Key objective findings
     a. Quadrant test (foraminal compression); reproduction of *arm* pain
     b. Upper extremity sensory, motor, and reflex tests. Neurologic deficit is confined to the involved segment.
        C5—Weak shoulder abduction or external rotation
           —Sensory changes over the radial aspect of the forearm
           —Diminished biceps or brachioradialis jerk
        C6—Weak elbow flexion or wrist extension
           —Sensory changes over the thumb or index finger
           —Diminished biceps or brachioradialis jerk
        C7—Weak elbow pronation, extension, or wrist flexion
           —Sensory changes over the index, middle, and ring fingers
           —Diminished triceps jerk
        C8—Weak thumb abduction, small finger abduction, or wrist ulnar deviation
           —Sensory changes over the little or ring fingers
D. *Frozen shoulder* (adhesive capsulitis)
  1. Typical subjective complaints include the following:
     a. Gradual onset of shoulder pain and stiffness, noted especially when combing hair, fastening buttons, bras, etc., behind the back, or reaching into the hip pocket
     b. Frequently there are problems with being awakened at night when rolling onto the painful side.
     c. The patient is more often a woman, usually 40 years old or older.
  2. Key objective findings: active shoulder movements with passive overpressure
     a. Considerable loss of external rotation and abduction, mild to moderate loss of flexion and internal rotation

    b. Pain at the extremes of shoulder movements, especially external rotation and abduction, with a capsular or muscle-spasm end feel.

E. *Shoulder tendinitis* (rotator cuff or biceps)

  1. Typical subjective complaints include the following:

    a. Gradual onset of lateral brachial pain, occasionally radiating into arm and forearm.

    b. The onset may be associated with increased use of the arm, such as in athletics.

    c. Painful twinges are felt with specific movements, such as putting on a jacket and reaching behind the back.

    d. The patient is likely to be 20 to 50 years old.

  2. Key objective findings: resisted shoulder, elbow, and forearm movements and pain on contraction of the involved muscle–tendon complex

    a. Supraspinatus: pain on resisted shoulder abduction

    b. Infraspinatus: pain on resisted external rotation

    c. Subscapularis: pain on resisted internal rotation

    d. Biceps (long head): pain on resisted elbow flexion or forearm supination

F. *Shoulder tendon rupture* (rotator cuff or biceps)

  1. Typical subjective complaints include the following:

    a. Gradual onset of inability to use the arm normally, especially above shoulder level if a rotator cuff tendon is involved. The onset may be sudden, especially in the case of a biceps rupture.

    b. History of intermittent shoulder pain over many years

    c. Possible history of repeated local corticosteroid injections

    d. Pain may or may not be a problem

    e. The patient is usually 50 years old or older

  2. Key objective findings

    a. Resisted movement tests

      i. Supraspinatus: resisted abduction is weak and painless

      ii. Infraspinatus: resisted external rotation is weak and painless

      iii. Biceps: resisted elbow flexion and forearm supination weak and painless

    b. Observable muscular atrophy

G. *Acute subdeltoid bursitis*

  1. Typical subjective complaints include the following:

    a. Gradual development of relatively intense, constant lateral brachial pain over a 48- to 72-hour period. Pain may radiate down the entire arm.

    b. Often a history of more minor, intermittent shoulder problems suggestive of preexisting tendinitis.

    c. Difficulty sleeping or using the arm at all because of intense pain.

    d. The patient is likely to be 30 to 50 years old.

  2. Key objective findings. Active shoulder movements with passive overpressure. Marked restriction of active flexion and abduction, with an empty end feel to passive overpressure. Mild-to-moderate restriction of internal and external rotation with the arm to the side.

H. *Elbow tendinitis*

  1. Typical subjective complaints include the following:

    a. Gradual onset of medial or lateral elbow pain that may radiate into the ulnar aspect of the forearm (medial tennis elbow) or into the dorsum of the forearm and hand and into the posterior brachial region (lateral tennis elbow)

    b. Onset may be associated with some activity such as playing tennis or golf or pruning shrubs

    c. Pain is aggravated by grasping activities such as hammering or carrying a suitcase and by prolonged fine finger activities such as knitting or sewing.

    d. The patient is usually 35 to 60 years old.

  2. Key objective findings

    a. Resisted wrist movements, performed with elbow extended

      i. Lateral tennis elbow (tendinitis at origin of extensor carpi radialis brevis): pain on resisted wrist extension

      ii. Medial tennis elbow (tendinitis at common flexor–pronator origin): pain on resisted wrist flexion

    b. Active wrist movements with passive overpressure, performed with elbow extended

      i. Lateral tennis elbow: pain on full wrist flexion with the elbow extended and forearm pronated

      ii. Medial tennis elbow: pain on full wrist extension with the elbow extended and forearm supinated

I. *Carpal tunnel syndrome* (pressure on the median nerve in the carpal tunnel)

  1. Typical subjective complaints include the following:

    a. Gradual onset of paresthesias into any or

all of the median nerve distribution of hand (thumb and middle three fingers). An aching sensation may be referred up the forearm and arm to the scapula and neck.

  b. Symptoms often awaken the patient at night and are aggravated by activities involving the finger flexors, such as writing, sewing, or knitting.

  c. Women are affected more often than men. The patient is usually 40 years old or older.

  2. Key objective findings. Three-jaw-chuck pinch with wrist held in sustained flexion (modification of Phalen's test). Reproduction of paresthesias into median nerve distribution of the hand (Fig. 18–25).

J. *De Quervain's disease* (tenosynovitis of the abductor pollicis longus and extensor pollicis brevis at the wrist)

  1. Typical subjective complaints include the following:

    a. Gradual onset of pain over the radial aspect of the distal radius that may radiate distally into the thumb or proximally up the radial aspect of the forearm.

    b. Pain is worse with activities involving thumb movements or wrist ulnar deviation.

    c. The patient is usually aged 40 or older.

  2. Key objective findings

    a. Resisted finger movements. Pain occurs over the radial styloid region on resisted thumb extension.

    b. Active wrist movements with passive overpressure. Pain occurs over the radial styloid region on full ulnar deviation with thumb held in patient's clenched fist.

K. *Carpal ligament sprain*

  1. Typical subjective complaints include the following:

    a. History of acute trauma, usually a fall on the dorsiflexed or palmarly flexed hand, followed by chronic wrist pain. The patient often has trouble localizing the pain to a particular aspect of the wrist.

    b. Pain is often felt only with specific activities, such as those requiring repeated wrist or weight movements or weight-bearing through the hand and wrist.

    c. The patient is usually a young or active person.

  2. Key objective findings

    a. Active wrist movements with passive overpressure

      i. Dorsal radiocarpal, dorsal lunocapi-

tate, or capitate – third metacarpal ligament: pain on full wrist flexion

      ii. Palmar radiocarpal or palmar lunocapitate ligament: pain on full wrist extension

    b. Upper extremity weight-bearing (through dorsiflexed wrist and straight arm). Pain is noted with either dorsal or palmar ligament sprains.

FORMAT OF THE CERVICAL – UPPER EXTREMITY SCAN EXAMINATION

The patient sits at the edge of the plinth with the neck, arm, and shoulder girdles exposed. The examiner briefly inspects the upper spine, shoulder girdles, and arms for obvious muscular atrophy or deformity (see Fig. 18–15 to 18–17).

  I. **Cervical tests.** Problems in the cervical spine can be ruled out by applying a series of joint-clearing tests.

    A. *Active cervical movements* (see Fig. 18–18). The patient is asked to perform each of the six cervical movements (flexion, extension, right and left lateral flexion, and right and left rotations), or the joints can be passively cleared by spring testing each cervical segment. If each active movement exhibits a full range of pain-free motion, then some passive overpressure is applied at the extreme of each movement.

      1. Tests for cervical joint restriction

      2. Overpressure to stress the noncontractile structures

    B. *Isometrically resisted movements.* Isometrically resisted movements at midrange are performed in each direction to stress the contractile units. One hand is placed on each side of the patient's head (without covering the auditory meatus). The forearms and elbows rest over the patient's trapezial ridges to help stabilize against trunk movements. From this position the examiner resists cervical rotation and sidebending to the left and right, without allowing movement of the head.

      To resist cervical extension, the examiner places one hand over the back of the patient's head such that the wrist lies over the patient's cervical spine and the forearm rests against the thoracic spine. The other hand reaches across the front of the patient to grasp the opposite shoulder. Extension of the patient's head and neck is resisted without allowing movement.

Flexion is resisted by approaching the patient from behind, resting the elbows against the back of the patient's shoulders, and placing both hands over the patient's forehead.

1. Tests the integrity of the upper cervical myotomes
2. Tests for lesions of the cervical muscles

C. *Quadrant test.* Position the patient's head in combined rotation, sidebending, and extension to one side. With the patient's head in this position, a gentle axial compression is applied through the neck by downward pressure to the top of the head.
1. Tests for localized capsular facet-joint tightness
2. Tests for interforaminal nerve root impingement

II. **Temporomandibular joint.** This joint is checked by palpation, by the patient actively opening and closing the mouth, and by tests of provocation.

A. *Active opening and closing of mouth.* While the examiner is palpating the temporomandibular joints, the patient is asked to carry out active opening and closing of the mouth to demonstrate the following:
1. Any localized swelling or tenderness
2. Abnormal dynamics of the joint or changes in range of motion
3. Clicking and pain during active motion or on closure

B. *Provocation tests.* If active movement exhibits a full range of pain-free motion, then provocation tests may be applied to stress the noncontractile structures of the temporomandibular joints by applying loading by forced biting or forced retrusion.

III. **Acromioclavicular joint**
A. *Inspection and palpation.* Inspection may show swelling and elevation of the clavicular end of this joint due to sprain. There will be a step deformity in the presence of a third-degree sprain or dislocation. Palpation is performed for normal positioning, tenderness, and crepitation.

B. *Active and passive movements.* Active ranges of depression, elevation, abduction, adduction, protraction, retraction, and circumduction are requested of the patient,

followed by passive motion by the examiner through these same ranges. The joint is palpated during active motion for crepitus and abnormal excursions. The patient is instructed to horizontally adduct the arm across the chest. If horizontal flexion exhibits a full range of pain-free motion, then passive overpressure is applied at the end of range to reproduce pain.
1. Tests for pain. If pain is elicited in any of these movements, the patient should be asked if it is the same type of pain that brought him or her to the clinician for examination.
2. Tests for range and symmetry of motion

IV. **Sternoclavicular joint**
A. *Inspection and palpation.* Synovitis is usually evident as a rounded soft-tissue swelling localized over the joint. Subluxation of the joint usually occurs in an anterosuperior direction and is best appreciated by looking down onto both joints. With anterior subluxation the clinician should be able to momentarily reduce the subluxation. On palpation there may be tenderness.

B. *Active and passive movements.* The same seven ranges as for the acromioclavicular joint are performed.
1. Tests for pain
2. Tests for restriction of motion. The sternoclavicular joint moves with movement of the shoulder girdle, but it is not practical to measure exact range. The examiner should observe range and note symmetry.
3. Tests for crepitus and abnormal excursions during motion

V. **Costosternal joints and ribs**
A. *Inspection and palpation.* Adjacent to the sternum the examiner should palpate the sternocostal and costochondral articulations, noting any swelling or tenderness. Swelling may indicate an inflammation or subluxation of the costosternal joint (costochondritis or Tietze's syndrome). The first rib on both sides is palpated for position and tenderness. Any differences on caudal pressure are noted.

B. *Active and passive motion.* There is normally little motion of these joints. Raising and lowering the arms and breathing deeply may elicit a click and produce pain if there is a subluxation. If manual compression of the ribs causes pain, the individual joint or joints should be palpated to determine which ones have abnormal motion.

1. Tests for abnormal motion
2. Tests for pain

VI. Scapulothoracic joint

A. *Inspection.* Inspection may reveal winging of the scapula if the long thoracic nerve has been injured.

B. *Active and passive motion.* Active motions are observed from behind: elevation, forward, sideways, horizontal abduction-adduction, external and internal rotation. Of particular importance is notation of scapular rotation for bilateral asymmetary and scapulohumeral rhythm. Passive motion testing (retraction, protraction, elevation, depression and mediolateral rotation [in side-lying]) is included with palpation.

1. Tests for excessive or reduced movement
2. Tests for contracture
3. Tests for pain or tenderness

VII. Costovertebral and costotransverse joints. Palpation may reveal tenderness if there is joint involvement. Deep breathing may induce pain and refer it to the shoulder or arm.

VIII. Upper thoracic spine

A. *Inspection and palpation.* Inspection may reveal a sharp kyphosis at the site of an injured vertebra or a flat back or reversal of the curve in a mobile spine. Injured vertebrae will usually be tender on compression of the spinous process.

B. *Active-passive movements.* Active range of flexion, extension, rotation, and lateral bending should be observed. If active motions are full and painless, overpressure is given to clear the joint.

1. Tests for limitation and asymmetrical movement
2. Tests for pain and muscle spasm

IX. Shoulder tests

A. *Active shoulder movements with passive overpressure.* The patient is asked to perform flexion of the arm (in the sagittal plane), abduction (in the frontal plane), and horizontal adduction (reaching across to behind the opposite shoulder); to touch the palm to the back of the neck and retract the elbow; and to crawl the thumb up the back as far as possible. If range of motion is full and painless, gentle passive overpressure is applied at the end point of each movement. Both arms are tested simultaneously for comparison, noting the presence of pain, muscle spasm, or loss of movement.

1. Tests for shoulder tendinitis: typically full range of motion with pain at the extremes of elevation and movements that stretch the involved tendon. A painful arc on abduction suggests rotator cuff tendinitis.
2. Tests for capsular restriction of the glenohumeral joint: considerable pain and restriction on external rotation and abduction, moderate restriction of flexion and internal rotation
3. Tests for acute bursitis: marked pain and restriction of elevation of the arm in any plane

B. *Resisted isometric shoulder movements.* The patient sits with the elbows close to the sides, the elbows bent to 90°, and the fingers pointed forward. Abduction is resisted with the arms held at about 30° abduction. External rotation and internal rotation are resisted with the elbows held tight against the sides, applying counterpressure just proxmal to the wrist. All movements are resisted bilaterally and simultaneously for easy comparison of one side with the other and for most efficient stabilization against trunk movements. Maximal contractions should be encouraged. Any joint movement should be prevented and the presence of pain or weakness noted.

1. Tests for the presence of tendinitis: the contraction of the involved muscle and tendon will be strong and painful.
2. Tests for the presence of a tendon rupture: the contraction will be weak and painless.
3. Tests the integrity of the C5 and C6 myotomes.

C. *Quadrant test and locking position of the shoulder if applicable.* Compare findings with those of the opposite side (see Ch. 10, The Shoulder).

X. Elbow tests

A. *Active movements with passive overpressure.* The patient is asked to fully flex and extend both elbows together. If this exercise is full and painless, passive overpressure is applied at the extremes of each movement and the patient is observed for pain, spasm, or restricted movement. These tests may be performed with the shoulder extended, in neutral, or flexed to test for involvement of the long head of the biceps or triceps.

1. Tests for capsular restrictions: Flexion is limited to about 90° to 100°, extension is lacking by 20° to 30°.
2. Tests for extracapsular pain or restrictions
   a. Loose body—extension is restricted; flexion is relatively free. Often there are painful twinges or crepitus noted during movement.
   b. Brachialis tightness—extension is limited; flexion is free. Tightness is felt anteriorly by the patient on forced extension. The restriction is unaffected by the position of the shoulder.
   c. Biceps tendinitis—pain may be reproduced with elbow extension performed with the shoulder extended.

B. *Resisted isometric movements.* The trunk is stabilized by placing a hand over the top of the patient's shoulder and resisting isometric flexion and extension of the elbow. Pronation and supination are resisted with the elbow bent to 90°. Pain or weakness is noted.

1. Tests the integrity of the C6 and C7 myotomes (biceps [C6], triceps [C7], and pronator teres [C7])
2. Tests for biceps tendinitis: resisted elbow flexion and forearm supination will be strong and painful.
3. Tests for biceps tendon rupture: flexion and supination will be weak and painless.

XI. **Wrist tests.** The patient's elbow is maintained in extension. The patient's arm is held snugly between the examiner's elbow and side, and the patient's forearm is cradled in the examiner's forearm and hand.

A. *Active movements with passive overpressure*

1. With the forearm pronated, the wrist is moved into full flexion and ulnar deviation. If movement is full and painless, passive overpressure is applied, once with the patient's fingers flexed, once with them relaxed. Pain or restricted motion is noted.
2. With the forearm supinated, the wrist is brought into full extension and radial deviation. If movement is full and painless, overpressure is applied, once with the fingers extended, once with them relaxed. Pain or restricted motion is noted.
   a. Tests for lateral tennis elbow: Elbow pain is reproduced on full wrist flexion and ulnar deviation with the forearm pronated and the fingers flexed.
   b. Tests for medial tennis elbow: Elbow pain is reproduced with full wrist extension with the fingers extended and forearm supinated.
   c. Tests for carpal ligament sprain: Pain on the movement that stretches the involved ligament.
   d. Tests for de Quervain's tenosynovitis: pain over the radial styloid region when the wrist is ulnarly deviated while the thumb is held flexed.
   e. Tests for capsular restriction of wrist movements: all wrist movements are limited.

B. *Resisted isometric wrist movements.* With the patient's arm held as described above and the patient's fist clenched, wrist flexion, extension, ulnar deviation, and radial deviation are resisted and pain or weakness is noted.

1. Tests the C6 (extension), C7 (flexion), and C8 (ulnar deviation) myotomes
2. Tests for tennis elbow: pain on resisted wrist extension
3. Tests for golfer's elbow: pain on resisted wrist flexion

C. *Modified Phalen's test* (see Fig. 18–25). The patient is asked to perform a "three-jaw-chuck" pinch with both hands and to maintain both wrists in extreme flexion by pressing the dorsum of the hands against one another. This position is held for 30 to 60 seconds. The production of pain or paresthesias is noted.

1. Tests for carpal tunnel syndrome: paresthesias into the thumb or index, middle and ring fingers are reproduced on the involved side.
2. Tests for dorsal carpal ligament sprain: Wrist pain is reproduced on full wrist flexion.

D. *Upper extremity weight-bearing.*

1. While he or she is still sitting, the patient is asked to place both hands to the side on the plinth and to attempt to raise the body off the plinth by pressing down with the hands.
2. Tests for carpal ligament sprain: This is often the only maneuver that will reproduce the wrist pain.

XII. Finger tests

A. *Grasp–release.* The patient is asked to squeeze two of the examiner's fingers, simultaneously with both hands, as hard as possible, and then to open the hands as wide possible. Pain, weakness, or joint restriction is noted.

1. Tests for the integrity of the T1 myotome: weakness will be noted on grasp.
2. Tests for tennis elbow: strong grasp may reproduce the elbow pain because the wrist extensors must contract to stabilize.
3. Tests for restriction of finger movement

B. *Resisted isometric abduction–adduction.* The patient attempts to keep the fingers spread apart as the examiner adducts the small finger and thumb simultaneously. Both hands are tested at the same time for comparison. Then the examiner interlaces his fingers between the patient's extended fingers and asks the patient to adduct the fingers. Pain or weakness is noted.

1. Tests the C8 myotome (thumb and small finger abduction) and the T1 myotome (finger adduction).
2. Tests for de Quervain's tenosynovitis: pain is produced with resisted thumb abduction.

XIII. Sensory tests. The patient sits with the forearms resting on the thighs, palms facing upward. Using a sharp pin or pinwheel, the examiner assesses sensation by applying the stimulus to a small area on one extremity and asking the patient if it feels sharp and then he repeats the test on the same area on the opposite extremity. Then the patient is asked if it feels the same on both sides. The key sensory areas in the hand are checked first, then various aspects of the forearms, arms and shoulder girdles, using the procedure described above. Asymmetries and reduction of sensation are noted. For more subtle testing, a wisp of cotton or tuning fork may be used.

A. Tests the integrity of the C4 through T1 dermatomes: rarely is a deficit noted proximal to the distal forearm in the case of nerve root lesions because of the extensive overlapping of dermatomes in all but the wrist and hand (see Fig. 18–23).

C4—Trapezial ridge to tip of shoulder

C5—Upper scapula, lateral brachial region, radial aspect of forearm

C6—Upper scapula, lateral brachial region, radiovolar aspect of forearm, thumb, and index finger

C7—Middle scapula, posterior brachial region, dorsum of forearm and hand, and palmar surface of index, middle, and ring fingers

C8—Middle to lower scapula, ulnar aspect of forearm, and palmar surface of ring and little fingers

T1—Ulnovolar aspect of forearm

B. Tests sensory integrity of upper extremity peripheral nerves

XIV. Deep tendon reflex tests. The patient sits with forearms resting on thighs.

A. *Jaw jerk* (V cranial nerve). With the mandible in the physiologic rest position, place the thumb over the mental area of the patient's chin. The examiner then taps the thumbnail with the reflex hammer; the reflex elicited will close the mouth. A brisk reflex may be due to an upper motor lesion.

B. *Biceps* (C5, C6—see Fig. 18–22A). As the patient maintains relaxation of the arm, the examiner places his or her thumb firmly over the patient's biceps tendon at the antecubital fossa and strikes the dorsum of the thumb with the reflex hammer to elicit the reflex. One should feel for tensing of the tendon and observe for contraction of the muscle and slight flexion of the elbow. Asymmetries in responses and clonic responses are noted.

C. *Triceps* (C7—see Fig. 18–22B). As the patient maintains relaxation of the arm, the examiner grasps the patient's upper arm (near elbow) and, while supporting the forearm at 90° elbow flexion, strikes the distal triceps tendon just above the olecranon. One should observe for triceps contraction and feel for slight elbow extension. Asymmetrical or clonic responses are noted.

D. *Brachioradialis* (C5, C6—see Fig. 18–22C). As the patient maintains relaxation of both arms, the examiner supports both forearms at about 90° elbow flexion by grasping both of the patient's thumbs in one hand (or the thumb of one hand, as illustrated). The brachioradialis tendon is struck just above the radial styloid process, slightly volarly. The brachioradialis muscle belly is observed for contraction and felt for slight elbow flexion and forearm pronation. Asymmetrical or clonic responses are noted. The integrity of the C5, C6, and C7 segments is tested.

XV. **Referred and related tissues**
   A. *Thoracic outlet syndrome* (see Ch. 18, The Cervical Spine). Because the thoracic outlet syndrome induces pain in the upper quadrant, specific tests should be used to rule out its causes. If applicable, hyperabduction tests, costoclavicular tests, scalenus anticus tests, neurovascular compression tests, overhead tests, and the Adson's maneuver may be carried out. Conditions that can cause or contribute to a thoracic outlet syndrome include the following: pseudoarthrosis of the clavicle, exostosis of the first rib and cervical rib, and fascial fusion of muscles.
   B. *Visceral conditions.* Pain may be referred to the upper quadrant from irritation of the diaphragm or peritoneum due to infection, the presence of free air or blood, an inflamed gallbladder, distended or inflamed stomach, or an injury to the liver or spleen. Cardiac ischemia may also cause shoulder pain.

SUMMARY OF STEPS TO CERVICAL– UPPER EXTREMITY SCAN EXAMINATION

In order for the scan examination to be of practical use, it must be performed within a very short period of time—5 minutes or less. Otherwise, one of its primary purposes, that of saving time in the clinic, is defeated. In order to perform the scan examination within a reasonable period of time, the clinician must sequence the tests so that they are performed as efficiently as possible. In doing so, care must be taken to avoid undue haste, which might lead to poor evaluatory technique and inaccurate findings. The scan examination condenses a number of tests within a short time period; in order to avoid confusion or the possibility of omitting crucial steps, the clinician must drill himself or herself on the sequencing of steps and the rationale for each step in order to be able to use the scan examination effectively in the clinic.

The steps to the scan examination in the order that they can be most efficiently performed are listed below:

1. Cervical resisted movements
2. Active cervical movements with passive overpressure
3. Quadrant test, left and right
4. Active shoulder movements with passive overpressure
   a. Flexion
   b. Abduction
   c. Hand to opposite shoulder
   d. Hand to back of neck, wing elbow back
   e. Hand behind and up back
5. Resisted shoulder movements
   a. Abduction (C5)
   b. Internal rotation
   c. External rotation
6. Active elbow and forearm movements with passive overpressure, resisted elbow and forearm movements
   a. Flexion (C6): passive overpressure, resist flexion
   b. Neutral: resist extension (C7), resist pronation (C7) and supination
   c. Extension: passive overpressure
7. Active forearm and wrist movements with passive overpressure
   a. Combined wrist flexion and ulnar deviation with the forearm pronated and elbow extended: passive overpressure with fingers flexed; passive overpressure with fingers relaxed
   b. Combined wrist extension and radial deviation with the forearm supinated and elbow extended: passive overpressure with fingers extended; passive overpressure with fingers relaxed
8. Resisted wrist movements
   a. Flexion (C6)
   b. Extension (C7)
   c. Radial deviation
   d. Ulnar deviation
9. Modified Phalen's test
10. Active and resisted finger movements
   a. Grasp–release
   b. Finger abduction (C6)
   c. Finger adduction (C7)
11. Upper extremity weight-bearing
12. Sensory tests
   a. C4–T1

13. Reflex testing
   a. Jaw jerk (V cranial nerve)
   b. Biceps (C5)
   c. Triceps (C6)
   d. Brachioradialis (C7)

RECOMMENDED READINGS

American Society for Surgery of the Hand: The Hand: Examination and Diagnosis. New York, Churchill-Livingstone, 1983

Corrigan B, Maitland GD: Practical Orthopaedic Medicine. London, Butterworths, 1985

Cyriax JH, Cyriax PJ: Illustrated Manual of Orthopaedic Medicine. Boston, Butterworths, 1983

Donatelli R (ed): Physical Therapy of the Shoulder. New York, Churchill Livingstone, 1987

Edwards BC: Combined movements of the cervical spine in examination and treatment. In Grant R (ed): Physical Therapy of the Cervical-Thoracic Spine, pp 125–152. New York, Churchill Livingstone, 1988

Grieves GP: Mobilisation of the Spine: Notes on Examination, Assessment and Clinical Methods, 5th ed. New York, Churchill Livingstone, 1988

Kenneally M, Rubenach H, Elvey R: The upper limb tension test: The SLR test of the arm. In Grant R (ed): Physical Therapy of the Cervical-Thoracic Spine, pp 167–194. New York, Churchill Livingstone, 1988

Magarey ME: Examination of the cervical thoracic spine. In Grant R (ed): Physical Therapy of the Cervical-Thoracic Spine, pp 81–110. New York, Churchill Livingstone, 1988

Magee DJ: Orthopedic Physical Assessment. Philadelphia, WB Saunders, 1987

Maitland GD: Vertebral Manipulations, 5th ed. Boston, Butterworths, 1986

Morrey BF: The Elbow and Its Disorders. Philadelphia, WB Saunders, 1987

Rocabado M: Diagnosis and treatment of abnormal craniomandibular mechanics. In Solbery W, Clark G (eds): Abnormal Jaw Mechanics: Diagnosis and Treatment. Chicago, Quintessence, 1984

Racobado M: The importance of soft tissue mechanics in stability and instability of the cervical spine: A functional diagnosis for treatment planning. J Craniomandibular Practice 5:130–138, 1987

Wadsworth CT: Wrist and hand examination and interpretation. J Orthop Sports Phys Ther 5:108–120, 1983

20 *The Lumbar Spine*

Darlene Hertling

EPIDEMIOLOGY

Backache ranks high as a cause of lost working days among Americans. Second only to the common cold as a reason for outpatient visits, it represents the single most common and most expensive industrial and occupational health problem.[104] Each year approximately 500,000 workers in the United States sustain back injuries, leading to lost time from work and financial compensation. Health care costs, disability payments, and lost productivity related to low back pain syndromes are estimated at some 20 billion dollars annually. Eight million Americans are estimated to suffer from chronic low back pain.[537] Each year more than 200,000 Americans undergo some sort of back surgery. About 30% of workers will at some time miss work because of a back ailment and 2% to 4% will actually change jobs at least once because of this problem, in addition to the ones who become disabled.[580] Studies reviewed by Kelsey and White in 1980 indicated that workers off the job more than 6 months with back pain have only a 50% chance of returning to work; this decreases to 25% after one year.[281]

An important brief paper is that of Nachemson in 1976, which is perhaps the most quoted paper in the field.[422] It states that 80% of society will suffer "back pain to some extent," men as often as women, "white collar as often as blue collar workers," with about 50 in 100 workers significantly affected each year, leading to 1400 to 2600 lost workdays per 1000 workers each year. Thus, back pain is the most expensive ailment in the 30- to 60-year-old age group.

The patient with acute low back pain presents different problems due to the self-limiting nature of the first episode: 88% will be asymptomatic in 6 weeks, 98% in 24 weeks, and 99% in 52 weeks; 97% of causes are unknown, 2% attributed to disk problems, and 1% to apophyseal joint disorders. No more than 29%

will require conservative measures, 1% surgery, and the remainder will recover spontaneously.[305]

According to Dagi and Beary, about 80% of all back cases can be attributed to soft-tissue conditions (i.e., muscular or ligamentous sprain, postural abnormalities, poor muscle tone, or neuromuscular disease) and 10% to intervertebral disk disease with or without radiculopathy.[104] The annual incidence of diagnosed disk prolapse is about 5% per year in 20- to 40-year-olds. These lesions occur most often at L4–L5 and L5–S1 segments. Thirty percent of all those who have back pain will have a syndrome consistent with radiculopathy at some time in their life.[580] Those operated on for disk herniation are usually 30 to 39 years old, tending to confirm the theory that partly degenerated disks are the most likely to herniate in such a way as to lead to surgery.

Roentgenographic evidence of disk-space narrowing and/or osteophytosis is found in 70% of men and 50% of women aged 55 to 64 years. Autopsy studies show that disk degeneration begins at 20 to 25 years of age.[281] With respect to facet joint disease, Kelsey and White state that disk and facet joint disease are closely but most inevitably linked.[281] Approximately 90% of autopsies in patients older than 45 years reveal lumbar facet osteoarthrosis, and more joints were affected as age increased. Most studies find that symptomatology is not significantly related to such findings.

The epidemiology of other specific diagnoses are not discussed thoroughly in the literature. For example, Shealy suggests that 20% of chronic unoperated back pain patients had sacroiliac joint symptoms as their major complaint, but did not further specify how this was demonstrated.[507] Travel and Simons make only scant reference to the epidemiology of myofascial pain and quote Kraft and associates as stating that the affected patients were most likely between the ages of 31 and 50 years.[299,570] The existence of a large number of soft-tissue–related anatomical and/or clinical syndromes (i.e., iliolumbar ligament strains, piriformis syndrome, lumbodorsal fascia tears, iliac crest syndrome) are described in the literature. However, few research studies or controlled tests have been conducted. Many of the more accepted terms used to describe these conditions, as Flor and Turk point out, are more descriptive than etiologic or useful, especially for consideration of treatment for individual patients.[164]

Recently a considerable amount of work has been done concerning risk factors, individual characteristics, and the natural history with respect to low back pain. Low back pain in general, and disk herniation specifically, are influenced by many factors including age and gender.[30,34,243,245,280,344,345,530,555,580] In general, low back pain is as frequent in females as in males.[243,555,580] When the work situation is taken into account however, the pattern changes. Magora found that 35% of women in physically heavy jobs had low back pain compared to 19.1% of males.[344,345] Strength factors could be a reason, or a mismatch between the physical strength of the worker and the job requirements.[13]

Repeated lifting of heavy loads is often considered a risk factor for back pain,[30,245-247,279,346,422] although others deny this.[245,246,381,580] Sudden unexpected maximal efforts were found by Magora to be particularly harmful.[346] Glover, Tichauer, and Troup express the same opinion about lifting in combination with lateral bending and twisting.[184,567,574] Magora's study is particularly interesting in that he found no relationship to heavy lifting while standing, but did find that those who handled materials while seated and bent over had a high incidence of back pain.[344,345]

In general, postural deformities, scoliosis–kyphosis, hypo- or hyperlordosis, and leg-length discrepancy do not seem to predispose to low back pain.[35,243,245,246,348,488,530] Although there is considerable disagreement, studies of static work postures indicate an increased risk of low back pain in subjects with predominantly sitting working postures.[245,246,301,312,346] Sitting with a bent-over working posture seems to carry a significant increased risk factor. Kelsey and Kelsey-Hardy found that men who spend more than half their workday in a car have a threefold increased risk of disk herniation.[279,280] This could be due to the combined effects of sitting and vibration.

Andersson reviewed the industrial epidemiology of the last 30 years and believed that physically heavy, static work postures, frequent bending and twisting, lifting and forceful movements, and repetitive work and vibrations had all been established as vocational factors in back pain.[12] He and others noted as well that tallness provides an increased risk of injury[12,279,312,561] and that sciatica is more frequent in the obese.[247]

Physical fitness and conditioning have been found to have significant preventative effects on the occurrence of back injuries. Weak trunk musculature and decreased endurance have come to be identified as significant risk factors in the development of back problems.[269] Cady and associates showed that among fire fighters muscle strength was an accurate prognostic indicator for the development of low back pain.[63] Chaffin and co-workers and Keyserling and associates have used pre-employment strength-testing procedures and found the risk of back injury increases threefold when the job requirements exceed capabilities on an isometric simulation of the job.[75,287]

Clinical observations led Rowe and Berquist-Ullman and Larsson to conclude that abdominal and spinal extensor muscle strength was decreased in patients with low back pain.[30,309,488] Many other investigators have established that patients with low back pain have lower mean trunk strength than healthy subjects.[4,7,31,221,253,386,444,448,469,500] Some investigators have found the extensors to be more influenced (weaker) than the flexors,[440,500] whereas others have identified relatively greater extensor strength.[35,36] Biering-Sorenson found that patients with recurrent back pain had weaker trunk muscles and diminished flexibility (particularly flexion) when compared with asymptomatic persons.[36] Conversely, good isometric endurance in men appears to prevent low back problems. Very little data concerning endurance capacity of the back muscles are to be found in the literature.[236,440] The most striking finding of Nicolaisen and Jorgensen in persons with early, serious low back trouble was decreased endurance capacity of the trunk extensors rather than muscle strength, when compared with normal subjects.[440]

Other factors identified as significantly associated with low back pain episodes include smoking and coughing.[180,555] Svenson speculated that coughing led to increased intradiskal pressure and thus to increased loading and low back pain.[555] Disk degeneration, osteoporosis, and spondylolisthesis are all associated with increased low back pain. The major risk for an episode of back pain is a previous history of back pain.[234]

Several reports give a fairly clear picture of how the patient with acute back pain fares.[15,30,123,573] Horal documented that 90% of acute symptoms will resolve in the 2 months following the first episode.[243] It is often suggested that little can be done in the way of treatment to alter this course. Some evidence exists, however, that short periods of bed rest (2 days), back school, and early and comprehensive care of the patient can speed up the return to work.[30,117] Thus, when initial history and physical examination suggest limited injury or abnormality, without significant neurological deficit, an initial trial of empirically based conservative treatment and early mobilization is warranted.[117] Nachemson has summarized a variety of data suggesting that motion, rather than rest, may be beneficial in healing soft tissues and joints.[423] For the patient who appears to have a herniated disk with a motor deficit, there is good biological rationale for recommending longer periods of bedrest (*i.e.*, reduction of intradiskal pressure).[420]

Some evidence exists that the risk for recurrence for the typical patient experiencing acute low back pain over the next couple of years is approximately 60%.[30,572] The next attack, however, may be shorter and have a more benign course. From a report of Troup and associates, attacks of accident-related pain take longer to subside, both during the first attack and with recurrence.[573] Other factors influencing recurrence include sciatic pain, alcoholism, specific job situations, sociopsychological stigmata, and general insurance benefits.[426]

Social problems are greatest in low back pain. Nachemson lists equally as many social or psychological findings as mechanical or occupational ones in considering the correlates of back pain.[422] He mentions abnormal profiles on the MMPI (Minnesota Multiphasic Personality Inventory), the most widely used psychological test, as well as alcoholism, history of divorce, educational level, and depression as some of the factors that may affect the interface between acute injury and/or pain and chronic back pain. Severe mental problems are no more common in low back patients, but changes in the MMPI are observed.[13]

Many different diseases can present as low back pain. The purpose of this chapter is not to classify the numerous known causes for low back pain but rather to deal with the more common types of back pain, including what has recently been termed as "idiopathic low back pain."[600] The reader is referred to other sources for an exhaustive encyclopedic classification of the etiology of low back pain.[8,341,383,426,505]

Musculoskeletal disorders are of primary importance because they represent the largest group of complaints that are most often seen by physical therapists and other health care practitioners. However, it is important to recognize systemic and visceral problems that may mimic low back pain.[52,196,518,607] Thus a thorough abdominal examination may direct attention away from the spine to a source of viscerogenic pain. It goes without saying that we are only interested here in minor mechanical derangements. This excludes fractures, dislocations, inflammatory disorders, and tumors.

APPLIED ANATOMY

THE THREE-JOINT SEGMENT

At any one level, the motion segment is made up of three distinct parts: the two facet (zygapophyseal) joints and the intervertebral joint (the disk) (Fig. 20–1). In a normal motion segment, these three joints are anatomically linked and mechanically balanced. With age or as a result of various pathologic processes, degeneration may affect the motion segment. The segment as a whole may be somehow programmed to fail, with the chondrocytes of the disk nucleus involuting at the same time that the subchondral bone fractures; or, by attrition, each component structure may succumb to stress in turn. Narrowing of the disk space, spondylolisthesis, and transitional vertebrae tend to apply abnormal stress to the posterior structures.[146] Conversely, dysplasia of the lumbosacral facet structures or degenerative changes in the facet joints can be the cause of spondylolisthesis.[437] The two major sites of pathological change—the intervertebral disks and facet joints—must not be considered independently of one another because dysfunction of one, if allowed to progress, will ultimately lead to dysfunction of the other. The disk depends on normal movement (and therefore adequate mobility at the facet joints) for its nutrition and for an even distribution of force to the annulus over time. On the other hand, normal arthrokinematics at the facet joints depend, in part, on a healthy disk. An inelastic disk at a given level tends to alter the normal centroid of movement for the respective facet joints, a factor likely to contribute to the initiation of a degenerative cycle of events, as discussed in Chapter 2, Arthrology.[152,153,415,602]

In considering joint dysfunction of the spine, as with the peripheral joints our conceptual model must include all of the anatomical and physiological structures of the joint. Only by looking at the whole picture is it possible to judge which tissues seem to be primarily affected in a particular disorder, as well as the probable or possible secondary effects on other joint tissues. In the spine, it is best to think more in terms of segmental dysfunction, rather than joint dysfunction, because of the intimate mutual dependency of the paired facet joints and the intervertebral joint. Therefore, it is important to consider a segment to include two vertebrae with their paired facet joints, the intervening intervertebral joint with its disk, the muscles and ligaments controlling the segment, the nerves supplying the segment, the nerve tissue within the vertebral canal at the segment, and the spinal nerves leading from the segment and the tissues which they innervate. From this it should be

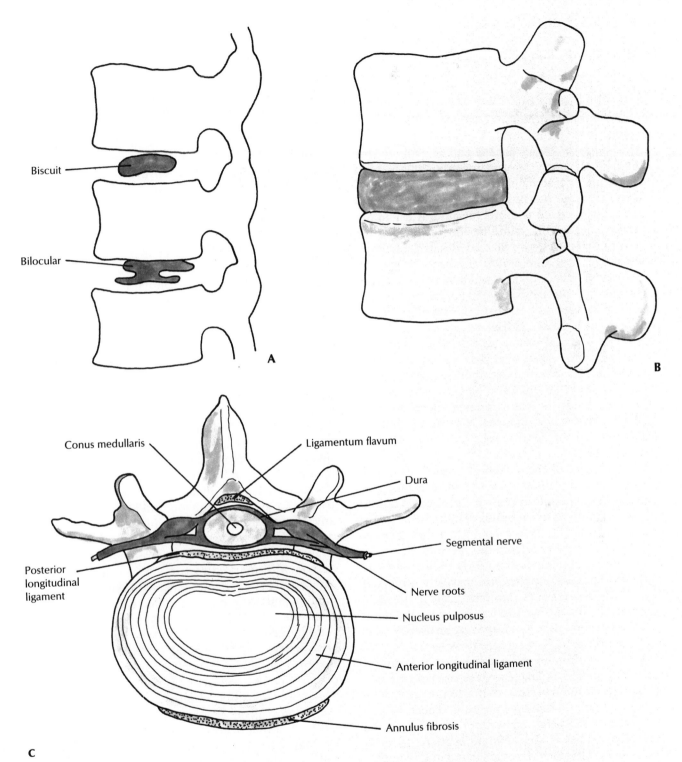

Fig. 20-1. *(A)* Some normal diskogram configurations. *(B)* A properly spaced lumbar vertebra. *(C)* Superior view of a normal intervertebral disk. *(A adapted from Finneson BE: Low Back Pain, 2nd ed, p. 104. Philadelphia, JB Lippincott, 1980)*

evident why spinal dysfunction is a much more complex phenomenon with which to deal than peripheral joint dysfunction.

Vertebrae

One of the more important aspects of the skeletal aging process is bone loss. A gradual decrease in cortical bone of 3% per decade can be expected for both sexes. In postmenopausal women a 9% rate of decrease in cortical bone per decade has been demonstrated. Trabecular bone (see Fig. 17–6) also decreases, but the rate is more variable. A 6% to 8% decrease in trabecular bone per decade can be expected to begin between 20 and 40 years of age in both sexes.[375]

These changes modify the load-bearing capacity of the vertebrae. Studies show that after age 40 the load-bearing capacity of cortical cancellous bone changes dramatically.[483] Before 40 years of age, about 55% of load-bearing capacity is attributed to cancellous bone, while after the age of 40 this decreases to about 35%. Bone strength decreases more rapidly than bone quantity.[26] This decrease in strength accounts for the end-plates bending away from the disk, wedge fractures of vertebral bodies, and end-plate fractures that are so common in osteoporotic spines.[128]

The end-plate of the vertebral body is the weak point of the disk. It is the site of failure when compressive loads become excessive. Between 23 and 40 years of age, there is a gradual demineralization of end-plate cartilage. By age 60, only a thin layer of bone separates the disk from the vascular channels. These nutrient channels are slowly obliterated and the arterioles and venules progressively thicken.[32] Such changes can have a significant role in the pathogenesis of lumbar disk disease. Because the adult disk has no blood supply, it must rely on diffusion for nutrition.[422]

In the upper lumbar spine, degeneration seems to start early with end-plate fractures and nuclear herniations (Schmorl's nodes) related to the essentially vertical loading of those segments.[153] Facet disease also starts first in the upper lumbar spine. In the lower lumbar spine, disk changes begin to occur in the late teens and facet changes in the mid-twenties. Both lesions typically are seen first at L5–S1, then at L4–L5. Degenerative changes of both synovial and vertebral joints seem to occur together, most often at the lumbosacral articulation.[196] Spondylitic and arthrotic change involving the whole segment are age-related and occur in about 60% of persons older than 45 years.[319]

Facet (Zygapophyseal) Joints

All of the pathologic considerations presented in Chapter 2, Arthrology apply to the posterior elements and the spinal facet joints. Primary inflammatory conditions affecting spinal joints are relatively rare, the two major exceptions being ankylosing spondylitis, affecting most often the young male, and rheumatoid arthritis, which primarily involves the upper cervical spine. Osteoarthrosis is probably the major joint condition affecting the spine, most frequently involving the lower cervical spine and the lower lumbar levels. In the lumbar region, development of degenerative changes of the facet joints can be said to be the rule rather then the exception in virtually every individual living beyond the third decade or so. This fact is attributable, in part, to the probability that the human spine has not completely adapted to the upright, weight-bearing position and to the fact that human life expectancy has been drastically extended, again a factor to which our spines are not adequately adapted. This normal degeneration should be considered a process that for the most part, progresses at such a gradual rate that only minor symptoms, if any, result. The person may, indeed, develop a "stiff spine" but usually not until an age at which the normal activity level does not require much mobility anyway. Again, because the process proceeds gradually over time, the joint tissues gradually adapt by means of fibrosis, bony hypertrophy, or even spontaneous ankylosis; thus, little if any inflammation or pain results. For this reason it is not unusual to see very marked joint narrowing with hypertrophic bony changes on roentgenograms in a person with marked restriction of spinal mobility, even if the person denies having had significant back pain or dysfunction over the years.

On the other hand, there are some persons who suffer a relative acceleration of the normal degenerative processes of the spinal joints. The reasons may include a genetic predisposition, such as asymmetry of facet planes in the lower lumbar spine; an occupational predisposition, such as a job involving abnormal compression of joint surfaces; or some other factor resulting in considerable alteration in normal joint mechanics, such as excessive muscle tension or sudden changes in disk mechanics (see The Intervertebral Disk, p 548). These persons eventually complain of spinal pain, the origin of pain being the facet joint capsule which undergoes abnormal stress from the alteration in normal mechanics. In such cases the altered joint mechanics occur suddenly enough, or to such a degree, that the joint tissues do not have time to adapt through fibrosis and bony hypertrophy. The painful condition continues unless joint stresses sufficient to cause pain are prevented through restoration of normal mechanics and avoidance of certain activities, or until the "condition runs its course," meaning that over the years the joint tissues will gradually adapt to the abnormal stresses placed on them. It must be emphasized that symptoms are likely to appear before significant radiographic changes and conversely, that roentgenographic "degenerative" changes cannot be reliably correlated with symptoms.[349] It must also be further emphasized that spinal joints, as with any synovial joint, are capable of referring pain into the relevant segments, or sclerotomes.[100,103] Pain of spinal joint origin tends to be a deep aching pain felt in an area that often does not correlate well to the skin overlying the site of the lesion; this is characteristic of pain of deep somatic origin.

Posterior element changes proceed from early degenerative joint disease (DJD) with articular erosion of the facet surfaces to fibrous dysplasia, loss of normal anatomical relationship of the facets, osteophyte formation (in an attempt to heal capsular injuries), synovial proliferations, and eventually hyper- or hypomobility of the joint.[153] Associated with this process are changes in the subchondral bone similar to those seen in DJD in other joints, but in the lumbar spine there is also frequently a fatty infiltration of the joint, revealing the "abnormal widening" and the lack of mechanical function of a fully degenerated joint.

The ligamentum flavum (see Fig. 17–8) becomes less elastic and thicker, although the thickness may result from shortening secondary to lost disk height, rather than the commonly implied "hypertrophy."[618] Thus, the ligament plays only a passive role in neural entrapment problems. Although the intimate association of the ligamentum flavum with the medial aspect of the facet joint capsule should retract the capsule and synovium when the capsule is slack, this system may not work well because the ligamentum flavum becomes shorter with age and disk height loss.[20] A number of works refer to the possibility of joint dysfunction and pain secondary to entrapment of the synovium, meniscoid bodies (or meniscoid inclusions), and/or capsule, or loose joint bodies, especially during re-extension after forward flexion.[299,456,459]

It has been suggested that in quick, poorly controlled movements or, for example, in the case of a relatively lax ligamentum flavum from segmental narrowing, a meniscoid may become entrapped with a resulting pinching of the innervated portion and a pulling on the capsule to which they attach. This re-

sults in a reflex, segmental muscle spasm that tends to prevent the spontaneous release of the entrapped structure. Clinically, the patient presents with a history of a sudden onset of localized pain and "spasm," usually accompanying a combined rotation and extension movement. The pain is immediate, persistent, and associated with rather marked spinal deformity in a direction of flexion, rotation, and sidebending away from the involved side. This must be distinguished from the patient who, while bent forward, feels an immediate pain in the back, which quickly subsides for the most part, then gradually builds to a constant, intense pain over a period of 8 to 12 hours; this is invariably an acute disk protrusion (see Intervertebral Disk Lesions, p 584).

It should be kept in mind that this dysfunction concept is highly theoretical. Its virtues lie in the fact that it is believed by many to be based on sound anatomical, physiological, and biomechanical principles. A review and anatomical study by Bogduk and Engel describes three types of meniscoid structures (connective tissue rim, adipose tissue pad, and fibroadipose meniscoid), which are in fact found in various percentages of lumbar facet joints.[42] A histologic study of the fibroadipose mensicoid (the only one long enough to be trapped between the articular surfaces) suggested to Bogduk and Engel that it is not strong enough to provide painful traction on the joint capsule in such circumstances.[42] There is a possibility of detachment of the meniscoid with resultant effusion, but that would not be relieved with manipulation, which has in the past been postulated to be effective in the facet joint meniscal syndrome. The authors concluded that it would be appropriate to consider other causes of "acute locked back" outside the lumbar facet joint.

Studies of intervention in the form of surgical fusion or surgical, chemical, or thermal denervation of the facets indicate that a substantial proportion of back pain cases may be of facet origin.[49,70,330,461,505] That impression is supported by the experiment of Mooney and Robertson, who produced typical sciatica, sometimes bilaterally, by facet joint injections with hypertonic saline in patients.[408]

Other proponents of the facet joint as a cause of pain have concentrated on root impingement caused by inflammatory hypertrophy of the joint margin, with resulting root compression or irritation. It has been noted that vertical subluxation of the superior facet occurs with loss of disk space, leading to superior articular facet syndrome and root impingement in the intervertebral foramen by the subluxated process.[145,486]

It has been the popular belief that damage to the

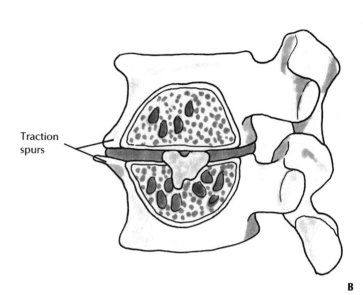

Fig. 20–2. Some abnormal diskogram-configurations. (A) Chronic lumbar degenerative joint disease. (B) Narrowing of the disk and foramina and hypertrophic changes at the vertebral margins. (B and C) Internal disruption of the disk. (A adapted from Finneson BE: Low Back Pain, 2nd ed, p. 104. Philadelphia, JB Lippincott, 1980)

facet joint is always secondary to disk failure. However, Farfan, Grieve, and others state that autopsy evidence clearly shows that facet damage, of varying degrees can and frequently does occur in the absence of disk failure.[152,153,196] Helfet and Lee maintain that lesions of the posterior element always have an effect on the disk and that disk lesions always have an effect on the posterior joints.[227]

The Intervertebral Disk

In a manner and at a rate not unlike those for the facet joints, human intervertebral disks (Fig. 20–2) undergo a normal process of degeneration. Early changes in the lumbar intervertebral disks are common as early as the second decade, when vascular channels begin to become obliterated. With the developing lumbar lordosis the posterior lamellae of the annulus become somewhat compressed vertically, and also horizontally, with an associated tendency toward posterior bulging of the annular fibers. The compaction of the posterior lamellae gives the posterior annulus the appearance of being thinner than the anterior annulus, although the number of lamellae remains the same. The nucleus remains a viscous, incompressible gel with a few collagen fibers imbedded within it.

The nucleus gradually changes from a gel to more

of a viscous, fibrous structure. Associated with this process is early breakdown of mucopolysaccharide (with a net loss of chondroitin sulfate); there is a resultant decrease in water-binding capacity, and a slight increase in collagen content (from 15% in the first decade to about 20% in the remaining years).[432] The original water content will decrease from 88% to about 70%.[432] Beginning at the third decade, there will be a 55% decrease in the glycosaminoglycan content of the nucleus pulposus.[219] There is a gradual increase in glycoprotein (noncollagen), particularly in the cross-beta form.[339] The posterior annulus gradually becomes more weight-bearing, probably owing in part to some loss in the preload condition of the nucleus and its ability to withstand vertical compression, but also because of the increasing lumbar lordosis. The posterior lamellae continue to compress posteriorly with an associated posterior bulging. The anterior annular lamellae, which have greater vertical height, remain comparatively loose but also begin bulging posteriorly. The posterolateral annulus becomes "dog-eared" in that it tends to compact and bulge considerably in the posterolateral direction. Between lamellae of the posterolateral annulus, clefts or gaps appear, perhaps secondary to a pressure atrophy from the combined vertical forces of weight-bearing and the horizontal pressure from the nucleus pulposus. Vascular channels have been shut off and have filled with fibrous scarring.

During the fourth decade, transformation of the nucleus from nearly a pure gel to a largely fibrous mass becomes complete. The nucleus gradually becomes less distinguishable from the surrounding annulus. A considerable portion of the nucleus, in addition to the invading collagen fibers, consists of pulpy debris left from the breakdown of the original protein–polysaccharide material. The water content continues to decrease, although the nucleus retains its volume. The cartilaginous end-plate begins to thin, and some of the scarred vascular channels tend to coalesce to form larger pits. It has been proposed that these weaker, pitted areas are often the site of Schmorl's nodes or invasion of the nucleus into the vertebral body (Fig. 20–2A). Clefting of the posterolateral annulus continues, spreading into the posterior annulus. Some of the clefts meet, forming even larger gaps in the posterolateral annulus. A few radial tears may begin to form across adjacent lamellae, especially in the inner layers of the posterolateral annulus.

Over the next 20 years, approximately from age 40 to 60, similar processes gradually continue. With continued loss of nuclear water content and collapse of annular lamellae, the "disk space" begins to narrow. The nucleus is now a pulpy, fibrous mass that is largely adhered to adjacent vertebral bodies (Fig. 20–2C). Clefts in the annulus continue to increase in number and distribution and to coalesce to form larger clefts. Radial tearing, especially posterolaterally, increases, often with rather large tears extending horizontally across the entire annulus, allowing the nucleus to protrude into the annular space. The annular fibers are correspondingly weaker and have lost their normal elasticity. With gradual narrowing, increased weight-bearing peripherally, and increased tension on the outer annular fibers attaching to the vertebral bodies at the periphery, the added stresses to the margins of the vertebral body result in a hypertrophic bony reaction with the development of spurs and osteophytes. These occur both anteriorly and posteriorly (Fig. 20–2B).

After the age of 60 years the disk space is essentially filled with a mass of relatively unorganized fibrous material connecting adjacent vertebral bodies. The area once occupied by the nucleus is virtually indistinguishable from the annular regions. The spaces are narrowed and bony changes at the periphery of the superior and inferior vertebral bodies are considerable.

Again, it must be emphasized that what is described above is a normal process that occurs in virtually every human spine. So long as the process continues gradually over the years, the involved tissues can be expected to adapt to the altered mechanics in such a manner that, while considerable changes occur, the individual suffers little pain or disability. For example, although the annulus weakens considerably, the nucleus, at the same time, becomes more fibrous and loses volume and therefore exerts less pressure upon the annulus, so that the annulus need not be as strong. Although the fibrosis of the disk space results in a very immobile segment, the individual, at the age at which this occurs, simply does not require much spinal mobility for activities of daily living.

As with the facet joints, we may consider pathologic disk changes to be those which occur prematurely, or at an accelerated rate, in such a fashion that either the individual or the related tissues are unable to adapt to the change, resulting in pain or disability. Such pathologic disk changes may result from several possible factors. Hyper- or hypomobility at the related facet joints may certainly cause changes in the normal stresses to the intervertebral disk, resulting in accelerated tissue change. For instance, at a segment in which a facet on one side lacks mobility but its mate moves freely, asymmetrical movement will result in increased pressure from the nucleus on an isolated portion of the annulus. This portion of the annulus would tend to degenerate and possibly tear

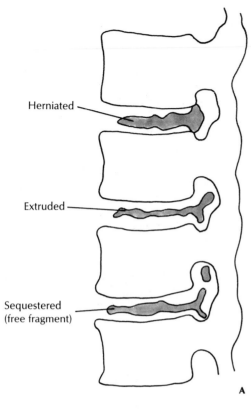

Herniated

Extruded

Sequestered
(free fragment)

A

Fig. 20–3. Abnormal diskograms, with contained and noncontained disks. *(A)* Lateral and *(B)* superior views. (Adapted from Finneson BE: Low Back Pain, 2nd ed, p. 104. Philadelphia, JB Lippincott, 1980)

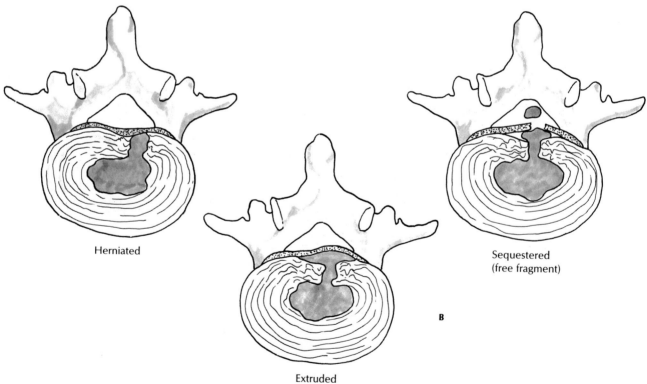

Herniated

Extruded

Sequestered
(free fragment)

B

prematurely, resulting in a herniation or protrusion of the nucleus into the torn portion of the annulus (Fig. 20–3). If an entire segment lacks mobility, the segment above or below might tend to become hypermobile, with added stresses on the disk at the hypermobile segment. Again, the annulus at this segment may not be able to withstand the increased horizontal forces applied to it by the nucleus, and may give way prematurely, allowing the nucleus to bulge into the space and applying pressure to the sensitive outer annular layers, posterior longitudinal ligament, or nerve root. Occupational factors may also play an important role. The person who must perform continual forward bending and lifting activities will, without question, place heavier and more frequent horizontal stresses to the inner layers of the posterior annulus than the more sedentary person. On the other hand, the sedentary person is likely to lose normal annular elasticity and movement between annular lamellae earlier. The annulus is then less able to yield to the relatively higher demand placed on it during more strenuous activities (e.g., occasional sports participation), with an increased likelihood of tearing.

No matter what factors predispose a person to early disk lesions, the age group between about 30 and 50 years is much more susceptible to suffering an acute, symptomatic disk injury. The reason is simply that at this age a person usually is still quite active, has a nucleus pulposus which is still of good volume and capable of imbibing fluid and exerting horizontal forces on the annulus, and has an annulus which is beginning to weaken and form clefts and is therefore more likely to tear. Before this age, the annulus is strong and elastic and capable of withstanding pressures transmitted to it by the nucleus. After this period, the nucleus loses volume and narrows and no longer has the capacity to bulge posteriorly into sensitive tissues. It must also be pointed out that the nucleus pulposus in the middle-aged person has been invaded by collagen tissue, which may be denser in some areas of the nucleus than in others. Because of this, the nucleus no longer exerts an even distribution of pressure on the posterior annulus, but rather areas of relatively high concentration of forces may result, again increasing the likelihood of an annular tear.

As implied above, the posterolateral annulus tends to weaken first, with earlier development of clefts and tears. This is perhaps because in the lumbar region, the posterior longitudinal ligament is stronger centrally, thinning out over the posterolateral disk in its characteristic hourglass shape. The central portion of the posterior annulus is, then, better reinforced by this ligament. Also, because functional movements of the trunk tend to be diagonal rather than pure saggital or coronal movements, the posterolateral annulus receives more pressure transmitted to it from the nucleus.

The person likely to experience symptoms of disk disease, then, is one in whom the inner layers of the posterior annulus tear in the presence of a nucleus pulposus is still capable of a bulging into the space left by the tear. If the tear is extensive enough, the nucleus may bulge sufficiently to cause increased pressure to the posterior longitudinal ligament or outer annular fibers, resulting in pain. This type of disk protrusion, in which the outer annulus and/or posterior longitudinal ligament remain intact, will be referred to herein as a *herniated nucleus (contained disk)*. If the outer annular and ligamentous fibers (posterior longitudinal ligament) also give way, allowing the nucleus to bulge into the neural canal, it will be referred to as a *prolapsed* or *extruded nucleus*. When the diskal material extrudes through the posterior longitudinal ligament, the condition is known as a *noncontained disk*. As long as the nuclear herniation is connected to the disk itself, a free protrusion is present. If the nuclear material has actually separated from the remaining nucleus, allowing it to be free in the neural canal, it will be called a *sequestration of nuclear material* (see Fig. 20–3). The term "disk protrusion" will be used in a general sense. It should be noted that a herniation is likely to result in a deep, somatic type of pain or scleratogenous pain, which is deeply, poorly localized and perhaps referred to part or all of the relevant scleratomal segment. Because the nucleus is still contained, the patient is likely to experience more pain in the morning after the nucleus has imbibed more fluid, because the added volume increases pressure on sensitive structures. A disk prolapse or sequestration (Figs. 20–3 and 20–4) is more likely to impinge on nerve tissue, resulting in "neurogenic" pain and perhaps a progressive nerve-root impingement syndrome, in which the symptoms change with prolonged pressure, as described in Chapter 3, Pain. Central prolapses, although relatively rare, may cause upper motor neuron disturbances if they occur in the cervical spine, with perhaps a plantar-flexion reflex response, lower extremity spasticity, and paresthesias into all four extremities. If the central prolapse occurs in the lumbar region, the lower sacral nerve roots may be compressed, resulting in bowel or bladder dysfunction.

PHASES OF DEGENERATION

Generally, three conditions are considered degenerative—spondylosis, osteoarthritis, and her-

Fig. 20–4. Pathologic processes of the lumbar spine. *(A)* Anteroposterior myelogram showing a large, central disk bulge. *(B)* Lateral myelogram and bilateral L4 showing disk bulges. Illustrations of *(C)* spondylolysis and *(D)* spondylolisthesis. Anatomical differences between *(E)* normal and *(F)* stenotic spinal canals. (From Finneson BE: Low Back Pain, 2nd ed, p. 141. Philadelphia, JB Lippincott, 1980)

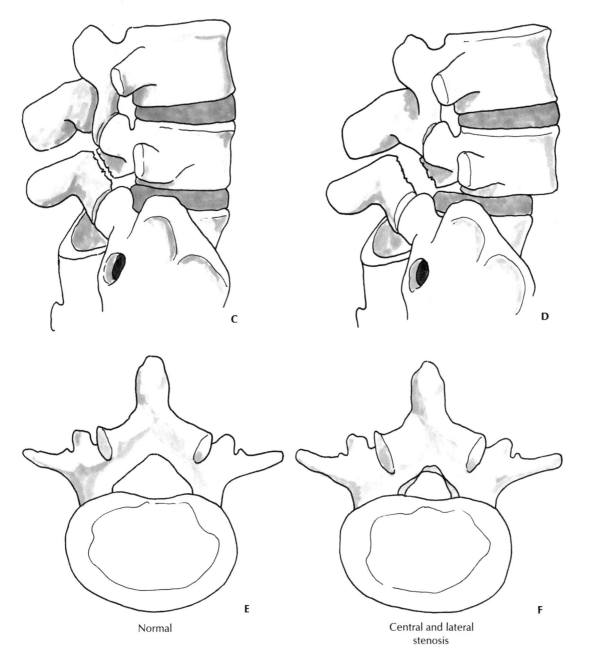

Normal

Central and lateral
stenosis

niated (or "slipped") disk (degenerative disk disease). Alone, or more often in combination, they can lead to spinal stenosis and nerve-root entrapment. One must understand that degenerative changes in general are the human body's attempt to heal itself. Thus, the human body will tend to stabilize an unstable joint by immobilizing the joint by the natural splintage of muscle spasms or by increasing the surface area of the joint.[128]

Kirkaldy-Willis has proposed a very reasonable system, based on our current understanding of the degenerating motion segment, to define this process more clearly.[288] The spectrum of degenerative change in the motion segment can be divided into three phases or levels of deterioration.

The first level is defined as an *early dysfunction phase*, with minor pathologic processes resulting in abnormal function of the posterior element and disk; damage has occurred in the motion segment but is reversible. Changes that occur in the facet joint during the dysfunction phase are the same as those that occur in any other synovial joint. The pathologic changes usually begin with synovitis. Chronic synovitis and joint effusion can stretch a joint capsule. The inflamed synovium may in turn project folds, which can become entrapped in the joint between the cartilage surfaces and initiate cartilage damage. Most often, this early dysfunction phase involves the capsule and synovium but can also involve the cartilage surface or supporting bone.

Disk dysfunction during this phase is less clear but probably involves the appearance of a number of circumferential tears in the annulus fibrosis. If these tears are situated in the outer layer, healing is possible because there is some vascular supply. In the deeper layers this is less likely to occur, because no blood supply is available. Slowly there is a progressive enlargement of the circumferential tears, which coalesce radial tears. The nucleus will begin to exhibit changes by losing proteoglycan content.

Next, an *intermediate instability phase* results in laxity of the posterior joint capsule and annulus; permanent changes of instability may develop because of chronicity and persistence of the dysfunction in earlier years.

Restabilization of the posterior segment takes the form of subperiosteal bone formation or bone formation along ligaments and capsular fibers, resulting in perifacetal osteophytes and traction spurs.[128] Finally, the disk is anchored by peripheral osteophytes that pass around its circumferences, producing a stable motion segment.

The *final stabilization phase* results in fibrosis of the posterior joints and capsule, loss of disk material,

and the formation of osteophytes.[288,596] Osteophytes form in response to abnormal motion to stabilize the affected motion segment.[341] Osteophyte formation around the three joints increases the load-bearing surface and decreases motion, resulting in a stiff and less painful motion segment.

Each of these categories defines a pattern of symptoms that may require varied treatment approaches.

Incidental Complications

Although degenerative changes in either the facet joint or the disk may in themselves produce painful syndromes, the pathologic interaction when both parts of the three-joint system are affected is most significant. Clinical experience has shown that it is indeed possible for the three-joint complex to go through these changes with very few symptoms. Pain is only a signal of impending or actual tissue damage and will become manifest only if the tissue failure threshold is reached. Thus, patients with minimal degenerative changes may present with chronic recurrent symptoms, while others with severe roentgenographic changes present with few or no symptoms.

Each phase carries a specific set of incidental complications that may result in painful clinical syndromes. In the phase of dysfunction, facet lesions may become manifest as painful facet syndrome. With increased formation of radial tears in the annulus a disk herniation may occur, often caused by minor trauma. Disk herniations most commonly occur at the end of the dysfunction phase or the beginning of the instability phase, but may occur during the stabilization phase.[288]

During the instability phase, dynamic degenerative spondylolisthesis (Fig. 20-4D) may occur when laxity predominates in the posterior restraining structures, or dynamic degenerative retrolisthesis when laxity predominates in the disk.[129] Both can produce dynamic lateral or central nerve entrapment.[472,581]

In the restabilization phase, narrowing of the central spinal canal at one level may be produced by osteophytic enlargement of the facet joints and circumferential osteophytes around the disk space, which can produce symptomatic central and/or lateral stenosis (Fig. 20-4F). Later, the degeneration process may spread to involve several levels.

An attempt should be made to correlate this spectrum of degenerative changes and symptoms with diagnosis and treatment. This natural history of disease enables the therapist to gain insight to the disease process, to make a more complete assessment, and to formulate a more rational regimen of treatment. An understanding of which forms of treatment are more likely to meet with success is obviously important.

MEDICAL MODELS AND DISEASE ENTITIES

INTERVERTEBRAL DISKS

Ever since Mixter and Barr delivered their paper in 1932, the disk has been thought to be the principal cause of all low back pain and pain referred from the back.[400] Because more research has been done on the intervertebral disk than any other structure, there is a tendency to attribute almost any type of backache to some type of disk disorder.[426] This often leads to tunnel vision because many disorders, both spinal and extraspinal, may simulate disk disease. Although the disk may cause most serious low back problems, it is rarely, if ever the initial cause of low back pain.

Disk protrusion seems to be regarded by most current orthopaedists and neurosurgeons as the most probable diagnosis only in cases of back pain with sciatica and evidence of nerve-root involvement suggested by physical examination, EMG, myelography, and other tests.[157,486,534,603] Cases not meeting these criteria are usually designated "mechanical" back pain, whereas, those that do meet them are treated conservatively (usually bedrest followed by flexion exercises if improved) and/or surgically by diskectomy or chemonucleosis alone, unless there is added indication for fusion.

Recently there seems to be a return within segments of the orthopaedic community to the concept that pain can arise from injured disk structures directly in cases of "annular tears."[153,288] A number of classifications of clinical syndromes now include pain due to disk degeneration itself (see "Hypomobility Lesions," p 590).[405,445,603]

Although established more than 35 years ago, the concept of primary disk pain is relatively unfamiliar to clinicians, having been overshadowed by the concept of disk prolapse.[326] Because the peripheral third of the annulus fibrosis of every lumbar disk is innervated, the disk is a potential source of pain.[39] The nerve endings in the disk can be stimulated by involvement of the innervated perimeter of the annulus by the autoimmune inflammatory processes of disk degeneration, by torsional strains of the annulus, or by a bulging nucleus straining the overlying annulus. In each case the pain is mediated by the nerves that supply the disk.

A wide variety of conservative and surgical means of treating intervertebral disk disorders has been proposed, including immobilization, manipulation, traction, therapeutic exercises, laminectomy, spinal fusion, and chemonucleolysis, to name but a few.[65,72,103,148,198,233,236,264,282,325,340,380,383,485] A frequently mentioned disk-based treatment approach is that of Cyriax, who believed that most back pain (95%) was secondary to disk disease and herniation. The diagnosis is mostly based on physical findings.[100] According to the Cyriax approach, back pain without sciatica is thought to be secondary to the blocking effect of a disk protrusion on the motion in the motion segment; back pain with local or buttock-referred symptoms is related to dural "involvement" or irritation by a protrusion that is not affecting a specific root. Muscular pain, sacral joint pain, and buttock pain are referral patterns and are not treated except by treating the disk lesion. Back pain with sciatica or sciatica alone is secondary to root compression or irritation by a disk fragment. Treatment recommended by Cyriax is manipulation for the so-called "hard" or annular protrusions, lumbar traction for "soft" or nuclear protrusions, and epidural steroids for persistent radiculopathy.

In addition to these procedures there is an emphasis on maintenance of a normal or exaggerated lumbar lordosis, especially in sitting, based on the theory that this will prevent or reduce disk protrusion of either the soft or hard type by compressing the disk forward rather than backward. Exercise, stretching, acupressure, and massage are not used for back pain, but prolotherapy (*i.e.*, the injection of sclerosants into connective tissue) is advocated for cases in which repeated attacks of pain are thought to indicate ligamentous laxity associated with and perhaps responsible for recurrent disk herniation. Patients are taught to avoid certain positions and stresses.

An increasingly popular conceptual system is that of McKenzie of New Zealand, who believes that the principle cause of back pain is disk disease manifested by abnormal mechanics resulting from the consequences of migration of the intact nucleus within the disk, not frank herniation.[383,384,506] Herniation is seen as a result of untreated, poorly treated, or unusually severe acute nuclear migration. A special case of nuclear migration is the "lateral shift phenomenon," which is a sciatic scoliosis caused by a lateral and/or posterior migration of the nucleus within the annulus.

The type of nucleus disk lesion is deduced through a program of prolonged or repeated stresses on the low back, to attempt to reproduce situations that the patient finds uncomfortable. The change in the pain during such procedures as repeated extension in standing, trunk extension in lying, and lateral bending is recorded and classified according to its peripheralizing or centralizing nature. The geographic pattern of the pain response (central or near the spine as opposed to peripheral) is held to be more important than its intensity. A series of positional self-mobilizations are then prescribed, based on the patterns found. Usually these self-mobilizations are in extension. When a "lateral shift" is found, it is first reduced by mobilizations by the therapist (and self-mobilizations) before extension is done to prevent possible peripheralization of symptoms. More conventional spinal manipulations are only recommended for certain situations.

McKenzie also describes a postural syndrome (derangement), characterized by mechanical deformation of the soft tissue as the result of prolonged postural stress that can lead to pain and a dysfunction syndrome that features pathologically involved muscles, ligaments, fascia, facet joints and the intervertebral disk.[383] The major factor is adaptive soft-tissue shortening (fixation) of the motion segment causing chronic mechanical deformation and loss of joint play. The precipitating causes are usually by-products of disk migration (derangement syndrome), spondylosis, or poor posture (postural syndrome). Based on the type of motion loss (flexion or extension), mobilization and home exercises are used. For example, when flexion loss is present a static supine position is used, progressing to sustained and active lumbar stretching into flexion.

Home therapy is key to the McKenzie approach to maintaining the corrective influences of therapy. McKenzie places a heavy emphasis on prevention of future attacks, usually by the use of lumbar rolls or special seating to maintain lordosis while sitting, and by instruction in body mechanics for daily activities and a daily program of exercise. McKenzie's text is extremely valuable and needs to be understood in depth. In context of this text it would be impossible to cover this field adequately herein, but other sources should be reviewed.[121,122,310,311,383,384,447,583]

FACET JOINTS

Despite earlier controversy, there is no doubt that the lumbar facet joints can be a source of both low back pain and referred pain.[39,149,377,408] Pathologically, the lumbar facet joints can be affected by a variety of disorders but most commonly they undergo degeneration, usually secondary to some form of injury or disk disease.[39] Facet joint pain can be referred to any part of the limb but most commonly it is the gluteal and proximal thigh or groin region.[39,149,377,407]

There are a number of clinicians who place great emphasis on pathologic processes of the facet joints in the genesis of back pain. Many manual therapists have tended to embrace views propounded by osteopaths,[398,542,544] a number of orthopaedists,[44,45,350,351,394,395,396] and physical therapists.[270,354,355,456,457]

Mennell produced a number of works elaborating the theory of "joint play" (see Chapter 6, Peripheral Joint Mobilization Techniques), a type of freedom or "slack" thought to be necessary for painless function of synovial joints in the spine and extremities.[395,396] Lack of joint play not only reduces motion at the joint but produces secondary effects including referred pain and the myofascial trigger point phenomena. Treatment is by mobilization of the restricted joints and procedures to break up the cycle of epiphenomena (spray and stretch, trigger-point injections, and contract–relax programs). Manipulations are often recommended. Determination of the level of the spine to be treated is by skin rolling, observation of gross and segmental movement abnormalities, and oscillations of the vertebral spine looking for hypersensitive levels, or as they are called by some, "facilitated segments."[357,457] Treatment is directed at an area of the spine that contains one or more symptomatic facet joints, in the expectations that joint mobilization will restore joint play.

Kaltenborn and Paris describe very detailed evaluation systems for locating individual hypo- or hypermobile joints.[270,271,456,459] Mobilizations are usually in the direction in which motion is "blocked" on examination, so that the facet motion is thus normalized.[457] In addition, Paris's patients are instructed in active abdominal exercises to reduce pelvic tilt and lumbar lordosis when standing and lifting. Instructions include positioning principles of Fahrni for specific control of the spine.[148]

In addition to Kaltenborn and Paris, Maitland (a physical therapist) and Maigne (an orthopaedic surgeon) are well known manual therapists who operate relatively empirically, attempting to avoid the argument about underlying lesions while using mobilization techniques similar to those of the osteopaths and the "facet school."[350,351,354,355] Maitland's evaluation system is closely linked to treatment and incorporates a widely used graphic record of range of motion and its restrictions.[352] He uses gentle, graded (I to IV), oscillating motions within or at the limit of the available range of motion of the joint in question, concentrating on end feel and tissue characteristics to guide the therapist (see Chapter 6, Peripheral Joint Mobilization Techniques).

Maigne employs "specific" mobilizations and manipulation techniques. Based on the evaluation, he implements therapy based on two major rules: (1) No painful manipulations should be performed, because they are unlikely in Maigne's experience to be successful; and (2) mobilizations or manipulations should be done initially in the direction of greatest mobility found on the examination; this rule would seem to be contradictory to other treatment systems.

Great importance has also been attached to the facets by clinicians who do not necessarily advocate manual therapy. Most recently Shealy, Mooney and Robertson, Rothman and Simeone, MacNab, Fairbank, and others have continued to place importance on facet pathology.[149,341,408,486,507] Following works by Kirkaldy-Willis and others, the role of the facet joint in radiculopathies is again becoming prominent, with a re-emergence of the facet joint syndrome theory that was popular between 1930 and 1945.[291]

Some authors believe that pathologic processes of the facet joints occur after and perhaps because of disk degeneration, while others believe that they occur with disk degeneration. Asymmetry of the facet joints is well documented and has been given particular significance by Farfan and Sullivan as a contributing factor to pathologic problems in the lower lumbar region. These authors suggest that facet asymmetry (by producing a camlike effect) may contribute to early degeneration of the L5–S1 intervertebral joint.[152]

POSTISOMETRIC RELAXATION TECHNIQUES

Grieve uses the term *postisometric relaxation techniques* to indicate the patient's active participation by muscle contraction and/or expiration during manual treatment.[44,45,147,188,315,319,321,398] These techniques rest on the prime importance of soft tissues, particularly muscles, in producing various moderately abnormal states of joint pain and movement limitation. The techniques may be used to decrease pain, mobilize restricted joints, stretch tight muscles and fascia, strengthen weak muscles, and improve local circulation. In postisometric techniques, the important consideration is the particular type of three-dimensional movement posture that will best localize the effect to a particular vertebral segment or rib joint. Many of these techniques employ modified proprioceptive neuromusclar techniques; the degree of resistance is very slight. Localization of force is more important than intensity of force. What is especially welcome about these methods is their substitution for manipulation procedures.[44,45]

To understand the principles and applications of *muscle energy techniques* and *functional techniques* (two forms of postisometric relaxation techniques), one must be familiar with the concepts of segmental facilitation proposed by Korr and with the work of Patterson and Sherrington on spinal reflexes.[296,463,510] According to Korr, when the gamma motoneuron discharge to the muscle spindle is excessive, less external stretch is required to fire the primary annulospiral ending, which reflexly fires the extrafusal muscle fiber via the alpha motoneuron.[296] The exaggerated spindle responses are provoked by motions which tend to lengthen the facilitated muscle and therefore create a restrictive spinal fault. The aim of both muscle energy and functional techniques is to restore the normal neurophysiology of the segment.

The *muscle energy* method was developed between 1945 and 1950 by Fred Mitchell, Sr, an osteopathic physician. His work has been documented by Mitchell, Jr, and associates.[398] The muscle energy method employs muscle contraction by the patient followed by relaxation and stretch of an antagonist and agonist. It is essentially a mobilization technique using muscular facilitation and inhibition.[321] The objective of therapy is to relax the abnormal muscle at the affected level, increase its length and movement, and thus increase the range of movement of the joint. It has been defined as a form of manipulative treatment in which the patient actively uses the muscles, on request, from a precisely controlled position in a specific direction, against a distinctly executed counterforce.[188]

The *functional method* was originated by Harold Hoover, an osteopathic physician.[306] The aim of functional techniques is to reduce the exaggerated spindle response from the facilitated segmental muscles and thus restore normal joint mobility.[47,314] Like combined movements,[137,138] and strain and counterstrain,[260,262] functional techniques seek combinations of movements to find the most pain-free starting position and superimpose on this starting position gentle, repetitive motions or sustained holding.[47,314] The goal of these approaches is to obtain an antalgic starting position—with subsequent reduction in the input from the depolarized nociceptors.[306]

SEGMENTAL INTERVERTEBRAL INSTABILITY

Instability may be defined as a loss of integrity of soft-tissue intersegmental control causing potential weakness and liability to yield under stress, according to Newman.[439] Lumbar instability, where a degenerating segment is functionally incompetent because of insufficient control (whether muscle, ligament, disk, or all three), can be an intractable problem.[137,197,198,317,410,436,438] According to Grieve and Paris, segmental hypermobility and ligamentous or disk insufficiency are not necessarily the same thing.[198,460] Paris defines hypermobility as a range of motion somewhat in excess of that expected for the particular segment, given the subject's age, body type, and activity status.[187] Simple hypermobility may be insignificant and need not result in instability. According to Paris, instability exists when, during the performance of active motion, there is a sudden aberrant motion such as a visible slip or shaking of the section.[460] Instability may be the end result of postural problems, congenital defects, severe trauma, disk degeneration (described by Kirkaldy-Willis and others, see p. 553), traumatic ruptures of ligaments with or without fractures, unsatisfactory results following disk surgery, overtreatment by manipulation, or excessive stretching related to certain sports.[288,289] In spondylolisthesis the spine sometimes is hypermobile. Hypermobility can also develop in areas adjacent to a hypomobile segment.

A lumbar segment is considered to be unstable when it exhibits abnormal movement in quality (abnormal coupling patterns) or in quantity (abnormal increased motion).[129] This instability can be asymptomatic or symptomatic, depending on the demands made on the motion segment. Instability (secondary) is seen in all ages — in the young, in spondylolithesis or following trauma; and in middle-aged or older patients, in degenerative conditions.[227]

With disk degeneration, vertebral motion becomes irregular, allowing rocking, gliding, and rotation of the adjacent vertebrae with excessive posterior excursion of facet joints. In degenerative spondylolisthesis or retrospondylolisthesis, degenerative subluxation of the facet joint allows posterior or anterior displacement of the vertebral body. The symptoms are those of instability and spinal and intervertebral canal stenosis consequent to secondary changes. Anterior displacement of a vertebral body on the one below causes nerve-root traction and compression. These patients (often elderly) may require decompression by laminectomy and stabilization by fusion.

Primary instability occurs chiefly in men in their thirties and forties, when they are vulnerable to such strains as heavy lifting, falls, and rotational injuries.[227,410] In a careful study, Morgan and King found "primary instability" of lumbar vertebrae to be the most common cause of low back pain.[413] This form of lumbar instability was labeled "pseudospondylo-

listhesis" by Jungham, because there is no neural arch defect.[267]

The disk may not be an unstable element in spondylolisthesis or after a ligamentous rupture, despite the fact that it is always involved. However, in some cases, a deranged disk is part of the complex of instability, whereas in others it is the only unstable element.

Instability may be present in extension, flexion, lateral tilt, lateral displacement, or rotation. The main effect of rotational injuries is on the intervertebral disk itself.[227] Hyperextension strains are the most frequent cause of back pain resulting from segmental instability. This disruption in the normal mechanism of the joint causes a constant position of hyperextension at the posterior facet joint. In this case there is no free play in the joint; it is held at its physiological limit constantly, so that even a slight hyperextension strain will cause irritation and pain.

The use of dynamic roentgenograms obtained both in flexion–extension and sidebending has proved to be a simple and reliable method to determine if motion segment laxity is present.[129] The mobility examination will reveal increased active and passive movement at the involved level. Some patients will describe a "slipping" or catching sensation or feeling of instability associated with movement (this is far from being a reliable or consistent finding). The segment involved will be tender to palpation.

Typically, the low back pain of patients with segmental instability is aggravated by both activity and inactivity. Prolonged sitting or standing causes aching, morning stiffness is common, and minor injury causes acute pain with diffuse radiation to the buttocks. One of the few clinical signs, according to Henderson, is restriction by pain of lumbar spine movement at the time of exacerbation.[228] The classic sign is lumbar insufficiency (reversal of the normal motion) when extending from the flexed position rather than extending the upper trunk over the buttocks and legs forward beneath the upper trunk in a ducking, irregular movement.

In the classic instability syndrome of spondylosis with a definable skeletal defect (common in adolescents), hamstring tightness (in defense of the instability) is the classical sign.[406] Transient neurologic signs, such as those arising from a spondylolisthesis and causing neurogenic claudication, are indicative of instability.[460] For example, a runner who clinically possesses an unstable spondylolisthesis may develop pain and neurological deficit after 5 to 10 miles. Conservative treatment consists of postural training, muscle strengthening to improve the power of the

Fig. 20-5. Strengthening exercises of the low back, with the lumbar joints in a neutral position. *(A)* The trunk is stabilized by straps around the ankles; the trunk is then raised to the horizontal and sustained in this position. *(B)* Another approach is to have the patient grasp the sides of the table, *(C)* then bring one or both legs to the horizontal. In both of these exercises the patient should breathe freely.

trunk both regionally and segmentally, lumbosacral supports (corsets and/or braces), and prophylactic guidance and adherence to good body mechanics.

Grieve proposes a basic scheme of progressive stabilization techniques for strengthening regional and segmental musculature.[195,198] Abdominal exercises and dynamic abdominal bracing may also be used.[284] Exercises are selected that avoid extreme positions (flexion, extension, or rotation) that are liable to exacerbate the condition. For example, a potent cause of aggravation of low back pain, due to hypermobility, is that of active forced extension in the neutral starting position of prone lying.

Mobilizations are used to relieve pain of the hypermobile segments within the normal range of accessory movement and to mobilize stiff segments as part of the treatment for lumbar instability (*i.e.*, where neighboring osteochondrotic segments have slowly induced hypermobility at the L5–S1 segment).[199] If the spinal extensor muscles are considered to be weak or to require extra strengthening, exercises to strengthen them should avoid inner range hyperextension movements. Therefore, the starting position should be selected so that the resisted movement occurs in middle range and the excursion ceases when normal postural length of the muscle is reached (Fig. 20–5*A,B*).[341] A segment held in hyperextension has no safety margin, so painful capsular lesions result.

Grimsby, Gustavsen, Holten, Johnson, and Batson employ similar schemes of progressive stabilization for strengthening regional and segmental musculature when the joints are hypermobile or painful.[21,22,23,202,207,240,259] Auto-stabilization exercises, with the patient's active participation, and training in synergies and developmentally, are looked upon as very useful from a prophylactic point of view. The prime importance of soft tissues, particularly muscles, as opposed to the skeletal elements of joint structures is underscored by selected exercises that not only emphasize pure strength training but also improve speed, endurance, and various combinations of these characteristics.[202,240]

Examples of stabilization exercises by strengthening regional and segmental musculature are illustrated in Figures 20–6 and 20–7. The examples are just a few of the voluntary exercises often necessary to complement passive movement techniques and at times comprise the main form of treatment. In seeking to stabilize the unstable segment and to avoid further stress, the aims are to:

1. Encourage the patient to recognize and maintain functional back positions during all activities and

teach avoidance of postures and activities known to aggravate the patient's specific back dysfunction.
2. Improve the strength of the trunk musculature and its function specific to the task demanded and the directional intent. The trunk muscles should be able to contract (isometrically), contract and shorten (concentrically), contract and lengthen (eccentrically), stretch, and—most importantly—rest, ideally at their resting length.

Other methods of stabilization include sclerosant injections and surgical fusions. Indications for surgical intervention include:

1. Lack of response to conservative measures.
2. Significant restriction of the patient's activities.
3. Neurologic findings which are progressing, or, in spondylolisthesis, progression of the slip itself.[48]

EFFECTS OF AGING

Intervertebral Joints

Spinal Stenosis. The term *spinal stenosis* includes narrowing of the spinal canal, nerve-root canals, and intervertebral foramina, all of which cause nerve-root entrapment.[46] Patients with spinal stenosis experience back pain, transient motor deficits, tingling, and intermittent pain in one or both legs; this is worsened by standing or walking (neurogenic claudication) and somewhat relieved by sitting.[480] Pain of neurogenic claudication, unlike claudication of vascular origin (which disappears quickly with rest), does not ease very readily with rest and may persist for several hours.

In some patients symptoms may be relieved by surgical correction.[82,126] Physical therapy is directed at increasing mobility (exercises and/or traction) and improving the patient's general posture to reduce lordosis. Lordosis tends to decrease the size of the intervertebral foramen and increase the patient's symptoms.[459]

Osteoporosis. Osteoporosis is the most common metabolic bone disease in adults.[158] Although loss of bone itself does not normally cause symptoms, associated fractures or collapse of vertebrae can bring about considerable pain. The pain produced is thought to be secondary to pressure on nerve roots or on sensory fibers in the periosteum. Women are more commonly affected than men, and it has been found that more than half of women aged 45 years and older have roentgenographic evidence of osteoporosis in the lumbar spine.[250] The exact cause is not known, but many theories have been proposed, in-

Fig. 20–6. Segmental stabilization exercises of the lower lumbar musculature. The therapist may use one hand on the lumbar region immediately above or below the involved segment. Moderate but increasing sustained pressure is applied to the patient's pelvis. *(A)* Rotation, *(B)* sidebending, and *(C)* flexion–extension techniques may be performed. Techniques may be modified to emphasize isometric, concentric, and eccentric control and to assist in stretching shortened tissues by using hold–relax techniques.

Fig. 20-7. Exercises for stabilization and strengthening. *(A)* Auto-resistance may be applied using posteroanterior or lateral pressures for strengthening the segmental musculature. Regional strengthening may be achieved through *(B)* standing exercises and *(C)* assuming the bridging position while maintaining a functional back position.

cluding lack of estrogen and long-standing calcium deficiency.

The most prominent manifestations of osteoporosis in terms of vertebral collapse are usually localized to the thoracic and upper lumbar region, with pain referred diffusely to the low back.[430,502]

Treatment is concentrated on pain reduction measures and increasing exercise and functional activities. In the presence of anterior compression fractures, active and passive exercises are stressed. All positions and activities involving flexion should be avoided.[492]

Kissing Lumbar Spinal Processes. Increased lordosis with disk collapse may lead eventually to the state of "kissing spines" (Baastrup's syndrome).[19] This condition may develop because of degenerative changes in many segments and lordotic postural stresses. The resulting chronic impaction of the spinous processes is accompanied by ligamentous changes and interferes considerably with vertebral mechanics. The flattening of the ligamentous system and disk may create an instability of the intervertebral joint and, in some cases, hypermobility of the joint.[267] Of the lumbar movements, extension is the most limited and painful in the low back.[196] Relief is gained by bending forward or by putting the knees to the chest.

The goal of treatment is to reduce the pressure and lordosis. According to Paris, the best method for this is to lessen the lordosis by stretching the tight myofascia and strengthening exercises for the abdominal muscles.[459]

Other Tissues and Structures

The most common diagnoses in patients with acute low back pain (0 to 3 months' duration) are nonspecific (*e.g.*, lumbosacral or ligamentous strains, muscular sprains, lumbar dorsal syndromes); only 10% to 20% can be given a precise pathologic diagnosis.[424] It would seem reasonable to assume that many of the acute temporary painful episodes of low back pain are caused by acute muscular, ligamentous, or capsular strains.[33,87,350] Practically all anatomical structures in the region of the motion segment have been cited as a source of pain and have had their proponents in the etiologic discussion. Conditions involving the soft tissues await, for the most part, further clinical attention and research. There is no clear way to ascribe low back pain to fasciitis, fibrositis, myositis, ruptured or degenerative ligaments, strains or sprains, synovitis of the facet joints, or hypertrophy of the ligamentum flavum.[210] It is clear, however,

that many of these structures do possess sensory innervation and are potential sources of pain. Hirsch and others have documented fine and complex encapsulated nerve endings in the lumbosacral fascia, supraspinous and interspinous ligaments, and vertebral periosteum.[233] The facet (apophyseal) joint capsules and outer third of the annulus are also innervated. Most cases of uncomplicated acute low back pain can be expected to subside within 3 weeks. Management should be directed at excluding other pathologic processes, providing relief of symptoms, and localized therapy. Treatment may progress to graduated activity with a maintenance exercise program and education in the care of the low back in working and recreational life.

Skin and Subcutaneous Tissue. In the skin and subcutaneous tissue, trigger points have been found that, when injected with a local anesthetic, sometimes reduce the pain.[25] Lumbosacral fascia fibrositis has been diagnosed clinically, although never proved by pathoanatomic pictures, according to Nachemson and Bigos.[426]

Ligaments. Ligaments have also been cited as a source of low back pain.[58,87,479,618] It is generally felt that ligamentous pain arises from a weakened ligament, which, when stretched, will produce pain and perhaps trigger muscle guarding. Traumatic ligamentous strains include flexion strains which exceed the limits of the interspinous and supraspinous ligaments.[39,58,87,196,209,539] A typical patient with this type of lesion is a middle-aged person who complains of sudden onset (after twisting) of one-sided back pain localized to the fourth or fifth level in the lumbar spine.[419] Pain sometimes radiates down over the gluteal region. Symptoms are increased by certain movements and relieved by rest. The patient particularly resents extension of the affected level, since this movement compresses an already acutely tender and edematous interspinous ligament between the spinous process of the sacrum and that of L5. The intervertebral space is acutely tender, but flexion of the lumbar spine in the supine position gives temporary relief because the injured ligament is no longer compressed.[87]

Ligamentous strains need time to heal. During the subacute stage, if mild mobilization and range of motion are used, normal mobility is likely to be achieved by the time complete healing has occurred. If the joint capsule or ligamentous structures are actually torn or overstretched during injury, the joints may be hypermobile (unstable) when healing is complete. Because ligamentous pain is known to arise from weakened ligaments, which when stretched will produce pain and perhaps trigger muscle guarding, it makes good sense to reduce the stress on these ligaments by correct or neutral postures supported by adequate muscle action and positions. In time, the ligaments should regain some of their integrity with less movement present on examination.

Muscles and Myofascial Structures. Myofascial restrictions may occur from overuse or overstrain and will also accompany any other type of injury in low back pain. These restrictions obviously limit function and may lead to adverse changes in other structures, such as the disk and/or facet joints.

Acute muscular strains, producing partial tears of muscle tissue attachments, typically are a young man's injury, where strong muscles are guarding a healthy spine.[228,277,341,395,396] Primary muscle disorders will probably heal in spite of the care given to them, but stiffness, weakness, and postural changes may occur during healing. To avoid loss of function and adaptive postural changes, the activity and mobilization treatment should be increased as the patient progresses. Despite the widespread use of exercises, there is little scientific information about their effectiveness in the management of acute low back pain. Kendall and Jenkins compared a variety of exercise regimens and concluded that isometric exercises were most effective.[282]

According to Wyke, myofascial pain is one of the common causes of primary backache resulting from irritation of the nociceptive system that is distributed through the muscle masses of the low back, their fascial sheaths, intramuscular septa, and the tendons that attach them to the vertebral column and pelvis.[615] Contrary to traditional opinions, inflammatory disorders of the back muscles and their related connective tissues are seldom the cause of low back pain. Far more often, backache of myofascial origin is the result of muscular fatigue, reflex muscle spasm, or trauma. According to Rovere and Keene, the most common cause of low back pain in the athlete is overuse, with resultant strains or sprains of the paravertebral muscles and ligaments.[277,487]

There are a number of muscular pain syndromes reported in the literature, for instance, the tenderness at motor points described by Gunn and Milbrandt,[204,205] which seem to fall within the myofascial pain and dysfunction group discussed by Travel and Simons.[570] A report by Gunn and Milbrandt and suggestions by others imply that sympathetic phenomena such as trophic changes, cutaneous and myalgic hyperalgesia, increased muscle tone, and piloerection can be seen early and late in patients with

"secondary" back pain caused by some degree of injury to the dorsal root ganglion or peripheral nerve.[205,512,513] Skin, connective tissue, and muscle may share in sensory disorders, and these detectable changes may be confusing in that their typical or unexpected distribution conforms more to a vasal rather than a neural topography. They are ascribed to early and reversible neuropathy rather than late and severe denervation.

Treatment of muscular back pain currently is the cause of some confusion, but major approaches include acupuncture, acupressure, spray and stretch, contract–relax techniques, soft-tissue mobilizations, dry needling, and anesthetic injections. There is some evidence that procaine is the least myotoxic agent and that steroids are not indicated for muscle use.[570]

It is generally agreed that spinal disorders primarily of muscle origin are uncommon. Although it is true that muscle guarding and/or intrinsic muscle spasm usually accompanies spinal pain regardless of the underlying cause, it is generally felt that there is no neurophysiologic reason for a normal muscle to spontaneously go into spasm. According to Wyke, type IV joint receptors in joint capsules, fat pads, and ligaments, when subject to sufficient irritation, will provoke intense nonadapting motor unit responses simultaneously in all muscles related to the joint, as well in more remote muscles elsewhere in the body.[614]

Dysfunction may lead to nociception (noxious stimulus) that will lead to a state of prolonged involuntary holding. Prolonged muscle guarding leads to circulatory stasis and the retention of metabolites. The muscle then becomes inflamed (myositis) and localized tenderness develops. This intrinsic muscle spasm adds additional pain and discomfort (see Fig. 9–4). Prolonged intrinsic muscle spasm tends to generate up and down the spine and may aggravate areas of degenerative joint and disk disease. During examination, muscle guarding and intrinsic muscle spasm may be noted during palpation or observation, and a positive weight-shift sign may be noted.

According to Nachemson and Bigos, although available data do not support the incrimination of muscle injury as a source of low back disorders, there is indirect evidence to warrant muscle rehabilitation.[426] Even if the musculature was not injured at the time of onset of low back pain symptoms, a subsequent decrease in activity would have an effect on endurance, stamina, and fitness. They advocate aerobic exercise. Aerobic exercise also provides other benefits: It has been documented as a means of treating depression, a common finding with at least chronic low back pain.[165,521] An increase in endorphins has been demonstrated in the cerebrospinal fluid[6] and in the blood stream[154] with aerobic training. Other benefits include positive effects of increased mental alertness,[131,619] sleep,[165,521] stamina,[275] improved self-image, and reversal of activity level compatible with chronic pain.[166,168]

Sacroiliac Joint. It is impossible to discuss management of the lumbar spine without reference to the sacroiliac joint. The pain felt at this joint is usually that of referred pain from the lumbosacral junction secondary to disk degeneration. However, subluxation (sprains) and dislocations do occur, especially before the age of 45 years, with typical presenting symptoms of pain on resistive hip abduction and weight-bearing, as well as tenderness of the symphysis pubis.

Osteopaths, followed by specialists in physical medicine and orthopaedists, have suggested that sacroiliac subluxations may be responsible for low back pain and even sciatica.[44,45,52,112,398,467] Management and evaluation of the lumbopelvic region and sacroiliac disorders have been well documented and will not be discussed in this text. However, involvement of this region needs to be ruled out when evaluating the lumbar spine. Treatment of this region and even the entire lower quadrant often need to be included in the total management of lumbar spine conditions.

Combined States

One of the greatest frustrations in the management of spinal pain is that the patient rarely has a single defined abnormality. The nature of degenerative or traumatic spinal disease is such that multiple joints in one or more segments can be involved and the patient can suffer pain from each component of the disease at different times. In cases of chronic spinal pain with little improvement, the patient usually presents with more than one syndrome.

Degenerative disk disease might not produce any symptoms, but the patient can have pain from secondarily affected facet joints or suffer from disk pain to complicate the dilemma. Any of these causes of pain can be superimposed on nerve root compression. All the elements of this lesion complex may require treatment.

Other conditions to be considered by the physician include viscerogenic pathologic processes, vascular lesions, ankylosing spondylitis, Scheuermann's disease, rheumatoid arthritis of the spinal joints, extraspinal lesions, and intraspinal lesions.

EVALUATION

An accurate history is the key component for successful treatment of the low back. The examination entails two modes of information. The first is subjective questioning of the patient regarding the onset of symptoms and their present status. The second mode is the physical examination, which consists of actual tests and measurements of the symptomatic area, whereby a data base is obtained. Evaluation of the soft tissues and a scan examination of the lumbar spine and lower extremity are covered in Chapter 4, Assessment of Musculoskeletal Disorders, and Chapter 21, The Lumbar–Lower Extremity Scan Examination. The lumbar spine–lower extremity scan examination is oriented toward detecting gross or subtle biomechanical abnormalities and toward determining the presence of common lumbar or lower extremity disorders.

Because of the strategic location of the lumbar spine, the examiner must remember that this structure should be included in any examination of the spine in terms of posture or in any examination of the lower extremity joints, particularly the hip and sacroiliac joints. Unless there is a definitive history of trauma it is difficult to know to which area to direct physical examination procedures after completing the history portion of the examination; thus, the lumbar spine, sacroiliac joints, and lower extremity joints should be examined in a sequential manner.

HISTORY

A general approach to history taking is described in Chapter 4, Assessment of Musculoskeletal Disorders; the concepts presented there all apply to the evaluation of the lumbar spine. History taking of the lumbar spine is probably best accomplished by a combination of written questionnaire and interview to assess reliability and to guarantee a thorough review.[533,587] All aspects in history taking are important because different conditions may be related to the patient's age group, sex, occupation, and family history. Previous history of trauma, accidents, or other episodes are considered with respect to recent history. Frequency and duration of each attack and knowledge of the exact mechanism of injury is often helpful and may give some clues as to which tissues may have been stressed. For example, disk lesions usually have an insidious onset caused by repeated activities related to slump sitting, lifting, and forward bending, whereas joint-locking is often caused by a sudden, unguarded movement. Inflammatory and systemic disorders usually present with a subtle onset,

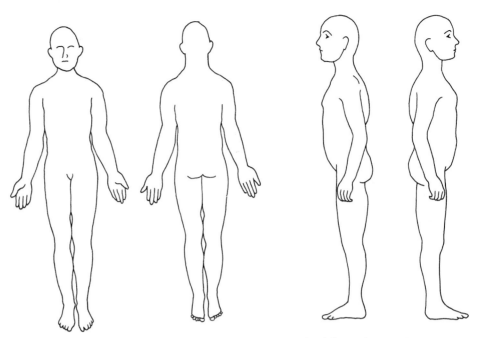

Fig. 20–8. Body chart for recording subjective and objective information.

whereas sprains and strains involve aggravation or trauma.

The history should include the chief complaints and a pain drawing. When using a body chart (Fig. 20–8) it is necessary to ascertain the area, type, depth, and intensity of pain, as well as to record areas and types of sensory disturbance. The pictorial record of information may by reference to sclertomes, myotomes, and dermatomes indicate which nerve root, if any, is involved. It also helps to distinguish organic pain from psychological pain fairly well.[74,407,478,593] If pain has been present for a significant time, other tests should be used for functional overlay.[435,533,600] The Oswestry function test and McGill Pain Questionnaire are helpful in trying to objectify the patient's perception of the quality of pain and its effect on function.[378,391]

Taking each symptomatic area separately, it is important to establish by questioning the severity and irritability of the symptoms and check the level of activity necessary to bring on the pain or other symptoms. It should also be ascertained how the patient eases the symptoms and how long this takes. It should be determined if there are any reliable historical clues to disease, by reviewing the following points:

A. *Signs and Symptoms*
    1. Are there any postures or actions that specifically increase or decrease the symptoms or cause difficulty? Patients suffering from me-

chanical problems affecting the low back (*i.e.*, herniated disks, osteoarthritic facet joints, or spondylolisthesis) know precisely which factors aggravate and which relieve their symptoms. For example, pain arising from the facet joints will often be relieved by sitting and forward bending, while walking is likely to be painful.

According to White, the diagnosis "annular tear" is suggested by pain that is aggravated by sitting, relieved by extension, and not stimulated by standing and walking (except prolonged standing).[599]

Classic radiculopathy causes radicular pain radiating into a specific dermatomal pattern with paresis, loss of sensation, and reflex loss. The classic history for radiculopathy resulting from disk herniation is back pain that progresses to predominantly leg pain. It is worsened by increases in intraspinal pressure such as coughing, sneezing, and sitting. Leg pain predominates over back pain and mechanical factors increase the pain.[505] Physical examination shows positive nerve stretch signs. A dermatomal distribution of leg pain that is made worse by straight-leg raising, sitting, or supine foot dorsiflexion, neck flexion, jugular compression, and direct palpation of the popliteal nerve is characteristic of radiculopathy.

Patients with mechanical problems do not

complain of symptoms being aggravated by "everything" they do. The person who develops spontaneous low back pain initially noted at night but later presenting constantly must be investigated for organic disease (*e.g.,* tumor, abdominal or pelvic disease). The possibility of any nonmechanical pathologic process may be exposed here, perhaps in the way of constant, unremitting pain which is made worse at night with the patient regularly having to get out of bed to find some relief.

2. It is necessary to establish whether there is any diurnal or nocturnal variation. Is the pain worse in the morning or evening? As the day goes on? For example, in chronic degenerative lumbar disk disease the history is of sudden catching pain in the back, morning stiffness that wears off to allow activity with "minimal pain"and a more prolonged (many hours) increase in pain after heavy use or abusive positioning. This is not sufficiently dissimilar to the history given by White for facet arthropathy (transient pain reproduced with certain motions and positions, including rotation, with "catching" pains and relief in neutral) to allow a diagnosis to be made from historical information alone.[599]

3. Which movements hurt? Which movements are stiff? Postural or static muscles tend to respond to pathologic processes by tightness in the form of spasm or adaptive shortening; dynamic or phasic muscles tend to respond by atrophy.[254,255] It is known that tightness of hamstrings or trunk erectors frequently develop in various back syndromes and similar postural defects, whereas abdominal and gluteal muscles show weakness. Janda suggests that just as we have a capsular pattern of joint restriction so may we have a typical muscle pattern.[254]

    a. Does the patient describe a painful arc of movement on forward or side flexion? If so, it may indicate a disk protrusion with a nerve root riding over the bulge.[100,542] The phenomenon of a painful arc throws light on intra-articular mechanics (see Chapter 17, The Spine—General Structure and Biomechanical Considerations), in which the nucleus tends to move backward during trunk flexion (see Fig. 17–13). According to Cyriax, as trunk flexion proceeds the movement comes to the half-flexed position when the surfaces have moved enough

to reverse the tilt.[100] At this point a mobile fragment of disk moves sharply backward, jarring the dura by pressure transmitted through the posterior longitudinal ligament. Pain may reappear at the extreme of trunk flexion if the loose part is squeezed even further backward.[100]

Pain associated with an acute injury and/or inflammation will often present if the joint is moved in any direction. Pain while resting suggests the presence of an inflammatory process.

    b. What position does the patient sleep in? Prone lying for a person with restricted extension will compress the posterior tissues and cause ischemia.

    c. Is there a change in symptoms in rising from a sitting position? Change may indicate possible ligamentous instability. The action of changing position is painful, but when an upright position is acquired the pain is diminished.

4. Does the patient describe a slipping, popping, or clicking sensation that is associated with certain movements? Popping that cannot be repeated every time is felt to be related to the vacuum effect that one experiences if the joint surfaces are separated suddenly.[88,493] This is a normal phenomenon and if a joint seems to pop quite easily it is indicative of a hypermobile joint.

B. *Special Considerations for the lumbar spine*
    1. Does the patient experience any tingling and numbness in the extremities, perineum (saddle), or pelvic regions? It should be remembered that the adult spinal cord ends at the bottom of the L1 vertebra, and becomes the cauda equina. The nerve roots extend in such a way that it is rare for the disk to pinch the nerve root of the same level (except when the protrusion is more lateral). For example, a herniated disk between L4–L5 will usually compress the fifth lumbar nerve root.
    2. Has there been any change in micturition habits associated with back trouble or sphincter disturbance (particularly urinary retention)? If so, the examiner should proceed with caution because this condition may involve more than the lumbar spine or may result from spinal stenosis or a disk problem. A disk derangement may cause total urinary retention, vesicular irritability, or loss of desire or awareness of the necessity to void.[342]

3. Is the patient taking any medications? Are anticoagulants or steroids being taken or have they been taken in the past? Long-term use of steroid therapy can lead to osteoporosis.
4. Is there any increase in pain with coughing, deep breathing, laughing, or the Valsalva maneuver? All of these actions increase the intrathecal pressure and suggest a pathologic process pressing on the theca (wrapping of the spinal cord).[242]
5. What is the status of the patient's general health? Is body weight stable?
6. Has the patient had a roentgenographic examination? If so, x-ray overexposure must be avoided; if not, roentgenograms may aid in the diagnosis.
7. Has the patient undergone any major surgery? If so, when was the surgery performed, what condition was being treated, and what was the site of operation?
8. Is there any history (or family history) of rheumatoid arthritis or ankylosing spondylitis, diabetes, or vascular disease? Previous treatment for malignant disease or osteoporosis may be a telltale clue to the current problem. Likewise, a brief systemic history might provide important information.

C. *History.* The history section completes the impression of the severity, irritability, and particularly the nature of the presenting condition. Putting the history at the end of the subjective examination facilitates constructive questioning.[74]

1. Recent history. A good method of taking a current pain history is to ask the patient to describe a typical 24-hour period. Some points in the recent history of the pain that may help to provide a clue to diagnosis include:
   a. When? Sudden or gradual onset?
   b. Cause, if any? If there is any obvious cause, obtain direction, amount, and duration of any forces involved.
   c. If no obvious cause, were there any predisposing factors?
   d. Where was the pain first felt? Did it spread to the leg and did any sensory disturbances develop?
   e. How have the symptoms varied and what has been the effect of any treatment?
   f. If the condition is improving or worsening, does the patient know why? Has a different activity or posture been used?

   Often a pain or symptom scale for better communication between patients and those treating them may be used. The scale is rated from 0 to 10. Zero is no pain at all and 10 is the worst pain that the patient has ever experienced. Patients may be asked to grade their pain on a graph throughout the day. Pain that does not go below a grade level of 3 with rest is suspected to be related to a psychological problem, cancer, or a disease process originating in a location other than a degenerative spinal segment.[603]

2. Past history. The patient's general history, especially of any past spinal symptoms or injury, should then be elicited. When was the first episode? Gradual or sudden? Cause? Site of pain? Any referral? Duration of first attack? What treatment was received and what was its effect? Did the patient completely recover after the attack?

3. From past to present. How many episodes and what frequency? Local or local and referred symptoms? How long do the attacks usually last? Is treatment usually necessary? If so, how treated and what is the effect? Is the patient symptom-free between episodes?

PHYSICAL EXAMINATION

Observation

The patient' posture, body type (*i.e.,* ectomorphic, mesomorphic, endomorphic, or mixed) and ability to move freely should be observed. Refer to Chapter 21, The Lumbar–Lower Extremity Scan Examination for common gait abnormalities and possible causes.

Functional Activities

An assessment of whether spinal movements are free or restricted may be made by observing the patient getting into or out of a chair, the position that is adopted while sitting, and in undressing before a more formal inspection of bony structures and alignment is undertaken.

Inspection

The patient should be asked to stand with the back, shoulders, and legs exposed for inspection. Features such as pelvic level, disturbances of spinal curves, or other deformities may be observed; the clinician should view the patient from the front, back, and sides. Record specific alterations in bony structure or alignment, soft-tissue configuration, and skin status.

I. **Bony Structure and Alignment.** The reader should refer to the section on assessment of structural alignment in Chapter 21, The Lumbar–Lower Extremity Scan Examination for a complete discussion of this part of the examination.

II. **Soft-Tissue Inspection**

    A. *Muscle contour.* Note obvious asymmetries in muscle bulk. The calves or hamstrings on one side may be atrophied in the presence of a chronic S1–S2 radiculopathy. Seek regions of muscle tightness and muscle spasm. Muscle spasm is noted as a tautness, particularly in the low back where the erector spinae stands in relief. One side may be tighter than the other, with subsequent listing of the torso.

III. **Skin and Markings.** Observe the skin for any local swelling or cutaneous lesions such as café-au-lait spots, patches of hair, areas of pigmentation, or any abnormal depression. A tuft of hair may indicate a spina bifida occulta or diastematomyelia.[364]

IV. **Selective Tissue Tension Tests—Active Movements.**

    A. *Active physiological movements of the spine.* With all movements, determine the range, rhythm, and quality of active movement. The examiner should watch the body contours and spinous processes carefully to observe whether the spinal joints move smoothly and evenly or whether there is any localized restriction of movement in the spinous processes between two or three vertebrae. Note disturbances of rhythm and the presence or absence of any protective deformity. Note any muscle guarding, a painful arc of motion, and whether the patient's symptoms are reproduced. It is important that the patient actively extend the movement as far as possible. As a general rule, facet joint restrictions are more noticeable during sidebending. Conversely, restrictions caused by muscular tightness will be proportionately more noticeable in forward bending.

    With the patient standing (feet a little apart and parallel), assess the following:

    1. *Extension* (backward bending). Kneeling behind the patient, support the patient's pelvis or shoulders for stability, while observing lumbar extension. Ask the patient to bend the head, shoulders, middle back, and lower back backward. The lumbar lordosis should be seen to increase from the resting position as the patient extends. Note the movement in relation to the painful site and any deviations toward one side. Observe the point on the spine at which extension originates.

        a. In the case of an acute spinal derangement, lumbar extension will be negligible, with most of the observable backward bending occurring at higher levels.

        b. With multisegmental capsular restriction, lumbar extension will also be markedly limited owing to premature close-packing of the facet joints.

        c. The spine may be seen to deviate away from the side of a localized unilateral capsular restriction.

        The normal range is about 20° to 35°. Extension is often the stiffest and most painful movement with lumbar problems. Suitable methods for measuring extension externally include the use of a kyphometer,[410] goniometer (spondylometer or hydrogoniometer),[127,171,335] and a tape measure.[162,342,402,403] The first two methods are based on a mathematical theory of angles outlined by Loebl and are expressed in degrees.

    2. *Lateral flexion* (sidebending). Ask the patient to sidebend the head, shoulders, middle back, and lower back first to one side and then to the opposite side. Symmetry of movement may be judged by comparing the distance from the fingertip to the fibular head on either side and by observing the degree of spinal curvature occurring with movements in either direction. Symmetry of movement, however, is only significant with respect to the starting position; if the resting position of the spine involves a right sidebending curve, then "normal" movement would be a greater degree of sidebending to the right than to the left. Also assess the continuity of segmental movement. Reproduction of pain on passive overpressure is most likely to occur when a capsular restriction exists

on the side to which the movement is performed.

a. In acute spinal derangements, such as a posterolateral disk protrusion or unilateral facet-joint derangement, lumbar sidebending may be absent on one side (usually toward the involved side), especially if a functional spinal deviation exists in the erect position.

b. With multisegmental capsular restriction, sidebending will be moderately restricted in both directions. All serious diseases of the lumbar spine (*e.g.*, malignancy, ankylosing spondylitis) result in equal limitation of both left and right sidebending.[103]

c. With localized unilateral capsular restrictions, sidebending will usually be only slightly limited toward the involved side. Unilateral restrictions are often difficult to detect.

Lateral flexion is approximately 15° to 20°. Suitable methods for measuring lateral flexion include the use of two Myrin goniometers and use of the tape measure method using either distraction or approximation.[189,401,498]

3. *Flexion* (forward bending) Forward flexion is an important movement and one most likely to be limited by a disk lesion. Ask the patient to bend the head forward, then the middle back, and finally the low back. A painful arc may be noted. Observe the level at which lumbar flexion originates. Reversal of normal spinal rhythm on attempting to regain the erect posture after forward flexion is characteristic of disk degeneration associated with a posterior joint lesion.[341] "Hitching" is sometimes seen in patients who have osteoarthritis of the facet joints; the patient first extends the lumbar spine, fixing it in lordosis, and then extends at the hips until the erect position is regained.[505] An instability problem may be present if there is a reversal of the normal pelvic rhythm, an arc or list through range, sharp catches of pain, or if the patient exhibits cogwheeling attempts to rise from the forward-bent position.[288,341,505]

a. If the patient has a relatively acute back problem and this movement is extremely difficult to perform—the patient may support his body weight by placing the hands on the thighs or a nearby plinth—a posterior disk prolapse should be suspected.

b. If the patient has a relatively acute back problem but is able to bend forward reasonably well, with only a mild discomfort and restriction, an acute facet-joint dysfunction or less severe disk prolapse might be considered. It is not unusual to see variations in lateral deviations of the spine as the patient bends forward in either instance. For example, the spine may start out deviated in the upright position and the deviations may disappear during forward bending. Or, the spine may be erect on standing and deviate as forward bending proceeds, and the deviation may or may not resolve by the end point of the movement. Such patterns may occur with movement abnormalities resulting from either disk or facet-joint derangements.

c. If the patient does not have an acute problem, the examiner should observe the spine during forward bending from the back, then from the side.

When viewing from behind, look for lateral deviation of the spine during movement. A deviated arc of movement is more likely to be secondary to an alteration of intervertebral disk mechanics, whereas a deviation that exists up to the end point of movement is more likely the result of a unilateral or asymmetrical capsular restriction or a fixed scoliosis. If a fixed scoliosis exists, a rotary component will be present; the side of the convexity will appear higher than the side of the concavity in the forward-bent position.

When viewing from the side, assess the continuity of movement at the various spinal segments. The overall spinal curve should be relatively smooth; flattened areas may reflect segmental hypomobility, whereas angular areas may be associated with segmental hypermobility.

With full forward bending of the lumbar spine, the normal lumbar lordosis should be straightened, but usually not reversed. Inadequate straightening of the lordosis may occur with localized or generalized capsular restriction. Reversal of the lumbar lordosis may suggest hypermobility.

The maximum range of motion is 40° to 60°. Suitable methods for measuring flexion include the kyphometer,[127,490] the goniometer (the spondylometer or hydrogoniometer), and the tape measure (including the Schober test employed to detect and then follow the loss of spinal motions in ankylosing spondylitis).[162,342,376,498]

4. *Lateral shift* (side-gliding). Lateral displacement of the pelvis on the thorax is a very important test movement, especially for the lower lumbar spine. McKenzie described its application fully.[383] Ask the patient to move the pelvis and shoulder simultaneously in opposite directions while keeping the shoulders parallel to the ground. Watch for unilateral restriction or blocking. When the patient has a lateral shift, movement is restricted in the opposite direction.

While maintaining a stabilized upper thoracic area, the patient is asked to allow the hips and pelvis to slide laterally in the horizontal plane to the left and right.[383]

Note: With the patient sitting, knees together, compare sitting posture to standing posture. Note any changes in bony structure and alignment.

5. *Rotation* With the arms held straight out in front and the hands together, ask the patient to turn toward the left and then the right side. In sitting, as rotation occurs in one direction, sidebending occurs in the opposite direction. The spinous processes move in the opposite direction of rotation. Symmetry of movement is assessed by observing the lateral curvature of the lower spine. The same considerations apply to assessment of rotation as discussed under sidebending. There is no significant rotation of the lumbar spine (3° to 18°),

but it is a useful test for the patient with nonorganic back pain.[418] Structural stresses could include torsional and shear stresses of the disk and neural arch. The contralateral facet is compressed, and the ipsilateral joint is stretched. Suitable methods for measuring lumbar spine rotation externally include the use of a tape measure and application of the rotometer developed by Twomey and Taylor.[403,568]

B. *Chest expansion and active peripheral joint tests*
  1. Chest expansion should be measured from normal expiration to maximal inspiration at the level of T4. An expansion of 3 cm is considered within the lower limits of normal.[403] Loss of chest expansion is usually a late finding in ankylosing spondylitis. Another late sign is decreased ability to extend the neck.
  2. Squatting on the heels from the standing position and returning to the erect position puts the peripheral joints through a full active range of motion. The ability to squat normally reflects the state of the hip joints as well as power of the quadriceps and gluteal muscles. A patient who complains of low back pain radiating down the anterior aspect of the thigh and who has difficulty in squatting may have a midlumbar disk lesion.[505] Changes in symptoms should be noted as well as where in the range they occur.

C. *Auxiliary tests* In most patients with symptoms arising from the lumbar spine, the active tests described above are sufficient to reproduce the patient's symptoms. If not, the following additional maneuvers may be used:
  1. Passive overpressure at the end range of the active physiological motions described above. The overpressure should be applied with care because the upper body weight is already being applied by virtue of gravity.
  2. Repeated motions. It may be helpful to do repeated physiological movements at various speeds.
  3. Sustained pressure. This is applied for approximately 10 seconds with the lumbar spine first in extension and then in lateral flexion, when necessary to reproduce the pain.

4. Combined motions.[55,137-139,505] These passive-movement tests are designed to position the joint under maximum stress. The combining of routine physiological movements to form test movements will either open or close one side of the intervertebral segment. In this way a pattern of painful movement may be found or a combination that relieves or increases symptoms. If pain is reproduced it should be determined whether the pain is felt in the midline, the same or opposite side, and if it radiates down the leg. Determine if patterns are regular or irregular. These motions may be applied with and without passive overpressure.

a. Active motions without overpressure include:

i. Lateral flexion combined with extension to the left and right
ii. Lateral flexion combined with flexion to the right and left

b. Combined movements with passive overpressure. The patient's pelvis is securely stabilized and maintained by the examiner. Once end range is reached the examiner applies passive overpressure.

i. Combined movements in flexion

A. Combined movement of forward flexion and right lateral flexion (Fig. 20–9). While maintaining a fully flexed position the patient laterally flexes to the right. At the end of range the therapist applies passive overpressure. Repeat to the left.

B. Combined forward flexion with rotation (Fig. 20–10). The patient is asked to bend forward in a fully flexed position. The patient's trunk is rotated to the right. Repeat se-

Fig. 20–9. Combined movement examination: lateral flexion in forward flexion.

Fig. 20–10. Combined movement examination: flexion and rotation.

quence with rotation to the left.

ii. Combined movements in extension. If it is thought that the pain may be coming from the lumbosacral level, it is advisable to have the standing patient first flex the pelvis (symphysis up), and then extend it.

A. Extension with lateral flexion to the right (Fig. 20–11). The patient first extends and lateral flexion is added to this position (the patient is now in a quadrant position). The examiner stands to the side (right) and places one arm across the chest so the hand grasps the patient's opposite shoulder, to which extension and lateral flexion will occur. The thumb and index of the examiner's opposite hand are placed over the transverse

process at the level of the lumbar spine to be examined. Following active extension, counterpressure is provided by the thumb while the upper arm is used to bring the patient's trunk into lateral flexion. Repeat this sequence on the left side.

B. Extension and rotation to the right (Fig. 20–12). The examiner places one arm across the chest so the hand grasps the opposite shoulder (left). The thumb and index finger of the opposite hand are placed over the transverse process at the level of the lumbar spine to be examined. The patient is encouraged to actively extend to the limit of the range. Using the upper hand (on patient's shoulder), the examiner guides the trunk into rotation as the thumb applies counter-

Fig. 20–11. Combined movement examination: lateral flexion in extension.

Fig. 20–12. Combined movement examination: extension and rotation.

pressure. Repeat this sequence on the left side.

The examining movements described above involve the combinination of two movements. However, three movements may also be combined and the sequence of performing movements may also be varied.[55,137–139,505] As a result of examining, analyzing, and treating using combined movements, a better appreciation of the mechanical presentation of spinal pathology and its application to treatment can be gained.

5. Positive heel-drop test. Have the patient stand on tiptoes, then drop heavily onto the heels. This will cause a jarring of the spine, which may be sufficient to reproduce the patient's symptoms.[505]

D. *Active segmental mobility* With the patient standing assess the following:

1. *Upper lumbar spine lateral flexion.* The patient is instructed to stride stand so that motion will be directed at the upper lumbar segments. With the weight transferred to the same side (right), the patient actively sidebends to the right. Repeat to the left.

2. *L5–S1 lateral flexion.* The patient is instructed to stride stand with weight transferred to the opposite side (left). The patient actively sidebends to the right. Repeat to the left.

3. *L5–S1 region.* The patient actively tilts the pelvis forward (symphysis up).

V. Selective Tissue Tension—Passive Movements

A. *Posture correction.* Posture correction is done to determine if return to normal posture is possible and if the patient's symptoms are altered. This may help find which structures are at fault and will also help the examiner determine to what extent the postural deformity is involved in the patient's current complaints. When an acute lumbar scoliosis is seen during an examination, an attempt should be made to correct it. If the scoliosis is caused by a moderate or mild disk protrusion (lateral shift) the correction procedure will often cause centralization of the pain in the lumbar region but no increase in peripheral symptoms.[383] If the scoliosis is a protective scoliosis, as described by Finneson, any attempt at correction will increase pain and other symptoms in the lower extremities.[156] The method is described below:

P—Stands with the elbow of the arm on the side of the lumbar convexity bent to 90°.

O—Contacts the lateral aspect of the patient's thorax with the clavicular region. The arms encircle the patient and the hands interlock to contact the lateral aspect of the patient's pelvis.

M—The sidebending deformity is very slowly reduced with a mild lateral pressure against the pelvis, toward the operator.

Note: See Figure 20-23, Nonspecific Spiral Mobilizations, for positioning of operator and patient.

B. *Quadrant testing.*[352] The quadrant test is a provocation test for a localized capsular restriction that may not cause an obvious restriction of motion or pain on active movement tests. The examiner stands to the patient's side and places one arm across the patient's chest to grasp the opposite shoulder and the other hand over the lower back, with the thumb over the region of the mammillary process of about L2 on the side closest to the examiner. Use the upper arm to bring the patient's trunk around into sidebending, rotation, and extension, while applying counterpressure forward and inward with the other thumb. When the limit of range is reached, hold the position for 20 seconds to allow for a delayed response. This maneuver localizes a close-packing movement to the facet joint immediately superior to the examiner's thumb and, therefore, localizes stress to the capsule of that joint. The remaining joints, caudal to the first segment tested, are examined in the same manner in an attempt to reproduce the patient's symptoms. The opposite side of the spine may then be tested. This test is less likely to reproduce nerve-root symptoms by reducing the size of the intervertebral foramen, as it may in the cervical spine, because the lumbar intervertebral foramina are quite large in diameter compared with the exiting nerve roots.

C. *Passive physiological movements of the spine.* Physiological movements of flexion, extension, rotation, and lateral flexion are tested by passive movements and compared with active motions.

1. *Flexion* (forward bending). The patient lies in supine with the knees bent. Forward bending is carried out by having the patient pull the knees to the chest. A general assessment of flexion is made and also compared with standing forward bending. Repeated motions may be used to determine if the symptoms change.

2. *Extension* (backward bending). Passive backward bending is checked with the patient lying prone. The patient is asked to press up with his arms, while letting his back sag. One should observe range, changes in pain (centralization or peripheralization), or other symptoms. The distance of the anterior-superior iliac spine (ASIS) from the table should be measured (approximately 2 inches is considered within normal limits).[493] Passive backward bending (press-ups) may also be repeated several times to determine if symptoms change with repeated motion (see Fig. 20-40).

3. *Lateral flexion* (sidebending). The patient lies supine with the knees bent. The examiner holds the patient's legs together with hips and knees bent to 90°. Spinal sidebending is produced by rotating the patient's pelvis about a vertical axis, using the patient's leg as a lever (see Fig. 20-21).

4. *Rotation.* The patient lies supine with the knees bent; the thorax is stabilized by placing the arm across the rib cage. The leg furthest from the examiner is grasped behind the knee and the hip brought to about 90° flexion. This leg is then pulled toward the operator, across the near leg. Repeat on the other side, and compare the two sides to each other (see Fig. 20-19).

D. *Passive physiological movements with segmental palpation.* Passive motion is also carried out with palpation to appreciate the movement of each individual segment. This is achieved by palpating between the spinous processes and comparing the movement obtained at each level.

Note the type of end feels. Normal end feels of the lumbar spine for flexion, extension, lateral flexion, and rotation are of tissue stretch. Determine if tissue tension limits movement before end of range. Abnormal end feel encountered may be boggy with greater than the expected movement (hypermobility), a rubbery rebound type of resistance, a fairly "hard" end feel (chrondro-osteophyte contact), or a block.[194] Seek abnormalities such as irritabilities. Does movement elicit spasm, pain and/or paresthesias locally and/or distally?

1. *Flexion–extension.* (forward and backward bending) (Fig. 20–13A,B). These movements may be tested by the operator flexing one or both of the patient's legs, but it is generally easier to use one leg. The patient lies on the side with the underneath leg slightly flexed at the hip and knee (a small, flat pillow under the waist will keep the lumbar spine in a neutral position). The examiner stands in front of the patient. The index or middle finger of the cranial hand rests between adjunct spinous processes, while the patient's upper leg is grasped at the knee (with the caudal hand) and passively flexed and released at the hip (extension). The movements of flexion and extension should be stretched to their limits. The amount of movement, noted as an opening and closing of the interspinous gap, is compared to other levels.

2. *Lateral flexion* (sidebending) (Fig. 20–13C). The patient lies on the side with the knees and hips bent so that the lumbar spine is relaxed midway between flexion and extension. The examiner (facing the patient), applies his caudal arm around the patient's upper pelvis and under the patient's ischial tuberosity. The examiner's cranial hand palpates between the interspinous spaces of the adjacent vertebrae (the pad of the palpating finger is placed facing upward in the underside of the interspinous space). The examiner firmly grasps the patient's pelvis and upper thigh with the caudal hand, then uses a rhythmical side sway of his own trunk toward the patient's head to produce a

Fig. 20-13. Passive physiological testing of (A) flexion, (B) extension, (C) lateral flexion, and (D) rotation between segments.

side-flexion movement from below upward by rocking the pelvis. Movement can be appreciated either as a gapping or approximation by the finger of the cranial hand. Repeat to the opposite side.

3. *Rotation* (Fig. 20–13D). Although active lumbar rotation does not provide much information, testing the small range of rotation is often of value. The positions of the examiner and patient are similar to those used for assessing lateral flexion or sidebending but with a flat pillow placed under the patient's waist to keep the lumbar spine in neutral. The examiner leans across the patient and places his cranial forearm along the lower thoracic spine with a reinforced finger resting against adjacent spinous processes from underneath. The caudal hand is placed over the patient's greater trochanter. As the examiner stabilizes the thorax with his cranial forearm, the patient's pelvis is rocked backward and forward so the pelvis and lumbar spine rotate. Repeat on the opposite side.

   Note: The three examination procedures above can be modified and used as mobility techniques, using appropriate grades of movement based on the findings found on the evaluation.[270,457]

E. *Segmental mobility* (T10–L5). The patient is in prone lying across the table, if necessary with a cushion under the abdomen to place the lumbar spine in neutral (resting position) (Fig. 20–14). The lower legs are supported on a stool (hips and knees in 90° flexion). The correct movements are achieved by moving the joint by thumb-tip pressure or with pisiform contact against the vertebral prominences. The examiner must take care to apply the pressure slowly and carefully so that the "feel" of movement can be recognized. This "springing test" may be repeated several times to determine the quality of the movement. The basic maneuvers include:

1. Posteroanterior pressure against the spinous processes (using the thumb or pisiform contact).
2. Transverse pressure against the lateral surface of the spinous process. Pressure should be applied to both sides of the spinous processes to compare the quality of movement.

Fig. 20–14. Position of the patient for palpation and segmental mobility testing of the lumbar spine.

3. Posteroanterior unilateral pressures over the mammillary process of the joint to be examined. The same anterior "springing pressure" is applied as in central pressure evaluation. Both sides should be evaluated and compared. For additional information:
   i. Alter the direction of posteroanterior pressure movements: cephalad (toward the head), caudally (toward the feet), and diagonally.
   ii. Exert counterpressure to the transverse process of the spinal process just below and over the spinous process above a tender segment to determine more precisely the location of the painful or involved segment.[350]

   These procedures may elicit pain, restricted movement and or spasm. If the range of movement is limited, the type of resistance—caused by either a sense of tightness or muscle spasm—is assessed. The direction of restriction and/or painful movement will determine the type of mobilization therapy to be used.

F. *Passive sacroiliac and peripheral joint tests* (see Passive Movement Techniques— Segmental Spinal Movements, page 607).

Painful joint conditions which may originate from the lumbosacral spine must be assessed. Pain from the spine can be referred to the hip, knee, and sacroiliac joints; pain originating in the hip or sacroiliac joint may be referred to the lumbar spine. Clearing tests of the peripheral joints include:

1. *Sacroiliac provocation/mobility tests.* These may reproduce pain from a sacroiliac disorder, and a snap might be elicited if the joint is abnormally mobile. (Little or no movement should occur at this joint.)

   a. Posterior rotation. The patient lies on the side with the side to be tested on top. The examiner flexes the upper knee toward the patient's abdomen, then holds it flexed with the examiner's upper thigh or pelvis in order to free the hands. One hand is placed over the patient's ASIS, the forearm directed diagonally in the posterocaudal direction with respect to the patient. The opposite hand is placed over the patient's ischial tuberosity, the forearm directed in an anterocephalad direction. The examiner then produces a force-couple movement to rotate the ilium backward on the sacrum while simultaneously moving the patient's hip and knee into more flexion with the examiner's pelvis or anterior thigh (see Fig. 20-36).

   b. Anterior rotation. The patient lies prone. The examiner stands at the side to be tested. The more cephalad hand is placed over the sacrum. With the opposite hand grasp around medially to the anterior aspect of the patient's knee. Push downward on the inferior aspect of the sacrum while simultaneously lifting the patient's leg into extension to move the ilium, by way of the hip joint capsule, into a forward position on the sacrum (see Fig. 20-37).

   c. Tests to demonstrate sacroiliac fixation as described by Kirkaldy-Willis are often included.[290]

2. *Hip joint.* A test that may be used to clear the hip joint and also assess the sacroiliac joint is the hip flexion–adduction test. This test uses the femur as a lever to stretch the posterolateral and inferior portions of the inferior capsule and compress the superior and medial portions of the capsule. With the patient in supine the examiner flexes the patient's knee and hip fully and then adducts the hip. As the knee is moved fully toward the patient's opposite shoulder, the examiner compresses the hip joint.

3. *Knee joint.* To clear the knee, the anterior drawer test (Lachman test) performed at 25° of knee flexion, and the valgus–varus stress test at 30° of knee flexion also may be used (see Chapter 14, The Knee).

VI. **Palpation.** This underused but important palpation examination should be incorporated in the assessment of every patient who has back pain. The aim of palpation is to detect abnormalities in bone structure (*e.g.,* spondylolisthesis), identify the level of the lesion, and determine the nature of the problem (*e.g.,* muscle spasm, stiffness or pain).

A useful test to assess muscle guarding in the lumbar spine is the weight-shift test.[493] With the patient standing, the examiner places his thumbs on the patient's lumbar paraspinals. The patient is then asked to shift the weight from one side to the other. Normally the paraspinals on the side of the stance foot will relax, but if muscle guarding or spasm is present, the muscle will not be felt to relax.

A. *Posterior Aspect.* For further palpation of the posterior aspect of the spine, the patient is placed in a relaxed prone position. This is best achieved in the 90–90 position of the hips and knees (Fig. 20–14). Standing behind the patient, the examiner places the fingers on the top of the iliac crests and thumbs at the same level on the midline of the back (the level of the fourth and fifth lumbar disk interspaces). Mark this reference point. Palpate the following:

1. *Ligaments.* The supraspinous ligaments are palpated for tenderness and consistency; the supraspinous ligament is normally springy and supple. If it is thick and hardened, the segment may be hypomobile. Tenderness is usually apparent over the involved intervertebral joint. Usually the interspinous ligament is also tender. This is found by applying exquisitely localized pressure with a key ring or the edge of a coin between the spinous processes.[350]

2. *Position of the transverse and spinous processes.* Note any alterations in the bony alignment, such as spondylolistheses and evidence of tenderness. Specific pain elicited in one segment is particularly helpful in patients with suspected instability.[426] If each spinous process is tapped sharply with a reflex hammer or fingertip, pain may be reproduced over the painful joint.

3. *Sacrum, sulcus, sacral hiatus, and coccyx.* Palpation of a the whole sacroiliac sulcus, hiatus, and coccyx should be included (Fig. 17-20). If indicated, a rectal examination of the coccyx may be performed. The sacroiliac joint should be palpated at its inferior extent in the region of the posteroinferior iliac spine. Acute unilateral tenderness is very common in painful sacroiliac conditions and, when well localized, is a useful confirmatory sign.[199] When palpating the joint, the patient's knee is flexed to 90° and the hip is passively medially rotated while the examiner palpates the sacroiliac joint on the same side. The procedure is repeated on the opposite side. A comprehensive examination of this joint should be regarded as an expanded section of the lumbar spine. Details of a comprehensive examination of this joint can be found in other sources and will not be covered here. [44,45,88,100–103,157,193–195,290,343,349,355,398,471,493,598]

4. *Iliac crest, ischial tuberosity, and hip joint.* Beginning at the posterosuperior iliac spine, the examiner moves along the iliac crest palpating for signs of pathologic processes such as Maigne's syndrome.[290] Pressure and friction over the iliac crest will often reveal a well-localized and actuely painful point (crestal point) at the gluteal level (8 to 10 cm from the midline). Pinching and rolling of the skin in the gluteal area will be painful as well as lateral pressure over the spinous processes (T11–L1). According to Maigne, referred pain may be mediated by the clunial nerves, the posterior rami of the T12 or L1 spinal nerves.[351] These nerves pass downward and outward on each side to supply the skin at the level of the iliac crest. The referred pain is experienced at this level. Irritation of these nerves may be responsible for low back pain, pseudovisceral pain, and pseudo hip pain. Because attention is usually directed to the site of referred pain, the source is frequently overlooked.[351] When Maigne's syndrome is suspected, the diagnosis is confirmed by alleviation of pain following manipulation or injections to the symptomatic posterior joints.[290]

Palpate the ischial tuberosities on both sides for any abnormalities. Do not forget the hip and greater trochanteric bursa, which sometimes mimics sciatica. It is often difficult to differentiate between hip and spine problems, because the symptoms may be similar.

5. *Muscles of the gluteal region and sciatic nerve.* Observe for apparent muscle atrophy, particularly of the gluteus maximus on one side. During palpation, it will often be found that one or several of the muscles will have hard, infiltrated fascicles which are at times cordlike. They may be very sensitive to pressure. According to Maigne, the gluteal muscle pain is responsible for a considerable number of instances of lumbar pain.[350] Deep pétrissage gives excellent results in this type of chronic pain.[350] Palpating midway between the ischial tuberosity and the greater trochanter, the examiner may be able to palpate the sciatic nerve. Deep to the gluteal muscles, the piriformis muscle should be palpated for potential pathologic processes.

6. *Skin and subcutaneous tissue.* The skin is palpated for tenderness, moisture, texture, and temperature changes. A quick wipe over the area with the back of the hand is used to register any apparent local changes in temperature or sweating. Any moles on the skin are examined to determine whether they are deep or superficial. Normally the skin can be rolled over the spine and gluteal region freely and painlessly. If there are subcutaneous pathologic changes, there will be tightness and pain when skin rolling is done.

B. *Anterior Aspect*

1. *Abdominal wall, iliac crest and symphysis pubis.* Palpate the abdominal wall, iliac crest, and symphysis pubis for tenderness. Palpate the symphysis pubis

bilaterally, over the superior aspect, to ensure that the two pubic bones are level and asymptomatic.

2. *Inguinal area and femoral triangle.* The general area within the triangle should be probed for enlarged lymph nodes (infections), symptoms of hernia, abscess, or other pathologic conditions.

3. *Arterial pulses.* Arterial supply to the legs is assessed by palpating the arterial pulses in the inguinal, popliteal, and dorsalis sites.

VII. **Neuromuscular Evaluation.** The neurologic portion of the musculoskeletal evaluation consists of a series of tests to determine if there is segmental interference of neural conduction. The most common cause of such findings is a disk extrusion in the lumbar spine. Other causes of neurologic deficits in the legs are rare but are usually more serious. Any multisegmental deficit should be viewed with some suspicion, because nerve-root impingement from a disk protrusion rarely involves more than one root, the occasional exception being an L5–S1 protrusion which may affect the L5 and S1 roots.

A. *Sensory (dermatomal) tests.* Subtle sensory deficits are best detected by assessing vibratory perception with a tuning fork. This is because pressure tends to affect the large, myelinated fibers that mediate vibratory and proprioceptive sensation first. Gross sensory testing may be carried out using a wisp of cotton or a pin.

The key sensory areas to test are in the distal part of the limb, because these are the areas where there is relatively little overlap of segmental innervation. These include:

L4 — Medial aspect of the big toe
L5 — Web space between the first and second toes
S1 — Below the lateral malleolus
S2 — Distal Achilles tendon region

These areas should be tested first; then test the various aspects of the leg and thigh. If a significant deficit is detected proximal to the foot, the clinician must be sure that more serious pathologic processes have been ruled out.

When performing sensory tests, test a small area of one limb. Ask the patient if the expected sensation is felt (*e.g.*, vibration, touch, or pinprick); then test the corresponding area on the opposite limb and ask the patient again if it is felt. Inquire if the intensity of stimulus felt is about the same on both sides. Proceed in this fashion for all of the areas to be tested. Sensory tests are most easily carried out with the patient supine.

B. *Resisted isometric tests* (motor, myotomal tests). Because most limb muscles receive innervation from more than one segment, only subtle motor dysfunction will be noted in the case of segmental deficits resulting from disk protrusions. Significant motor loss should suggest a more serious pathologic process. Key muscles should be tested for each segment. Large muscle groups, such as the quadriceps and calf muscles, must be tested by repetitive resistance against a load, because even in the presence of loss of segmental input to such muscles, sufficient tension may still be produced to prevent the examiner from detecting weakness by overcoming the contraction. Key muscle groups may be tested for each of the segments contributing to the limb.

In general, isometric tests are used to test for any muscle weakness that may result from nerve-root compressions. However, plantar flexion of the foot cannot be adequately tested by an isometric contraction. Instead, weight-bearing ankle plantar flexion is tested by repeated toe-raises. When testing muscles (and reflexes), look for unusual fatigue. Always compare both sides. Tests that are of clinical significance are listed below.

1. Tests with patient in supine
   a. L2 — Hip flexion (iliopsoas). The patient holds the flexed hip and knee at 90° while resistance is applied just above the knee.
   b. L3 — Knee extension (quadriceps). Test by repetitive one-legged half-squats in the standing position or in supine using an isometric contraction. The examiner supports the thigh with one arm underneath it, with the examiner's hand supported on top of the opposite thigh. Resistance is applied to the lower leg while the patient holds the leg just short of full extension.
   c. L4 — Ankle dorsiflexion and inversion (tibialis anterior). Test bilater-

ally. The patient holds the feet in dorsiflexion and inversion as resistance is applied against the dorsal-medial aspect of the foot.

    d. L5—Great toe extension (extensor hallucis longus). Toe extension is tested bilaterally. The patient holds the foot and toes dorsiflexed as resistance is applied against the dorsal aspect of the great toe.

    e. L5–S1—Extension of the toes (extensor digitorum longus). The patient holds the foot and toes dorsiflexed as resistance is applied against the dorsum of the toes.

    f. S1—Ankle eversion (peroneus longus and brevis). The patient is asked to keep the heels together with the feet everted as resistance is applied to the lateral borders of the feet, pushing them together.

2. Tests with patient in prone

    a. S2—Knee flexion (hamstrings). The hamstrings are tested bilaterally as the patient holds the knees flexed to 90° as resistance is applied behind the patient's heels.

    b. S1—Hip extension (gluteus maximus). The patient holds the hip extended with the knee bent while the examiner applies resistance just above the knee with one hand while palpating the gluteal mass with the other hand to assess firmness.

3. Tests with patient standing

    a. S1—Plantar flexion (gastrocnemius). The patient stands on one leg and plantar flexes by rising on the toes through a full range of motion. Repeat 6 to 10 times for each side. Plantar flexion can also be tested by having the patient walk on the toes.

    b. L3—Knee flexion (quadriceps). Unilateral half squats. Repeat 6–10 times. The girth of the limbs above and below the knee is measured to document any muscle wasting.

C. *Dural mobility tests.* The dura, nerve-root sleeves, and nerve roots are sensitive to pain. Their irritants are many, as are the pathologic processes that induce them. Included are disk prolapse,[51,549,578] adhesions (*e.g.*, post-traumatic or postsurgical epidural fibrosis, subarachnoid adhesions),[578]

hypertrophic changes in the facet joints and margins of the vertebral bodies,[408,145] and indirect compressions from ischemic changes secondary to chronic progressive compression (*e.g.*, enlarged masses, thickening of the ligamentum flavum, apophyseal joint swelling).[352]

Dural mobility tests (sciatic nerve, straight-leg raising) may reproduce symptoms (usually pain) in the case of a disk prolapse, in which a bulging disk may approximate the anterolateral aspect of the dural sac of the cauda equina, or in the case of a disk extrusion, in which the protruded disk material may be adjacent to some part of the dural investment of a nerve root. The dura can be moved in a cephalad direction by flexing the neck or in a caudal direction by applying tension to the femoral or sciatic nerves. The femoral nerve and its contributing nerve roots are stretched by side-lying or prone knee flexion and hip extension; the sciatic nerve and its roots by straight-leg raising. Additional tension is applied to the sciatic nerve by dorsiflexion of the ankle.

1. Dural mobility tests for the sciatic nerve roots may be done sitting or supine. It is often best to perform them in both positions and to compare the results. Sitting increases the likelihood of obtaining a positive test in the case of a minor prolapse, because it is a position of relatively high intradiskal pressure. However, to judge improvement, the tests performed are best in the supine position, measuring the distance from the lateral malleolus to the plinth at which pain is produced on straight-leg raising.

    A true-positive dural mobility test will reproduce back pain, hip girdle pain, leg pain, or some combination thereof, and pain should be felt somewhere between 30° and 60° of straight-leg raising. At angles less than 30° there is very little movement of the nerve roots, and by 60° the dura will have already moved sufficiently to have caused reproduction of pain. Also, above 60° there is the possibility that reproduction of pain is caused by movement of the spinal column as the pelvis tilts backward. The examiner must be prepared to differentiate between pulling on tight hamstrings and reproduction of leg pain from dural impingement. Possible mechanical effects from movement of the spine or sacroiliac joint can be ruled out by seeing if ankle dorsiflexion further accentuates the pain produced; if so, it is likely to be a true-positive dural sign.

a. The sitting tests are done with the patient sitting at the edge of the plinth. First move one knee toward extension, noting any guarding of the movement and inquiring as to reproduction of symptoms. If pain is produced, the leg is held just up to the painful point and the effects of ankle dorsiflexion and neck flexion are assessed. The opposite leg is similarly tested.

b. The supine tests are carried out in a similar manner by moving first one leg and then the other into flexion with the knee straight. Again, the effects of ankle dorsiflexion and neck flexion are assessed. Test straight-leg raising with the hip in neutral rotation and slightly adducted straight-leg raising of the asymptomatic leg. Positive straight-leg raising of the opposite leg can be more important than ipsilateral straight-leg raising, and a discussion of this sciatic traction test would be incomplete without mention of what is called the "well leg test" or the crossed straight-leg raising test. This test has a high correlation with large central disk protrusions that impale on the root in its axilla.[130,244,530,613] The pattern of positive results yields some clues as to the relationship between the protrusion and the pain-sensitive structure (*e.g.*, dura or dural covering of a nerve root).

i. In the case of prolapsed or extruded material that is anterior to the pain-sensitive tissue, ipsilateral leg raising, contralateral leg raising, and neck flexion may all hurt.

ii. If the protruded material is medial to the nerve root as it exits from the dural sac (rare), leg raising may hurt bilaterally, but neck flexion may be painless.

iii. If the protrusion is lateral to the existing nerve root, ipsilateral leg raising may reproduce symptoms, neck flexion may or may not be painful, and contralateral leg raising will be painless.

Another aspect relevant to the straight-leg raising test is that there is an increase in intradiskal pressure when the patient sits or stands, as compared with lying.[428] This may effect a discrepancy in the degree of limitation of straight-leg raising performed in the standing and lying positions. Tests in both positions can therefore be of value.[354]

c. The slump test is an excellent test for a disk lesion and dural tethering; it is performed on the patient who has low back pain with or without leg pain.[354,418] Maximum tension can be exerted on the canal structures with the patient's chin on the chest.[354] With the patient sitting erect on the examination table, the patient is asked to do the following:

i. Let the back slump through its full range of thoracic lumbar spine flexion

ii. Having established full range of the hip and spine from T1 to the sacrum, flex head and neck fully

iii. Straighten first the unaffected leg and actively dorsiflex the ankle and then the affected leg.

Note and record the pain response after each step. There are many variations of this test, including passive and sustained overpressure of the head and neck while in the slump position, releasing the neck flexion component, raising the head to neutral, neck extension in the slump position, and performance of the test in long sitting. According to Maitland, in making a judgment as to the findings of this test, the pain response, particularly in relationship to releasing the neck flexion component, is most important.[353] Maitland has described the slump test very clearly and its significance fully.[353,354]

2. Femoral-nerve traction test.[130] The patient lies on the unaffected side with the lower limb flexed at both the hip and knee joints to stabilize the trunk. The head is flexed slightly to increase ten-

sion on the cauda equina. The test has two components:

    a. The uppermost part of the thigh is first passively extended just short of provoking lumbar spine extension to create tension in the iliopsoas, and hence traction on the upper lumbar nerve root.

    b. Next, the knee is progressively flexed to increase femoral nerve tension by stretching the quadriceps femoris muscle.

In the presence of an L3 radiculitis, pain radiates down the medial thigh to the knee. When the L4 root is involved, the pain is more anterior on the thigh and extends to the midtibial portion of the leg.[130]

D. *Reflex Tests.* Plantar responses and deep tendon reflexes are tested for any evidence of an upper motor neuron lesion.

    1. *Plantar reflex test.* With the patient's leg extended, stimulate the lateral border of the sole with a blunt object. The stroke begins on the lateral aspect of the heel, moves distally, and then across the metatarsals just proximal to the toes. Plantar flexion is a normal response, but dorsiflexion (a positive Babinski response) is pathologic and indicates spinal cord injury (upper motor neuron lesion).

    2. *Deep-tendon reflexes.* Segmented neurologic deficits may result in diminution of deep-tendon reflexes (DTRs) on the involved side. When examining DTRs, primarily observe for asymmetry of responses from one side to the other. Difficulty eliciting reflexes on both sides is not an indication of a pathologic process, so long as there is no asymmetry in response. Look for unusual fatigue. Elicit reflex at least six times; always compare sides.

        a. Knee jerk reflex—L3, L4

        b. Ankle jerk reflex—S1, S2

        c. Great toe reflex—L5[562]

        Note: The medial (L5, S1) and the lateral (S1) hamstring reflexes are not routinely tested but may at times assist in decisions about involvement of those roots.[199]

Superficial reflex (upper motor neuron) testing may be indicated and include the abdominal, cremasteric, and anal reflexes.[242,343]

E. *Test for ankle clonus.* A test to determine if the patient has clonus may be included here. A hyperactive stretch reflex is the mechanism that supports clonus. Ankle clonus is elicited by quickly stretching the gastroc–soleus muscle group by dorsiflexing the foot and then maintaining moderate stretch to the plantar flexors. The clonus response is alternating plantarflexion and dorsiflexion of the foot.

F. *Balance testing.* Based on the information provided by Wyke, balance testing is conducted to appraise the receptor integrity in the joints of the lower extremities and lumbar spine.[615,616] The Romberg test, "stork standing," or digital balance boards can be used to assess balance.

If a mechanical lesion of the low back is suspected the above tests are generally sufficient. However, if neurologic disease is suspected (*e.g.,* diabetic neuropathy), motor performance, temperature, and proprioception should be tested as well.

VIII. General Physical Examination. A general physical examination, including the abdomen and chest, may be necessary. In cases of suspected pelvic lesions, a rectal examination is necessary. These tests will help the examiner to determine the severity of the back pain, the level of the lesion, the presence of nerve-root pressure, and the authenticity of the patient's pain. Based on the literature reviewed by the Quebec Task Force (1987), a history and physical examination are usually sufficient to identify the majority of patients for whom specific therapy is required.[475] Because of the drawbacks of routine roentgenography, many authors have proposed selective studies based on clinical findings.

IX. Other Studies

A. *Roentgenograms and other imaging studies.* The examiner may review any imaging studies that have been done.[262,397] In addition to basic roentgenograms, other special techniques may be used.

    1. Myelograms. A radiopaque dye is placed within the epidural space and allowed to flow to different levels of the spinal cord. This technique carries a sufficient morbidity and is usually reserved for patients with suspected spinal canal stenosis or spinal tumor, or it is used to demonstrate the level of a prolapsed disk. With disk prolapse, the column of dye should be indented or distorted with evidence of compression or shortening of the nerve-root dural sheath (see Fig. 20-4A,B).

2. Diskography. This test involves injecting a water-soluble radiopaque dye under roentgenographic control into the nucleus pulposus in order to reproduce signs of disk disease and localize the level of impingement. The injection should reproduce the patient's pain before the test can be considered positive (see Figs. 20-1A and 20-2A).

3. Computed axial tomography (CAT scan). Tomography has become a common technique. It involves a computerized display that recreates a three-dimensional image of the spine. It provides a noninvasive alternative to the techniques described earlier. Plane tomograms or computer isotomograms have improved the capability to outline both bony and soft tissues. CAT scans are most useful in outlining structural spinal deformities such as lumbar canal stenosis, abnormalities in the facet joints, vertebral disease, and disk prolapse.[71]

4. Bone Scanning. This noninvasive, sensitive technique employs chemicals labeled with isotopes such as technetium pyrophosphate, which is taken up by bone and bound to hydroxyapatite crystals. The isotope may be localized where there is a high level of activity relative to the rest of a bone. Its major role is in identifying pathologic changes such as stress fractures, tumors, and metabolic bone disease.

5. Other techniques include radiculography, epidural blocks, magnetic resonance imaging (MRI), and venography.[603]

B. *Electromyography.* Electromyography may be used to localize the level of a spinal lesion with nerve-root pressure. Evidence of denervation may be found as early as 2 weeks after the onset of nerve damage.[88]

C. *Laboratory tests.* Among the laboratory tests used to investigate spinal disease are a complete blood count (CBC). Urine analysis should be performed routinely.

X. **Tests for Nonorganic Back Pain.** Several tests are useful in the differentiation of organic and nonorganic back pain (*e.g.,* that seen in patients suffering from depression, emotional disturbance, or anxiety states).[88,283,486,488,489] Great difficulty will be encountered in assessing a patient who has or has had an organic back lesion but whose symptoms are exacerbated or prolonged by psychological factors. In those patients symptoms are usually out of proportion to signs (*i.e.,* inconsistent joint findings, abnormal postures or gait). Tests include the following:

A. *Distraction test* (leg test or flip test).[283,587] A positive physical finding is demonstrated in a routine manner; this finding is then checked while the patients attention is distracted. For example, after performing the usual straight-leg-raising test in supine, ask the patient to sit up, swing the legs over the end of the table and repeat leg raising. If marked improvement is noted, the patient's response is inconsistent. Leg raising is a most useful distraction test.

B. *Stimulation tests.* These tests should not be uncomfortable: if pain is reported, a nonorganic influence is suggested.
   1. Axial loading employs manual pressure through the standing patient's head. Few patients whose lumbar pain is organic will suffer discomfort on this test.[283,587]
   2. Hip and shoulder rotation.[283,587] With the patient standing, examine for pain by passively rotating the patient's hips or shoulders while the feet are kept on the ground. This maneuver is usually painless for patients with organic back disorders.
   3. Kneeling on a stool (Burns test).[88,283] The patient kneels on a stool or chair and is asked to bend over and try to touch the floor. Even with a severely herniated disk, most patients will attempt the task to some degree. Persons with nonorganic pain will often refuse on the ground that it would cause great pain or else may tend to overbalance them on the chair.

C. *Other methods.* Other tools for assessing nonorganic physical signs include regional disturbances, which involve a divergence from the accepted neuroanatomy (*i.e.,* atypical motor and sensory disturbances), overreaction during examination (*i.e.*, disproportionate verbalization, muscle tension, and tremor), and tenderness.[589,592] Tenderness, when related to physical disease is usually localized to a particular skeletal or neuromuscular structure. Nonorganic tenderness is nonspecific and diffuse. Further verification is possible by use of pain drawings, as recommended by Ransford and associates (Fig. 20-8).[478]

A number of other psychopathic signs and observations have been described by Mooney, Carins, MacNab, Melzack, Pheasant, and Spengler.[341,391,407,466,533] These signs should alert the therapist that further psychological evaluation is indicated and to guard against potential overtreatment.[466,535,606]

Other types of investigation such as the Minnesota Multiphasic Personality Inventory (MMPI)[24,38,50,105,106,113,166,389,533,539] and other psychological tests have been used for lumbar spine problems; these include the Cornell Medical Index, Diagnostic Drives, Mooney Problem List, Quick Test, Rorschach Sentence Completion, and the Weschsler Adult Intelligence Scale.[59,385,390,391] Since its development in 1940 by Hathaway and McKinley, the MMPI has become one of the most widely used personality screening tests.[222]

XI. **Activities of Daily Living.** A formal exercise obstacle course may be used to evaluate the patient's ability to perform activities of daily living.[603] Activities to be assessed include sitting, standing, walking, bending, lifting, pushing, pulling, climbing, and reaching. Endurance may be evaluated while the patient is walking or on a stationary bicycle. Quantitative functional capacity measurements can give objective evidence of the patient's physical abilities and degree of effort and can significantly guide the clinician in administering an effective treatment program.[370]

XII. **Computerized Tests.** Isokinetic forms of resisted muscle testing are felt to be the most effective and yield reliable measurements of muscular strength, power (at slow as well as fast speeds), and endurance; these measures can be recorded in graphic form for comparison later in rehabilitation.[140] The potential value of objective measurement of spinal function has been recognized for some time, although practical and clinically useful technology has not been generally available.[35,163,420,554]

The increasing understanding of disuse and deconditioning syndromes as a factor in long-term disability and the recent development in qualification of true spinal range of motion,[371,372,374] trunk muscle strength,[109,307,359,565,566] endurance, and lifting capacity bring a new dimension to low back pain management.[226,292,373,471]

COMMON LESIONS AND MANAGEMENT

INTERVERTEBRAL DISK LESIONS

It is now apparent that sciatica is caused by many intraspinal abnormalities other than disk prolapse.[3,81,192,201,238,322,469,531] For example, decrease in size of the lateral bony nerve-root canal can result from degenerative hypertropy of the lumbar facets or a trefoil canal (a congenital variant in cross-sectional geometry).[17,289] Other less common causes of sciatica include congenital anomalies of the lumbar nerve roots, "hip-pocket" sciatica, the piriformis syndrome, and even viral infections. Space does not permit a discussion or differentiation from other possible causes of acute spinal dysfunction. Despite the extensive differential diagnosis, intervertebral disk prolapse is the most common diagnosis of sciatica. Ninety eight percent of intervertebral disk prolapse cases involve the L4–L5 or L5–S1 lumbar disk space.[531] Older patients have a relatively increased risk of disk prolapse at the L3–L4 and L2–L3 levels.[177]

The sensitive spinal cord has an elaborate protective mechanism comprising a most pain-sensitive anterior dural sheath and the posterior longitudinal ligament. The following can occur with a prolapsed disk.

1. The disk bulges against the ligament and the dura. This produces a dull, deep, poorly localized pain in the back and over the sacroiliac region because the dura does not have specific dermatomal localization.
2. The disk bulges posterolaterally against the nerve root. This is a natural route because the annulus fibrosus is no longer reinforced by the posterior ligament. The result is sharp nerve root pain (*e.g.*, sciatica).
3. The disk ruptures and the thick gelatinous fluid of the nucleus pulposus flows around the dura and nerve roots. This is an extremely irritating substance causing a reaction around the nerve-sensitive tissue. It is the most likely cause of agonizing persistent back pain. When the disk ruptures, fragments of the harder annulus fibrosus may

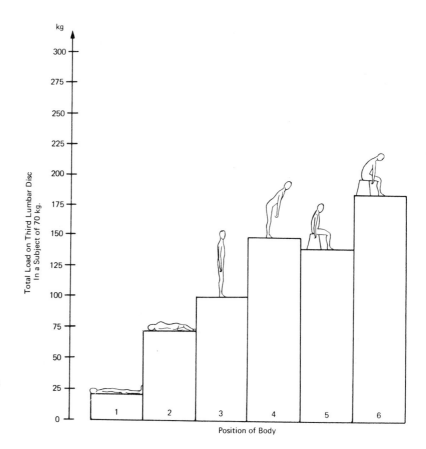

Fig. 20–15. Intradiskal pressures (relative) as they relate to body positions. (Finneson BE: Low Back Pain, 2nd ed. Philadelphia, JB Lippincott, 1980)

protrude into the spinal canal; this usually requires surgical intervention.

Experiments on human volunteers by Nachemson and Morris in 1964, which measured the interdiskal pressures in the lumbar spine with a diskogram, and subsequent studies have enhanced our understanding of the intervertebral disk (Figs. 20–15 and 20–16).[422,428] Obviously, bending forward while lifting

increases the pressure. The situation is aggravated by sitting when the lumbar lordosis is reduced by leaning forward.

Disk Prolapse

Some of the known clinical features associated with disk prolapse include:

1. Age—The peak age is in the 20- to 45-year age

Fig. 20–16. Intradiskal pressures (relative) as they relate to activities. (Adapted from Nachemson AL: The lumbar spine: An orthopedic challenge. Spine 1:59–71, 1976)

group. Prolonged work posture of lumbar flexion is a frequent factor in the history.

2. Sex—Males are more commonly affected than females by approximately 3:2.

3. Site—In 1000 cases of lumbar disk operations, Armstrong found that 46.9% occurred at the lumbosacral disk, 40.4% at the L4–L5 disk, and 2.1% at the upper three disks; in 10.7% of the cases double lesions were present.[16]

History. Back pain may occur for no apparent reason—rather, it may be caused by the accumulative effects of months or even years of forward bending, lifting, or sitting in a slumped, forward-bent position.[76,110,114,383,441,461,528,531,600] There may be a history of attacks of back pain, sometimes associated with a sensation of back locking. Many patients tend to relate it to some minor traumatic incident or after a strain, such as bending, lifting, or twisting which may be associated with a tearing sensation.[88]

In the early stages, the patient will complain of pain, usually in the lower back, but sometimes in the posterior buttocks or thigh. As a general rule, leg pain indicates a larger protrusion than does back pain alone.[383] Pain may be described as a dull ache or knifelike. Onset of pain may be sudden and severe or may develop more gradually. Pain at first may be intermittent and relieved by rest, standing, lying, or changing position. Spinal pain tends to be greater on one side than the other. Bilateral spinal pain is probably secondary to a connecting branch of the sinuvertebral nerve, which joins the right and left portions of that nerve.[158] Pain is aggravated by straining, stooping, sneezing, coughing, car travel, and sitting. The patient will also often report that prolonged sitting will cause pain to move from the lower back into the leg. Difficulty in assuming an erect posture after lying down or sitting may also be described. Ultimately, pain usually becomes severe and may disturb sleep.

Back pain may be followed by leg pain, which is almost always unilateral but usually is severe. The back pain may disappear when the leg pain begins. The distribution of the leg pain will vary according to the nerve root involved.

Clinical Examination. Signs consist of varying combinations and degrees of mechanical derangement of the lumbar spinal joints and evidence of nerve-root involvement. Mechanical derangement is evidenced by alterations in posture, muscle spasms, disturbance of movements, and alterations in the spinal contours.

Gait and movement are guarded and restricted. Gait may also be antalgic, with as little weight as possible being transferred to the painful side. Transfer activities, such as rising from a sitting position and moving about on the plinth, are performed guardedly, with the lumbar spine being reflexively protected from compressive loading or movement.

Regarding posture and alterations in spinal contours, the clinical picture will reveal a patient who sits in a slumped posture or who insists on standing in the waiting room because of increased intradiskal pressure caused by sitting. In erect standing, patients may be unable to bear any weight on the painful leg and so stand with the hips and knees flexed and the back held rigid. The patient may have loss of the normal lordosis and flattening of the thoracic spine and shoulder-girdle retraction as well.[88,100,383,590] The patient may have a lateral shift (lumbar scoliosis) away from the side of pain (contralateral, 85% of cases), but occasionally toward the painful side (ipsilateral, 15% of cases).

Inspection. To evaluate active movement, the physiological movements of the spine are tested to determine their range, whether pain is reproduced, the behavior of the pain with movement, whether an arc of pain is present, and the presence of any deformity.

Lumbar forward bending (flexion) is sometimes limited because of the severity of the pain, and the degree of its loss usually reflects the severity of the disk prolapse. The patient often tends to compensate by bending at the hips and knees and may guard the spine against excessive compression by placing the hands on the thighs. In less severe cases, where forward bending is possible, the bending may be associated with a deviated arc of movement in which the spine shifts out of and back toward the midline as movement proceeds. When tested in the standing position, flexion may cause the pain to move peripherally. This is especially true if forward flexion is repeated several times.[383]

Movement into lateral flexion varies. There may be full and painless range to each side, or there may be painful limitation to one side. This occurs more commonly toward the side of pain; lateral flexion to the other side is then usually full. If a lateral shift is present, it should be corrected before testing extension.

Loss of backward bending (extension) is not as common as loss of flexion. In patients with a loss of the normal lordosis, extension or backward bending (after the lateral shift has been corrected) will almost always be restricted and will cause increased pain. The patient usually compensates by extending the thoracic spine and retracting the shoulder girdle. It is important to note whether the increase in pain centralizes or becomes peripheral from the center of the spine into the leg.

The spine is reflexly splinted in a position that compromises between minimizing interdiskal pressure, reducing tension on the dural material, and preventing impingement of the protruded materials. Lordosis is lost because the posteriorly protruded disk material forces the segment toward forward bending, and backward bending would tend to compromise the prolapse. Forward bending is difficult because the marked increase in intradiskal pressure it causes would tend to increase the pressure against the pain-sensitive structures.[11,420] Lateral bending is restricted because of increased intradiskal pressure and because of impingement of the protrusion when performed to the involved side. McKenzie maintains that 50% of patients with this disorder have a lateral shift because of the tendency of the nuclear gel to shift posterolaterally.[383] As the gel moves posteriorly, the patient tends to shift the body weight in an anterior direction, flattening the lumbar spine. When the patient shifts the shoulder away from the side of the nuclear movement, a lateral shift occurs.[88,151,158,285,446] Usually the protrusion is lateral to the existing nerve root, in which case a lateral shift away from the defect minimizes the dural impingement. Less often the bulge is located at the axilla formed by the root stemming from the dural sac. The spine is shifted toward the ipsilateral side or painful side (15% of cases). The presence of a lateral shift may be noted while the patient is standing or flexing or extending the lumbar spine. It is not rare for a patient with only unilateral pain and a contralateral list to have this change under treatment to an ipsilateral list or *vice versa*.[196]

Passive movements—both physiological and accessory—are found to be limited because of spasms, stiffness, and pain. Passive physiological restriction is usually less because of reduced compression imposed on the spine in a reclining position. Accessory movements are usually compromised by protective muscle guarding.

Nerve-root involvement is indicated by the loss of freedom of movement of the nerve root in the spinal canal or its intervertebral foramen. It is characterized by the fact that true neurologic signs and symptoms are produced. The patient will have all the signs and symptoms previously discussed, with the addition of positive neurologic signs such as strength loss, decreased muscle stretch reflexes, loss of sensation, and positive dural mobility signs. Tests should include straight-leg raising and the femoral nerve traction test. Neurologic assessment to determine the nerve root involved and the degree of compression is essential. The most important clinical features are the localization of pain to an affected nerve root and the reproduction of the pain by a positive nerve-root tension sign.[495]

Palpation. The affected spinal level is usually tender to palpation in the midline or in the paravertebral area on the same side as the disk prolapse. The sciatic nerve may also be tender. If the patient has had pain for more than 1 or 2 days, the muscles may be tender from guarding and muscle spasm. Positional changes can occasionally be felt by palpating the spinous processes. For example, if the segment is locked in rotation and sidebending, the superior spinous process will not be in alignment with the adjacent inferior spinous process.

Clinical Variations. Many clinical variations of the pain pattern and neurologic involvement are possible. The most common pain pattern is back pain followed by leg pain, but the patient may present with back pain alone, sciatic pain alone, or simultaneous back and leg pain. Pain may radiate into both legs simultaneously and consecutively. A large posterior prolapse may implicate two nerve roots on either side at the same level or at different levels.[88]

Acute nerve-root compression, represents a severe back problem, usually caused by an advanced disk protrusion, and must be handled with care. The disorder has a protracted course of 6 to 12 weeks. More than 50% of patients recover in 6 weeks.[14] Rarely is surgical treatment required, thus delaying surgery is appropriate in most cases.

Conservative Treatment. In the *acute stage*, the nonsurgical treatment of acute symptomatic disk prolapse includes bedrest, medications, epidural steroids, and minimizing the lesion by reducing intradiskal pressure. The therapist must be aware of those positions and activities known to increase intradiskal pressure so as to carefully instruct the patient to avoid situations that may cause the protrusion to progress (see Figs. 20–15 and 20–16).[10,11,91,92,420,423]

How much bedrest is optimal remains to be established, but Deyo and associates observed no differences in outcome between patients with 2 days of bedrest and those treated with 1 week of bed rest.[117] In patients with a demonstrated radicular compression, bedrest is efficacious, as shown in Weber's study of 2 weeks of bed rest.[594] This does not mean absolute bed rest, however, because with prolonged recumbency, the disk tends to imbibe fluid from the adjacent verterbral bodies. Activities related to feeding and personal hygiene may actually be more difficult to achieve in bed than out of bed.

Prospective, randomized trials of autotraction,[183] phenylbutazone, and indomethacin have demonstrated that these treatment procedures moderate a decrease in pain.[27]

Epidural infiltrations of cortisone and local anesthetics have been the topic of a number of clinical studies with variable results, and their utility remains controversial.[46,95,527] Epidural steroids reduced pain and increased function in one randomized study,[120] but a recent comparison of epidural steroid therapy and placebo (saline) demonstrated no differences 24 hours after injections.

Traction can be applied by means of autotraction, inversion traction, gravity reduction, 90/90 traction and motorized techniques, including three-dimensional lumbar traction.* Some clinical studies have compared the effects of different types of traction, but no controlled study has demonstrated their relative efficacy.[333,475,495,627] At least 60% of the body weight must be applied for dimensional changes in the lumbar disk to occur.[177] Claims that disk prolapse can be reduced are unproven. Studies have shown autotraction and gravity axial traction and positional traction to have a short-lived benefit in acute low back pain and sciatica.[60,183,456]

When treating an acute disk protrusion with spinal traction, the treatment time should be short. The patient may feel less pain while the distractive force is applied, but as the traction is released a marked increase in pain often is experienced.[495] Such an effect is probably secondary to absorption of additional fluid by the nucleus while the traction is applied and the development of a high intradiskal pressure as the distractive force is relaxed. This adverse reaction has not been observed if treatment times are kept under 10 minutes for intermittent and under 8 minutes for sustained traction.[491]

Braces and lumbar corsets remain controversial. In separate studies, Morris and associates and Nachemson and Morris have shown that when a garment such as a lumbosacral corset which compresses the abdomen is worn, intradiskal pressure is diminished by approximately 25%.[414,428] Significant unloading of the disk occurs in both the standing and sitting positions.

Certainly, the first step in any treatment program for acute low back pain should be education. The following points should be considered with respect to reduction of intradiskal pressure:

1. Sitting (see Fig. 20–15), especially with the lumbar part of the spine in a forward-bent position, causes very high intradiskal pressure.[422] Sitting with the knees and hips flexed is especially contraindicated. The patient must be taught to sit and rise to standing without bending forward at the lumbar part of the spine. Sitting for a bowel move-

---

* References 60, 61, 89, 97, 103, 115, 141, 241, 309, 318, 325, 360, 362, 417, 431, 443, 451, 462, 489, 491, 493, 519, 576

ment may cause a marked increase in intradiskal pressure because of the Valsalva maneuver. The patient must be taught to sit leaning back, with a wide base of support, with one or both legs outstretched. Use of a raised toilet seat and of a laxative also may be advisable.

2. Most patients are more comfortable while standing than sitting, which confirms Nachemson's findings that on standing interdiskal pressure is decreased by 29%.[428] The normal lumbar curve should be maintained. If the patient is fixed in some degree of forward bending, walking should only be allowed with the aid of crutches to reduce weight-bearing compressive forces to the disk.[485]

3. Isometric abdominal contractions and pelvic tilt exercises that increase intradiskal pressure should not be instituted in the early acute stage.

Physical Therapy. Oscillatory techniques may relieve pain by increasing large-fiber proprioceptive input, which in turn relieves some of the protective muscle spasm. Physical programs that use such modalities as ultrasound, hot packs, cold packs, and diathermy cannot be expected to make any impact on the disease process, but only serve to placate the patient by providing temporary pain relief.[88,422]

Perhaps the most controversial form of treatment is *manipulative therapy,* which Haldeman has divided into manipulation, mobilization, manual traction, soft-tissue massage, and point-pressure massage.[214,215] Brewerton, Deyo, Haldeman, and Ottenbacher and DeFabio have evaluated multiple critical trials that have compared manipulative therapy with other treatment such as medications and sham therapy, and concluded that short-term manipulative treatment may temporarily decrease pain and improve function.[53,116,214,449] Although sciatica is not viewed as a contraindication to manipulation by its proponents, there are reports of forceful manipulations causing new or increased neurologic deficits.[107]

Total management often involves passive exercises as soon as they can be done without increasing peripheral signs and symptoms. An organized form of exercise, termed "the McKenzie program," has been found to be effective against both chronic and acute low back pain.[582] This program uses a series of individualized, progressive exercises to localize, and ultimately to eliminate, the patient's pain. A comparative study found the McKenzie protocol twice as effective in alleviating low back pain as traction and back schools.[121,582] More than 40 different exercise regimens are available. The appropriate exercise regimen must be individualized to each patient, incorporating only those movements (done in the proper sequence and with or without the effects of gravity) that bring about symptom centralization.[121] Typically, McKenzie advocates correction of any lateral shift and passive extension exercises to move the nucleus of the disk centrally.[383] He also advocates constant maintenance of the correction to allow healing of the annular fibers. There is evidence that healing of the disk can occur.[153,220,232,331] The key is to reduce the bulge and then to maintain the posterior aspect of the disk, in close approximation, so the scar that is formed will protect it from further protrusion.[97,383,462] The patient must absolutely avoid positions and activities that increase the intradiskal pressure or cause a posterior force on the nucleus (*i.e.*, slump sitting, forward bending, and flexion exercises). Restoration of full mobility is a necessary component of treatment as soon as the protrusion is stable. Passive exercises and joint mobilization are indicated if mobility is restricted. Finally, a full fitness program should be implemented.

DISORDERS OF MOVEMENT

Disorders of spinal movement may be classified as acute mechanical derangement, hypomobility, and hypermobility lesions.

Acute Mechanical Derangement

The *acute locked back, sudden backache, facet syndrome, facet blockage, subluxation* or *fixation*, and *acute lumbago* are all terms used to describe sudden pain in the back. This condition may be regarded as an acute form of mechanical derangement and locking of the intervertebral joint complex. Several theories have been proposed to explain its occurrence. These include ligamentous tears,[33,58] a primary muscle lesion,[341,547] apophyseal-joint (facet) lesions (including subluxation—an overriding or shifting of the facet joint out of its normal congruous relationship),[504] synovitis, an impacted synovial fringe or intra-articular structure such as a meniscoid body,[297,299] acute nuclear prolapse of the disk, acute hydrops of the disk,[80] and an annular tear.[82]

This form of acute backache (lumbago) should be regarded as a syndrome in which more than one condition can produce a typical attack.[195] The term *lumbago* is used here to describe a lumbar spinal syndrome characterized by sudden onset of severe persistent pain, marked restriction of lumbar movements, and a sensation of "locking" in the back. Attacks may vary in severity from severe and incapaci-

tating to more minor discomfort. During an attack it is not possible to know the exact mechanism, and one can only speculate.

Lumbago can occur at any age but is most frequently seen between the ages of 20 and 45 years.[504] The mechanism of injury is usually a sudden, unguarded movement involving backward bending, forward bending, sidebending, and/or rotation. If the attack is severe, the patient presents with an onset of sudden, intense lower lumbar pain, which may be bilateral but typically is unilateral. The pain and sensation of back locking may render the patient immobile with the back "stuck" in one position. There are some instances where the patient may even fall down or have had to crawl on hands and knees off a tennis court or into bed from the bathroom. Not all attacks are severe. The patient may be aware only of a mild discomfort in the low back after the triggering movement. The symptoms are initially mild but within a few hours or after having gone to bed, the patient awakens to find that he or she is unable to get out of bed because of agonizing pain in the low back. Some examples of sudden back pain, which may serve as a guide when planning initial treatment, are described below.

Impacted Synovial Mensicoid.[195] The patient with sudden backache caused by a presumed locking of a facet joint by an impacted synovial menisicoid is often a young person with a degree of hypermobility. Lumbar synovial joint locking typically results during some activity involving reaching up (*e.g.*, to open a window) or after a forward-flexion movement, which may have been slight (*e.g.*, picking up a piece of paper or a tennis ball), in which a hypermobile segment undergoes additional distraction.

Examination reveals the following:

1. Marked paraspinal muscle spasm, more prominent on one side than the other. A spinal deformity is present.
2. Physiological movements. Extension and lateral flexion toward the painful side may be nearly full, with pain near the extremes of range; lateral flexion toward the painless side is restricted early in the range and is more painful. Flexion is cautious and limited.
3. Straight-leg raising is limited by pain, with movement of the contralateral (painless) leg equally restricted. Straight-leg raising usually provokes acute discomfort in the region of the posterosuperior iliac spine.
4. Negative neurologic signs.

Locking of arthrotic facet joint.[197] A typical patient

is middle-aged or older, with a degree of presupposed degenerative joint disease, who complains of sudden onset (after twisting) of one-sided back pain localized to the fourth or fifth level in the lumbar spine. The history is that of a simple, nonstressful daily activity such as getting out of a bathtub, bending over to tie a shoe, leaning over a bathroom sink, coughing, sneezing, or lifting a weight. Sudden pain to one side fixes the patient in a flexed posture, and a vertical position can only be regained with some difficulty. The patient may present with a kyphosis or a reversal of the normal lumbar curve.

Examination reveals the following:

1. Pain is unilateral, extension and lateral flexion away from the side of pain are the most painful.
2. Flexion may not appear to be limited and may be painless, but is performed with the lumbar spine fixed in lordosis. Passive overpressure may provoke localized lumbosacral pain.
3. There are no neurologic signs. Straight-leg raising is usually negative; there may be localized pain at the extreme of leg raising on the painful side.

Most cases of acute mechanical derangement can be expected to subside within 3 weeks; spinal mobilizations will shorten that time. One mobilization technique that is useful in early treatment is gentle, rhythmical manual traction applied to the patient's legs (see Passive Movement Techniques section, p. 598). As the patient improves, other mobilization techniques may be added. Specific and non-specific rotational manipulations are appropriate (see p. 602). Vertebral manipulation is probably the therapeutic modality most frequently studied in controlled trials. A few studies have shown that short-term manipulative treatment may temporarily decrease pain and improve function.[53,90,116,119,185,191,210,214,239,257,351,363,449,475]

Traction can be applied by manual, auto-traction, gravity reduction, and motorized methods. It is often wise to precede mobilization or traction with ice or heat and massage in order to relieve the muscle guarding and spasm that may accompany acute mechanical derangement. Finally, the restoration of normal mobility of the lumbar spine, particularly in patients who have had several attacks, seems to be facilitated by appropriate therapeutic exercise.

This condition cures itself in most cases when enough time is allowed to pass and when rest (relative) is prescribed. Nevertheless, mobilizations shorten the duration of pain in a manner which is frequently dramatic.

Hypomobility Lesions

Localized Restriction. Facet joint capsular tightness and/or degenerative changes in the disk result in localized hypomobility lesions.

The chronic form of a mechanical derangement, usually of the intervertebral joint complex, is the result of prolonged immobilization secondary to injury or poor posture. Often there is a history of acute low back dysfunction.

The onset of pain may be gradual or sudden; the patient may relate it to bending, twisting, or a traumatic event. Pain varies in degree from minor to severe and is usually described as a dull aching in the lumbosacral region or referred into the buttocks, leg, or abdominal region. Symptoms are aggravated by long periods of standing, walking, or activity involving prolonged or repetitive lumbar extension. Symptoms are worse in the evening than in the morning.

When evaluating a patient it is often difficult, if not impossible, to determine if pain is coming from the disk or the facet joints. The mechansim of aggravation and analysis of the most painful position may give reliable clues. If extension (standing and walking) is the most aggravating, the facets are most likely involved. If the pain is diskogenic in nature, it may be because of mechanical irritation or inflammation of the outer wall of the annulus.[493] In this case, flexion (sitting and forward bending) is the most painful movement or is the mechanism of aggravation.

The clinician should consider the following points and tests in evaluating the patient:

1. Possible subtle predisposing biomechanical factors such as leg-length discrepancy.
2. Physiological motions may appear normal but usually show some evidence of restricted motion only in certain directions (*e.g.*, minor restriction of sidebending to the involved side; deviation of the spine toward the involved side on forward bending and away from the involved side on extension). When motions are restricted they should also reproduce the patient's pain. The normal, rhythmical pattern of lumbar movement may also be disturbed. This is best appreciated by standing behind the patient to observe spinal movement.
3. In most cases there will be loss of the normal passive joint-play movements that reproduce the patient's pain. However, because degenerative joint/disk disease can develop because of hypermobility or instability of the joint, accessory movements are sometimes excessive. Pain may

occur within the limited range, but most often at the limits of the range. The examination consists of direct pressure over the spinous process, lateral pressure over the spinous process, pressure over the facet joints, and pressure over the interspinous and supraspinous ligaments. Pain may be referred and is usually unilateral.

4. Special tests may be indicated if the above tests fail to reproduce symptoms. The quadrant test or combined movements are used in attempt to reproduce the symptoms at the appropriate level. Examination using combined movements and recognition of regular (or irregular) patterns of movement can be most helpful in the selection of treatment techniques.[138]
5. The involved level will be tender to palpation. Often, a thickened supraspinous ligament can be palpated.
6. Roentgenograms should be normal for the patient's age.

Manipulations, segmental distraction techniques, and mobilizations (including muscle energy techniques and combined movements) are the manual treatments of choice. On the whole, mobilization techniques are most effective because of the variety of joint responses which can be facilitated.[306] A vast array of mobilization techniques are at the disposal of the therapist. In spite of a variety of names, they are linked by similarities (see Medical Models and Disease Entities, p. 554).

In the presence of hypermobility, localized stabilization techniques should be used instead. At times both mobilization and stabilization techniques may be indicated. Mobilizing exercises are indicated if the condition has been present for a long time. Based on the evaluation, the home program should include localized segmental auto-mobilization and/or stabilization techniques (see Figs. 20-6 and 20-7). Prolonged rest and use of supports are contraindicated, because they tend to increase the restrictions.

Multisegmental Bilateral Capsular Restriction.   Degenerative joint/disk disease, osteoarthritis, lumbar spondylosis, and facet arthritis are all included in this category (see Applied Anatomy, page 554).

A variety of terms, including spondylosis, is used to describe osteoarthritic changes in the spine that may lead to back pain, which is more common among middle-aged or older persons. Although degenerative joint/disk disease is a natural process of aging and is often asymptomatic, symptoms sometimes develops as the result of hypomobility and repeated trauma. (Hypermobility can also contribute

to the development of degenerative joint/disk disease.) Patients with symptomatic degenerative joint disease will frequently have difficulty bending because of stiffness and aching in the low back. On stooping over a wash basin they usually lean on one arm to support the body weight. After simple loosening-up exercises or a hot shower, the discomfort eases tremendously. As the condition progresses, the patient tends to get worse as the day goes on, but at times the pain may be more pronounced after a night rest and then ease as the patient becomes more mobile. Patients also may note discomfort with increasing sports activities and may even cut down on sports as they become aware that pain and stiffness tend to be more pronounced the following day.

A striking symptom relates to many patients' avocations or occupational activities[504]—they do not like to hold their backs in a flexed positon. Homemakers, carpenters, plumbers, and others who must frequently work in a stooped position find their symptoms increased. They do not like standing for lengthy periods because this increases the lumbar lordosis. Aching is relieved if one foot is placed on a stool or step while standing. Where facet arthrosis is more advanced, turning over in bed becomes increasingly difficult because of movement imposed on the facet joints.

Because degenerative changes involve both the anterior and posterior portions of the intervertebral joint complex, it is not possible to implicate the exact mechanism of symptom production. The most likely basis for attacks of mechanical derangement is recurrent episodes of synovitis in the facet joints after overuse, such as excessive bending (as in gardening), stressful unaccustomed activity, or abrasive positioning with resultant strain of the joints. After several hours of heavy use, pain develops that can last for hours. Pain is typically at the lower lumbar midline but, may radiate out to the groin or buttock. Degenerative joint/disk disease may also occur with neurologic complications (*i.e.,* lateral spinal stenosis). Pain may be experienced in one or both legs and three mechanisms may be involved: (1) Pain may be referred with stimulation of the sinuvertebral nerve; (2) sciatica may result from nerve-root pressure; or (3) leg pain my be caused by the pressure of a spinal canal stenosis.[88]

The clinician should consider the following in evaluating a patient:

1. Aggravating–relieving symptoms. Some loss of normal lordosis may be noted. Pain may increase if the patient tries to sit up straight or slumps.

Symptoms are decreased with the back in a neutral or functional position. Pain is increased when upright (standing and walking). One test that Seimon has found positive in almost all of these patients is to stand semistooped and to maintain this position for 1 to 2 minutes.[504] This increases the tension in the disks and also strains the capsular ligaments of the facet joints.

2. **Physiological movements.** Early on, spinal motions may appear normal. Remember that most of the discomfort and stiffness occurs early in the day and may have subsided by the time of the physical assessment. With advanced chronic degeneration, restriction of active and passive motions occurs in a generalized capsular pattern: marked restriction and equal limitation of side flexion, and moderate restriction of rotation, forward bending, and backward bending.

3. Moderate to marked restriction of all accessory motions may be noted.

4. With reference to the neurological assessment, the findings in uncomplicated degenerative disease are normal. Patients who complain of pain on coughing, sneezing, jarring movements, or turning over in bed will frequently have a positive heel-drop test (see p. 573).

5. Degenerative changes are observed on roentgenograms, affecting the disk and facet joints. The severity of pain is not proportional to the extent of the roentgenographic findings.[504]

With advanced degenerative joint/disk disease, movements will be stiff in all directions, so treatment will require a combination of several techniques in different directions, including intermittent variable lumbar traction, mobilization, and a program of exercises. There may also be attacks of mechanical derangement; it is important to first take care to have settled any localized single joint signs superimposed on an otherwise stiff spine by local treatment, or these will be worsened by a generalized regimen. The facet joints are more vulnerable to facet impingement, sprains, and inflammation when degenerative joint disease is present.

Nonsteroidal anti-inflammatory drugs are used in patients with evidence of the more severe degrees of degenerative joint disease in an attempt to reduce any associated synovitis.[418]

Passive movements (*i.e.*, flexion, extension, and sidebending) play a major role in the management of patients with multisegmental involvement. Starting in the direction opposite that of pain aggravation, exercises are progressed to include motions in all directions. Manual and mechanical lumbar tractions

and spinal-mobilization techniques may be expected to increase mobility and to relieve pain. Caution should be used with joint mobilization and exercise in the presence of nerve-root irritation because it may increase symptoms. Postural training and carefully instituted isometric exercises to strengthen the abdominal and back muscles may be indicated. Patients with this condition may be overweight and their type of work may aggravate the disorder. The overweight patient should be encouraged to lose weight and to exercise by walking or swimming within the limits of pain. It is often found that brisk walking (in patients who are bothered by standing) often relieves their pain.

CHRONIC LOW BACK PAIN

After 3 months of low back pain, only 5% to 10% of patients have persisting symptoms,[177,426] yet it is this population that accounts for 85% of the costs in terms of compensation and loss of work related to low back pain.[178,529] In these patients the presence of a treatable active disease has been carefully eliminated. Pain, with its consequences, has become the patient's main preoccupation, limiting daily activity.[475] It is important to reach a definitive diagnosis if possible, and to rule out any of the known causes for back pain for which specific treatment exists. No study in the medical literature demonstrates a specific method of treatment for chronic idiopathic low back pain.[426]

The differential diagnosis of chronic low back pain includes all the conditions previously discussed, which may be overlooked or neglected during the acute and subacute phases. The additional diagnostic possibilities include a variety of degenerative conditions, spondyloarthropathies, and ill-defined syndromes of fibrositis. Some psychologists[166] maintain that this pain represents a behavior reaction, whereas neurophysiologists lean toward the hypothesis that nervous structures irritated for a prolonged period generate new mechanisms of pain generation. Chronic pain has also been described as a variant of depression. In a study of patients with chronic low back pain, a structured diagnosis was possible in 50%, whereas no diagnosis could be determined in the remainder.[468]

Degenerative Spinal Stenosis

Included in this diagnostic category are degenerative spondylolisthesis[580] and degenerative lumbar stenosis,[17,289,290] affecting either the central canal or the lateral recesses, or consisting of isolated disk resorption (see p. 559).[93]

Other Causes of Chronic Low Back Pain

A second group of degenerative conditions characterized by predominant low back pain has less certain criteria.[177] Included in this group are facet syndromes,[408] disk-disruption syndrome,[94] segmental instability,[180,198,291,410,425,546] idiopathic vertebral sclerosis,[601] diffuse idiopathic skeletal hyperostosis,[180] inflammatory spondyloarthropathy,[66] myofascial syndromes,* fibrositis,[1,67,234,298,569,570,610–612] and primary fibromyalgia.[67,69,273,569,612,620,621,623–625] Recent investigations have shown that primary fibromyalgia is a characteristic clinical entity with pathologic changes in the muscle.[621]

According to Maigne, in many cases of chronic distal lumbago and sciatica, there is often a cellulomyalgic syndrome present, revealed by the presence of myalgic cordlike structures in the muscles of the external iliac fossa (*i.e.*, the gluteus medius, tensor fasciae latae, gluteus maximus, or piriformis).[350] In the syndromes of sciatica, in addition to the muscles of the iliac fossa, the distal portion of the biceps femoris, lateral gastrocnemius (S1), and the anterior lateral aspect of the leg (L5), may be involved. With joint manipulation, tenderness often disappears but in some cases pain remains. In addition to procaine injections of trigger points, treatment by slow, deep massage and long, continued stretching can be quite helpful.

Evaluation

A definitive diagnosis requires careful history taking to identify the distribution of back and leg pain as well as such aggravators of pain as poor posture, mechanical loads, and walking. The physical examination should include observation of gait, trunk mobility, deformities, leg-length inequalities, and assessment of coordination, endurance, and function. The examination should include a careful search for neurosensory and motor loss and signs of nerve-root tension. The neurologic examination may be confusing and show no anatomical sensory losses in patients with spinal stenosis.[190] In addition to a detailed neuromuscular examination, abdominal and vascular evaluations should be included, particularly in the elderly and those with symptoms suggesting neurogenic claudication. The degenerative conditions that may be causing the pain can be classified according to the clinical history, roentgenographic findings, diagnostic blocks, and imaging studies. Psychological testing should be used to determine the psychological status of the patient and to explore for systematic relationships between pain behavior and reinforcing consequences.

The results of a physical examination in such patients are often nonspecific, except for demonstration of restricted motion and muscle spasm. However, many degenerative conditions can be strongly suggested by roentgenographic studies. When segmental instability is suspected, flexion and extension films may demonstrate abnormal displacements.[180,288,410] If nerve-root symptoms or claudication are present, myelography is the most sensitive study for identifying the level of neural encroachment, followed by CT scanning. CT and magnetic resonance imaging (MRI) are rapidly surpassing myelograms as the imaging technique of choice in the majority of patients with radiculopathies. Electromyography may also be used to provide additional confirmation of the levels of nerve-root involvement.[143] In patients with suspected facet syndrome, a CT scan may reveal degeneration, but a definitive diagnosis is based on the relief of symptoms by the injection of local anesthetics into the affected joints.[149,404,407] In patients with suspected internal disruption, diskography is thought to be diagnostic, particularly when combined with CT scans, but this remains controversial.

Treatment

Most patients with chronic low back pain can be treated with anti-inflammatory medications and exercise programs.[177] As in other nonmalignant chronic pain syndromes, narcotic analgesics are to be avoided. Alternative therapeutic modalities have been used, including biofeedback, acupuncture, transcutaneous nerve stimulation, implanted neurostimulators and ablative neurosurgical procedures. These methods have resulted in varying degrees of success, and all are fraught with methodologic problems.[116] For selected patients, trigger-point injections may be beneficial.[480]

Soft-Tissue Mobilization Techniques, Massage, and Relaxation. Soft-tissue techniques, which have the specific purpose of improving vascularity and extensibility of the soft tissues, represent another approach to pain management. Massage and a variety of soft-tissue mobilization techniques are being used now more than ever before and are at the disposal of the manual therapist.[28,78,102,133,304,315,351,388,453,454,519,544,597] There is no dispute that these techniques are beneficial, although research has been lacking in this area for hundreds of years.[214,215] The effectiveness is attributed in part to increased

---

* References 18, 29, 68, 159, 160, 186, 211, 237, 358, 376, 452, 509, 514–517, 527, 570, 610, 611, 622

circulation to the area, release of muscle spasm, stretching of abnormal fibrous tissue (connective tissue), increased proprioception, and extensibility of the soft tissues. An increase in extensibility may also allow for a secondary increase in circulation.[83] Acupressure massage presumably elicits some of the same beneficial effects as acupuncture and acupuncture-like transcutaneous electrical nerve stimulation (TENS).[79,560,617] Rocking chair therapy and mechanical vibration are other forms of sensory stimulation that have been reported to relieve both chronic and acute pain.[99,217,218,336-338,393,450,666] Relaxation techniques can affect the pain cycle by directly eliciting relaxation and gain the secondary effects of an increase in circulation and a decrease in pain (see Chapter 9, Relaxation). Stress and tension influence strongly the perception of pain and pain tolerance.

Exercise. Currently, aerobic exercise is a popular form of treatment. The bases for these exercise programs have been extensively reviewed with respect to their effects on disk nutrition, pain modulation, and spinal mechanics.[107,251,424] Knowledge of the body's endogenous chemical pain-modulating capability, the endorphin system, continues to increase.[6,429,503,619] It has been shown that activity in large muscle groups yields an increased amount of endorphins in both the blood stream and the cerebrospinal fluid.[6,154] This in turn lessens the pain sensitivity.[367,429,503,619] Johansson and associates have demonstrated in ten patients with chronic back pain a significantly lower amount of endorphins in the cerebrospinal fluid, a finding recently corroborated by Pug and co-workers.[258,474] Aerobic exercise also provides other bonuses: It has been documented as a means of relieving depression,[165,521] a common finding with at least chronic low back pain. Other benefits include positive effects of increased mental alertness,[131,619] sleep,[165,521] stamina,[275] improved self-image, and reversal of activity level compatible with chronic pain.[166,521] With respect to aerobic activity, walking and jogging on soft, even ground are recommended; indoor cross-country skiing machines are preferable to stationary bikes and water aerobics are preferable to swimming.

Most authorities agree that some exercise is useful and its role has been summarized by Jackson and Brown.[251] It has been shown that high levels of physical fitness reduce the risk of further injury and speed rehabilitation. It has also been demonstrated that the more physically fit a person is, the more pain he or she can tolerate.[86,172,503.] But there is little agreement about what form the exercise should take. As in most spheres relating to this subject, the problem seems to be that treatment is not tailored to the diagnosis. A plea for selectivity of exercise based on a thorough clinical evaluation is made by Jackson and Brown, and is supported here.[251]

Anterior Element Pain. Anterior element pain has been defined as pain made worse by sustained flexion of the lumbar spine.[511] Characteristically, anterior element pain is made worse by sitting and is relieved by standing. Patients assume the hyperlordotic posture to relieve their pain. Fracture of the vertebral body and prolapsed intervertebral disks produce anterior element symptoms. In young patients in whom anterior element pain is the most common presentation, extension exercises and press-ups are more likely to produce remission than flexion exercises.[282] This is borne out by the tendency of many flexion exercises to increase intradiskal pressure, whereas extension exercises unload the disk.[251] Therefore, the hyperextension principles advocated by Cyriax and McKenzie are logical for patients with anterior element pain.[100,311,383,384] Lesions resulting in chronic anterior pain are obscure; it is tempting to assume that anterior element pain is diskogenic in origin, but there is no evidence for this. Unlike the acute group, patients with chronic anterior element pain may respond to manipulative techniques.[310,511]

Posterior Element Pain. Pain is worsened by increasing the lumbar lordosis, standing, and walking. It is eased by maintained forward flexion, sitting, and hip flexion (with or without the knees extended). Patients who have structural or postural hyperlordosis, who have facet arthropathy, and who suffer from foraminal stenosis show features of posterior element pain.[511] Pain from extension and rotation are usually of facet origin.[603] Flexion treatment frequently improves facet disease, spondylolysis, flexion dysfunction, and certain types of derangement.[121,122,383,603] Prescription of hyperextension exercises may make the condition worse.[282]

Movement-Related Pain. Patients with movement-related pain are most comfortable at rest; pain is precipitated only by activity or jarring. Heavy manual work, repeated twisting, fast walking or running (especially on hard surfaces), and traveling in cars over rough ground all precipitate pain. Movement-related pain occurs in association with traumatic fracture–dislocations, in symptomatic spondylolysis or spondylolisthesis, and as a result of chronic degenerative segmental instability as described by MacNab. Diagnosis may be confirmed by obtaining lateral flexion and extension roentgenograms of the lumbar spine and noting abnormal translational movements. A basic scheme of progressive stabilization by strengthening regional and segmental musculature isometrically should be considered.[198-200] According to Grieve, mature patients and those in most pain may need to start abdominal exercises with knees bent and progress more slowly. Sidelying stabilization techniques and dynamic abdominal bracing also may be used.[284] Home exercises must be efficiently monitored and the patient taught the avoidance of posture and activities known to constitute his or her "specific" additional stimuli.[497]

Mechanical Pain Without Postural or Movement Exacerbations (Static-Sensitive). Patients with static-sensitive low back pain have an inability to maintain any one position (other than lying) for a normal length of time and obtain relief by changing position and moving. Many of these patients appear to have discrete structural disease, such as scoliosis.[54]

Altered patterns of muscle recruitment in chronic low back pain have been clearly delineated by Janda.[253-256,265] One of the most common of these is the overuse and early recruitment of the low back muscles.[387] Another common pattern associated with low back pain is overuse of the hip flexors (psoas) and weakness of the abdominals. It is frequently important to retrain the gluteal muscles and inhibit overuse of lumbar extension, a maladaptive pattern.

The dynamic trunk stabilizers, aside from the gluteus maximus, which originate or insert into the lumbodorsal fascia, are the latissimus dorsi, transverse abdominus, and internal oblique muscles. The main purpose for strengthening these muscles is to produce a force-couple that is designed to stabilize the trunk and effectively control the antigravity weight line or the way in which this area bears weight.

There are many types of isometric exercises, and Grieve provides some good examples to improve the power of the gluteal and abdominal muscles in the treatment of chronic low back pain, including abdominal wall and abdominal bracing exercises.[199] These exercises avoid high interdiskal pressures and emphasize eccentric control, free breathing, and the maintenance of the functional position of the spine. When performing exercises for the upper abdominals, the feet should be plantar flexed to inhibit action of the psoas.[254]

Isotonic exercise can be helpful for some patients and may be used in all patients as a progression of the exercise program, with or without manual or mechanical resistance.[64,124,181,206,207,240,350,551,552]

Spinal Bracing. A number of lumbar supports have been advocated. Spinal bracing seems justified in patients with osteoporotic compression fractures, spondylolisthesis, or segmental instability, and in some patients with spinal stenosis—although no controlled studies have demonstrated its efficacy precisely. Approximately 80% to 90% of patients wearing a simple support describe some benefit when interviewed.[426] The mechanical effects include prevention of excessive motion and a reminder to the wearer not to exaggerate the lumbar load.

Educational Programs

Educational programs have become an essential part of the care of chronic low back pain patients.* It is imperative that all patients be educated in learning how to live with their discomfort. Advice regarding everyday activities must be individualized and in many instances is the most important aspect of treatment. Educational programs have been shown to be more effective than flexion exercises, although some studies have questioned the effectiveness of low back schools. Historical surveys have demonstrated that only 40% of patients who have been disabled for 6 months can be successfully rehabilitated; at 1 year, the figure drops to 20%; and 2 years after injury the chances for rehabilitation are virtually nil. In the context of this text it would be impossible to cover the various intervention programs; the reader is therefore directed to the references in each section. General approaches are outlined below.

Functional Training. These structured programs include the identification of routine daily living and work postures and activities, re-education exercises for required performance, and instruction to acquire a safe mode of function.[475] Mayer and associates have devised a functional program that emphasizes restoration of muscle strength and aerobic capacity, vocational assessment, and short-term psychological intervention with careful qualification of progress.[368,369] One year after this 3-week intervention, 85% of patients have returned to work.

Back Schools. These structured intervention programs are aimed at groups of patients and include the provision of general information on the spine, recommended posture and physical activities, preventive measures, and exercises for the back.[2,30,161,170,216,224,293,308,329,332,365,382,603,608,626] The main objective of these programs is to transmit information to the patient on anatomy and disorders of the spine and to teach the principles underlying healthy posture, daily activities, and sports. The content of the programs varies considerably from place to place. Overall patient satisfaction with back

* References 73, 84, 101, 148, 161, 173, 223, 224, 293, 300, 302, 316, 323, 341, 368, 369, 381, 382, 492, 499, 504, 546, 548, 551, 586

schools is 75% to 96%, and 70% to 90% find their pain is at an acceptable level after attending back school, according to White.[603]

One American program forms the basis for White's book on back schools.[603] This book entails a hospital back school for acute back pain and incorporates education with progressive remobilization. White includes McKenzies's protocol and techniques in his school. Acute back schools and education can often keep patients out of the hospital and return many of them to a normal life-style in a matter of days.[603] Back schools in the home, work environment, and an athletic back school for chronic low back patients are also described.

Work-hardening or work-capacity training is considered the "Superbowl" of back schools. Contributing factors for a higher rate of recurrent low back injury and for poor work tolerance are possible underlying pathologic processes and incomplete rehabilitation prior to return to work. With the work endurance program there has been significant improvement of work tolerance and a decreased rate of recurrent injury.[316,323,369,604]

Specialized Centers. Series of exercises and therapeutic activities may be prescribed, directed, and/or supervised by a health professional.[181,240,284,382,411,412] Generally exercises are done in a specialized center for a limited time only, mainly to instruct the patient, and then are continued at home by the patient. Sometimes specific rehabilitation demands prolonged therapy in a specialized environment.

In most of these programs the *functional position* of the spine is emphasized. This position has been described by Morgan and Vollowitz as "the optimal position in which the spine functions." These positions vary depending on the physical condition of the spine and the stresses it must withstand. There is no one position for all functional tasks, and the best functional position varies from person to person. It is often near the midrange of all available movement. The functional position should not be confused with the theoretical "neutral" position of the spine.[340]

The spinal control method (stabilization) is a form of body mechanics which trains and uses any or all of the muscles associated with body alignment to place a given spinal segment in its functional balanced position and hold it there while other joints and muscle groups accomplish a specific task. Thus, the involved spinal segment is stabilized to whatever degree is necessary to allow pain-free activity.[412]

Pain Clinics. A polyvalent therapeutic approach that focuses principally on behavioral adaptations of patients to help them withstand and control their condition over the long term is the basis of pain clinics.[475] This form of intervention is recommended solely to evaluate the factors that modify the patient's perception of pain and to support the patient. Improved understanding of the relationship between pain and activity has resulted in a change in management from a negative philosophy of treatment for pain to more active restoration of function. Fordyce and other behavioral psychologists have investigated the relationship between chronic pain and physical activity.[168,329] They suggest that pain behaviors are influenced and modified by their consequences.[167,169]

Occupational Interventions. Advice based on knowledge of a specific work environment and a functional evaluation of a worker can help to ensure a better balance between job assignments and capabilities.[475] Information is available only on chronic conditions for which ergonomic interventions represent an integral component of the therapeutic program. Ergonomists seek to create a harmonious balance between workers and the equipment they use, the patterns of work, and the total working environment—both at work and in the home.

Manual handling and lifting has received more attention from ergonomists[76,77,111,178,179,346,347,556] than virtually any other topic. Since Brackett first identified the possible dangers of lifting a heavy load from the ground with the back in a fully flexed position,[49] ergonomists have sought to identify safer lifting techniques and load limits.[110,223–225,420,421,547,549]

Another aspect of back pain that has interested ergonomists is work postures, particularly the seated work posture. Several epidemiologic studies point to the relationship between sitting and back pain, and clinicians use the increase of pain in sitting as a diagnostic indicator.[279,280] Many authors as early as Staffel in 1884 made recommendations about seating design.[43,56,223,356] The importance of the design of the backrest was underlined by Akerblom in 1948.[5,276] More recently Andersson and associates measured changes in interdiskal pressure at the L3–L4 disk in different sitting positions and for different configurations of the backrest and lumbar support. In order to reduce the interdiskal pressure, they recommended a positive lumbar support maintaining the lumbar spine in lordosis.

Published information about seating and driving positions in the past has demonstrated a confusing lack of agreement. Until recently concepts of correct design appear to have been based more on aesthetics, ethics, and wishful thinking than on science. Fortunately that is beginning to change. The chair is a principal adjunct in industrialized labor. The results of numerous studies confirm the necessity to integrate seating design not only in the whole of the work space but also the job design. It is also hoped that, in the future, car seat manufacturers will propose alternative designs which will aim at substantially reducing stresses on the spine.

Modern ergonomists have a much broader understanding of the topic of back pain, based on physiological, biomechanical, environmental, and psychological factors.

LUMBAR SPINE TECHNIQUES — PASSIVE MOVEMENTS

The following are representative examples of passive movement techniques. Although these techniques are not all-inclusive, they should be useful in treating properly selected patients when they are applied according to the guidelines already presented. For complete descriptions and illustrations of the great variety of mobilizations and passive movements available, other appropriate texts should be consulted.[101,270,350,354,383,394-396,398,544] Although some of McKenzie's techniques are briefly described (see pp. 599 and 608), the reader should refer to his textbook to adequately plan a treatment program.[383] Determination of the tissue type involved is critical.

HYPOMOBILE JOINTS

The principles set out in Chapter 6, Peripheral Joint Mobilization Techniques, also hold true for the spinal column. There are, however, some specific technical points to be mentioned with respect to the spine; for instance, because it is not possible to move a single segment actively, passive movement represents, as it were, joint play. Because of this relative difficulty in moving single joints, both specific and nonspecific techniques are described. One way of achieving a specific effect is to apply "locking" techniques. If leverage is used, this is to great advantage when moving the legs and pelvis to mobilize the lumbar spine (see Fig. 20–28). To make such a technique specific, the clinician must try to lock all segments except for the one to be mobilized. The principle of locking consists in bringing into an extreme position the segments that are not to be moved, under a certain degree of tension. The mechanism is either tension of ligaments or opposition of bony structures (facet locking). Ligamentous locking involves taking up of all the slack in the soft tissues. When using ligamentous tension-locking techniques for localization, it is desirable to use direct contact to achieve some degree of specificity. For example, a vertebra may be fixed by direct contact in at least one direction (e.g., fixation of a spinous process from the side prevents rotation in the opposite direction).

Facet locking is achieved mainly by a careful combination of sidebending and rotation, making use of combined motions to achieve bony opposition. One positions the patient just short of complete fixation so that a small range of movement is possible in the joint in question, but less in the adjacent joints above and below. To achieve the maximum specific effect, a combination of leverage and locking techniques with direct contact and fixation is commonly used.

There are also nonspecific techniques that can be useful in mobilizing larger sections of the spinal column, such as traction along the long axis of the spine. Whereas lumbar traction along the long axis acts on the intervertebral disk, distraction of the apophyseal joints is produced by rotation around that same axis. Another type of nonspecific method is represented by soft-tissue mobilization and massage techniques.

HYPERMOBILE JOINTS

One must also consider the hypermobile joint, which often coexists with hypomobile segments. The hypermobile joint should be considered abnormal when it gives rise to pain of ligamentous origin. Further stretching must be avoided and support must be given to enable the ligaments to regain their normal strength. The supporting structures, particularly the muscles that move the affected joint, must be strengthened and stability achieved. Finally, adjacent hypomobile joints must be mobilized so an even distribution of movement is achieved.

It should be kept in mind that assessment continues throughout the treatment period and the response to what is done initially and subsequently provides guidance for the next step in treatment. For example, the aim to make the hypomobile joint able to sustain a grade IV movement (a small-amplitude movement, conducted at the very end of the range of motion without pain) is not always possible nor advisable. If symptoms have been relieved, it is often better not to attempt to influence joint limitations that are clearly the result of adaptive shortening. *Do not overtreat;* when signs and symptoms are cleared, stop. Passive movement treatments should be adapted according to presenting signs and symptoms; as these change, so should the treatment. For mobilization to be effective a sense of "feel" of movement is required. The movements taking place are often not seen but sensed.[88]

Many passive movements have been described for

the lumbar spine; only a few of the more commonly used techniques will be presented here.

Note: P—patient; O—operator; M—movement

NONSPECIFIC SPINAL MOBILIZATIONS

1. *Flexion* (Fig. 20–17)
   P—Lies supine with the knees bent
   O—Grasps across the anterior aspect of both proximal tibias and approximates the patient's knees to the axillae.
   M—Traction may be employed by passing the left arm behind the knees and the right arm in front of the thighs. The hands are interlocked; by lifting and pulling with the arms, the knees are flexed toward the chest. A certain amount of traction is carried out along the line of the femurs by lifting the pelvis with the left arm as the knees are flexed.
   Use—Global stretching into flexion is used for patients with a generally tight (particularly with loss of flexion) back, or to assist apprehensive patients in beginning a home stretching program. Large-amplitude oscillations can increase general mobility, stimulate joint motion, or reduce active muscle guarding. Gentle, small-amplitude oscillations can relieve pain.
2. *Extension* (Fig. 20–18)
   P—Lies prone
   O—Grasps across the anterior aspect of the patient's distal femurs. The spine is extended by extension of the patient's legs and hip girdle.
   This technique is used as in flexion above and to prepare patient for more specific techniques. Occasionally this method is better tolerated than specific, more vigorous techniques.

Fig. 20–18. Nonspecific long-lever extension mobilization of the lumbar spine.

3. *Rotation* (Fig. 20–19)
   P—Lies supine with knees bent
   O—Stabilizes the patient's thorax by placing an arm across the lower rib cage. The leg further from the operator is grasped behind the knee and the hip is brought to about 90° flexion. This leg is then pulled toward the operator, across the near leg. Be sure some knee and hip flexion of the near leg is maintained to prevent overextension of the spine.
4. *Rotation* (Fig. 20–20)
   P—Sidelying, hips and knees slightly flexed. Localization of this movement to one area is obtained by the degree of rotation by positioning of the patient's pelvis and thorax. For the lower lumbar spine, rotation is used with the spine toward flexion; for the upper lumbar spine, rotation is used with the spine in minimal extension

Fig. 20–17. Nonspecific long-lever flexion mobilization of the lumbar spine.

Fig. 20–19. Nonspecific long-lever rotational mobilization of the lumbar spine.

Fig. 20–22. Alternative method for nonspecific long-lever lateral flexion mobilization of the lumbar spine.

Fig. 20–20. Alternative method for nonspecific long-lever rotational mobilization of the lumbar spine.

O—Stands behind patient. Simultaneously rotates patient's top shoulder toward and hip away until all slack is taken up. Then positioned directly over patient with both elbows straight, applies firm pressure down and cranially against shoulder, and down and caudally against greater trochanter, taking up additional slack.

M—An oscillation movement is produced by the therapist's caudal hand, which rotates the pelvis while the cranial hand is used to stabilize the thorax (grade III). Additional stretch or thrust (given through shoulder and hip) may be performed (grade IV).

This is a very useful technique for unilateral back or leg pain. Gentle, small-amplitude oscillations can relieve pain, and large-amplitude oscillations

Fig. 20–21. Nonspecific long-lever lateral flexion mobilization of the lumbar spine.

can increase general mobility or reduce active guarding.

5. *Lateral Flexion* (sidebending) (Fig. 20–21)
   P—Lies supine with knees bent
   O—Holds patient's legs together with hips and knees bent to 90°
   M—Spinal sidebending is produced by rotating the patient's pelvis about a vertical axis, using the patient's legs as a lever.

6. *Lateral Flexion* (sidebending) (Fig. 20–22)
   P—Lies on the side toward which sidebending is to occur. A small, soft roll may be placed under the lumbar spine region to create a greater excursion of movement. The hips and knees are comfortably flexed.
   O—Contacts the lateral aspects of the patient's hip girdle and shoulder girdle with the forearms. The fingertips contact the far sides of the spinous processes
   M—Movement is produced by pressing outward the downward with the forearms and pulling upward on the spinous processes. Additional leverage is gained by caudal pressure of the operator's chest on the patient's top hip and thigh.

This technique is useful for global stretching and pain relief. Its potential for separating vertebral bodies and opening intervertebral foramen may be valuable in relieving nerve-root entrapment.

7. *Correction of Acute Lateral Deviation* (Fig. 20–23)
   P—Stands, with elbow bent to 90° and resting on side to which thorax deviates (see Fig. 20–23A)
   O—Contacts patient's thorax and arm with shoulder or chest. Operator's arms encircle

Fig. 20–23. Correction pressure to the patient's trunk for lateral deviation. *(A)* The initial contact and *(B)* with slight "overcorrection" at the end.

the patient and hands interlock to contact the lateral aspect of the patient's pelvis.

M—The lateral deviation is *very slowly* (may take several minutes and/or attempts) reduced with a simultaneous pressure against thorax and hips.

Fig. 20–24. Correction pressure to the patient's trunk for flexion deformity.

—Small-amplitude oscillations may be superimposed on slow pressure, for patient comfort.

—Original deviation should be slightly "overcorrected" (see Fig. 20–23B).

Note: The patient may be taught to perform this maneuver at home (see Fig. 20-41). In performing this technique, original or more central back discomfort is acceptable, whereas more distal pain is not. This technique is useful for acute disk prolapse and is more successful if radicular signs/symptoms are not present.[380,383] This procedure is usually followed by technique 8 below.

8. *Correction of Flexion Deformity in Standing* (Fig. 20–24)

P—Standing, as relaxed as possible

O—Contacts the low lumbar spine with the thenar eminence of one hand (if the level at which blockage occurs can be identified, the thenar eminence should contact the spinous process below that level). The opposite arm reaches across the front of the patient's thorax to grasp the shoulder on the opposite side.

M—Extension is slowly and gradually produced with a mild forward pressure of the contacting hand, while the thorax is gently moved backward.

Note: The patient may be taught to perform this maneuver at home (see Fig. 20-39).

SEGMENTAL SPINAL MOVEMENTS

1. *Posteroanterior Central Vertebral Pressure* (Fig. 20–25)
   P—Prone. The spine may be prepositioned in the desired degree of extension by placing a pillow under the abdomen (for more flexion) or the chest and/or thighs (for more extension).
   O—Contacts the spinous process of the vertebra to be mobilized with the thumb pads of

A

B

Fig. 20–25. Posteroanterior central vertebral pressure on the spinous processes.

both hands. The fingertips or knuckles are used to stabilized the handhold by placing them alongside the spine on both sides.
   M—Segmental movement is localized by downward pressure through the arms, forearms, and thumbs. Graded oscillations are used.

2. *Posteroanterior Central Vertebral Pressure* (Fig. 20–26)
   P—Prone; may be prepositioned as described above.
   O—Contacts spinous process of vertebra to mobilize with ulnar border of hand closest to patient's head (see Fig. 20-26A). The other hand is used for support, as shown (see Fig. 20-26B).
   M—Same as for technique 1, above
      —If patient is prepositioned in flexion, overpressure may be applied cranially, into more flexion.
   This is a technique of choice for pain reduction or gentle, specific mobilization, for stretching stiff segments and for helping patients with disk prolapse to achieve greater extension.

3. *Posteroanterior Unilateral Vertebral Pressure* (Fig. 20–27)
   P—Prone with the spine prepositioned in the desired degree of initial extension
   O—Places both thumb pads over the mammillary process of the joint to be mobilized. These are located approximately level with the spaces between the spinous processes and perhaps an inch to the side.
   M—Movement is produced with a downward pressure, in an oscillatory manner through the arms, forearms, and thumbs in a direction perpendicular to the contour of the spine.

Note: Isometric exercises for strengthening the segmental musculature related to a hypermobile joint may be carried out in a similar fashion as the preceding segmental spinal movements (see Figs. 20-25 to 20-27). The patient is instructed to prevent displacement of the spinous or mammillary process at the level of the hypermobile segment. The direction of the applied sustained pressures may be altered (diagonally, transversely, posteroanteriorly, caudally, and cephalad) to recruit the appropriate musculature. Progression is made by increasing the pressure being sustained and the duration of the hold.

4. *Extension* (Fig. 20–28)
   P—Prone
   O—Ulnar border of cranial hand contacts

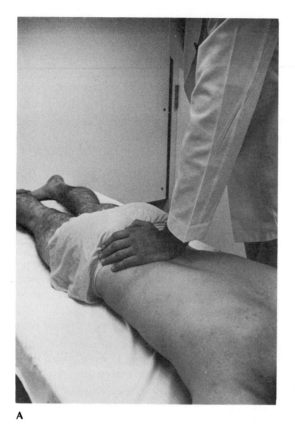

A   **B**

Fig. 20–26. Alternative method for posteroanterior central vertebral pressure on the spinous processes, with *(A)* ulnar border contact and *(B)* support of the other hand.

spinous process of segment to be mobilized (see Fig. 20–28A). Other hand grasps firmly around patient's near thigh, just above knee, and raises (extends) that leg until motion occurs at the desired segment.

— Alternatively, the pad of the thumb contacts

Fig. 20–27. Posteroanterior unilateral vertebral pressure.

the mammillary process on near side for unilateral extension (see Fig. 20–28B).

M — Movement is produced by pressing downward on spinous process or mammillary process, and/or extending the leg.

Because of the long lever arm (the patient's leg), a significant amount of force can be applied with this technique. It is, therefore, a technique of choice for patients with chronic lumbar stiffness. At the same time, it may be too vigorous for patients with more acute disorders and should be used with caution.

5. *Rotation* (Fig. 20–29)

  P — Prone

  O — Grasps across to the opposite anterosuperior iliac spine with the more caudal hand. Contacts on far side of spine over mammillary process of upper vertebra of segment to be mobilized with ulnar border or pisiform of opposite hand (see Fig. 20–29A).

  — Alternatively, thumb or pisiform contacts near side of spinous process of upper vertebra of segment to be mobilized (see Fig. 20–29B).

  M — Movement is performed by simultaneously

A

B

Fig. 20–28. Long-lever extension mobilization of the lumbar spine with *(A)* ulnar border contact or *(B)* thumb contact with the supporting or mobilizing hand.

lifting up on the pelvis and pressing downward with the contacting hand. This produces rotation (of spine) away from side of pelvis contacted.

An effective stretching (Grade IV) and pain-reducing (Grades I–III) technique. Also useful for disk prolapse (without neurologic deficit), usually with painful side toward operator.

6. *Rotation* (Fig. 20–30)

P—Prone, knees flexed to 90°

O—Cranial hand contacts upper vertebra of segment to be mobilized at far side (mammillary process) using pisiform contact. Other hand grasps patient's ankles and lowers them until movement just occurs at desired segment (see Fig. 20–30A).

—Alternatively, contact is made on near side of spinous process of upper vertebra with pisiform or thumb (see Fig. 20–30B).

M—Movement is produced by lowering the

ankles and/or pressing downward and laterally with contacting hand.

7. *Rotation* (Fig. 20–31)

P—Lies on side opposite that to which movement will occur. Hips and knees are comfortably flexed, head and neck slightly flexed, and arms rest in front of patient.

O—Flexes upper hip, keeping knee level with plinth, until movement just occurs at segment below that to be moved (palpate motion with middle finger). Position dorsum of patient's foot behind opposite knee or thigh.

—Rest patient's upper arm across lateral aspect of thorax.

—Grasp lower arm at distal humerus, gaining a purchase on the humeral epicondyles. Third finger of opposite hand palpates between spinous processes at level above that to be moved. Patient relaxes and spine is

A

B

Fig. 20-29. Rotational mobilization using (A) ulnar border or (B) thumb contact with the lumbar spine.

rotated until movement just occurs at segment palpated by pulling outward on patient's arm.

—Forearm is placed across posterolateral aspect of patient's pelvis, and opposite forearm across deltopectoral groove. Middle finger of caudal hand hooks underneath to opposite side of spinous process of more caudal vertebra of segment to be moved. Opposite middle finger or thumb contacts near side of spinous process of more cranial vertebra.

—Slack is taken up in shoulder girdle by pushing down and away with forearm, and in hip girdle by pulling down and toward operator.

M—Movement is produced by pulling up on caudal spinous process while continuing to move pelvic girdle (as above), and simultaneously pushing down on the cranial spinous process while moving the shoulder girdle (as above). Use body weight to complete end range distraction. One may also use oscillations.

Note: In selected cases a gentle thrust is performed at the end point of movement or a contract–relax technique may be employed to facilitate maximum range of motion. Positioning for this variation is similar to that illustrated under technique 14 (see Fig. 20-38).

8. *Sidebending* (Fig. 20–32)

P—Prone

O—Cranial hand makes thumb or pisiform contact at near side of upper spinous process of segment to be mobilized. Other hand grasps patient's near thigh just above knee. Patient's leg is abducted, which sidebends lumbar spine, until motion reaches desired level.

A   B

Fig. 20–30. Alternative method for rotational mobilization using *(A)* pisiform contact on the far side or *(B)* thumb contact on the near side of the lumbar spine.

M—Overpressure is applied at spine through thumb and/or at leg (into more abduction). Because of the long lever arm employed, a significant amount of force can be used. It is, therefore, a technique of choice for patients with chronic joint stiffness.

9. *Traction* (Fig. 20–33)
   P—Supine, knees and hips flexed
   O—Sits or stands at patient's feet (and thus secures them with his buttocks or thighs). Grasps behind patient's knees.
   M—Operator leans backward, exerting a longi-

Fig. 20–31. Alternative method for rotational mobilization of the lumbar spine.

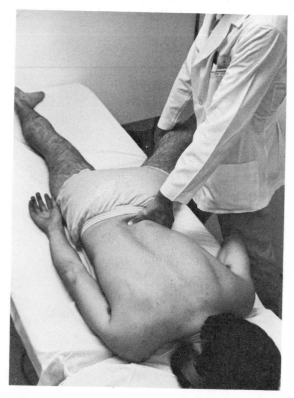

Fig. 20-32. Lateral flexion mobilization of the lumbar spine with transverse vertebral pressure and leg abduction.

tudinal movement through his arms and patient's legs to patient's spine. Movement can be graded, depending on patient tolerance and desired result.

This technique provides gentle traction to relieve pressure on disk and also comfortable stimulation and movement to painful segments

which may not tolerate more vigorous techniques. Belt traction may be used.[417] The belt is placed around the patient's upper calves with a pad interposed for comfort. The therapist places the clasped loop of the adjustable belt around his upper back. By leaning the trunk in the desired direction, lumbar traction is applied. A foam pad may be placed under the patient's trunk and next to his skin to prevent slipping.

10. *Traction* (Fig. 20-34)
   P—Supine, at end of plinth
   O—Assumes a walk-standing position at the foot of the table, facing the patient. Places patient's crossed legs over his shoulder and clasps his hands around patient's proximal thighs, keeping elbows in tight to chest.
   M—Operator draws patient's hips toward him, thus distracting spine, by simultaneously rocking his body backward and tucking (flexing) his trunk.

11. *Unilateral Traction* (Fig. 20-35)
   P—Supine or prone
   O—Grasps distal tibia on side to be distracted, gaining a purchase on malleoli. Patient's leg is flexed and adducted just until movement occurs at spinal level below that at which movement is desired.
   M—Movement is produced by a longitudinal pull through the leg, leaning backward with body weight. Counter-movement is provided against sole of patient's opposite foot with anterior aspect of operator's thigh. The opposite leg may be placed in a hook position (hip and knee flexed, with the feet flat on the plinth) or held in the Thomas position, to flatten out the lumbar spine.

Fig. 20-33. Traction mobilization of the lumbar spine, using the legs.

Fig. 20-34. Alternative method for traction mobilization of the lumbar spine, using the hips.

Fig. 20-35. Unilateral traction mobilization of the lumbar spine, using the leg.

12. *Sacroiliac Posterior Torsion* (Fig. 20-36)

P—Lies on side opposite the joint to be moved

O—Flexes patient's hip and knee as far as possible and holds leg in that position by contacting anterior aspect of patient's leg around operator's waist. Patient's other leg is extended, and dorsum of foot is secured at far edge of plinth. Operator's more cranial hand contacts patient's anterosuperior iliac spine and opposite hand contacts ischial tuberosity. Forearms are situated parallel to each other in a direction to create a force-couple around the joint axis.

M—Movement is produced by a force-couple, pushing the anterosuperior iliac spine backward and the ischial tuberosity forward. Further pressure is placed against patient's leg with operator's abdomen.

This is an effective technique for correcting anterior sacroiliac dysfunction. Contract–relax or muscle energy techniques may be used.

13. *Sacroiliac Anterior Torsion* (Fig. 20-37)

P—Prone

O—Places cranial hand directly over patient's sacrum. Opposite hand reaches around to grasp anterior aspect of distal thigh of near leg.

M—Movement is produced by simultaneously pressing downward on the distal sacrum with the heel of the hand and lifting leg upward, thus rotating the proximal ilium forward (anteriorly).

This is an effective technique for correcting posterior sacroiliac dysfunction.

Note: An example of how this technique might employ an isometric relaxation or muscle-energy technique is described.[44,398] The leg is elevated in extension and usually slight abduction and rotation to loose-pack the sacroiliac joint (operator monitors sulcus with fingers). Pressure is exerted on the iliac crest slightly above the posterior iliac spine. The leg is elevated in extension, until the restrictive barrier at the limit of passive range of motion is engaged. The patient is then instructed to pull the leg down toward the table against the resistance of the therapist's hand. The patient relaxes and additional slack in the joint motion is taken up until a new restrictive barrier is engaged. This process is repeated three or four times.

14. *Positional Distraction* (Fig. 20-38)

P—Sitting on side of plinth, with soft roll

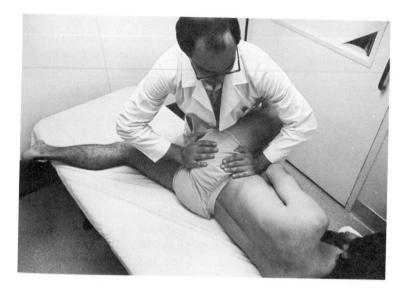

Fig. 20–36. Posterior rotation of the ilium on the sacrum.

placed at the side, between pelvic crest and chest wall (see Fig. 20–38A)

M—Patient is carefully assisted into sidelying position. Sidebending occurs due to roll. Patient's hips and knees are slightly flexed, for comfort (see Fig. 20–38B).

—Operator palpates between spinous processes at level where maximal positional traction is desired. Grasping patient's top knee, operator slides it up edge of plinth, flexing hip and spine until movement just occurs at level palpated. Dorsum of patient's foot is secured behind other knee or thigh (see Fig. 20–38C).

—Operator then palpates at next highest level, with third finger of other hand. Opposite hand grasps patient's distal humerus and pulls up and out, rotating upper spine, until motion just occurs at the level palpated (see Fig. 20–38D).

—Patient's arm is placed across chest. This position is maintained as long as tolerable by the patient (usually 5 to 25 minutes).

This technique is used primarily to relieve pressure on lumbar nerve root in patients with radicular signs and symptoms.

AUTOMOBILIZATION

1. *Standing Extension* (Fig. 20–39)
   a. *General*—Place hands on hips, thumbs forward. Keeping knees straight, bend back over hips, extending lumbar spine. Keep cervical spine neutral.

Fig. 20–37. Anterior rotation of the ilium on the sacrum.

A

B

C

D

E

Fig. 20–38. Positional distraction technique. Beginning with the patient (A) sitting on the side of the plinth, (B) assist him into sidelying. While palpating the level where maximal positional traction is desired, the hip and spine are flexed (C), the upper spine is rotated (D), and the position is maintained (E).

Fig. 20–39. Automobilization. *(A)* Specific bilateral and *(B)* unilateral extension techniques for localized acute back pain with some loss of normal lumbar lordosis.

A

B

Fig. 20–40. *(A)* Prolonged and *(B)* intermittent prone extension.

Fig. 20–41. Self-correction of lateral deviation using *(A)* hand pressure and *(B)* wall contact. (*Note:* In both *A* and *B*, a *left* lateral deviation has been slightly overcorrected so that the patient is shown in a slight *right* lateral deviation.)

A   B

b. *Specific*—Place hands on hips, thumbs making contact with lower spinous process of segment to be mobilized. Extend lumbar spine, maintaining pressure with thumbs and localizing force at desired level (see Fig. 20–39*A*).

c. *Unilateral*—As above, with single general or specific contact (thumb just lateral to spinous process) only. Bend back and to side of hand contact.

2. *Prone Extension* (Fig. 20–40)
   a. *Prolonged*—Lie prone with elbows and shoulders flexed approximately 90°, cervical spine neutral. Relax back and abdomen, allowing spine to stretch into extension (see Fig. 20–40*A*)
   b. *Intermittent*—Lie prone with hands at shoulder level. Push shoulders up until motion is halted by stiffness or discomfort. Back and abdomen remain completely relaxed (see Fig. 20–40*B*).

Use—Prolonged or intermittent, vigorous stretch into extension for stiffness, or to allow patient with acute disk prolapse to achieve desired extension.

3. *Self-Correction of Lateral Deviations*[382] (Fig. 20–41)
   a. Standing, hands contact protruding hip and chest (lateral chest wall to same side as trunk deviation, and pelvic crest on opposite side).

Hand pressure slowly forces spine into straight, then slightly "overcorrected" position (see Fig. 20–41*A*).
   b. Alternatively, elbow to side of deviations is held at 90° against lateral chest wall. Contact wall with that arm and shoulder. Slowly move hips toward wall, eventually assuming a slightly overcorrected position (see Fig. 20–41*B*).

REFERENCES

1. Abel OJR, Siebert WJ: Fibrositis. J Missouri Med Assoc 36:435–437, 1939
2. Aberg J: Evaluation of an advanced back pain rehabilitation program. Spine 7:317–318, 1982
3. Adams MA, Hutton WC: Gradual disc prolapse. Spine 10:524–531, 1985
4. Addison R, Schultz A: Trunk strength in patients seeking hospitalization for chronic low back disorders. Spine 5:539–544, 1980
5. Akerblom B: Standing and Sitting Posture with Special Reference to the Construction of Chairs. Thesis. Stockholm, Nordiska Bockhandeln, 1948
6. Almay BG, Johansson F, Von Knorring L, et al: Endorphins in chronic pain: I. Differences in CSF endorphin levels between organic and psychogenic pain syndromes. Pain 5:153–162, 1978
7. Alston W, Carlson KE, Feldman DJ, et al: A quantitative study of muscle factors in chronic low back syndrome. J Am Geriatr Soc 14:1041–1047, 1966

8. American Academy of Orthopaedic Surgeons: A Glossary on Spinal Terminology. Chicago, American Academy of Orthopaedic Surgeons, 1981

9. Andersson BJ, Murphys RW, Ortengren R, et al: The influence of back rest inclination and lumbar support on lumbar lordosis. Spine 4:52–58, 1979

10. Andersson BJ, Ortengren R, Nachemson A, et al: Lumbar disc pressure and myoelectric back muscle activity during sitting: I. Studies on an experimental chair. Scand J Rehabil Med 6:104–114, 1974

11. Andersson BJ, Ortengren R, Nachemson A, et al: The sitting posture: An electromyographic and discometric study. Orthop Clin North Am 6:105–120, 1975

12. Andersson GBJ: Epidemiologic aspects on low back pain in industry. Spine 6:53–60, 1981

13. Andersson GBJ, Pope MH: The patient. In Pope MH, Frymoyer JW, Andersson G (eds): Occupational Low Back Pain, pp 137–156. New York, Praeger, 1984

14. Andersson GJB, Sevensson HO, Oden A: The intensity of work recovery in low back pain. Spine 8:880–884, 1983

15. Andersson JAD: Back pain and occupation. In Jayson M (ed): The Lumbar Spine and Back Pain, pp 57–82. London, Pittman Medical, 1980

16. Armstrong JR: Lumbar Disc Lesions. London, Livingstone, 1967

17. Arnoldi CC, Brodsky AE, Cauchoix J, et al: Lumbar spinal stenosis and nerve root entrapment syndromes: Definitions and classification. Clin Orthop 115:4–5, 1976

18. Awad EA: Interstitial myofibrositis: Hypothesis of mechanism. Arch Phys Med Rehabil 54:449–453, 1975

19. Baarstrup C: On the spinous processes of the lumbar vertebrae and soft tissues between them and on pathological changes in that region. Acta Radiol 14:52, 1933

20. Badgley CE: The articular facets in relation to low-back pain and sciatica radiation. J Bone Joint Surg 23(A):481–496, 1941

21. Batson G: Balancing mobility with stability for dynamic spine function: Part I. Mobility. Kinesiology for Dance. 9:8–10, 1987

22. Batson G: Balancing mobility with stability for dynamic spine function: Part II. Stability. Kinesiology for Dance 9:12–15, 1987

23. Batson G: Balancing mobility with stability for dynamic spine function: Part III. Strengthening the trunk. Kinesiology for Dance 10(1):12–16, 1987

24. Beals RK, Hickman NW: Industrial injuries of the back and extremities. J Bone Joint Surg 54(A):1593–1611, 1972

25. Becker DP, Gluck H, Nulsen FE, et al: An inquiry into neurophysiological basis for pain. J Neurosurg 30:1–13, 1969

26. Bell GH, Dunbar O, Beck SJ, et al: Variation in strength of vertebrae with age and their relation to osteoporosis. Calcif Tissue Res 1:75–86, 1967

27. Bell GR, Rothman RH: The conservative treatment of sciatica. Spine 9:54–56, 1984

28. Benjamin BE: Are You Tense? The Benjamin System of Muscular Therapy: Tension Relief Through Deep Massage and Body Care. New York, Pantheon Books, 1978

29. Bennet RM: Fibrositis: Misnomer for a common rheumatic disorder. West J Med 134:405–413, 1981

30. Berquist-Ullman M, Larsson U: Acute low back pain in industry: A controlled prospective study with specific reference to therapy and vocational factors. Acta Orthop Scand (Suppl) 170:1–117, 1977

31. Berkson M, Schultz A, Nachemson A, et al: Voluntary strengths of male adults with acute low back syndromes. Clin Orthop 129:84–95, 1977

32. Bernick S, Caillet R: Vertebral end-plate changes with aging of human vertebrae. Spine 7:97–102, 1982

33. Bianco AJ: Low back pain and sciatica: Diagnosis and indications for treatment. J Bone Joint Surg 50(A):170–181, 1968

34. Biering-Sorensen F: Low back trouble in a general population of 30-, 40-, 50- and 60-year-old men and women: Study design, representativeness and basic results. Dan Med Bull 29:289–299, 1982

35. Biering-Sorensen F: A prospective study of low back pain in a general population: I. Occurrence, recurrence and aetiology. Scand J Rehabil Med 15:71–78, 1983

36. Biering-Sorensen F: Physical measurement as risk indications for low back trouble over a one-year period. Spine 9:106–118, 1984

37. Biering-Sorensen F, Hilden J: Reproducibility of the history of low-back trouble. Spine 9:280–286, 1984

38. Blumett AE, Modesti LM: Psychological predictions of success or failure of surgical intervention for intractable back pain. In Bonica JJ, Albefessard D (eds): Advances in Pain Research and Therapy, Vol I, pp 323–326. New York, Raven Press, 1976

39. Bogduk N: Lumbar dorsal ramus syndrome. Med J Aust 2:537–541, 1980

40. Bogduk N: The innervation of the lumbar spine. Spine 8:286–293, 1983

41. Bogduk N: Lumbar dorsal ramus syndrome. In Grieve GP (ed): Modern Manual Therapy of the Vertebral Column. New York, Churchill Livingstone, 1986

42. Bogduk N, Engel R: The menisci of the lumbar zygopophyseal joints. Spine 9:454–460, 1984

43. Boothby B: Seating by design. Physiotherapy 70:44–47, 1984

44. Bourdillion JF: Spinal Manipulation, 3rd ed. New York, Appleton–Century–Crofts, 1982

45. Bourdillion JF, Day EA: Spinal Manipulations, 4th ed. Los Altos, CA, Appleton and Lange, 1987

46. Bourne IHJ: Treatment of chronic back pain comparing corticosteroid–lignocaine injections with lignocaine alone. Practitioner 228:333–338, 1984

47. Bowles CH: Functional technique: A modern perspective. J Am Osteopath Assoc 80:326–331, 1981

48. Boxall D, Bradford DS, Winter RB, et al: Management of severe spondylolisthesis in children and adolescents. J Bone Joint Surg 61(A):479–495, 1979

49. Brackett EG: Low back strain with particular reference to industrial accident. JAMA 83:1068–1075, 1924
50. Bradley LA, Prokop CK, Margolis R, et al: Multivariate analyses of the MMPI profiles of low back pain patients. J Behav Med 1:235–272, 1978
51. Braunarski DT: Clinical trials of spinal manipulations: A critical appraisal and review of the literature. J Manipulative Physiol Ther 7:243–249, 1984
52. Breig A, Troup JDG: Biomechanical considerations in straight-leg-raising test. Spine 4:242–250, 1979
53. Brewerton DA: The doctor's role in diagnosis and prescribing vertebral manipulations. In Maitland GD (ed): Vertebral Manipulations, 5th ed, pp 14–17. London, Butterworth, 1986
54. Brinckmann P: Injury of the annulus fibrosus and disc protrusions: An in vitro investigation on human lumbar disc. Spine 11:149–153, 1986
55. Brown L: An introduction to the treatment and examination of the spine by combined movements. Physiotherapy 74:347–353, 1988
56. Brunswic M: Ergonomics of seat design. Physiotherapy 70:40–43, 1984
57. Buckle PW, Kember PA, Wood AD, et al: Factors influencing occupational back pain in Bedfordshire. Spine 5:254–258, 1980
58. Burnell A: Injection techniques in low back pain. In Twomey LT (ed): Symposium: Low Back Pain, pp 111. Perth, Western Australian Institute of Technology, 1974
59. Buros OK: Eighth Mental Measurements. Lincoln, University of Nebraska Press, 1978
60. Burton CV: Conservative management of low back pain. Post Grad Med 70:168–183, 1981
61. Burton CV, Nida G: The Sister Kenny Institute gravity lumbar reduction therapy program. Minneapolis, Sister Kenny Institute, 1976 (Pub no 7311)
62. Bush HD, Horton WG, Smare DL, et at: Fluid content of the nucleus pulposus as a factor in the disk syndrome. Br Med J 2:831–832, 1956
63. Cady LD, Bischoff DP, O'Connell ER, et al: Strength and fitness and subsequent back injuries in fire fighters. J Occup Med 21:269–272, 1979
64. Cailliet R: Low Back Pain Syndrome, 3rd ed. Philadelphia, FA Davis, 1981
65. Cairns D, Thomas L, Mooney V, et al: A comprehensive treatment approach to chronic low back pain. Pain 2:301–308, 1976
66. Calin A, Porta J, Fries JF, et al: Clinical history as a screening test for ankylosing spondylitis. JAMA 237:2613–2614, 1977
67. Campbell SM, Clarks, Tindall EA, et al: Clinical characteristics of fibrositis: I. A "blinded" controlled study of symptoms and points. Arthritis Rheum 26:817–824, 1983
68. Caro XJ: Immunofluorescent studies of skin in primary fibrositis syndrome. Am J Med (Suppl 3A) 81:43–48, 1986
69. Caro XJ, Wolfe F, Johnston WH, et al: Controlled and blinded study of immunoreactant deposition at dermal–epidermal junction of patients with primary fibrositis syndrome. J Rheumatol 13:1086–1092, 1986
70. Carrera GF: Lumbar facet arthrography and injection in low back pain. Wis Med J 78:35–37, 1979
71. Carrera GF, Haughton VM, Syversten A, Williams AL: Computerized tomography of the lumbar facet joints. Radiology 134:145–148, 1980
72. Carvin PJ, Jennings RB, Stern IJ: Enzymatic digestion of the nucleus pulposus: A review of experimental studies with chymopapain. Orthop Clin North Am 8:27–35, 1977
73. Chadwick PR: Advising patients on back care. Physiotherapy 65:277–278, 1979
74. Chadwick PR: Examination, assessment and treatment of the lumbar spine. Physiotherapy 70:2–7, 1984
75. Chaffin DB: Human strength capacity and low back pain. J Occup Med 16:248–253, 1974
76. Chaffin DB: Manual materials handling: The case of overexertion injury and illness in industry. J Environ Pathol Toxicol Oncol 2:31–36, 1979
77. Chaffin DB, Herrin GD, Keyserling WM: Pre-employment strength testing: An updated position. J Occup Med 20:403–408, 1978
78. Chamberlain GJ: Cyriax's friction massage: A review. J Orthop Sports Phys Ther 4:16–22, 1982
79. Chan PC: Finger Acupressure. Los Angeles, Price/Stern/Sloan Publishers, 1982
80. Charnley J: Orthopaedic signs in the diagnosis of disc protrusion with specific reference to straight leg raising test. Lancet 1:186–192, 1951
81. Chrisman DO, Mittnacht A, Snook GA: A study of the results following rotatory manipulation in the lumbar intervertebral disc syndrome. J Bone Joint Surg 46(A):517–524, 1964
82. Ciric I, Milhael MA, Tarkington JA, et al: The lateral recess syndrome: A variant of spinal stenosis. J Neurosurg 53:433–443, 1980
83. Clelland J, Savinar E, Shepard KF: The role of the physical therapist in chronic pain management. In Burrows GD, Elton D, Stanley GV (eds): Handbook of Chronic Pain Management, pp 243–258. New York, Elsevier, 1987
84. Clements L, Dixon M: A model role of occupational therapy in back education. Can J Occup Ther 46:161–163, 1979
85. Cloward RB: The clinical significance of the sinu-vertebral nerve of the cervical spine in relation to the cervical disc syndrome. J Neurol Neurosurg Psychiatry 23:321–326, 1960
86. Colt EWD, Wardlaw SL, Frantz AG: The effect of running on plasma B-endorphin. Life Sci 28:1637–1640, 1981
87. Coplans CW: The conservative treatment of low back pain. In Helfet AJ, Gruebel LDM (eds): Disorders of the Lumbar Spine, pp 135–183. Philadelphia, JB Lippincott, 1978
88. Corrigan B, Maitland GD: Practical Orthopaedic Medicine. Boston, Butterworth, 1985

89. Cottrell GW: New, conservative and exceptionally effective treatment for low back pain. Compr Ther 11:59–65, 1985

90. Coulehan JL: Chiropractic and the clinical art. Soc Sci Med 21:383–390, 1985

91. Coventry MB, Ghormley RK, Kernohan JW: The intervertebral disc: Its microscopic anatomy and pathology: 2. Changes in the intervertebral disc concomitant with age. J Bone Joint Surg 27(B):233–247, 1945

92. Coventry MB, Ghormley RK, Kernohan JW: The intervertebral disc: Its microscopic anatomy and pathology: 3. Pathological changes in the intervertebral disc. J Bone Joint Surg 27(B):460–474, 1945

93. Crock HV: Isolated lumbar disk resorption as a cause of nerve root canal stenosis. Clin Orthop 115:109–115, 1976

94. Crock HV: Internal disc disruption: A challenge to disc prolapse fifty years on. Spine 11:650–653, 1986

95. Cuckler JM, Bernini PA, Wiesel SW, et al: The use of epidural steroids in the treatment of lumbar radicular pain: A prospective, randomized, double-blind study. J Bone Joint Surg 67(A):63–66, 1985

96. Cummings GS, Routon JL: Validity of unassisted pain drawings by patients with chronic pain (abstr). Phys Ther 5:668, 1985

97. Cyriax J: Treatment of lumbar disk lesions. Br Med J 2:1434–1438, 1950

98. Cyriax J: Conservative treatment of lumbar disc lesions. Physiotherapy 50:300–303, 1964

99. Cyriax J. Deep friction. Physiotherapy 63:60–61, 1977

100. Cyriax J: Textbook of Orthopaedic Medicine, 8th ed, Vol 1: Diagnosis of Soft Tissue Lesions. London, Bailliere Tindall, 1982

101. Cyriax J: The Slipped Disc. New York, Charles Scribner's Sons, 1980

102. Cyriax JC, Coldham M: Textbook of Orthopaedic Medicine, 11th ed, Vol 2: Treatment by Manipulation, Massage and Injection. Philadelphia, Bailliere Tindall, 1984

103. Cyriax J, Cyriax P: Illustrated Manual of Orthopaedic Medicine. Boston, Butterworths, 1983

104. Dagi FT, Beary JF: Low back pain. In Beary JF (ed): Rheumatology and Outpatient Orthopedic Disorders: Diagnosis and Therapy, 2nd ed, pp. 97–103. Boston, Little, Brown, & Co, 1987

105. Dahlstrom WG, Welsh GS, Dahlstrom LE: An MMPI Handbook, Vol I. Minneapolis, University of Minnesota Press, 1975

106. Dahlstrom WG, Welsh GS, Dahlstrom LE: An MMPI Handbook, Vol 2. Minneapolis, University of Minnesota Press, 1975

107. Dan NG, Saccason PA: Serious complications of lumbar spine manipulations. Med J Aust 2:672–673, 1983

108. Davidson EA, Woodhall B: Biochemical alterations in herniated intervertebral disks. J Biol Chem 234:2951–2954, 1959

109. Davies G, Gould J: Trunk testing using a prototype: Cybex II isokinetic stabilization system. J Orthop Sports Phys Ther 3:164–170, 1982

110. Davis P: Reducing the risk of industrial bad backs. Occup Health Saf, May/June: 45–47, 1979

111. Dehlin O, Lindberg B: Lifting burden for a nursing aide during patient care in a geriatric ward. Scand J Rehabil Med 7:65–72, 1975

112. Delmas A: Fonction sacro-iliaque et statique du corps. Rev Rhum 17:475–481, 1950

113. Dennis MD, Greene RL, Farr SP, et al: The Minnesota Multiphasic Personality Inventory: General guidelines to its use and interpretation in orthopaedics. Clin Orthop 150:125–130, 1980

114. DePalma A, Rothman RH: The Intervertebral Disc. Philadelphia, WB Saunders, 1970

115. deVries HA, Cailliet R: Vagotonic effect of inversion therapy upon resting neuromuscular tension. Am J Phys Med 64:119–129, 1984

116. Deyo RA: Conservative therapy for low back pain: Distinguishing useful from useless therapy. JAMA 250:1057–1062, 1983

117. Deyo RA, Diehl A, Rosenthal M: How many days of bed rest for acute low back pain? N Engl J Med 315:1065–1070, 1986

118. Deyo RA, Diehl AK: Lumbar spine films in primary care: Current use and the effects of selective ordering criteria. J Gen Intern Med 1:20–25, 1986

119. DiFabio RP: Clinical assessment of manipulation and mobilization of the lumbar spine: A critical review of the literature. Phys Ther 66:51–54, 1986

120. Dike TFW, Burry HC, Grahame R: Extradural corticosteroid injection in management of lumbar nerve root compression. Br Med J 2:635–637, 1973

121. Dimaggio A, Mooney V: Conservative care of low back pain: What works? J Musculoskel Med 4:27–34, 1987

122. Dimaggio A, Mooney V: The McKenzie program: Exercise effective against back pain. J Musculoskel Med 4:63–74, 1987

123. Dixon ASJ: Progress and problems in back pain research. Rheumatol Rehabil 12:165–175, 1973

124. Dominguez RH, Gajda R: Total Body Training. New York, Warner Books, 1982

125. Dontigny RL: Function and pathomechanics of the sacroiliac joint: A review. Phys Ther 65:35–44, 1985

126. Dorwart RH, Volger JB III, Helms CA: Spinal stenosis. Radiol Clin North Am 21:301–325, 1983

127. Dunham WF: Ankylosing spondylitis. Measurement of hip and spine movements. Br J Phys Med 12:126–129, 1949

128. Dupuis PR: The natural history of degenerative changes in the lumbar spine. In Watkins RG, Collis JS (eds): Principles and Techniques in Spine Surgery, pp. 1–4. Rockville, MD, Aspen Publications, 1987

129. Dupuis PR, Yong-Ling K, Cassidy JD, et al: Radiologic diagnosis of degenerative lumbar spinal instability. Spine 10:262–276, 1985

130. Dyck P: Sciatic pain. In Watkins C (ed): Lumbar Dis-

cectomy and Laminectomy. Rockville MD, Aspen Publications, 1987

131. Eastmond CJ, Woodrow JC: The HLA system and the arthropathies associated with psoriasis. Ann Rheum Dis 36:112, 1977

132. Ebner M: Connective Tissue Massage. Physiotherapy 64:208–212, 1978

133. Ebner M: Connective Tissue Manipulations, Therapy and Therapeutic Application. Malabar, FL, Robert Kreiger, 1985

134. Echternach JL: Evaluation of pain in the clinical environment. In Echternach JL (ed): Pain, pp 39–72. New York, Churchill Livingstone, 1987

135. Eckert C, Decker A: Pathological studies of intervertebral discs. J Bone Joint Surg 29:447–454, 1947

136. Edgar MA, Park WM: Induced pain patterns on passive straight leg raising in lower disc protrusion. J Bone Joint Surg 56(B):658–667, 1974

137. Edgar MA: Backache. Br J Hosp Med 32:290–301, 1984

138. Edwards BC: Combined movements of the lumbar spine: Examination and significance. Aust J Physiother 25:147–152, 1979

139. Edwards BC: Combined movements in the lumbar spine: Examination and treatment. In Grieves GP (ed): Modern Manual Therapy of the Vertebral Column, pp 561–566. New York, Churchill Livingstone, 1986

140. Edwards BC: Clinical assessment: The use of combined movements in assessment and treatment. In Twomey LT, Taylor JR (eds): Physiotherapy of the Low Back, pp 81–109. New York, Churchill Livingstone, 1987

141. Eggart JS, Leigh D, Vergamini G: Preseason athletic physical evaluations. In Gould JA, Davies GJ (eds): Orthopaedic and Sports Physical Therapy, pp 605–642. St Louis, CV Mosby, 1985

142. Eggertz AM: Auto-traction, a nonsurgical treatment of low back pain and sciatica. In Grieve GP (ed): Modern Manual Therapy of the Vertebral Column, pp 796–804. New York, Churchill Livingstone, 1986

143. Ehard R, Blowling R: The recognition and management of the pelvic component of low back and sciatic pain. Presented at the annual meeting of the American Physical Therapy Association (Orthopaedic Section), July 2, Miami FL, 1967

144. Eisen A, Hoirch M: The electrodiagnostic evaluation of spinal root lesions. Spine 8:98–106, 1983

145. Epstein JA, Epstein BS, Lavine LS, et al: Lumbar nerve root compression at the intervertebral foramina caused by arthritis of the posterior facets. J Neurosurg 39:362–369, 1973

146. Epstein JA, Epstein BS, Lavine LS, et al: Surgical treatment of nerve root compression caused by scoliosis of the lumbar spine. J Neurosurg 41:449–454, 1974

147. Evjenth O, Hamberg J: Muscle Stretching in Manual Therapy: A Clinical Manual, Vol 1: The Extremities; Vol 2, The Spinal Column and the TMJ. Alfta, Sweden, Alfta Rehab Forlag, 1980

148. Fahrni WH: Conservative treatment of lumbar disc degeneration: Our primary responsibility. Orthop Clin North AM 6:93–103, 1975

149. Fairbanks JCT, Park WN, McCall JW, et al: Apophyseal injection of local anesthetic as a diagnostic aid in primary low back syndromes. Spine 6:598–605, 1981

150. Fajersztajn J: Uber das gekreuzte ischiasphanomen. Wien KlinWochenschr 14:41–47, 1901

151. Falconer MA, McGeorge M, Begg AC: Observation on the cause and mechanism of symptom production and low back pain. J Neurol Neurosurg Psychiatry 11:13–26, 1948

152. Farfan HF, Sullivan JD: The relation of facet orientation to intervertebral disc failure. Can J Surg 10:179–185, 1967

153. Farfan HF: Mechanical Disorders of the Low Back. Philadelphia, Lea & Febiger, 1973

154. Farrell PA, Gates WK, Maksud MG: Plasma beta-endorphin/beta lipotropin immunoreactivity increases after treadmill exercise in man (abstr). Med Sci Sports 13:134, 1981

155. Feinstein B, Langton J, Jameson R: Experiments on pain referred from deep skeletal structures. J Bone Joint Surg 36(A):981–997, 1954

156. Finneson B: Low Back Pain. Philadelphia, JB Lippincott, 1973

157. Finneson BE: A lumbar disc surgery predictive score card: A retrospective evaluation. Spine 4:141–144, 1979

158. Finneson BE: Low Back Pain. Philadelphia, JB Lippincott, 1980

159. Fischer AA: Documentation of myofascial trigger points. Arch Phys Med Rehabil 69:286–291, 1988

160. Fischer AA, Chang CH: Temperature and pressure threshold measurements in trigger points. Thermology 1:212–215, 1986

161. Fisk J, Dimonte P, Courington S: Back Schools. Clin Orthop 179:18–23, 1983

162. Fitzgerald KG, Wynveen KJ, Rhealt W, et al: Objective assessment with establishment of normal values for lumbar spinal range of movement. Phys Ther 63:1776–1781, 1982

163. Flint M: Effect of increasing back and abdominal strength on low-back pain. Res Q 29:160–171, 1955

164. Flor H, Turk DC: Etiological theories and treatments for chronic back pain: Somatic models and interventions. Pain 19:105–121, 1984

165. Folkins CH, Sime WE: Physical fitness training and mental health. Am Psychol 36:373–389, 1981

166. Fordyce WE: Behavioral Methods for Chronic Back Pain and Illness. St Louis, CV Mosby, 1976

167. Fordyce WE, Fowler RS, Lehmann JF, et al: Some implications of learning in problems of chronic pain. J Chronic Dis 21:179–190, 1968

168. Fordyce WE, McMahon R, Rainwater G, et al: Pain–compliant-exercise performance relationship in chronic pain. Pain 10:311–321, 1981

169. Fordyce WE, Shelton JL, Dundore DE: The modification of avoidance learning pain behaviors. J Behav Med 5:405–414, 1982
170. Forsell MZ: The back school. Spine 6:104–106, 1981
171. Fox RF, Van Breemer J: Chronic Rheumatism: Causation and Treatment. London, Churchill, 1934
172. Fraioli F, Moretti C, Paulucci D, et al: Physical exercise stimulates marked concomitant release of B-endorphins and adrenocorticotrophic hormones (ACTH) in peripheral blood in man. Experientia 36:987–989, 1980
173. Fredrickson BE, Trief PM, Van Beveren P, et al: Rehabilitation of the patient with chronic back pain. Spine 13:351–353, 1987
174. Friberg S, Hirsch C: Anatomical and clinical studies on lumbar disc degeneration. Acta Orthop Scand 19:222–242, 1949
175. Fries JF, Mitchell DM: Joint pain or arthritis. JAMA 233:199–204, 1976
176. Frymoyer JW: Basics for all (abstr). Challenge of the Lumbar Spine: Ninth Annual Meeting, New York, October 7–10, 1987
177. Frymoyer JW: Back pain and sciatica. N Engl J Med 318:291–300, 1988
178. Frymoyer JW, Pope MH, Clements JH, et al: Risk factors in low back pain: An epidemiological survey. J Bone Joint Surg 65(A):213–218, 1983
179. Frymoyer JW, Pope MH, Clostanza MC, et al: Epidemiologic studies of low-back pain. Spine 5:419–423, 1980
180. Frymoyer JW, Selby DK: Segmental instability: Rationale for treatment. Spine 10:280–286, 1985
181. Garrett R: Back strength and fitness programme using Norsk and sequence training. Physiotherapy 73:573–575, 1987
182. Gatchel RJ, Mayer TG, Capra P, et al: Qualification of lumbar function: VI. The use of psychological measures in guiding physical functional restoration. Spine 11:36–42, 1986
183. Gillstrom P, Ehrnberg A: Long-term results of autotraction in the treatment of lumbago and sciatica: An attempt to correlate clinical results with objective parameters. Arch Orthop Trauma Surg 104:294–298, 1985
184. Glover JR: Back pain and hyperaesthesia. Lancet 1:1165–1169, 1960
185. Godfrey CM, Morgan PR, Schatzker J: A randomized trial of manipulations for low back pain in a medical setting. Spine 9:301–304, 1984
186. Goldenberg DL: Psychologic studies in fibrositis. Am J Med (Suppl 3A) 81:67–81, 1986
187. Gonnella C, Paris S, Kutner M: Reliability in evaluating passive intervertebral motion. Phys Ther 62:437–444, 1982
188. Goodridge JP: Muscle energy technique: Definition, explanation, methods of procedure. J Am Osteopath Assoc 81:249–254, 1981
189. Gorman HO, Gwendolen J: Thoracic kyphosis and mobility: The effect of age. Physiotherapy Practice 3:154–162, 1987
190. Grabias S: The treatment of spinal stenosis. J Bone Joint Surg 60(A):308–313, 1980
191. Greenland S, Reisbord LS, Haldeman S, et al: Controlled clinical trials of manipulation: A review and proposal. J Occup Med 22:670–676, 1980
192. Grieve GP: Sciatica and the straight-leg-raising test in manipulative treatment. Physiotherapy 6:337–346, 1970
193. Grieve GP: The sacroiliac joint. Physiotherapy 62:384–400, 1976
194. Grieve GP: Mobilization of the Spine, 3rd ed. New York, Churchill Livingstone, 1979
195. Grieve GP: Common patterns of clinical presentation. In Grieve GP: Common Vertebral Joint Problems, 2nd ed, pp 355–458. New York, Churchill Livingstone, 1988
196. Grieve GP: Clinical features. In Grieve GP: Common Vertebral Joint Problems, 2nd ed, pp 159–209. New York, Churchill Livingstone, 1988
197. Grieve GP: Pathological changes: Combined regional degenerative. In Grieve GP: Common Vertebral Joint Problems, 2nd ed, pp 197–248. New York, Churchill Livingstone, 1988
198. Grieve GP: Lumbar instability. Physiotherapy 68:2–9, 1982
199. Grieve GP: Mobilization of the Spine: Notes on Examination, Assessment and Clinical Methods, 4th ed. New York, Churchill Livingstone, 1984
200. Grieves GP: Lumbar instability. In Grieve GP (ed): Modern Manual Therapy of the Vertebral Column, pp 416–441. New York, Churchill Livingstone, 1986
201. Grieve GP: Diagnosis. Physiotherapy Practice. 4:73–77, 1988
202. Grimsby O: Advanced course: Lumbar–thoracic spine. Continuing education course. Institute of Graduate Health Sciences, Nashville, Tennessee, 1976
203. Grimsby O: Advanced extremity mobilizations. Continuing education course. Sorlandet's Institute, Portland, Oregon, 1979
204. Gunn CC, Milbrandt WE: Tenderness at motor points: A diagnostic and prognostic aid for low back injury. J Bone Joint Surg 58(A):815–825, 1976
205. Gunn CC, Milbrandt WE: Early and subtle signs in low back sprain. Spine 3:267–281, 1978
206. Gunnari H, Evjenth O, Brady MM: Sequence Exercise. Oslo, Breyers Forlag, 1983
207. Gustavsen R: Fra aktiv avspenning. Oslo, Olaf Norlis Bokhannel, 1977
208. Guymer AJ: Proprioceptive neuromuscular facilitation for vertebral joint conditions. In Grieve GP (ed): Modern Manual Therapy of the Vertebral Column, pp 622–634. New York, Churchill Livingstone, 1986
209. Hackett GS: Referred pain from low back ligament disabilities. Arch Surg 73:878–883, 1956
210. Hadler NM: Legal ramifications of the medical definition of back disease. Ann Intern Med 89:992–999, 1978
211. Hadler NM: Regional back pain. N Engl J Med 315:1090–1092, 1986

212. Hadler NM: A critical reappraisal of the fibrositis concept. Am J Med 81:26–30, 1986

213. Hadler NM: A benefit of spinal manipulations as adjunctive therapy for acute low back pain: A stratified controlled trial. Spine 12:703–706, 1987

214. Haldeman S: Spinal manipulative therapy as a status report. Clin Orthop 179:62–70, 1983

215. Haldeman S: Soft tissue techniques. Challenge of the Lumbar Spine, Ninth Annual Meeting, New York, October 7–10, 1987

216. Hall H, Iceton JA: Back school: An overview with specific reference to the Canadian Back Education Units. Clin Orthop 179:10–17, 1983

217. Hansson P, Ekblom A: Acute pain relieved by vibratory stimulation (letter). Br Dent J 151:213, 1981

218. Hansson P, Ekblom A: Transcutaneous electrical nerve stimulaton (TENS) as compared to placebo: TENS for the relief of acute orofacial pain. Pain 15:157–165, 1983

219. Happey T, Pearson CH, Palframan J, et al: Proteoglycans and glycoproteins associated with collagen in the human intervertebral disc. Z Klin Chem 9:79, 1971

220. Harris RI, MacNab I: Structural changes in the lumbar intervertebral disc. Their relationship to low back pain and sciatica. J Bone Joint Surg 36(B):304–322, 1954

221. Hasue M, Fujiwara M, Kikuchi S: A new method of quantitative measurement of abdominal and back muscle strength. Spine 5:143–148, 1980

222. Hathaway SR, McKinley JC: A multiphasic personality schedule (Minnesota): I. Construction of the schedule. J Psychol 10:249, 1940

223. Hayne CR: Ergonomics and back pain. Physiotherapy 70:9–13, 1984

224. Hayne CR: Back schools and total care programs. Physiotherapy 70:14–17, 1984

225. Hayne CR: Prophylaxis and ergonomic considerations. In Grieve GP (ed): Modern Manual Therapy of the Vertebral Column, pp 860–872. New York, Churchill Livingstone, 1986

226. Hazard RG, Reid S, Fenwick J, et al: Isokinetic trunk and lifting strength measurements: Variability as an indicator of effort. Spine 13:54–57, 1988

227. Helfet AJ, Gruebel Lee DM: Disorders of the Lumbar Spine. Philadelphia, JB Lippincott, 1978

228. Henderson I: Low back pain and sciatica: Evaluation and surgical management. Aust Fam Phys 14:1149–1159, 1985

229. Hendler N: Psychological tests for chronic pain. In Hendler N: Diagnosis and Nonsurgical Management of Chronic Pain, p 101–120. New York, Raven Press, 1981

230. Hendry NGS: The hydration of the nucleus pulposus and its relation to intervertebral disc derangement. J Bone Joint Surg 40(B):132–144, 1958

231. Hirsch C: Studies on the mechanism of low back pain. Acta Orthop Scand 20:261–273, 1951

232. Hirsch C: The reaction of the intervertebral discs to compressive forces. J Bone Joint Surg 37(A):1188–1196, 1955

233. Hirsch C, Ingelmark BE, Miller M: The anatomical basis for low back pain: Studies on the presence of sensory nerve endings in ligamentous, capsular and intervertebral disc structures in the human lumbar spine. Acta Orthop Scand 33:1–17, 1963

234. Hirsch C, Jonsson B, Lewin T: Low-back symptoms in a Swedish female population. Clin Orthop 63:171–176, 1969

235. Hirsch C, Nachemson A: The reliability of lumbar disc surgery. Clin Orthop 29:189–195, 1963

236. Hirschberg GG: Treating lumbar disc lesions by prolonged continuous reduction of intradiscal pressure. Tex Med 70:58–68, 1974

237. Hirschberg GG, Froetscher L, Naem F: Iliolumbar syndrome as a common cause of low back pain: Diagnosis and prognosis. Arch Phys Med Rehabil 60:415–419, 1979

238. Hitselberger WE, Witten RM: Abnormal myelograms in asymptomatic patients. J Neurosurg 28:204–206, 1968

239. Hoehler FK, Tobin JS, Buerger AA: Spinal manipulations for low back pain. JAMA 245:1835–1838, 1981

240. Holten O: Medisinsk Trenigsterapi Trykk Fugseth and Lorentzen, Medical Training Course, Salt Lake City, March 1–4, 1984

241. Hood LB, Chrisman D: Intermittent pelvic traction in the treatment of the ruptured disc. Phys Ther 48:21–30, 1968

242. Hoppenfeld S: Physical Examination of the Spine and Extremities. New York, Appleton–Century–Crofts, 1976

243. Horal J: The clinical appearance of low back pain disorders in the city of Goteborg, Sweden: Comparison of incapacitated probands and matched controls. Acta Orthop Scand (Suppl 118):1–109, 1969

244. Hudgins WR: The crossed–straight leg raising test. N Engl J Med 297:1127, 1977

245. Hult L: The Munfors investigation: A study of the frequency and causes of the stiff neck–brachalgia and lumbago–sciatica syndromes as well as observation on certain signs and symptoms from the dorsal spine and the joints of the extremities in industrial and forest workers. Acta Orthop Scan (Suppl 16):1–76, 1954

246. Hult L: Cervical, dorsal and lumbar spinal syndromes. A field investigation of a non-selected material of 1200 workers in different occupations with special reference to disc degeneration and so-called muscular rheumatism. Acta Orthop Scand (Suppl 17):1–102, 1954

247. Ikata T: Statistical and dynamic studies of lesions due to overloading on the spine. Shikoku Acta Med 21:262–286, 1965

248. Ingham JG: A method of observing symptoms and attitudes. Br J Soc Clin Psychol 4:131–140, 1965

249. Ingham JG: Quantitative evaluation of subjective symptoms. Proc R Soc Med 62:492–494, 1969

250. Iskrant AP, Smith RW: Osteoporosis in women 45

years and over related to subsequent fracture. Public Health Rep 84:33–38, 1969

251. Jackson CP, Brown MD: Is there a role for exercise in the treatment of patients with low back pain? Clin Orthop 179:39–45, 1983

252. Jackson HC, Winkelmann RK, Bichel WH: Nerve endings in ligamentous, capsular and intervertebral disc structures in the human lumbar spine. J Bone Joint Surg 48(A):1272–1281, 1966

253. Janda V, Schmid HJA: Muscles as a pathogenic factor in back pain. Proceedings 4th Conference of International Federation of Orthopaedic Manipulative Therapists. Christ-Church, New Zealand, 1980

254. Janda V: Muscles, central nervous motor regulation and back problems. In Korr I (ed): The Neurobiologic Mechanisms in Manipulative Therapy, pp 27–42. London, Plenum Press, 1978

255. Janda V: Muscle Function Testing. Boston, Butterworths, 1983

256. Janda V: Muscle weakness and inhibition (pseudoparesis) in back pain syndromes. In Greive GP (ed): Modern Manual Therapy of the Vertebral Column, pp 197–201. New York, Churchill Livingstone, 1986

257. Jayson MIV, Sim-Williams H, Young S, et al: Mobilization and manipulations for low back pain. Spine 6:409–416, 1981

258. Johansson F, Almay BG, von Knorring L, et al: Predictors for the outcome of treatment with high-frequency transcutaneous electrical nerve stimulation in patients with chronic pain. Pain 9:55–61, 1980

259. Johnson G: Functional orthopaedics II: Advanced techniques of soft tissue mobilizations for evaluation and treatment of the extremities and trunk. Continuing education course, San Francisco, November 21–24, 1985

260. Jones LH: Spontaneous release by positioning. Doctor Osteopathy 4:109, 1964

261. Jones LH: Strain and Counterstrain. Colorado Springs, American Academy of Osteopathy, 1981

262. Jones MD: Basic Diagnostic Radiology. St Louis, CV Mosby, 1969

263. Jorgensen K: Back muscle strength and body weight as limiting factors for work in the standing slightly-stooped position. Scand J Rehabil Med 2:149–153, 1970

264. Judovich B, Nobel GP: Lumbar traction therapy: A study of resistive forces. Am J Surg 93:108–114, 1957

265. Jull GA: Examination of the lumbar spine. In Greive GP (ed): Modern Manual Therapy of the Vertebral Column, pp 547–560. New York, Churchill Livingstone, 1986

266. Jull GA, Janda V: Muscles and motor control in low back pain: Assessment and management. In Twomey LT, Taylor JR (eds): Physical Therapy of the Low Back, pp 253–278. New York, Churchill Livingstone, 1987

267. Jungham H: Spondylolisthesen ohne Spalt im Zwischengelenkstuck (pseudospondylolisthesen). Arch Orthop Unfall Chir 29:118–123, 1930

268. Jungham H: Die wirbelsaule in der Arbeitmedizin. Wirbel saule Forch Praxis 79:1–395, 1979

269. Kahanovitz N, Nordin M, Verderame R, et al: Normal trunk muscle strength and endurance in women and the effect of exercises and electrical stimulation: Part 2. Comparative analysis of electrical stimulation and exercise to increase trunk muscle strength and endurance. Spine 12:112–118, 1987

270. Kaltenborn FM: Test Segment: Moblis Columbia Vertebris. Oslo, Freddy Kaltenborn, 1975

271. Kaltenborn FM: Manual Therapy for the Extremity Joints. Oslo, Olaf Norlis Bokhandel, 1976

272. Kaltenborn FM: Manual Mobilizations of the Extremity Joints: Vol II. Advanced Treatment Techniques. Oslo, Olaf Norlis Bokhandel, 1986

273. Kalyan-Raman UP, Kalyan-Raman K, Yunus MB, et al: Muscle pathology in primary fibromyalgia syndrome: Light microscopic, histochemical and ultrastructural study. J Rheumatol 11:808–813, 1984

274. Kane RL, Craig L, Olsen D, et al: Manipulating the patient: A comparison of the effectiveness of physician and chiropractor care. Lancet 1:1333–1336, 1974

275. Kavanagh T: Exercise: The modern panacea. Ir Med J 72:24–27, 1979

276. Keegan JJ: Alterations to the lumbar curve related to posture and seating. J Bone Joint Surg 35(A):589–603, 1953

277. Keene JS, Drummond DS: Mechanical back pain in the athlete. Compr Ther 11:7–14, 1985

278. Kellgren JH: On the distribution of pain arising from deep somatic structures with charts of segmental pain areas. Clin Sci 4:35, 1939

279. Kelsey JL: An epidemiological study of the relationship between occupations and acute herniated lumbar intervertebral discs. Int J Epidemiol 4:197–205, 1975

280. Kelsey JL, Hardy RJ: Driving of a motor vehicle as a risk factor for acute herniated lumbar intevertebral disc. Am J Epidemiol 102:63–73, 1975

281. Kelsey JL, White AA: Epidemiology and impact of low-back pain. Spine 5:133–142, 1980

282. Kendall PH, Jenkins JM: Exercises for backache: A double blind controlled study. Physiotherapy 54:154–157, 1968

283. Kenna O, Murtagh A: The physical examination of the back. Aust Fam Physician 14:1244–1256, 1985

284. Kennedy B: An Australian programme for management of back problems. Physiotherapy 66:108–111, 1980

285. Kessler RM: Acute symptomatic disc prolapse: Clinical manifestations and therapeutic considerations. Phys Ther 59:978–987, 1979

286. Keyes DC, Compere EL: The normal and pathological physiology of the nucleus pulposus of the intervertebral disc. J Bone Joint Surg 14(A):897–938, 1932

287. Keyserling WM, Herrin GD, Chaffin DB: Isometric strength testing as a means of controlling medical

incidents on strenuous jobs. J Occup Med 22:332–336, 1980

288. Kirkaldy-Willis WH: The three phases of the spectrum of degenerative disease. In Kirkaldy-Willis WH: Managing Low Back Pain, pp 75–90. New York, Churchill Livingstone, 1983

289. Kirkaldy-Willis WH: The relationship of structural pathology to the nerve root. Spine 9:49–52, 1984

290. Kirkaldy-Willis WH (ed): Managing Low Back Pain, 2nd ed. New York, Churchill Livingstone, 1988

291. Kirkaldy-Willis WH, Wedge JH, Yong-Hing K, et al: Lumbar spinal nerve entrapment. Clin Orthop 169:171–178, 1982

292. Kishino ND, Mayer TG, Gatchell J, et al: Qualification of lumbar function IV: Isometric and isotonic lifting simulation in normal subjects and low-back dysfunction patients. Spine 10:921–927, 1985

293. Klaber Moffett JA, Chase SM, et al: A controlled prospective study to evaluate the effectiveness of a back school in low back pain. Spine 11:120–122, 1986

294. Knott M, Voss DE: Proprioceptive Neuromuscular Facilitation, 2nd ed. New York, Harper & Row, 1968

295. Kopala B, Matassarin-Jacobs E: Sensory–perceptual pain assessment. In Bellack JP, Banford PA (eds): Nursing Assessment: A Multidimensional Approach. Belmont, CA, Wadsworth, 1984

296. Korr IM: Proprioceptive and somatic dysfunction. J Am Osteopath Assoc 74:123–135, 1975

297. Kos J, Wolf J: Intervertebral menisci and their possible role in intervertebral blockage. Bulletin of the Orthopaedic Section of the American Physical Therapy Association 1:8, 1976

298. Kraft GL, Johnson EW, La Ban MM: Fibrositis syndrome. Arch Phys Med Rehabil 49:155–162, 1968

299. Kraft GL, Levinthal DH: Facet synovial impingement. Surg Gynecol Obstet 93:439–443, 1951

300. Kramer J: Intervertebral Disc Disease. Chicago, Year Book Medical Publishers, 1987

301. Kroemer KHE, Robinette JC: Ergonomics in the design of office furniture. Ind Med Surg 38:115–125, 1969

302. Kvien TK, Nilsen H, Vik P: Education and self-care of patients with low back pain. Scand J Rheumatol 10:318–320, 1981

303. La Freniere JG: The Low-Back Patient: Procedures for Treatment by Physical Therapy. New York, Masson, 1979

304. La Freniere JG: La Freniere Body Techniques. Chicago, Year Book Medical Publishers, 1984

305. Lageard P, Robinson M: Back pain: Current concepts and recent advances. Physiotherapy 72:105, 1986

306. Lamb DW: A review of manual therapy for spinal pain with reference to the lumbar spine. In Grieve GP (ed): Modern Manual Therapy of the Vertebral Column, pp 605–621. New York, Churchill Livingstone, 1986

307. Langrana N, Lee C, Alexander H, et al: Quantitative assessment of back strength using isokinetic testing. Spine 9:287–290, 1984

308. Lankhorst GL, Vanderstadt RJ, Vogelaar JW, et al: The effect of the Swedish back school in chronic idiopathic low back pain. Scan J Rehabil Med 15:141–145, 1983

309. Larsson V, Choler V, Lidstrom A, et al: Autotraction for treatment of lumbago–sciatica. Acta Orthop Scand 51:791–798, 1980

310. Laslett M: The role of physical therapy in soft tissue rheumatism. Patient Management 15:57–68, 1986

311. Laslett M: Use of manipulative therapy for mechanical pain of spinal origin. Orthop Rev 16:65–73, 1987

312. Lawrence JS: Rheumatism in coal miners. Part III. Occupational factors. Br J Ind Med 12:249–261, 1955

313. Lee CL: Work hardening: Return to work and work hardening (abstr). Challenge of the Lumbar Spine, ninth annual meeting. New York, October 7–10, 1987

314. Lee D: Principles and practice of muscle energy and functional techniques. In Grieve GP (ed): Modern Manual Therapy of the Vertebral Column, pp 640–655. New York, Churchill Livingstone, 1986

315. Lee HM, Whincup G: Chinese Massage Therapy: A Handbook of Therapeutic Massage. Boulder, CO. Shambhala, 1983

316. Lee SLK, Wesers B, McInnis S, et al: Analysing risk factors for preventive back education approaches: A review. Physiother Can 40:88–98, 1988

317. Lettin AWF: Diagnosis and treatment of lumbar instability. J Bone Joint Surg 49(B):520–529, 1967

318. Levernieux J: Traction Vertebrale. Paris, Expansion Scientifique, 1960

319. Lewin T: Osteoarthrosis in lumbar synovial joints. Gottesborg, Orstadius Bokryckeri Aktiebolag, 1964

320. Lewit K: Manipulative Therapy in Rehabilitation of the Motor System. London, Butterworth, 1985

321. Lewit K, Simons DG: Myofascial pain: Relief by postisometric relaxation. Arch Phys Med Rehabil 65:452–456, 1984

322. Leyshon A, Kirwan E, Wynn–Parry GB: Is it nerve root pain? J Bone Joint Surg 62(B):119, 1980

323. Lichter R: Work hardening: Simulated job training using work performances for worker rehabilitation and testing (abstr). Challenge of the Lumbar Spine, Ninth annual meeting, New York, October 7–10, 1987

324. Lichter RL, Hewson JK, Radke S, et al: Treatment of chronic low-back pain. Clin Orthop 190:115–123, 1984

325. Lind G: Auto-traction: Treatment of Low Back Pain and Sciatica. Thesis, University of Kinkopinj, 1974

326. Lindblom K: Technique and results in myelography and disc puncture. Acta Radiol 34:321–330, 1950

327. Lindblom K: Technique and result of diagnostic disc puncture and injection (discography) in the lumbar region. Acta Orthop Scand 20:316–326, 1951

328. Lindblom K: Intervertebral disc degeneration considered as a pressure atrophy. J Bone Joint Surg (A):39:933–945, 1957

329. Linton SJ: The relationship between activity and chronic pain. Pain 21:289–294, 1985

330. Lippit AB: The facet joint and its role in spine pain management with facet joint injections. Spine 9:746–750, 1984

331. Lipson SJ, Muir H: Proteoglycans in experimental intervertebral disc degeneration. Spine 6:194–210, 1981

332. Liston CB: Back schools and ergonomics. In Twomey LT, Taylor JR (eds): Physical Therapy of the Low Back, pp 279–303. New York, Churchill Livingstone, 1987

333. Ljunggren AE, Weber H, Larson S: Autotraction with prolapsed lumbar intervertebral discs. Scand J Rehabil Med 16:117–124, 1984

334. Llewellyn RLJ, Jones AB: Fibrositis. London, Heinemann, 1915

335. Loebl WY: Measurement of spinal posture and range of spinal movement. Ann Phys Med 7:103–110, 1967

336. Lundeberg T: Vibratory stimulation for alleviation of chronic pain. Acta Physiol Scand (Suppl) 523:8–51, 1983

337. Lundeberg T: Long-term results of vibratory stimulation as a pain relieving measure for chronic pain. Pain 20:13–23, 1984

338. Lundeberg T, Nordemar R, Ottoson D: Pain alleviation by vibratory stimulation. Pain 20:25–44, 1984

339. Lyon HE, Jones E, Quinn FE, Sprunt DH: Changes in the protein–polysaccharide fractions of the nucleus pulposus from human intervertebral disc with age and disc herniation. J Lab Clin Med 68:930–939, 1966

340. MacNab I: Chemonucleolysis. Clin Neurosurg 20:183–191, 1973

341. MacNab I: Backache. Baltimore, Williams & Wilkins, 1977

342. MacRae IF, Wright V: Measurement of back movement. Ann Rheum Dis 28:584–589, 1969

343. Magee DJ: Orthopedic Physical Assessment. Philadelphia, WB Saunders, 1987

344. Magora A: Investigation of the relation between low back pain and occupation: 1. Age, sex, community, education and other factors. Ind Med Surg 39:465–471, 1970

345. Magora A: Investigation of the relation between low back pain and occupation: 2. Work history. Ind Med Surg 39:504–510,1970

346. Magora A: Investigation of the relation between low back pain and occupation: 3. Physical requirements: Sitting, standing and weight lifting. Ind Med Surg 41:5–9, 1972

347. Magora A: Investigation of the relation between low back pain and occupation: 4. Physical requirements: Bending, rotation, reaching, and sudden maximal effort. Scand J Rehabil Med 5:186–190, 1973

348. Magora A: Investigation of the relation between low back pain and occupation: 7. Neurologic and orthopedic conditions. Scand J Rehabil Med 7:146–151, 1975

349. Magora A, Schwartz A: Relation between the low back pain syndrome and X-ray findings: I. Degenerative osteoarthritis. Scand J Rehabil Med 8:115–125, 1976

350. Maigne R: Orthopaedic Medicine. Springfield IL, Charles C Thomas, 1976

351. Maigne R: Manipulation of the spine. In Rogoff JB (ed): Manipulations, Traction and Massage, 2nd ed, pp 59–120. Baltimore, Williams & Wilkins, 1980

352. Maitland GD: Vertebral Manipulation, 4th ed. Boston Butterworths, 1977

353. Maitland GD: Movement of pain-sensitive structures in the vertebral canal in a group of physiotherapy students. South African Journal of Physiotherapy. 36:4–12, 1980

354. Maitland GD: Vertebral Manipulations, 5th ed. Boston, Butterworths, 1986

355. Maitland GD: The Maitland concept: Assessment, examination and treatment by passive movements. In Twomey LT, Taylor JR (eds): Physical Therapy of the Low Back, pp 135–156. New York, Churchill Livingstone, 1987

356. Mandal AC: The correct height of school furniture. Physiotherapy 70:48–53, 1984

357. Mannheimer JS, Lampe GN: Clinical Transcutaneous Electrical Nerve Stimulation. Philadelphia, FA Davis, 1984

358. Masi AT, Muhammad B, Yunus MD: Concepts of illness in populations as applied to fibromyalgia syndromes. Am J Med (Suppl 3A)81:19–25, 1986

359. Matheson L, Ogden L: Work Tolerance Screening. Trabues Canyon, CA, Rehabilitation Institute of Southern California, 1983

360. Mathews J: Dynamic discography: A study of lumbar traction. Ann Phys Med 9:275–279, 1968

361. Mathews J: The effects of spinal traction. Physiotherapy 58:64–66, 1972

362. Mathews JA, Hickling J: Lumbar traction: A double-blind controlled study for sciatica. Rheumatol Rehabil 14:222–225, 1975

363. Mathews JA, Mills SB, Jenkins VM, et al: Back pain and sciatica: Controlled trials of manipulation, traction, sclerosant and epidural injections. Br J Rheumatol: 26:416–423, 1987

364. Matson DD, Woods RP, Campbell JB, et al: Diastematomyelia (congenital clefts of the spinal cord). Pediatrics 6:98–112, 1950

365. Mattmiller AW: The California back school. Physiotherapy 66:118–121, 1986

366. Maxwell TD: The piriformis muscle and its relation to the long-legged syndrome. J Can Chir Assoc 51:10–24, 1978

367. Mayer DJ, Price DD: Central nervous system mechanisms of analgesia. Pain 2:379–404, 1976

368. Mayer H, Mayer TG: Functional Restoration: New concepts in spinal rehabilitation. In Kirkaldy-Willis WH (ed): Managing Low Back Pain. New York, Churchill Livingstone, 1988

369. Mayer TG, Gatchel RJ: Functional Restoration for Spinal Disorders: The Sports Medicine Approach. Philadelphia, Lea & Febiger, 1988

370. Mayer TG, Gatchel RJ, Kishino N, et al: Objective assessment of spine function following industrial injury: A prospective study with comparison and one-year follow-up. Spine 10:482–493, 1985

371. Mayer TG, Kishino N, Kedy J, et al: Using physical measurements to assess low back pain. J Musculoskel Med 2:44–51, 1985

372. Mayer TG, Smith SS, Keeley J, et al: Qualification of lumbar function: II. Sagittal plane trunk strength in chronic low-back pain patients. Spine 10:765–772, 1985

373. Mayer TG, Smith SS, Tencer A, et al: Measurement of isometric and multispeed isokinetic strength of lumbar spine musculature using a prototype Cybex testing device on normal subjects and patients with chronic low back pain. Proceedings of the International Society for Study of the Lumbar Spine, Montreal, Canada, 1983

374. Mayer TG, Tencer AF, Kristoferson S, et al: Use of noninvasive techniques for qualification of spinal range of motion in normal subjects and chronic low-back dysfunction patients. Spine 9:588–595, 1984

375. Mazess RB: On aging bone loss. Clin Orthop 165:237–252, 1983

376. McCain GA: Role of physical fitness training in the fibrositis/fibromyalgia syndrome. Am J Med (Suppl 3A) 81:73–77, 1986

377. McCall IW, Park WM, O'Brien JP: Induced pain referral from posterior lumbar elements in normal subjects. Spine 4:441–448, 1979

378. McCarthy RE: Coping with low back pain through behavioral change. Orthopedic Nursing 3:30–35, 1983

379. McKenna O, Murtagh A: The physical examination of the back. Aust Fam Physician 14:1244–1256, 1985

380. McKenzie RA: Manual correction of sciatic scoliosis. NZ Med J 76:194–199, 1972

381. McKenzie RA: Prophylaxis in recurrent low back pain. NZ Med J 89:22–23, 1979

382. McKenzie RA: Treat Your Own Back. Waikanae, New Zealand, Spinal Publications Ltd, 1980

383. McKenzie RA: The Lumbar Spine: Mechanical Diagnosis and Therapy. Waikanae, New Zealand, Spinal Publications Ltd, 1981

384. McKenzie RA: Mechanical diagnosis and therapy for low back pain: Toward a better understanding. In Twomey LT, Taylor JR (eds): Physical Therapy of the Low Back, pp 157–174. New York, Churchill Livingstone, 1987

385. McKinley JC, Hathaway SR: The identification and measurement of the neuroses in medical practice. JAMA 23:161–167, 1943

386. McNeill T, Warwick D, Andersson G, et al: Trunk strengths in attempted flexion, extension and lateral bending in healthy subjects and patients with low back disorders. Spine 5:529–538, 1980

387. McQuarrie A: Physical therapy. In Kirkaldy-Willis WH (ed): Managing Low Back Pain, pp 345–354. New York, Churchill Livingstone, 1988

388. Meagher J, Boughton P: Sports Massage. New York, Doubleday, 1980

389. Meikle JCE: The Minnesota Multiphasic Personality Inventory (MMPI) and back pain. Clinical Rehabilitation 1:143–145, 1987

390. Melzack R: The Puzzle of Pain. New York, Basic Books, 1973

391. Melzack R; The McGill pain questionnaire: Major properties and scoring methods. Pain 1:277–299, 1975

392. Melzack R, Vetere P, Finch L: TENS for low back pain Phys Ther 63:489–493, 1983

393. Melzack R, Wall PD: The Challenge of Pain. New York, Basic Books, 1983

394. Mennell JB: The Science and Art of Joint Manipulation, Vol 2. London, Churchill, 1952

395. Mennell J MCM: Back Pain. Boston, Little, Brown & Co, 1960

396. Mennell J MCM: Joint Pain. Boston, Little, Brown & Co, 1960

397. Miller WT: Introduction to Clinical Radiology. New York, MacMillian, 1982

398. Mitchell FL: An Evaluation and Treatment Manual of Osteopathic Muscle Energy Procedures, 1st ed. Valley Park, MO, Mitchell, Moran, Pruzzo, 1979

399. Mitchell PEG, Hendry MGC, Billewicz WZ: The chemical background of intervertebral disc prolapse. J Bone Joint Surg 43(B):141–151, 1961

400. Mixter WJ, Barr JS: Rupture of the intervertebral disc with involvement of the spinal canal. N Engl J Med 211:210–215, 1934

401. Moll JMH, Liyanange SP, Wright V: An objective clinical method to measure lateral spine flexion. Rheumatol Rehabil 11:225–239, 1972

402. Moll JMH, Liyanange SP, Wright V: An objective clinical method to measure spinal extension. Rheumatol Rehabil 11:293–312, 1972

403. Moll JMH, Wright V: Measurement of spinal movement. In Jayson M (ed): The Lumbar Spine and Back Pain, pp 93–112. New York, Grune & Stratton, 1981

404. Mooney V: Alternative approaches for the patient beyond the help of surgery. Orthop Clin North Am 6:331–334, 1975

405. Mooney V: The syndromes of low back disease. Orthop Clin North Am 14:505–515, 1983

406. Mooney V: Evaluation and guidelines for nonoperative care of the low back. Instr Course Lect 34:3–16, 1985

407. Mooney V, Cairns D, Robertson JA: A system for evaluating and treating chronic back disability. West J Med 124:370–376, 1976

408. Mooney V, Robertson J: The facet syndrome. Clin Orthop 115:149–156, 1976

409. Moore M: Endorphins and exercise: A puzzling relationship. Physician Sports Med 10:111–114, 1982

410. Moran FP, King T: Primary instability of the lumbar vertebrae as a common cause of low back pain. J Bone Joint Surg 39(B):6–22, 1957

411. Morgan D: Concepts in functional training and pos-

tural stabilization for low back injured. Topics in Acute Care and Trauma Rehabilitation: Industrial Back Injury: Part II. Clinical Applications. Aspen, CO, Aspen, Pub, 1988

412. Morgan D, Vollowitz E: Training the Patient with Low Back Dysfunction. Course notes, February 27–28, Folsom Physical Therapy Education Division. Folsom, CA, 1988

413. Morgan FP, King T: Primary instability of the lumbar vertebrae as a common cause of low back pain. J Bone Joint Surg 39(B):6–22, 1957

414. Morris JM, Lucus DB, Besler B: The role of the trunk in the stability of the spine. J Bone Joint Surg 43(A):327–351, 1961

415. Morris JM, Markoff KL: Biomechanics of the lumbar spine. In American Academy of Orthopaedic Surgeons: Atlas of Orthotics, pp 312–331. St Louis, CV Mosby, 1975

416. Mottice M, Goldberg D, Bennr EK, et al: Soft Tissue Mobilization. Monroe Falls, Ohio, JEMD Publications, 1986

417. Mulligan BR: Belt techniques. In Grieves GP(ed): Modern Manual Therapy of the Vertebral Column, New York, Churchill Livingstone, 1986

418. Murtagh J, Findlay D, Kenna C: Low back pain. Aust Fam Physician 14:1214–1224, 1985

419. Murtagh JE, McKenna OJ: Muscle energy therapy. Aust Fam Physician 15:756–765, 1987

420. Nachemson AL: The load on lumbar discs in different positions of the body. Clin Orthop 45:107–122, 1966

421. Nachemson A: Towards a better understanding of low back pain. A review of the mechanics of the lumbar disc. Rheumatol Rehabil 14:129–143, 1975

422. Nachemson AL: The lumbar spine: An orthopedic challenge. Spine 1:59–71, 1976

423. Nachemson AL: Work for all: For those with low back pain as well. Clin Orthop 179:77–85, 1983

424. Nachemson AL: Recent advances in the treatment of low back pain. Int Orthop 9:1–10, 1985

425. Nachemson AL: Lumbar instability: A critical update and symposium summary. Spine 10:290–291, 1985

426. Nachemson A, Bigos SJ: The low back. In Cruess RL, Rennie WRJ (eds): Adult Orthopedics, Vol 2, pp 843–938. New York, Churchill Livingstone, 1984

427. Nachemson A, Lindh M: Measurement of abdominal and back muscle strength with and without low back pain. Scand J Rehabil Med 1:60–65, 1965

428. Nachemson A, Morris JM: In vivo measurement of intradiskal pressures. J Bone Joint Surg 46(A):1077–1092, 1964

429. Nagi SZ, Riley LE, Newby LG: A social epidemiology of back pain in a general population. J Chronic Dis 26:769–779, 1973

430. Nassim R, Burrows HJ (eds): Modern Trends in Diseases of Vertebral Column. London, Butterworth, 1959

431. Natchev E: A Manual on Autotraction Treatment for Low Back Pain. Stockholm, E Nachev, 1984

432. Naylor A: The biophysical and biochemical aspects of intervertebral disc herniation and degeneration. Ann R Coll Surg 31:91–114, 1962

433. Naylor A: Intervertebral disc prolapse and degeneration. Spine 1:108–114, 1976

434. Naylor A, Happey F, MacRae T: The collagenous changes in the intervertebral disc with age and their effect on its elasticity. Br Med J 2:570–573, 1954

435. Nelson MA, Allen P, Clamp SE, et al: Reliability and reproducibility of clinical findings in low back pain. Spine 4:97–101, 1979

436. Newman PH: "Sprung back." J Bone Joint Surg 34(B):30–37, 1952

437. Newman PH: The etiology of spondylolisthesis. J Bone Joint Surg 45(B):39–59, 1963

438. Newman PH: The spine, the wood and the trees. Proc R Soc Med 61:35–41, 1968

439. Newman PH: Surgical treatment for derangement of the lumbar spine. J Bone Joint Surg 55:7–19, 1973

440. Nicolaisen T, Jorgensen K: Trunk strength, back muscle endurance and low-back trouble. Scand J Rehabil Med 17:121–127, 1985

441. Norby E: Epidemiology and diagnosis in low back injury. Occup Health Saf 50:38–42, 1981

442. Nordin M, Kahanovitz N, Verderame R, et al: Normal trunk muscle strength and endurance in women and the effect of exercise and electrical stimulation: Part I. Normal endurance and trunk muscle strength in 101 women. Spine 12:105–111, 1987

443. Nosse LJ: Inverted spinal traction. Arch Phys Med Rehabil 59:367–370, 1978

444. Nummi J, Jarvinen T, Stambej U, et al: Diminished dynamic performance capacity of back and abdominal muscles in concrete reinforcement workers. Scand J Work Environ Health (Suppl 4) 1:39–46, 1985

445. O'Brian JP: The role of fusion for chronic low back pain. Orthop Clin North Am 14:639–647, 1983

446. O'Connell JEA: Protrusion of lumbar intervertebral discs: A clinical review based on five hundred cases treated by excision of the protrusion. J Bone Joint Surg 33(B):8–30, 1951

447. Oliver JO, Lynn JW, Lynn JM: An interpretation of the McKenzie approach to low back pain. In Twomey LT, Taylor JR (eds): Physical Therapy of the Low Back, pp 225–251. New York, Churchill Livingstone, 1987

448. Onishi N, Nomara H: Low back pain in relation to physical work capacity and local tenderness. J Human Ergol 2:119–132, 1973

449. Ottenbacker K, Defabio RP: Efficacy of spinal manipulations/mobilization therapy: A meta-analysis. Spine 10:833–837, 1985

450. Ottoson D, Ekblom A, Hansson P: Vibratory stimulation for the relief of pain of dental origin. Pain 10:37–45, 1981

451. Oudenhoven RC: Gravitational lumbar traction. Arch Phys Med Rehabil 59:510–512, 1978

452. Pace JB, Nagle D: Piriformis syndrome. West J Med 124:435–439, 1976

453. Palastanga N: The use of transverse frictions of the

soft tissue. In Grieve GP (ed): Modern Manual Therapy of the Vertebtal Column, pp 819–826. New York, Churchill Livingston, 1986

454. Palastanga N: Connective tissue massage. In Grieve GP: Modern Manual Therapy of the Vertebral Column, pp 827–833. New York, Churchill Livingstone, 1986

455. Paris SV: The theory and technique of specific spinal manipulations. NZ Med J 62:320–321, 1963

456. Paris SV: The Spinal Lesion. New Zealand, Degasus Press, 1965

457. Paris SV: Mobilization of the spine. Phys Ther 59:988–995, 1979

458. Paris SV: Anatomy as related to function and pain. Orthop Clin North Am 14:475–489, 1983

459. Paris SV: Clinical decision: Orthopaedic physical therapy. In Wolf SL (ed): Clinical Decision Making in Physical Therapy, pp 215–254. Philadelphia, FA Davis, 1985

460. Paris SV: Physical signs of instability. Spine 10:277–279, 1985

461. Park WM: Radiological investigation of the intervertebral disc. In Jayson MIV (ed): The Lumbar Spine and Back Pain, 2nd ed, pp 185–230. Kent, England, Pitman, 1980

462. Parson W, Cummings J: Mechanical traction in the lumbar disc syndrome. Can Med Assoc J 77:7–11, 1957

463. Patterson MM: A model mechanism for spinal segmental facilitation. J Am Osteopath Assoc 76:121–131, 1976

464. Pederson OF, Peterson R, Staffeldt ES: Back pain and isometric back muscle strength of workers in a Danish factory. Scand J Rehabil Med 7:125–128, 1975

465. Peltier LF: The classic back strain and sciatica. Clin Orthop 219:4–6, 1987

466. Pheasant HC: Sources of failure in laminectomies. Orthop Clin North Am 6:319–329, 1975

467. Piedalla P: Problemes sacroiliaques. Home Sain II. Bordeaux, Biere, 1952

468. Pope MH, Rosen JD, Wilder DG, et al: The relation between biomechanical and psychological factors in patients with low back pain. Spine 5:173–178, 1980

469. Porter RW, Hibbert C, Evans C: The natural history of the root entrapment syndrome. Spine 9:418–421, 1984

470. Porterfield JA: The sacro-iliac joint. In Gould JA, Davies GJ (ed): Orthopaedic and Sports Physical Therapy, pp 550–580. St Louis, CV Mosby, 1985

471. Porterfield JA, Mostardi RA, King S, et al: Simulated lift testing using computerized isokinetics. Spine 12:683–687, 1987

472. Posner I, White AA, Edwards WT, et al: A biomechanical analysis of the clinical stability of the lumbar and lumbosacral spine. Spine 7:374–389, 1982

473. Pritzker KPH: Aging and degeneration in the lumbar intervertebral discs. Orthop Clin North Am 8:65–75, 1977

474. Pug MM, Laorden ML, Miralles FS, et al: Endorphin levels in cerebrospinal fluid of patients with postoperative and chronic pain. Anesthesiology 57:1–4, 1982

475. Quebec Task Force on Spinal Disorders: Report of the Quebec Task Force on Spinal Disorders. Spine (Suppl) 12(7):S1–S54, 1987

476. Rae PS, Waddell B, Verner RM: A simple technique for measuring lumbar flexion. J R Coll Surg Edinb 29:281–284, 1984

477. Ramani PS, Perry RH, Tomlinson BE: Role of ligamentum flavum in the symptomatology of prolapsed lumbar intervertebral disc. J Neurol Neurosurg Psychiatry 38:550–557, 1975

478. Ransford AO, Cairns D, Mooney V: The pain drawing as an aid to the psychologic evaluation of patients with low back pain. Spine 1:127–134, 1976

479. Rasmussen GG: Manipulation in the treatment of low back pain: A randomized clinical trial (abstr). Man Med 1:8–21, 1979

480. Reuler JB: Low back pain. West J Med 143:259–265, 1985

481. Ritchie JH, Faharni WH: Age changes in intervertebral discs. Can J Surg 13:65–71, 1970

482. Rockey PH, Tomkins RK, Wood RW: The usefulness of x-ray examination in the evaluation of patients with back pain. J Fam Pract 7:455–465, 1978

483. Rockoff SD, Sweet E, Bluestein J: The relative contribution of trabecular and cortical bone to the strength of human lumbar vertebrae. Calcif Tissue Res 3:163–175, 1969

484. Roofe PG: Innervation of annulus fibrosis and posterior longitudinal ligaments: Fourth and fifth lumbar level. Arch Neurol Psych 44:100–103, 1940

485. Rothman RH: Indications for lumbar fusion. Clin Neurosurg 20:215–219, 1973

486. Rothman RH, Simeone FA: The Spine. Philadelphia, WB Saunders, 1982

487. Rovere GD: Low back pain in athletes. Physician Sports Med 15:105–117, 1987

488. Rowe ML: Low back pain in industry: A position paper. J Occup Med 11:161–169, 1969

489. Salib R: Gravity lumbar reduction traction: The results for documented lumbar disc herniation. Presented at the meeting of the Society for the Study of the Lumbar Spine, Sydney, Australia, November 23–24, 1985

490. Salisbury PJ, Porter RW: Measurement of lumbar sagittal mobility: A comparison of methods. Spine 12:190–193, 1987

491. Saunders DH: Use of spinal traction in the treatment of neck and back conditions. Clin Orthop 179:31–37, 1983

492. Saunders DH: Educational back care programs. In Saunders DH: Evaluation, Treatment and Prevention of Musculoskeletal Disorders, pp 297–324. Viking Press, Minneapolis, 1985

493. Saunders DH: Evaluation, Treatment and Prevention of Musculoskeletal Disorders. Minneapolis, Viking Press, 1985

494. Sawyer WM: The role of the physical therapist before and after lumbar spine surgery. Orthop Clin North Am 14:649–659, 1983

495. Scham SM, Taylor TKF: Tension signs in lumbar disc prolapse. Clin Orthop 75:195–204, 1971

496. Schatzker J, Pennal GF: Spinal stenosis: A cause of cauda equina compression. J Bone Joint Surg 50(B):606–608, 1968

497. Schmorl G, Jungham H: The Human Spine in Health and Disease, 2nd ed. New York, Grune & Stratton, 1971

498. Schned ES: Ankylosing spondylitis. In Beary JF, Christian CL, Johanson MA (eds): Manual of Rheumatology and Outpatient Orthopedic Disorders: Diagnosis and Therapy. Boston, Little Brown & Co, 1987

499. Schuchmann JA: Low back pain: A comprehensive approach. Compr Ther 14:14–18, 1987

500. Schultz A, Andersson G, Ortengren R, et al: Loads on the lumbar spine, validation and biomechanical analysis by measurements of intradiscal pressures and myoelectric signals. J Bone Joint Surg 64(5):713–720, 1982

501. Scott J, Huskisson EC: Graphic representation of pain. Pain 2:175–184, 1976

502. Scott ME: Spinal osteoporosis in the aged. Aust Fam Physician 3:281, 1974

503. Scott V, Gijsbers K: Pain perception in competitive swimmers. Br Med J 283:91–93, 1981

504. Seimons LP: Low Back Pain: Clinical Diagnosis and Management. Norwalk, CT, Appleton–Century–Crofts, 1983

505. Selby DK, Paris SV: Anatomy of facet joints and its correlation with low back pain. Contemporary Orthopedics 31:1097–1103, 1981

506. Shah JS: Structure, morphology and mechanics of the lumbar spine. In Jayson M (ed): The Lumbar Spine and Low Back Pain, pp 359–406. London, Pittman Medical, 1980

507. Shealy CN: Facet denervation in the management of back and sciatic pain. Clin Orthop 115:159–164, 1976

508. Shealy CN, Shealy M: Behavioral techniques in control of pain: A case for health maintenance vs disease treatment. In Weisenberg M, Tursky B (eds): Pain: New Perspectives in Therapy and Research, pp 21–34. New York, Plenum Press, 1976

509. Sheon RP: Regional myofascial pain and the fibrositis syndrome (fibromyalgia). Compr Ther 12:42–52, 1986

510. Sherrington C: The integrative action of the nervous system. New Haven, Yale University Press, 1961

511. Sikorski JM: A rationalized approach to physiotherapy for low-back pain. Spine 10:571–579, 1985

512. Simons DG: Muscle pain syndromes: Part I. Am J Phys Med 54:289–311, 1975

513. Simons DG: Muscle pain syndromes: Part II. Am J Phy Med 55:15–42, 1976

514. Simons DG, Travell JG: Myofascial origins of low back pain: 1. Principles of diagnosis and treatment. Post Grad Med 73:66–77, 1983

515. Simons DG, Travell JG: Myofascial origins of low back pain: 2. Torso muscles. Post Grad Med 73:81–92, 1983

516. Simons DG, Travell JG: Myofascial origins of low back pain: 3. Pelvic and lower extremity muscles. Post Grad Med 73:99–108, 1983

517. Simons DG, Travell JG: Myofascial pain syndromes. In Wall PD, Melzack R (eds): Textbook of Pain, pp 263–276. New York, Churchill Livingstone, 1984

518. Sims FH, Dahlin DC: Primary bone tumors simulating lumbar disc syndrome. Spine 2:65–74, 1977

519. Smidt G: Inversion traction: Effects on spinal column, heart rate and blood pressure (abstr). Presented at the meeting of the International Society for the Study of the Lumbar Spine, Sydney, Australia, November 23–24, 1985

520. Smidt GL, Blanpied PR, Anderson MA, et al: Comparison of clinical and objective methods of assessing trunk muscle strength: An experimental approach. Spine 12:1020–1024, 1987

521. Smith AE: Physical activity: A tool in promoting mental health. J Psychiatr Nurs 11:24–25, 1979

522. Smith SS, TG Mayer, Gatchel RJ, et al: Qualification of lumbar function: I. Isometric and multispeed isokinetic trunk strength measures in sagittal and axial planes in normal subjects. Spine 10:757–764, 1985

523. Smyth MJ, Wright V: Sciatica and intervertebral disc: An experimental study. J Bone Joint Surg 40(A):1401–1418, 1958

524. Smythe HA: Non-articular rheumatism and the fibrositis syndrome. In Hollander JL, McCarty DJ (eds): Arthritis and Allied Conditions, 8th ed, pp 874–884. Philadelphia, Lea & Febiger, 1972

525. Smythe HA: Nonarticular rheumatism and psychogenic musculoskeletal syndromes. In McCarty DJ (ed): Arthritis and Allied Conditions: Textbook of Rheumatology, 9th ed, pp 1083–1094. Philadelphia, Lea & Febiger, 1979

526. Smythe H: Referred pain and tender points Am J Med (Suppl 3A) 81:90–98, 1986

527. Snoek W, Weber H, Jorgensen B: Double-blind evaluation of extradural methylprednisolone for herniated lumbar disc. Acta Orthop Scand 48:635–641, 1977

528. Snook SH: The design of manual handling tasks. Ergonomics 21:963–985, 1978

529. Snook SH: Low back pain in industry. In White AA, Gordon SL (eds): American Academy of Orthopaedic Surgeons Symposium on Idiopathic Low Back Pain, pp 23–48. St Louis, CV Mosby, 1980

530. Sorensen KH: Scheuermann's juvenile kyphosis. Thesis, Copenhagen, Munksgaard, 1964

531. Spangfort EV: The lumbar disc herniation: A computer-aided analysis of 2,504 operations. Acta Orthop Scand (Suppl) 142:1–95, 1972

532. Spencer DL, Irwin GS, Millar JAA: Anatomy and significance of fixation of the lumbosacral nerve roots in sciatica. Spine 8:672–679, 1983

533. Spengler DM, Freeman CW: Patient selection for lumbar discectomy: An objective approach. Spine 4:129–134, 1979

534. Spengler DM, Freeman CW: Low Back Pain: Assessment and Management. New York, Grune & Stratton, 1982

535. Staffel F: Zur Hygiene des Sitzens Gesundheitspflege 3:403–421, 1983

536. Steindler A, Luck JV: Differential diagnosis of pain low in the back. JAMA 111:106–112, 1938

537. Steiner C, Staubs C, Ganon M, et al: Piriformis syndrome: Pathogenesis, diagnosis, and treatment. J Am Osteopath Assoc 87:318–323, 1987

538. Steinmetz ND: MRI of the Lumbar Spine: A Practical Approach to Image Interpretation. Thorofare, NJ, Slack, 1987

539. Sternbach RA: Pain Patients: Traits and Treatment. New York, Academic Press, 1974

540. Stewart ML: Measurement of clinical pain. In Jacox AK (ed): Pain: A Source Book for Nurses and Other Health Professionals. Boston, Little, Brown & Co, 1977

541. Stoddard A: Conditions of the sacro-iliac joints and their treatment. Physiotherapy 44:97, 1958

542. Stoddard A: Manual of Osteopathic Technique. London, Hutchinson, 1959

543. Stoddard A: Cervical spondylosis and cervical osteoarthritis. Man Med 2:31, 1970

544. Stoddard A: Manual of Osteopathic Techniques, 1st ed. London, Hutchinson, 1980

545. Stokes IAF, Frymoyer JM, Lunn RA: Segmental motion and segmental instability (abstr). Orthop Trans 10:517–518, 1986

546. Strachan A: Back care in industry. Physiotherapy 65:249–251, 1949

547. Strange FG: Debunking the disc. Proc R Soc Med 9:952–956, 1966

548. Stubbs DA, Buckle PW, Hudson MP, et al: Back pain in the nursing profession: I. Epidemiology and pilot methodology. Ergonomics 26:755–765, 1983

549. Stubbs DA, Buckle PW, Hudson MP et al: Back pain in the nursing profession: II. The effectiveness of training. Ergonomics 26:767–779, 1983

550. Sugiura K, Yoshida T, Mimatsu T: A study of tension signs in lumbar disc hernia. Int Orthop 3:225–228, 1979

551. Sullivan PE, Markos PD, Minor MAD: Low back. In Sullivan PE, Markos PD, Minor MAD (eds): Approach to Therapeutic Exercise: Theory and Clinical Application pp 333–351. Reston, VA, Reston Pub Co, 1982

552. Sullivan PE, Markos PD: Therapeutic exercise for the patient with low back disorders. In Sullivan PE, Markos PD: Clinical Procedures in Therapeutic Exercise, pp 211–218. Los Altos, CA, Appleton & Lange, 1987

553. Sunderland S: The anatomy of the intervertebral foramen and mechanism of compression and stretch of nerve roots. In Haldemann S: Modern Developments in Principles and Practice of Chiropractics, pp 297–299. New York, Appleton–Century–Crofts, 1980

554. Suzuki N, Endo S: A quantitative study of trunk muscle strength and fatigability in low-back syndrome. Spine 8:69–74, 1983

555. Svensson HL, Andersson GBJ: Low back pain in 40- to 47-year-old men: I. Frequency of occurrence and impact on medical services. Scand J Rehabil Med 14:47–53, 1982

556. Svensson HL, Andersson GBJ: Low back pain in 40- to 47-year-old men. Spine 8:272–276, 1983

557. Svensson HL, Vedin A, Wihelmsson C, et al: Low back pain in relation to other diseases and cardiovascular risk factors. Spine 8:277–285, 1983

558. Sylven B: On the biology of nucleus pulposus. Acta Orthop Scand 20:275–279, 1951

559. Tanigawa M: Comparison of the hold–relax procedure and passive mobilization in increasing muscle length. Phys Ther 52:725–735, 1972

560. Tappan FM: Healing Massage Techniques: A Study of Eastern and Western Methods. Reston VA, Reston Pub Co, 1978

561. Tauber J: An unorthodox look at backaches. J Occup Med 12:128–130, 1970

562. Taylor TKF, Weiner M: Great-toe extensor reflexes in the diagnosis of lumbar disc disorder. Br Med J 2:487, 1969

563. Terenius L: Endorphins and pain. Front Horm Res 8:162–171, 1981

564. Thompson NN, Gould JA, Davies GJ, et al: Descriptive measures of isokinetic trunk testing. J Orthop Sports Phys Ther 3:164–170, 1982

565. Thompson NN, Gould JA, Davies GJ, et al: Descriptive measures of isokinetic trunk testing. J Orthop Sports Phys Ther 7:43–49, 1985

566. Thorsteinsson A, Nilsson J: Trunk muscle strength during constant and velocity movements. Scand J Rehabil Med 14:61–68, 1982

567. Tichauer ER: The Biomedical Basis of Ergonomics: Anatomy Applied to the Design of The Work Situation, New York, Wiley Inter-Sciences, 1978

568. Twomey LT, Taylor JR: A description of two new instruments measuring the ranges of sagittal and horizontal plane motions in the lumbar region. Aust J Physiother 31:106–112, 1985

569. Traut FF: Fibrositis. J Am Geriatr Soc 16:531–538, 1968

570. Travel JG, Simons DG: Myofascial Pain and Dysfunction: The Trigger Point Manual. Baltimore, William & Wilkins, 1983

571. Trott PH, Grant R, Maitland GD: Manipulative therapy for the low lumbar spine: Technique, selection, and application to some syndromes. In Twomey LT, Taylor JR (eds): Physical Therapy of the Low Back, pp 199–224. New York, Churchill Livingstone, 1987

572. Troup JDG: Causes, prediction and prevention of back pain at work. Scand J Work Environ Health 10:419–428, 1984

573. Troup JDG, Martin JW, Lloyd DCEF: Back pain in industry: A prospective survey. Spine 6:61–69, 1981

574. Troup JDG, Roantree WB, Archibald RM: Survey of cases of lumbar spinal disability. A methodological study. Med Officers Boardsheet, National Coal Board, 1970

575. Tursky B: The development of a pain perception pro-

file: A psychophysical approach. In Weisenberg M, Tursky B (eds): Pain: New Perspectives in Therapy and Research, pp 171–194. New York, Plenum Press, 1976

576. Twomey LT: Sustained lumbar traction: An experimental study of long spine segments. Spine 10:167–169, 1985

577. Twomey LT, Taylor JR: A description of two new instruments measuring the ranges of sagittal and horizontal plane motions in the lumbar region. Aust J Physiother 31:106–112, 1985

578. Urban LM: The straight-leg-raising test: A review. J Orthop Sports Phys Ther 2:117–133, 1981

579. Urban LM: The straight-leg raising test: A review. In Grieve GP (ed): Modern Manual Therapy of the Vertebral Column, pp 567–575. New York, Churchill Livingstone, 1986

580. Valkenberg HA, Haanen HCM: The epidemiology of low back pain. In White AA, Gordon SL (eds): American Academy of Orthopaedic Surgeons Symposium on Idiopathic Low Back Pain, pp 9–22. St Louis, CV Mosby, 1982

581. Van Akkerveeken PF, O'Brien JP, Park W: Experimentally induced hypermobility in the lumbar spine. Spine 4:236–241, 1979

582. Vanharanta H, Videman T, Mooney V: McKenzie exercise, back track and back school in lumbar syndrome (abstr). Orthop Trans 10:533, 1986

583. Van Wijmen PM: The management of recurrent low back pain. In Grieve GP (ed): Modern Manual Therapy of the Vertebral Column, pp 756–776. New York, Churchill Livingstone, 1986

584. Vollowitz E: Furniture prescription for the conservative management of low back pain. In Topics in Acute Care and Trauma Rehabilitation. Industrial Back Injury: Part II. Clinical Applications. Aspen, CO, Aspen Publications, 1988

585. Voss DE, Ionta MK, Myer BJ: Proprioceptive Neuromuscular Facilitation, 3rd ed. Philadelphia, Harper & Row, 1985

586. Waddell G: A new clinical model for treatment of low back pain. Spine 12:632–644, 1987

587. Waddell G, Main CJ, Morris EW, et al: Normality and reliability in the clinical assessment of backache. Br Med J 284:1519–1523, 1982

588. Waddell G, Main CJ, Morris EW, et al: Chronic low back pain, psychological distress and illness behavior. Spine 9:209–213, 1984

589. Waddell G, McCulloch JA, Kummel EG, et al: Nonorganic physical signs in low back pain. Spine 5:117–125, 1980

590. Waitz E: The lateral bending sign. Spine 6:388–397, 1981

591. Walker JM: Deep transverse frictions in ligament healing. J Orthop Sports Phys Ther 6:89–94, 1984

592. Walters A: Psychogenic regional pain alias hysterical pain. Brain 84:1–18, 1961

593. Watkins R, O'Brien J, Drauglis R, et al: Comparison of preoperative and postoperative MMPI data in chronic back patients. Spine 11:385–390, 1986

594. Weber H: Lumbar disc herniation: A controlled prospective study with ten years of observation. Spine 8:131–140, 1983

595. Weber H, Ljunggren AI, Walker L: Traction therapy in patients with herniated lumbar intervertebral disc. J Oslo City Hosp 34:61–70, 1984

596. Wedge JH: The natural history of spinal degeneration. In Kirkalady-Willis WH (ed): Managing Low Back Pain, pp 3–8. New York, Churchill Livingstone, 1983

597. Weintraube A: Soft tissue mobilization of the lumbar spine. In Grieve GP (ed): Modern Manual Therapy of the Vertebral Column, pp 750–755. New York, Churchill Livingstone, 1986

598. Wells PE: The examination of the pelvic joints. In Greive GP (ed): Modern Manual Therapy of the Vertebral Column, pp 590–564. New York, Churchill Livingstone, 1986

599. White AA: Injection technique for the diagnosis and treatment of low back pain. Orthop Clin North Am 14:553–567, 1983

600. White AA, Gordon SL: Synopsis workshop on idiopathic low-back pain. Spine 7:141–149, 1982

601. White AA, McBride ME, Wiltse LL, et al: The management of patients with back pain and idiopathic vertebral sclerosis. Spine 11:607–616, 1986

602. White AA, Panjabi MM: Clinical Biomechanics of the Spine. Philadelphia, JB Lippincott, 1978

603. White AH: Back Schools and Other Conservative Approaches to Low Back Pain. St Louis, CV Mosby, 1983

604. White AA: Work hardening: General conditioning (abstr 91). Challenge of the Lumbar Spine, Ninth annual meeting, New York, October 7–10, 1987

605. Wiberg G: Back pain in relation to the nerve supply of the intervertebral disc. Acta Orthop Scand 19:211–221, 1949

606. Wiesel SW, Bernini P, Rothman RM, et al: Effectiveness of epidural steroids in the treatment of sciatica: A double-blind clinical trial. Presented at meeting of the International Society for the Study of the Lumbar Spine, Toronto, June 6–10, 1982

607. Wilkinson M: A neurological perspective. Rheum Rehabil 14:162–163, 1975

608. Williams SJ: The back school. Physiotherapy 63:90, 1977

609. Wiltse LL, Rocchio PD: Preoperative psychological tests as predictors of the success of chemonucleolysis in treatment of low back syndrome. J Bone Joint Surg 57(A):478–483, 1975

610. Wolfe F: The clinical syndrome of fibrositis. Am J Med (Suppl 3A) 81:99–104, 1986

611. Wolfe F: Development of criteria for the diagnosis of fibrositis. Am J Med (Suppl 3A) 81:99–104, 1986

612. Wolfe F, Hawley DJ, Cathey MA, et al: Fibrositis: Symptom frequency and criteria for diagnosis: Evaluation of 291 rheumatic disease patients and 58 normal individuals. J Rheumatol 12:1159–1163, 1985

613. Woodhall B, Hayes GJ: The well leg raising test of Fajersztajn in the diagnosis of ruptured lumbar inter-

vertebral disc. J Bone Joint Surg 32(A):786–792, 1950

614. Wyke B: The neurological basis of thoracic spinal pain. Rheum Phys Med 10:356–367, 1970

615. Wyke B: The neurology of low back pain. In Jayson, MIV (ed): The Lumbar Spine and Back Pain, 2nd ed, pp 265–340. London, Pitman Medical, 1980

616. Wyke B: Articular neurology and manipulative therapy. In Idezak RM (ed): Aspects of Manipulative Therapy. Carlton, Australia, Lincoln Institute of Health Sciences, 1980

617. Yao J: Acutherapy: Acupuncture, TENS and Acupressure. Acutherapy. Libertyville IL, Postgraduate, 1984

618. Young-Hing K, Reilly J, Kirkaldy-Willis WH: The ligamentum flavum. Spine 1:226–234, 1976

619. Young RJ: The effect of regular exercise on cognitive functioning and personality. Br J Sports Med 3:110–117, 1979

620. Yunus MB: Primary fibromyalgia syndrome: Current concepts. Compr Ther 10:21–28, 1984

621. Yunus MB, Kalgan-Raman UP, Kalyan-Raman K: Primary fibromyalgia syndrome and myofascial pain syndrome: Clinical features and muscle pathology. Arch Phys Med Rehabil 69:451–454, 1988

622. Yunus MB, Kalgan-Raman UP, Kalyan-Raman K, et al: Pathologic changes in muscle in primary fibromyalgia syndrome. Am J Med (Suppl 3A) 81:38–42, 1986

623. Yunus MB, Masi AT: Association of primary fibromyalgia syndrome (PFS) with stress-related syndrome. Clin Res 33:923A, 1985

624. Yunus MB, Masi AT, Aldag JC: Criteria studies of primary fibromyalgia syndrome (PFS). Arthritis Rheum 30(Suppl):S50, 1987

625. Yunus MB, Masi AT, Calabro JJ, et al: Primary fibromyalgia (fibrositis): Clinical study of 50 patients with matched normal controls. Semin Arthritis Rheum 11:151–171, 1981

626. Zachrisson Forsell M: The back school. Spine 6:104–106, 1981

627. Zylbergold RS, Piper MC: Cervical spine disorders: A comparison of three types of traction. Spine 10:867–871, 1985

21 The Lumbar–Lower Extremity Scan Examination

Randolph M. Kessler and Darlene Hertling

A common problem in the clinical examination of patients presenting with chronic, insidious musculoskeletal problems of the low back and lower extremities is not knowing to which area to direct physical examination procedures after completing the history portion of the examination. The reason for this is twofold: (1) chronic musculoskeletal disorders affecting the low back and the various regions of the lower limbs often present with similar pain patterns, and (2) biomechanical disorders affecting the back and various lower extremity regions often coexist. The former is a result of the common phenomenon of referred pain that is characteristic of most common musculoskeletal disorders; localized pain arising from deep somatic tissues is usually perceived in an area not corresponding well to the exact pathologic site. Thus, patients with "low-back pain" usually feel discomfort primarily in the upper buttock or sacroiliac regions, patients with trochanteric bursitis often have significant pain in the posterior hip and lateral thigh areas, and those with chondromalacia patellae frequently feel pain over the medial aspect of the distal thigh and upper leg. Also, as the severity of the pathologic process increases, there is greater likelihood that pain may be perceived throughout a distribution corresponding to any or all of the relevant sclerotome. So, if a relatively acute disorder affects a tissue innervated primarily by the L5 segment, the patient may feel pain in any or all of those regions also innervated by L5.

A typical example would be the patient with moderate to advanced degenerative hip disease who invariably experiences pain in the groin, spreading into the anterior thigh and to the knee—the L3 sclerotome. This occurs because the anterior aspect of the hip joint capsule, from which the pain primarily arises, is innervated largely by the L3 segment.

Similarly, the patient with involvement of the L3 segment of the spine from, for example, facet joint or disk, may feel pain that spreads in the same distribution as that described for hip joint disease. It may not be obvious from subjective information alone whether the hip, the low back, or both are involved. Likewise, it is often difficult to determine on the basis of subjective information alone whether a patient has trochanteric bursitis, an L5 spinal disorder, or both; the trochanteric region is innervated primarily by L5, and pain arising in conjunction with trochanteric bursitis is often felt down the lateral aspect of the thigh and dorsum of the leg (the L5 sclerotome), as may be the case with pain originating at the L5 spinal level.

Another classic example of localization of pain to distant regions of a relevant sclerotome occurs in the child with a hip joint disorder, such as a slipped capital femoral epiphysis, who feels pain primarily in the knee; both the hip and the knee joints are innervated largely by L3. Because delocalization and reference of pain are common phenomena, the subjective account of pain distribution does not provide a reliable indication of the true site of the pathologic process. Additional objective information is often required.

The prevalence of coexistent disorders or abnormalities of the low back and lower extremity regions is largely a result of the biomechanical interdependency of the weight-bearing joints in the closed kinetic chain. Normal attenuation of the energy introduced to the weight-bearing joints by the vertical displacement of the center of gravity requires that the overall displacement of the center of gravity be minimized, which in turn requires normal movement of the weight-bearing joints during stance phase of gait. Loss of critical movement at any of the weight-bearing joints will cause increased energy input to the entire weight-bearing skeleton from the force of the body weight acting over a greater distance, with the result being added vertical compressive loading during stance phase. Similarly, energy input to the weight-bearing joints in a horizontal plane is normally attenuated by joint movements. With the foot fixed to the ground, in order for the body to be normally moved through space in the presence of reduced critical movement at any joint, compensation is required at some other joint. Such an alteration in function is likely to result in added stresses to the compensating joint. Thus, the patient with loss of hip extension tends to walk with greater extension of the lower lumbar joints and the person with loss of ankle dorsiflexion undergoes greater-than-normal extension movements at the knee. Since the close-packed positions of the spine and knee are extension, these abnormalities are likely to cause increased subchondral compressive stresses and increased capsular tensile stresses to the knee and spinal joints.

Less obvious are the results of abnormalities in transverse rotation of the weight-bearing joints during stance phase of gait. From heel-strike to foot-flat the pelvis, thigh, and leg normally undergo internal rotatory movements, the distal segments more so than their supradjacent neighbors. The segments of the leg similarly undergo external rotation during foot-flat to toe-off. Since the foot is relatively fixed to the ground, however, it does not rotate. This means that the ankle–foot complex must absorb the rotatory movements imposed from above—internal rotation is absorbed by pronation of the foot, and external rotation is transmitted to the foot as a supinatory movement. The reader should observe the result of rotating the leg over the foot that is fixed to the ground; internal rotation causes the calcaneus to shift into valgus position and the medial arch to lower (pronation of the hindfoot), whereas external rotation brings the heel into varus position and raises the arch (supination of the hindfoot). It should also be noted that internal rotation of the thigh with the knee slightly bent causes an increased valgus angulation at the knee. This is of practical significance because the knee remains slightly bent during all phases of the gait cycle.

Again, because attenuation of the forces of the body weight moving over the fixed foot requires a normal contribution of movement from all weight-bearing joints, abnormalities of function at any one joint may affect the function of one or more of the others in the chain. A common example occurs in the person with increased femoral anteversion, who tends to walk with excessive internal rotation during stance phase of gait. This results in abnormal valgus angulation at the knee and increased foot pronation. The former may predispose to patellar tracking

problems, while the latter may lead to a variety of problems, including plantar fasciitis, heel spurs, hallux valgus, metatarsalgia, and fatigue of the intrinsic foot musculature (see Chapter 15, The Ankle and Hindfoot). On the other hand, a primary problem of abnormal foot pronation may lead to excessive internal rotatory and valgus stresses to the knee and increased internal rotation of the hip during gait. It should be clear that the best approach to management of pathologic lesions resulting from such biomechanical derangements would be one that takes into consideration primary etiologic factors. This often requires that evaluating procedures be directed to areas other than simply the primary region of involvement.

The above considerations should help emphasize the need to evaluate all of the weight-bearing joint regions in many, if not most, chronic musculoskeletal disorders affecting the low back or lower limb. A further factor to consider in this regard is the common phenomenon of summation of otherwise subliminal afferent input from coexistent minor disorders involving tissues innervated by the same or adjacent spinal segments. A common example is the person who stresses the joint capsules of the low back excessively throughout the day and who also has some low-grade inflammation of the trochanteric bursa. Noxious input from both areas may summate at the dorsal horn of the spinal cord, and other central neural connections, to cause more low-back pain as well as more lateral thigh pain than would be present if either disorder existed by itself. In this particular example the clinician must differentiate between the possibility of one lesion referring pain into another part of the relevant segment and two distinct pathologic processes within the same segment. This cannot be determined without evaluating both the low-back and the hip regions. Pain arising from the summation of input from different sites of the same segment will, of course, be more likely to occur in the patient with multisegmental restrictions of motion of the lower spine, since with daily activities the soft tissues (joint capsules and ligaments) of the spine will be stressed more, causing an increase in afferent input to the relevant spinal levels. In such cases, the threshold of pain arising from minor disorders affecting tissue in the lower limbs innervated by the corresponding spinal segments is probably reduced. Any back pain is likely to be enhanced by such segmentally related pathologic processes. Most persons, by middle age or later, develop some lower-lumbar facet-joint capsular restriction secondary to disk narrowing or other causes. Thus, middle-aged or older persons with chronic low-back or lower-limb pain should always be examined for coexistent segmental disorders that may be contributing to the amount of pain the person experiences.

In summary, the low back–lower extremity scan examination may be used to:

1. Determine the area of involvement in cases in which relatively vague subjective information fails to suggest the site of the pathologic process. This is not an uncommon occurrence and is related to the fact that pain of deep somatic origin may be referred to any or all of the relevant sclerotome.
2. Examine for the presence of some distant biomechanical derangement that may be related, in cause or effect, to the patient's primary physical lesion that causes his or her pain.
3. Rule out the possibility of some segmentally related disorder that may, by the mechanism of summation of segmentally related afferent input, contribute to the patient's pain perception.

The scan examination is oriented, then, toward detecting gross or subtle biomechanical abnormalities and toward determining the presence of common lumbar or lower extremity musculoskeletal disorders. Essential to the detection of significant biomechanical derangements are careful assessment of function (gait analysis), evaluation of bony structure and alignment, and examination of joint mobility. These examination procedures are combined with the key objective tests for the common chronic disorders affecting the lower back and lower extremities, to constitute the lumbar–lower extremity scan examination. A discussion of the common pathologic processes and their primary clinical manifestations will facilitate understanding and interpretation of the examination procedures involved in the scan examination.

COMMON LESIONS OF THE LOW BACK AND LOWER EXTREMITIES AND THEIR PRIMARY CLINICAL MANIFESTATIONS

THE LUMBOSACRAL REGION

I. **Acute (severe) posterolateral disk prolapse (outer annulus or posterior longitudinal ligament still intact)**
  A. *Subjective complaints*
    1. Sudden onset of unilateral lumbosacral pain, often with gradual buildup of pain intensity. Occasionally the patient denies a sudden onset and notes first experiencing pain on rising in the morning. There may be some aching in the leg.
    2. Worse with sitting and on rising from a long period of recumbency; somewhat relieved with recumbency
  B. *Key objective signs*
    1. Functional lumbar deformity, with a loss of lordosis and usually a lumbar scoliosis with the convexity to the involved side
    2. Marked, painful restriction of spinal movement, especially forward and backward bending
    3. Positive dural mobility tests; usually positive leg-raising tests bilaterally

II. **Acute facet-joint derangement**
  A. *Subjective complaints*
    1. Sudden onset of lumbosacral pain and deformity; little or no leg discomfort
    2. Pain is aggravated by being up and about and relieved by sitting or recumbency.
  B. *Key objective findings*
    1. Marked lumbar deformity; loss of lordosis and lumbar scoliosis with convexity to side of involvement
    2. Lumbar extension and sidebending to the side of involvement are painfully restricted. Forward bending and contralateral sidebending are slightly restricted.
    3. Negative dural signs

III. **Localized unilateral facet-joint capsular tightness**
  A. *Subjective complaints*
    1. Often a history of past episodes of acute low-back dysfunction
    2. Aching in the lumbosacral region, aggravated by long periods of standing, walking, or activities involving prolonged or repetitive lumbar extension; also worse with increased muscular tension, such as during periods of emotional stress, and worse in the evening than in the morning.
  B. *Key objective findings*
    1. Possible subtle predisposing biomechanical factor such as a leg-length disparity
    2. Possible minor restriction of sidebending to the involved side and deviation of spine toward the involved side on forward bending and away from the involved side on extension
    3. Discomfort on quadrant tests when localized to the involved segment

IV. **Multisegmental bilateral capsular restriction of lumbar facet joints — degenerative joint disease (DJD)**
   A. *Subjective complaints*
      1. The patient is middle-aged or older.
      2. Often there is a long history of intermittent back problems.
      3. Aching across the lower back and hip girdles is made worse with long periods of standing or walking. The back is stiff in the morning, somewhat better at midday, and aching again by evening. Some intermittent aching in one or both legs may occur.
   B. *Key objective findings*
      1. Some loss of the normal lumbar lordosis
      2. Restriction of spinal motion in a generalized capsular pattern of limitation: marked restriction of spinal extension, moderate restriction of sidebending bilaterally, and mild to moderate restriction of rotations and forward bending

V. **Lower lumbar disk extrusion with nerve root impingement**
   A. *Subjective complaints*
      1. Sudden or gradual onset of lumbosacral pain and unilateral leg pain. The patient may describe an onset suggestive of an acute posterolateral prolapse (see above) with progressive loss of back pain and increase in leg pain.
      2. The leg pain may be relatively sharp and is usually felt down the posterolateral thigh and into the anterolateral or posterior aspect of the lower leg. The leg pain may be aggravated by sitting or by being up and about and is relatively relieved by rest.
   B. *Key objective findings*
      1. Mild to moderate loss of lumbar movement, usually toward extension and in movements toward the side of involvement; it occasionally occurs away from the involved side.
      2. Mild segmental neurologic deficit
      3. Positive dural mobility signs

VI. **Acute sacroiliac dysfunction**
   A. *Subjective complaints*
      1. Sudden onset of unilateral sacroiliac pain, often associated with some twisting motion
      2. Occasional spread of pain to the posterior thigh

3. Pain is usually aggravated by activities involving combined hip and spine extension, such as standing erect (posterior torsional displacement). Less often it is aggravated by combined hip and spine flexion, such as sitting (anterior torsional displacement).
   B. *Key objective findings*
      1. Posterior torsional displacement (most common)
         a. Tendency to stand with the hip, knee, and low back slightly flexed on the involved side. If so, the knee landmarks and the greater trochanter will be lower on the involved side than on the uninvolved side. The posterior-superior iliac spine and iliac crest will also be lower on the involved side, more so than the knee landmarks and trochanter. The anterior-superior iliac spine will not be as low on the involved side as the knee and trochanteric landmarks. The pelvis will be shifted away from the involved side.
            If the patient stands with the legs straight, all of the landmarks up to and including the trochanters will be level. The posterior-superior iliac spine and iliac crest will be lower on the involved side than on the uninvolved side, but the anterior-superior iliac spine will be higher. The pelvis will appear to be rotated forward on the involved side.
         b. The anterior rotation test will be quite painful; the posterior rotation test will be less painful.
         c. Contralateral straight-leg raising may cause some pain, which is relieved when the involved leg is raised.
      2. Anterior torsional displacement (rare)
         a. Tendency to stand with the hip and knee in more extension on the involved side than on the uninvolved side. The pelvis may be shifted toward and inclined away from the involved side. If the patient stands in this manner, the knee landmarks and trochanter will be lower on the uninvolved side. The posterior-superior iliac spine and iliac crest will also be lower on the uninvolved side, more so than the knee landmarks and tro-

chanter. The anterior-superior iliac spine will not be as low on the uninvolved side as the other landmarks.

If the patient can stand erect, the trochanters and landmarks below will be level. The posterior-superior iliac spine and iliac crest will be higher on the involved side; the anterior-superior iliac spine will be lower on the involved side.

    b. Posterior rotation test will be quite painful; anterior rotation test will be less painful.

    c. Ipsilateral straight-leg raising test may cause some pain, which is relieved when the opposite leg is raised.

VII. Chronic sacroiliac hypermobility
  A. *Subjective complaints*
    1. History suggestive of intermittent acute sacroiliac dysfunction with gradual progression to more chronic sacroiliac and posterior thigh pain. Development may be associated with past pregnancy.
    2. Pain is aggravated by prolonged or repetitive activities involving
      a. Combined hip and spine extension or hip extension with contralateral hip flexion
      b. Combined hip and spine flexion or hip flexion with contralateral hip extension
  B. *Key objective findings*
    1. Possible signs of sacroiliac asymmetry on assessment of structural alignment (see above under acute sacroiliac dysfunction)
    2. Pain or crepitus on one or more sacroiliac stress tests

THE HIP

I. Degenerative joint disease
  A. *Subjective complaints*
    1. Gradual, progressive onset of hip pain and dysfunction
    2. Pain is felt first and most in the groin region. With progression, pain may spread to the anterior thigh, posterior hip, and lateral hip regions.
    3. Pain is first noticed after long periods of weight-bearing activities. Later, pain and stiffness are noted on rising in the morning, easing somewhat by midday, and then increased again by evening.

  B. *Key objective findings*
    1. Tendency to stand with hip and knee flexed and lumbar spine hyperextended; pelvis is shifted toward the involved side
    2. Gait abnormality characterized by tendency to incline the trunk toward the involved side during stance phase
    3. Painful limitation of hip motions in a capsular pattern of restriction; marked limitation of internal rotation and abduction; moderate restriction of flexion and extension; mild to moderate restriction of adduction and external rotation

II. Trochanteric bursitis
  A. *Subjective complaints*
    1. Insidious onset of lateral hip pain, often spreading into the lateral thigh, aggravated most by climbing stairs or, occasionally, by sitting with the involved leg crossed over the uninvolved leg.
    2. Occasionally an acute onset is described, associated with a "snap" felt in the hip region (the iliotibial band snapping over the greater trochanter).
  B. *Key objective findings*
    1. Pain on resisted hip abduction
    2. Pain on approximation of the knee on the involved side to the opposite axilla
    3. Possible pain on stretch of the iliotibial band
    4. Possible pain on full passive hip abduction

III. Iliopectineal bursitis
  A. *Subjective complaint.* Gradual, usually nontraumatic, onset of anterior hip pain, made worse by activities involving extreme or repetitive hip extension
  B. *Key objective findings*
    1. Pain on resisted hip flexion
    2. Pain on full passive hip extension
    3. Possible pain on full hip flexion

THE KNEE

I. Acute medial ligamentous injury
  A. *Subjective complaints*
    1. Sudden onset of knee pain, usually associated with some athletic activity. There may or may not have been some external force acting on the knee at the time of injury in the case of a partial tear.
    2. Gradual buildup of swelling over several hours in the case of a partial tear; there is

little swelling in the case of a complete rupture.

3. The patient often attempts to continue the activity in which he was engaged in the case of a complete rupture, but much less so in the case of a partial tear.

B. *Key objective findings*

1. Antalgic, toe-touch gait in the acute phase of a partial tear; less severe gait disturbance or no gait disturbance in a complete rupture

2. Effusion with limitation of motion in a capsular pattern in the case of a partial tear; little swelling and relatively free range of motion if a complete rupture

3. Pain and spasm on valgus and external rotary stress if a partial tear; painless hypermobility in the case of a complete rupture

II. Acute meniscus tear

A. *Subjective complaint.* Essentially the same as for a partial ligamentous tear. The patient is very hesitant to continue to engage in the activity.

B. *Key objective findings*

1. The same as for a partial ligament tear except no pain on stress tests

2. Point tenderness over the anteromedial joint line

3. Disproportionate loss of extension (*e.g.,* locked knee) if a mechanical block to movement is created by a displaced piece of the meniscus

III. Lateral patellar tracking dysfunction (chondromalacia patellae)

A. *Subjective complaints*

1. Gradual onset of medial knee pain aggravated especially by descending stairs and sitting for long periods of time

2. The onset may be associated with an increase in some activity involving repeated loaded knee extension

B. *Key objective findings*

1. There may be some predisposing structural factor such as anteversion of the hip, genu valgum, a small patella, a high-riding patella, or a diminution in the prominence of the anterior aspect of the lateral femoral condyle.

2. There may be some atrophy of the vastus medialis.

3. Lateral glide of the patella may cause some medial discomfort.

4. Palpation of the medial aspect of the back side of patella may cause discomfort.

5. Femoropatellar crepitus may be noted on weight-bearing knee flexion–extension.

IV. Chronic coronary ligament sprain (adhesion)

A. *Subjective complaint.* Sudden medial knee pain associated with some weight-bearing twisting movement, followed by persistent aching or twinging of pain over the medial knee region. There is usually no significant disability.

B. *Key objective findings*

1. Point tenderness over the anteromedial joint line

2. Pain on passive external rotation of the tibia on the femur; no pain on valgus stress

V. Tendinitis—biceps, iliotibial, or pes anserinus

A. *Subjective complaint.* Gradual onset of pain, almost always associated with long-distance running or some other athletic activity. The pain is lateral for biceps or iliotibial tendinitis and medial for pes anserinus tendinitis. There is little that reproduces the pain except the activity that caused the problem.

B. *Key objective findings*

1. Pain on resisted knee flexion and external tibial rotation in the case of biceps tendinitis

2. Pain on resisted knee extension and external tibial rotation in the case of iliotibial tendinitis

3. Pain on resisted knee flexion and internal rotation for pes anserinus tendinitis

4. Pain on straight-leg raising for biceps tendinitis

5. Point tenderness over the site of the lesion, usually at the tenoperiosteal junction

6. Pain on iliotibial band extensibility test for iliotibial tendinitis

THE ANKLE AND FOOT

I. Acute ankle sprain

A. *Subjective complaints*

1. Sudden onset of lateral ankle pain, associated with plantar flexion–inversion strain, usually during some athletic activity. Continued participation in the activity, at the time of injury, is usually not possible.

Table 21–1. Effects of Common Pathologic Conditions on Gait—Sagittal Plane (Patient Viewed From the Side)

	PAINFUL OR RESTRICTED ANKLE PLANTAR FLEXION	PAINFUL OR RESTRICTED ANKLE DORSIFLEXION	PAINFUL OR RESTRICTED KNEE EXTENSION	PAINFUL OR RESTRICTED HIP EXTENTION	PAINFUL OR RESTRICTED LOW-BACK EXTENSION
Nature of Gait Disturbance	1. Capsular restriction (*e.g.,* postimmobilization) 2. Traumatic arthritis (*e.g.,* post–ankle sprain)	1. Capsular restriction (*e.g.,* postimmobilization) 2. Heel-cord tightness (*e.g.,* postimmobilization) 3. Traumatic arthritis, (*e.g.,* post–ankle sprain)	1. Capsular restriction (*e.g.,* DJD or postimmobilization) 2. Traumatic arthritis (*e.g.,* post-sprain) 3. Locked knee (*e.g.,* bucket-handle meniscus tear)	1. Capsular restriction (*e.g.,* DJD) 2. Iliopectineal bursitis	1. Multisegmental capsular restriction (*e.g.,* DJD) 2. Posterior disk prolapse 3. Acute facet-joint dysfunction
Pattern of Gait Disturbance					
Loss of heel-strike a. Toe-touch gait			X (if painful or locked)		
b. Flatfooted gait	X		X (if stiff)		
Loss of plantar flexion following heel-strike with accelerated stance phase	X		X (if stiff)		
Loss of dorsiflexion during foot-flat stage of stance → premature heel-rise, exaggerated hip and knee flexion during early swing phase		X	X (if stiff)		
Loss of push-off and heel-rise	X		X	X	
Shortened stance phase on involved side	X	X	X	X	X (stance shortened bilaterally)
Tendency toward increased knee extension during stance		X (if stiff)			
Trunk lurch forward during stance		X	X	X (if painful)	
Knee held in increased flexion during stance	X (early and late stance)		X	X	X
Loss of hip extension during stance		X	X	X	X
Loss of low-back extension during stance; trunk held in forward position				X (if painful)	X
Tendency toward inreased low-back extension during stance				X (if stiff)	

2. Gradual development of lateral ankle swelling over the subsequent several hours with continued difficulty in weight-bearing

B. *Key objective signs*

1. Obvious limp associated with traumatic arthritis of the ankle mortise joint (Table 21-1)
2. Swelling and often marked ecchymosis over the lateral aspect of the ankle
3. Pain is reproduced on
   a. Plantar flexion–inversion stress
   b. Anterior glide of the talus in the mortise

II. Chronic recurrent ankle sprains

A. *Subjective complaint.* History of acute ankle sprain (see above) followed by one or more episodes of the ankle's giving way during activities involving jumping or quick lateral movements. Pain, swelling, and dysfunction associated with subsequent episodes are usually not as severe as that occurring with the original injury.

B. *Key objective findings.* These are variable, depending on the causative factors. Consider the following possible causes and the related clinical manifestations.

1. True structural instability (rare)—hypermobility of anterior glide of the talus in the mortise
2. Residual ligamentous adhesion—hypomobility or pain on anterior glide of the talus in the mortise
3. Alteration in proprioceptive neuromuscular protective response—poor balance reactions on one-legged standing

III. Achilles tendinitis and bursitis

A. *Subjective complaint.* Usually a gradual onset of posterior ankle pain that may be associated with some increase in activity level. The pain is made worse when wearing lower-heeled shoes and is improved with wearing higher heels.

B. *Key objective findings*

1. Pain on strong resisted or repetitive resisted ankle plantar flexion
2. Pain on extreme hindfoot dorsiflexion
3. Tenderness to palpation over the distal Achilles region

IV. Medial metatarsalgia

A. *Subjective complaint.* Pain over the first two metatarsal heads after long periods of weight-bearing. The onset is usually insidi-

ous, occasionally associated with a change in foot wear.

B. *Key objective findings*

1. Pressure metatarsalgia
   a. Often associated with a pronated or pronating foot.
   b. The first metatarsal may be abnormally short.
   c. The medial metatarsal heads may be tender to deep palpation.
2. Tension metatarsalgia (from increased tension on the distal insertion of the plantar fascia)
   a. Usually associated with a pronating foot.
   b. The pain may be reproduced by everting the hindfoot while supinating the forefoot and dorsiflexing the toes.

THE SCAN EXAMINATION TESTS

GAIT ANALYSIS

The reader should refer to Tables 21-1 and 21-2 for an overview of the primary gait abnormalities associated with various common lumbar or lower extremity disorders or structural deviations. These tables emphasize the biomechanical interplay among the weight-bearing regions. A careful assessment of gait is an essential component of the evaluation of chronic low back and lower extremity disorders, since it is, of course, the most important functional requirement of these regions and also because many biomechanical abnormalities will not be evident on other parts of the examination.

When evaluating chronic disorders, most of which are the result of stress overloads, it is important to realize which functional abnormalities are present and to appreciate that these are not always mainifest as obvious static deviations or deformities. For example, a person's foot may undergo excessive pronation while walking but the foot may not necessarily appear "pronated" on assessment of bony structure and alignment during standing. Experience in gait analysis is invaluable in understanding the pathomechanics and, in some instances, the etiologies of many common chronic disorders. For this reason it also leads to greater sophistication in devising and implementing treatment strategies, since many chronic disorders are temporarily relieved by "symptomatic" treatment but will inevitably recur unless the underlying causes are dealt with.

Tables 21-1 and 21-2 are organized to serve as a

Table 21-2. Effects of Common Pathologic Conditions on Gait—Frontal Plane and Transverse Planes (Patient Viewed From the Front or Back)

	PRONATION DEFORMITY OR FUNCTIONAL PRONATION DEVIATION OF HINDFOOT	PAINFUL OR RESTRICTED ANKLE OR KNEE FLEXION OR EXTENSION	VARUS DEFORMITY OR VALGUS DEFORMITY DEVIATION OF KNEE	VARUS DEFORMITY OR DEVIATION OF KNEE	EXTERNAL TIBIAL TORSION
Nature of Gait Disturbance	1. Congenital hypermobility of foot (flexible deformity) 2. Tarsal coalition (fixed deformity) 3. Increased femoral anteversion (functional) 4. Genu valgum (functional) 5. Loss of hindfoot dorsiflexion (*e.g.,* tight heel cord)	See Table 21–1	1. DJD of lateral knee (deformity) 2. Increased femoral anteversion (function → structural) 3. Increased foot pronation (functional) 4. Tight iliotibial band (functional)	1. DJD of medial knee (deformity) 2. Increased femoral retroversion (functional)	1. Congenital (structural) 2. Acquired compensation for femoral anteversion
Pattern of Gait Disturbance					
Toeing inward					
Lowered navicular (flatfoot)	X				
Valgus deviation of heel	X		X		
Toeing outward		X			X (uncompensated)
Patella facing outward during swing phase				X (if 2° retroversion)	
Patella facing inward during swing phase					
Patella facing inward during stance	X		X (if 2° anteversion)		X (if compensated)
Patella facing outward during stance					
Pelvis rotates excessively externally (contralateral side forward) during stance					
Pelvis shifted ipsilaterally					
Pelvis shifted contralaterally					
Trunk inclined ipsilaterally during stance					
Trunk inclined contralaterally during stance					

Table 21-2. Continued

INTERNAL TIBIAL TORSION	INCREASED FEMORAL ANTEVERSION OR FUNCTIONAL INTERNAL ROTARY DEVIATION OF FEMUR	INCREASED FEMORAL RETROVERSION OR FUNCTIONAL EXTERNAL ROTARY DEVIATION OF FEMUR	PAINFUL OR RESTRICTED HIP ABDUCTION AND INTERNAL ROTATION	RESTRICTED HIP ADDUCTION	PAINFUL OR RESTRICTED LUMBAR LATERAL DEVIATION
Nature of Gait Disturbance					
1. Congenital (structural) 2. Acquired compensation for femoral retroversion	1. Congenital (structural) 2. Increased foot pronation (functional) 3. External tibial torsion (compensatory)	1. Congenital (structural) 2. Internal tibial torsion (compensatory)	Capsular restriction (*e.g.*, hip DJD)	Tight iliotibial band	1. Posterolateral disk protrusion 2. Acute facet joint dysfunction (unilateral)
X (uncompensated)	X (uncompensated)				
	X (if compensated for by external torsion)				
	X (if compensated for by external torsion)				
		X (uncompensated)	X		
		X			
	X				
	X				
X (if compensated)		X			
	X				
			X		
				X	
			X		X (rare)
					X

guide to the clinical assessment of gait abnormalities associated with the common disorders affecting the low back and lower extremities. After having documented the salient features of some abnormal gait pattern, the clinician may consult the tables to estimate what the underlying physical dysfunction may be and to see what the common causes are. This information should then be correlated with findings from the remainder of the physical examination.

ASSESSMENT OF STRUCTURAL ALIGNMENT

Static alterations in skeletal alignment are significant if they are relatively pronounced or if they are acquired. In either case, they affect a considerable reduction in the stresses that may be imposed on related tissues without pain or degenerative changes. Congenital skeletal deviations, as long as they fall within relatively normal limits, are usually insignificant under normal activity levels, since the related tissues automatically adapt to the various stresses they must withstand as the musculoskeletal system develops. However, such "normal" deviations may make the patient more susceptible to certain stress-overload disorders under conditions of increased activity, such as recreational or competitive athletics. To avoid omitting crucial assessments, the examination of structural alignment may be organized into the following three components: (1) frontal alignment, (2) sagittal alignment, and (3) transverse (rotary) alignment. The primary assessments of each are carried out with the patient in a relaxed standing position, the low back and lower extremities well exposed (shorts are best), and the feet at a normal base width and pointed slightly (about 5° to 10°) outward. The patient is instructed to look straight ahead and to keep arms to the side.

I. **Frontal alignment.** The patient is viewed from behind.
   A. *Horizontal asymmetry* is best detected by use of a plumb bob. The plumb bob is hung so that it barely clears the ground, and the patient is positioned as close as possible to the plumb line, without touching it, and with the plumb bob bisecting the heels.
      1. It should be noted, first, whether the plumb line bisects the legs, pelvis, and lower spine. If there is a lateral shift of the pelvis with respect to the plumb line, consider the following possibilities:
         a. A shorter leg on the side of the shift;

this will be checked for later during assessment of vertical symmetry.
         b. Tight hip abductors (almost always the iliotibial band) on the side opposite the shift. This is often associated with a valgus deviation of the knee on the tight side. Iliotibial band extensibility should be checked later.
         c. Loss of hip abduction on the side of the shift. The most common cause is a capsular restriction secondary to degenerative hip disease. Hip range of motion should be assessed later to determine if a capsular pattern of restriction exists.
      2. Note obvious valgus/varus deviations or asymmetries.
         a. Bilateral genu valgum (knock knees) is often associated with femoral anteversion, foot pronation, or both.
         b. Unilateral genu valgum is often associated with iliotibial band tightness, lateral compartment DJD of the knee, unilateral femoral anteversion, or unilateral foot pronation.
         c. Bilateral genu varum (bowed legs) is often associated with femoral retroversion.
         d. Unilateral genu varum is often associated with medial degenerative knee disease or unilateral femoral retroversion.
         e. Tibial varum or valgum should be differentiated from genu varum or valgum.
         f. Calcaneal valgum is usually associated with foot pronation, genu valgum, femoral anteversion, or some combination thereof. It is evidenced by inward bowing of the Achilles tendon.
         g. Calcaneal varum may be present with foot supination, femoral retroversion, genu varum, or some combination and is seen as outward bowing of the Achilles tendon.
      3. Note obvious asymmetries in muscle bulk. The calves or hamstrings on one side may be atrophied in the presence of a chronic S1 or S2 radiculopathy.
      4. Note lateral spinal curvatures. A lumbar scoliosis may be associated with
         a. A lateral pelvic inclination. The lumbar convexity will be toward the side on which the pelvis is lower.

b. A lateral pelvic shift. The convexity will be on the side toward which the pelvis is shifted.

c. Acute spinal derangements (disk prolapse or facet-joint dysfunction). The lumbar convexity is usually toward the side of the problem, except in some prolapses in which protruding disk material is medial to the sensitive structure (*e.g.*, the nerve root).

d. Asymmetrical lumber degenerative changes, with asymmetrical disk narrowing and facet-joint tightness. The convexity is usually away from the side of the degeneration.

e. A structural thoracolumbar scoliosis. The patient is asked to bend forward to observe for a fixed rotary component, typical of structural curves. The lumbar convexity is usually to the left, with a left rotary component; the thoracic convexity is to the right, with a right rotary component. These curves, unless severe, are generally asymptomatic.

B. The presence of segmental vertical asymmetries (leg-length disparities) is best determined by comparing the heights of the key bony landmarks listed below. This is usually done by palpating similar prominences or contours with the same finger of both hands, then assessing the relative heights of the palpating fingers. For each of the landmarks, it is not so important that the examiner feel some precise point as it is that he or she feel the same prominence or contour with both palpating fingers.

1. Medial malleoli. The most common cause of one being lower than the other is a foot that is more pronated on the lower side. The examiner should check transverse alignment later and correlate this with the position of the calcaneus, since with foot pronation the calcaneus will tend to be in a valgus position.

2. Fibular heads and popliteal folds. If the malleoli are level and these not level, disparity in tibial length should be suspected. One should inquire about a previous fracture or other possible causative factors.

3. Greater trochanters. If the ankle and knee landmarks are level but the trochanters are not level, the shaft of one femur is probably shortened, barring severe de-

generative changes of the knee. Again, one should inquire about previous fractures.

4. Posterior-superior iliac spines. If the ankle and knee land-marks as well as the trochanters are level, but the posterior-superior iliac spines are not, the following are possible: (1) torsional asymmetry in the sacroiliac joints, (2) valgus–varus asymmetry in the proximal femur, and (3) advanced degenerative changes of one hip joint.

a. The most common torsional displacement at the sacroiliac joint is a backward torsion of the ilium on the sacrum, in which case the posterior-superior iliac spine on the involved side will be lower than the one on the opposite side, but the anterior-superior iliac spine on the involved side will be higher. One should, then, check the relative heights of the anterior-superior iliac spines.

b. In the case of femoral valgus or varus asymmetry, both the posterior-superior and the anterior-superior iliac spines will be higher on the side that is in relative valgus position. Nélaton's line may be used to confirm the existence of valgus–varus asymmetry. The position of the greater trochanter is assessed with respect to a line formed from the anterior-superior iliac spine to the ischial tuberosity; with a valgus femur the trochanter will fall more inferiorly with respect to Nélaton's line compared with a varus femur. It should be realized that valgus angulation of the femur is usually associated with increased anteversion and a relatively mobile hip joint, whereas a varus femur is usually associated with retroversion and a more stable hip joint.

c. Advanced degenerative changes of a hip joint, sufficient to cause noticeable lowering of the pelvis on the involved side, will invariably be associated with a capsular restriction of motion at the hip. Internal rotation and abduction are markedly restricted, flexion and extension are moderately restricted, and adduction and external rotation are somewhat limited.

5. Iliac crests. If these are not level, the

cause of asymmetry should be looked for at some lower segment (see above). **Note:** Asymmetry in the height of landmarks at any level should result in a corresponding asymmetry of all landmarks situated more superiorly. If not, combined segmental asymmetries must be suspected (one asymmetry compensating for, or adding to, another).

II. **Sagittal alignment.** The patient is viewed from the side. Obvious abnormalities or asymmetries in flexion–extension positioning of the lower extremity joints and spine are noted. It should be realized that a fairly broad range of "normal" variation exists in sagittal alignment. For some persons, it is normal to stand with the ankles, hips, and knees slightly flexed and the spinal curves somewhat flattened. For others it might be normal to stand with the lower extremity joints well extended and with more accentuation of the spinal curves. Any "deviation" must be considered in light of other findings. Asymmetries can be considered to be more reliably significant.

  A. *Abnormal extension* (e.g., hyperextension) of the knee and other weight-bearing segments is most often the result of restricted ankle dorsiflexion, as from a tight heel cord or capsular ankle restriction. A less common and more serious cause of severe "back knee" is neuropathic arthropathy such as may occur with tertiary syphilis.

  B. *Abnormal flexion* of the knee and other segments occurs with a greater variety of disorders, including

  1. Restricted ankle plantar flexion (rare), the most common cause of which is capsular restriction following immobilization.

  2. Restricted extension of the knee from
     a. Capsular restriction, occurring acutely with traumatic arthritis (effusion) or chronically following immobilization or surgery.
     b. An internal derangement, such as a bucket-handle meniscus tear, causing a mechanical block to knee extension.

  3. Restricted hip extension, most commonly resulting from degenerative hip disease and the associated capsular pattern of restriction

  4. Restricted low-back extension caused by
     a. An acute spinal derangement, such as

a posterior disk prolapse or acute facet-joint dysfunction.
     b. Multisegmental capsular restriction associated with degenerative spinal changes.

III. **Transverse rotary alignment.** The patient is viewed from the front. The stance width should be normal and the feet slightly (5° to 10°) pointed outward. Obvious foot deformities, such as hallux valgus, should be noted. Hallux valgus is often associated with abnormal foot pronation, which, in turn, often occurs in conjunction with transverse rotary abnormalities of more proximal segments. Assessment of segmental rotary alignment is performed, working upward from the feet, by examining the positioning and symmetry of the following landmarks:

  A. *Navicular tubercles.* The positions of the navicular tubercles are assessed compared with a line from the medial malleolus to the point where the first metatarsal contacts the ground. The tubercle should fall just on, or below, this line. The person with a static (*i.e.,* resting) pronation deviation of the foot will have a navicular tubercle that falls well below the line. This is a true flatfoot and will invariably be associated with a valgus heel. Abnormality in bony alignment must be confirmed since many persons have considerable bulk of the medial soft tissues of the foot, which gives the foot a flattened appearance. When a true flatfoot is detected, one must determine whether it is structural (fixed) or functional (mobile). To do so, the patient is asked to raise up on the balls of the feet or to attempt to externally rotate the legs over the stationary foot; in both cases, the arch will be seen to rise significantly if the pronated position of the foot is functional. The common cause of a structurally pronated foot is tarsal coalition. The common causes of a mobile flatfoot are congenital ligamentous laxity and femoral anteversion. It must be appreciated that a person who does not have static pronation deviation of the foot, as evidenced on examination of structural alignment, may still have a problem from abnormal foot pronation during gait. On the other hand, it should be realized that a person with a static pronation deviation of the foot does not necessarily have a pronation problem, especially if the deviation has existed since childhood. The tissues of the foot will have adapted to the increased pronatory stresses during development.

B. *Intermalleolar line.* A line passing through the tips of the medial and lateral malleoli should make an angle, opening laterally, of about 25° with the frontal plane when the knee axis is situated in the frontal plane (*i.e.*, when the patellae are facing straight forward). **Note:** Twenty-five degrees corresponds to the lateral malleolus being about 4 cm posterior to the medial malleolus when the intermalleolar distance is 10 cm, or about 3.5 cm posterior for a 9-cm intermalleolar width, or about 3 cm posterior for an 8-cm width.

   1. If the angle is excessive, the examiner must suspect increased external tibial torsion or increased femoral anteversion. It is not unusual for these to coexist, the two having a mutual compensatory effect to cancel abnormal toeing inward (from femoral anteversion) or toeing outward (from external tibial torsion). Compensation would occur during development. The presence of femoral anteversion is best determined clinically by assessing hip rotational range of motion in the prone position. An anteverted hip is a very mobile hip that appears to have an increase in internal rotation at the expense of a loss of external rotation.

   2. Similarly, if the angle the intermalleolar line makes with the frontal plane is diminished when the patellae face straight forward, there may be an increase in femoral retroversion or abnormal internal tibial torsion. A retroverted hip is a less mobile hip that will appear to have a loss of internal rotation, with external rotation perhaps somewhat increased.

C. *Patellae.* With the feet pointed slightly outward the patellae should face straight forward.

   1. If the patellae face inward, suspect increased femoral anteversion, increased external tibial torsion, or both (see above).

   2. If the patellae face outward when the feet are in a normal position, the cause may be femoral retroversion, internal tibial torsion, or both (see above).

D. *Anterior-superior iliac spines.* These should

be positioned in a frontal plane. If the pelvis is rotated (one iliac spine more anterior than the other) the common causes to be considered are

   1. A fixed (structural) spinal scoliosis, the rotary component of which is transmitted to the pelvis through the sacrum by way of the lumbar spine

   2. Torsional asymmetry of the sacroiliac joints. The pelvis will appear to be rotated forward on the side on which the ilium is in more anterior torsion with respect to the sacrum.

REGIONAL TESTS

I. **Lumbosacral tests**

   A. With the patient standing, the examiner demonstrates the movement to be performed as verbal instructions are given. The examiner is looking for the patient's willingness to do the movements, for limitation of motion, and for its possible causes such as pain, stiffness, or spasm. When viewing from behind, one should note if movements are asymmetrical and should watch for the levels affected. The examiner can determine if any deviations are painful or painless when corrected. When viewing the patient from the side, the examiner should assess the continuity of movement at the various spinal segments and look for reversal of the lumbar lordosis. The most painful movements should be done last. The following active movements are carried out in the lumbar spine:

   1. Extension (backward bending)
   2. Lateral flexion (sidebending) (left and right)
   3. Flexion (forward bending)
   4. Lateral shift (side glide)
   5. Rotation (patient sitting, knees together with the arms folded or held in 90° flexion and hands together) (left and right)

   B. *Active auxiliary tests.* If the patient's symptoms have not been reproduced the following additional maneuvers may be conducted (patient standing).

   1. Passive overpressure at end range of active physiological spinal motions
   2. Repeated physiological motions at various speeds

3. Sustained pressure at end range of extension and lateral flexion
4. Combined motions without overpressure (left and right)
   a. Flexion (forward bending) with rotation
   b. Lateral flexion with flexion (forward bending)
5. Combined motions with passive overpressure (left and right)
   a. Flexion (forward bending) and lateral flexion
   b. Flexion (forward bending) with rotation
   c. Extension (backward bending) with lateral flexion (forward bending)
   d. Extension with rotation

C. *Active segmental mobility.* With the patient in stride-standing, the examiner can assess the following:
   1. Upper lumbar spine—lateral flexion
   2. L5–S1—lateral flexion
   3. Active pelvic tilt (L5–S1—painful or painless?)

D. *Passive movements*
   1. Is posture correction painful or painless?
   2. Quadrant test (standing)—passive auxiliary test for segmental involvement
   3. Passive physiological movements (non-weight-bearing).
      a. Flexion (forward bending)
      b. Extension (backward bending)
      c. Lateral flexion (side bending—left and right)
      d. Rotation (left and right) ·
   4. Passive physiological movements with segmental palpation. Note type of end feel and seek abnormalities.
      a. Flexion–extension (forward and backward bending)
      b. Lateral flexion (side bending—left and right)
      c. Rotation (left and right)
   5. Segmental mobility
      a. Posteroanterior central pressures—T10–L5
      b. Transverse pressures—T10–L5
      c. Posteroanterior unilateral pressures—T10–L5

For the fullest information, one should alter the direction of posteroanterior pressure; counterpressures are exerted to the spinous process of the segment above and below, and posteroan-

terior pressures may be applied diagonally in caudal and cephalad directions—T10–L5.

E. *Passive movements of the sacroiliac and peripheral joints*
   1. Sacroiliac auxiliary (provocation) and mobility tests
      a. Posterior rotation test
      b. Anterior rotation test
   2. Hip joint: Hip flexion–adduction test
   3. Knee joint
      a. Anterior drawer (Lachman) test
      b. Valgus–varus stress test at 30° knee flexion

F. *Neuromuscular tests*
   1. Key sensory areas (L4–S2)—stroking test and sensibility to pinprick, if applicable.
   2. Resisted isometric (myotomal) tests (L2–S2). Compare both sides.
   3. Dural mobility testing
      a. Straight-leg raising (sciatic nerve)—sitting and supine, with and without cervical spine flexion)
      b. Slump test (sciatic nerve)
      c. Femoral nerve traction test
   4. Reflexes
      a. Knee jerk (L3) and plantar response
      b. Ankle jerk (S1)
      c. Great toe jerk (L5)
      d. Test for ankle clonus

II. **Hip tests**
A. *Active movements.* The emphasis is on assessing functional activities involving the use of the hip. If the patient is able to do active flexion (knee to chest), extension in standing, and abduction and rotation in non-weight-bearing with little difficulty, the examiner may use a series of functional tests to see if increased intensity of activity produces pain or other symptoms (*i.e.*, squatting, going up and down stairs, running and jumping).

B. *Passive movements.* Passive movements should be performed to determine the end feel and the degree of passive range of motion.
   1. Perform passive hip flexion–extension, abduction–adduction, internal-external rotation, and combined flexion, adduction, and rotation.
   2. If indicated, the assessment of muscle lengths is included; the Thomas test to detect a hip flexion contracture, Ely's test

for the iliopsoas and rectus femoris, 90°-90° straight-leg raising for hamstring, and the Ober test for the iliotibial band.

C. *Resisted isometric movements*
1. Resisted hip flexion–extension, adduction, and internal-external rotation are tested isometrically in the supine position to determine which muscles may be at fault or for the presence of a possible bursitis. Resisted hip flexion is also done as a test for the integrity of the L2 myotome.
2. Resisted hip abduction is tested with the patient in the prone position for the presence of possible trochanteric bursitis or gluteus medius tendinitis.

III. Knee tests
A. *Active movements*. Flexion–extension can be assessed at the same time as hip flexion and extension and, in a weight-bearing situation, while testing the L3 myotome.
1. During weight-bearing movements, the examiner should palpate at the femoropatellar joint and at the femorotibial joint for crepitus that may indicate degenerative changes. Snapping and popping during movement is common, but a continuous grinding, suggestive of sand in the joint, is more significant.
2. During non-weight-bearing, the knee is assessed for loss of dynamic tibial function and for any evidence of quadriceps lag. These tests allow the examiner to detect subtle abnormalities that may predispose to chronic knee pain and perhaps progressive degeneration. These patients often respond well to manual therapy techniques.
3. Functional tests. If the preceding tests are performed with little difficulty, the examiner may put the patient through a series of functional tests to see if these activities reproduce the patient's symptoms or pain.

B. *Passive physiological movement with passive overpressure*. More information may be derived by testing passive ranges of extension, flexion, and axial rotation in cardinal planes and combined motions.

C. *Patellar glide*. The patella is moved passively, posteriorly, medially, and laterally. At the extremes of medial movement, the underside of the medial patella is palpated for tenderness.

D. *Resisted isometric movements*
1. Internal-external rotation with the knee bent. Resisted internal rotation will reproduce pain from pes anserinus; resisted external rotation may reproduce pain from iliotibial band tendinitis.
2. Knee flexion (also tests for the S2 myotome). This may reproduce pain from pes anserinus tendinitis or biceps tendinitis.
3. Knee extension (L3). Pain may be reproduced in patellar tendinitis.

IV. Ankle and foot tests
A. *Active motion and passive movements*
1. Flexion–extension. The patient lies prone with the feet over the edge of the table. With the foot in subtalar neutral, active and passive dorsiflexion is assessed and then repeated with the knee bent to 90°. Pain from Achilles tendinitis may be reproduced at the extremes of dorsiflexion. Pain from an anterior talofibular ligament sprain or adhesion may be reproduced on plantar flexion–inversion with passive overpressure.
2. Hindfoot inversion–eversion. With the patient sitting, the range of passive calcaneal inversion–eversion is assessed.
3. Forefoot supination–pronation. With the subtalar joint maintained via the calcaneus in subtalar neutral, the examiner should maximally supinate (untwist) and pronate (twist) the forefoot. With the foot held untwisted, the toes are moved into sustained dorsiflexion. Untwisting of the foot may reproduce pain from a calcaneocuboid ligament sprain; sustained toe dorsiflexion may reproduce pain from plantar fasciitis or calcaneal periostitis, since this stretches the plantar fascia.
4. Anterior glide of the talus in the mortise. Hypermobility will be present in the case of chronic anterior talofibular ligament rupture. Pain will be reproduced from a talofibular ligament sprain or adhesion.
5. Functional tests. If the patient is able to do the preceding activities with little difficulty, functional tests may be performed to see whether these activities reproduce the symptoms or pain (*i.e.,* standing and walking on the toes, standing on one foot at a time, running and jumping). These activities should be selected and geared to the individual patient.

B. *Resisted isometrics.* With the patient in the supine position, the presence of pain and weakness is assessed. Movements tested isometrically include the following:

1. Knee flexion (S2)
2. Tibialis anterior (L4) (dorsiflexion–inversion)
3. Tibialis posterior (L5) (plantar flexion–inversion)
4. Peroneus tertius (dorsiflexion–eversion)
5. Peroneus longus and brevis (S1) (plantar flexion–eversion)
6. Toe flexion-extension: extensor digitorum (L5–S1) and hallucis longis (L5)

CLINICAL IMPLEMENTATION OF THE LUMBAR—LOWER EXTREMITY SCAN EXAMINATION

Gait analysis and a comprehensive assessment of structural alignment should be included in the assessment of virtually all chronic disorders of the low back and lower extremities. It is rare, however, to include all of the regional tests discussed during any one examination; tests are chosen as indicated by subjective information and findings on gait analysis and inspection of structural alignment. The clinician must be prepared to judge which tests might be relevant in a particular case—a judgment that is facilitated by experience.

In order for the scan examination to be of practical use in a busy clinical setting, the clinician must be able to perform the examination within a reasonable period of time, for example, 15 minutes or less. This requires knowledge of which tests are to be performed, understanding of the rationale for each test, skill in appropriately carrying out each test, and ability to interpret the results.

Clinically, the tests of the scan examination must be carried out according to the patient's position in order to minimize time requirements and to prevent omission of crucial tests. The following is a summary of the tests included in a complete lumbar-lower extremity scan examination, according to the position of the patient. This format should be followed in the clinical implementation of the scan examination.

I. **Standing**
 A. *Gait analysis*
  1. Sagittal
  2. Frontal
  3. Transverse
  4. Equilibrium. The patient stands on one leg with the eyes closed. Check stabilization efficiency of each hip.
 B. *Inspection of structural alignment and soft tissue*
  1. Frontal—from behind
  2. Sagittal—from the side
  3. Transverse (rotatory)—from the front
  4. Posture correction
 C. *Functional tests*
  1. Active lumbar (physiological) movements
   a. Extension (backward bending)
   b. Lateral flexion (sidebending)
   c. Flexion (forward bending)
   d. Lateral shift (side gliding)
  2. Active lumbar segmental movements
   a. Upper lumbar
   b. L5–S1
  3. Active peripheral joint movements
   a. Hip flexion–extension
   b. Standing unilateral half squats (L3)
   c. Standing unilateral toe raises (S1–S2)
  4. Auxiliary tests (if indicated) to clear.

II. **Sitting**
 A. *Alignment*
  1. Compare sitting posture to standing.
  2. Position of the patellae
  3. Rotatory position of the tibia
 B. *Function*
  1. Active lumbar spine rotation
  2. Resisted isometrics—hip flexion (L2)
  3. Tibial rotatory mechanics
  4. Dural mobility
 C. *Resisted isometrics*
  1. Resisted hip flexion (L2)
  2. Resisted knee extension (L3)

III. **Supine**
 A. *Functional tests*
  1. Passive tests—hip, knee, ankle, and foot ranges compared with other limb with assessment of end feel and overpressure if applicable. One should seek regions of muscle tightness: hamstrings, hip adductors, and gastroc-soleus.
   a. Hip and knee flexion–extension range
   b. Hip adduction–abduction range
   c. Knee internal-external rotation
   d. Patellar glide, medially and laterally
   e. Ankle dorsiflexion–plantar flexion
   f. Hindfoot inversion–eversion and forefoot twisting and untwisting. Dorsiflex toes when untwisted.
 B. *Resisted isometrics*
  1. Resisted hip abduction

2. Resisted dorsiflexion (L4)–plantar flexion—tibialis posterior (L5)
3. Resisted large toe extension (L5)

C. *Sensation*—include vibratory perception, stroking test, and sensibility to pinprick, if applicable

D. *Dural mobility*

E. *Reflexes*
   1. Knee jerk (L3–L4)
   2. Great toe jerk (L5)
   3. Test for ankle clonus
   4. Plantar response

IV. Sidelying — Function

A. *Passive physiological movements with segmental palpation*—Lumbar spine
   1. Flexion–extension (forward-backward bending)
   2. Lateral flexion (side bending)
   3. Rotation

B. *Sacroiliac posterior rotation*

C. *Iliotibial band extensibility*

V. Prone

A. *Functional tests*
   1. Sacroiliac anterior rotation
   2. Hip internal-external rotation range of motion

B. *Resisted isometrics*
   1. Resisted hip extension (S1)
   2. Resisted knee rotations
   3. Resisted knee flexion
      a. Assess strength—S1, S2, myotomes
      b. Assess irritability—biceps or pes anserinus tendonitis
   4. Reflexes—ankle jerk—S1, S2

RECOMMENDED READINGS

Corrigan B, Maitland GD: Practical Orthopaedics Medicine. London, Butterworths, 1985

Cyriax JF, Cyriax PJ: Illustrated Manual of Orthopaedic Medicine. Boston, Butterworths, 1983

Edward BC: Clinical assessment: The use of combined movements in assessment and treatment. In Twoney LT, Taylor JR (eds): Physiotherapy of the Low Back, pp 175–198. New York, Churchill Livingstone, 1987

Edwards BC: Combined movements in the lumbar spine: Their use in examination and treatment. In Grieve GP (ed): Modern Manual Therapy of the Vertebral Column, pp 561–566. New York, Churchill Livingstone, 1986

Finneson BE: Low Back Pain. Philadelphia, JB Lippincott, 1981

Grieve GP: Mobilisation of the Spine: Notes on Examination and Clinical Methods, 5th ed. New York, Churchill Livingstone, 1988

Grueber-Lee DM: Disorders of the Hip. Philadelphia, JB Lippincott, 1983

Hunt GC: Examination of lower extremity dysfunction. In Gould JA, Davies GJ (eds): Orthopedics and Sports Physical Therapy, pp 408–436. St. Louis, CV Mosby, 1985

Hunt GC (ed): Physical Therapy of the Foot and Ankle. New York, Churchill Livingstone, 1988

Jahss MH (ed): Disorders of the Foot. Philadelphia, WB Saunders, 1982

Magee DJ: Orthopedic Physical Assessment. Philadelphia, WB Saunders, 1987

Maigne R: Orthopedic Medicine. Springfield, IL, Charles C Thomas, 1976

Maitland GD: Vertebral Manipulations, 5th ed. Boston, Butterworths, 1986

Markolf KL: Quantitative examination for anterior cruciate laxity. In Jackson DW, Drez D (eds): The Anterior Cruciate Deficient Knee: New Concepts in Ligament Repair. St. Louis, CV Mosby, 1987

McKenzie R: The Lumbar Spine: Mechanical Diagnosis and Therapy. Waikanae, New Zealand, Spinal Publications, 1981

Nicholas JA, Hershmann EB (eds): The Lower Extremity and Spine in Sports Medicine. St. Louis, CV Mosby, 1986

Paulos LE: Knee and leg: Soft tissue trauma. In American Academy of Orthopaedic Surgeons: Orthopaedic Knowledge Update 2, 1987

Root ML, Orien WP, Weed JH: Biomechanical Examination of the Foot and Ankle, vol I. Los Angeles, Clinical Biomechanics Corp, 1971

Sonzogni JJ: Physical assessment of the injured knee. Emergency Med April 1988, pp 74–92

Wells PE: The examination of the pelvic joints. In Grieve GP (ed): Modern Manual Therapy of the Vertebral Column. New York, Churchill Livingstone, 1986

Appendix A: Component Motions, Close-Packed Positions, Loose-Packed Positions, Rest Positions, and Capsular Patterns

Component motions are joint motions taking place in the joint complex or related joints that accompany, and are necessary for, full active range of motion. For example, inferior glide of the head of the humerus into the lower portion of the glenoid fossa during active movement of the shoulder is a component motion.

The most stable position of a joint is called the *close-packed position*.[5] In this position the tension on the articular capsule and ligaments is maximal, with the joint surfaces often temporarily locked together. The locking together is frequently performed by a screw-home component. The close-packed configuration usually occurs at a position that is the extreme of the most habitual position of the joint. For example, the close-packed position for the wrist joint is full extension. The other extreme position of the joint that is less commonly assumed is also very congruent and is called the potential close-packed position.[2,12,16,19]

In the close-packed position, the joint capsule and major ligaments are twisted, causing the joint surfaces to become firmly approximated. This is a direct result either of the conjunct rotation that necessarily accompanies a diadochal movement into this position or of the spin that accompanies an impure swing into the position. From this it follows that movement into or out of a close-packed position is never accomplished by a pure chordate swing alone. **Note:** Habitual movements of daily activities usually involve motions that move a joint closer to or farther from a close-packed position. A typical example would be the motions occurring at the hip when walking.

Consider the relationship between the close-packed position at a particular joint and the capsular pattern of restriction, as described by Cyriax,[5] at the same joint: The more intimate the anatomical and functional relationship between the joint capsule and major supporting ligaments, the more likely the close-packed position will be the most restricted position of the joint in a capsular pattern of restriction. Thus, in the hip and shoulder joints, in which the major ligaments blend with the joint capsule, movements into the close-packed position are the first to be lost with a capsular pattern of restriction. In the knee, however, in which the ligaments are easily distinguished from the capsule, flexion may be the most limited in a capsular restriction, whereas extension constitutes the close-packed position.

In any position of the joint other than the close-packed position of the joint, the articular surfaces are non-congruent and some part of the joint capsule is lax; in these positions, the joint is said to be *loose-packed*. In many cases there is sufficient laxity in mid-range to allow distraction of the joint surfaces by an externally applied force. The laxity of the capsule in the loose-packed position allows for the elements of spin, glide, and roll, which are present in most joint movements in various degrees. The *resting position* is the maximum loose-packed position and is the ideal position for evaluation and early treatment procedures used in restoring joint play. The resting position is also the position in which the joint capsule had its greatest capacity and where the joint is under the least amount of stress. Determination of accessory movement, traditionally part of the joint mobilization examination, is necessary if the therapist is to restore the normal roll-glide action that takes place during joint movements: joint-play and component motions.

THE TEMPOROMANDIBULAR JOINT

Note: Both temporomandibular joints are involved in every jaw movement, forming a bicondylar arrangement.

Component Motions

Opening of the Mouth

1. The head of the mandible first rotates around a horizontal axis (rolls dorsally) in relation to the disk (lower compartment).
2. This movement is then combined with gliding of the head anteriorly (and somewhat downward) in contact with the lower surface of the disk.
3. At the same time, the disk glides anteriorly (and somewhat downward) toward the articular eminence of the glenoid fossa (upper compartment). The forward gliding of the disk ceases when the fibroelastic tissue attaching to the temporal bone posteriorly has been stretched to its limits.
4. Thereafter there is some further hinging and gliding anteriorly of the head of the mandible until it articulates with the most anterior part of the disk and the mouth is fully opened.

Closing of the Mouth. The movements are reversed.
Protrusion. The disks glide anteriorly in the upper compartment (simultaneously on both sides). Both condyles glide anteriorly and slightly downward but do not rotate.
Retraction. The movements are reversed.
Lateral Movements. Anterior gliding occurs in one joint while rotation around a cranial-caudal axis occurs in the other joint. One condyle glides downward, forward, and inward, while the other condyle in, the fossa rotates and glides ipsilaterally.
Note: When the jaw is moved from side to side (as in chewing) a movement involving a shuttling of the condylar-disk assembly occurs in the concave parts of the fossa.

Resting Position

The mouth is slightly open. The teeth of the mandible and maxillae are not in contact but slightly apart.

Close-Packed Position

Unlike other joints both temporomandibular joints become nearly "close-packed" with full occlusion of the dental arches.[11] It remains questionable whether these joints truly possess a close-packed position, since the restraining capsule and ligaments are not maximally tightened during the maximum occlusion of the dental arches.[16]

Potential Close-Packed Position

This is full or maximal opening. **Note:** The potential close-packed position is one in which the joint is also very congruent and stable but is less commonly assumed. The ligaments, in particular the temporomandibular ligament and capsular constraints of the craniomandibular articulation, seem particularly tightened during maximum opening.[11]

Capsular Pattern of Restriction

In bilateral restriction, lateral movements are most restricted; opening of the mouth and protrusion are both limited; closing of the mouth is most free. **Note:** In unilateral capsular restrictions, contralateral excursions are most restricted. In mouth opening, the mandible will deviate toward the restricted side.

UPPER EXTREMITY

THE SHOULDER (GLENOHUMERAL JOINT)

Component Motions

Flexion (Elevation in the Sagittal Plane)

1. At full elevation of the humerus, whether accomplished through coronal abduction or sagittal flexion, the humerus always ends up back in the plane of the scapula, *as if* it had been elevated through a pure swing; that is, at an angle midway between the sagittal and coronal planes. Since sagittal flexion is an impure swing, the humerus tends to undergo a lateral conjunct rotation on its path to full elevation. If this were allowed to occur, however, the humerus would end up such that the medial condyle pointed backward, rather than forward, with the capsule of the glenohumeral joint completely twisted. This essentially would involve a premature close-packing that would prevent full elevation. To avoid this, the humerus must rotate medially on its long axis during the complete arc of sagittal flexion. The rotation occurs because the anterior aspect of the joint capsule pulls tight on flexion, while the posterior capsule remains relatively lax.
2. Downward (inferior) glide of the head of the humerus on the glenoid.

Abduction

1. Lateral rotation of the humerus on its long axis to counter the medial conjunct rotation that tends to occur during this impure swing (see *Flexion*). In this case, the posterior capsule pulls tight during abduction, effecting a lateral rotation of the humerus.
2. Inferior glide of the humeral head on the glenoid.

   External Rotation — Anterior glide of the head of the humerus.
   Internal Rotation — Posterior glide of the head of the humerus.
   Horizontal Adduction — Posterior glide of the humeral head.
   Horizontal Abduction — Anterior glide of the humeral head.

Resting Position

Semiabduction: 55° abduction, 30° horizontal adduction.

Close-Packed Position

Horizontal abduction and external rotation are combined.

Capsular Pattern of Restriction

External rotation is most limited; abduction, quite limited; internal rotation and flexion, somewhat limited (relatively free).

ACROMIOCLAVICULAR JOINT

Component Motions

1. Allows widening and narrowing of the angle (looking from above) between the clavicle and the scapula. Narrowing occurs during protraction; widening occurs during retraction (about 10° total, according to Kapandji). This occurs about a vertical axis.
2. Allows rotation of the scapula *upward*, such that the inferior angle of the scapula moves away from the midline; or *downward*, such that it moves toward the midline. This occurs about a horizontal axis lying in the sagittal plane. Actually, very little acromioclavicular joint motion is involved in this rotation of the scapula. While about 30° occurs with elevation of the clavicle at the sternoclavicular joint, much of the remaining 30° occurs because of axial rotation of the clavicle; since the clavicle is S-shaped anteroposteriorly, an axial rotation converts the S to a superoinferior

attitude, the distal end pointing more or less upward. This occurs as a result of tightening of the coracoclavicular ligaments as the scapula begins to rotate upward (the coracoid rotating downward).
3. Allows rotation of the scapula such that the inferior angle swings anteriorly and posteriorly. As the scapula moves upward and forward on the thorax, the inferior angle swings posteriorly. This occurs about an axis lying horizontally in the frontal plane and probably is accompanied by considerable length rotation at the sternoclavicular joint as well.

Resting Position

Arm rests by the side in the normal physiological position.

Close-Packed Position

Upward rotation of the scapula relative to the clavicle is combined with narrowing of the angle between the scapula and clavicle as seen from above. This occurs during elevation of the arm and during horizontal adduction (see Fig. 10–3).

Capsular Pattern

Primarily there is pain into the close-packed position, such as when horizontally adducting the arm.

STERNOCLAVICULAR JOINT

Component Motions

1. Allows length rotation of the clavicle, as discussed under Acromioclavicular Joint: about 50° total. This occurs during elevation of the arm and somewhat during protraction and retraction.
2. Allows upward and downward swing of the clavicle such as during shoulder shrugging or elevation of the arm. This occurs about an axis passing through the costoclavicular ligament, so that with elevation the clavicular articular surface slides inferiorly on the sternum and, with depression, superiorly: about 30° total.
3. Allows forward and backward swing of the clavicle, such as with protraction and retraction. This occurs about an axis lying somewhat medial to the joint, so that the clavicular articular surface slides forward on protraction: about 45° to 60° total.

Resting Position

Arm rests by the side in the normal physiological position.

Close-Packed Position

Full or maximum rotation of the clavicle occurs when the arm is fully elevated.

Capsular Pattern

Pain occurs at the extremes of motion. **Note:** To emphasize the interplay of all joints involved with shoulder movements, the components of shoulder abduction in the frontal plane, which is one of the more complex shoulder movements, are reviewed here.

With the arm at the side in the resting position, the glenoid faces almost equally anteriorly and laterally. The humerus rests in the "plane of the scapula," or in alignment with the glenoid, such that the medial humeral condyle points about 45° inward and backward (see Fig. 10–2).

During the first 30° or so of abduction what happens to the scapula is variable, but during this time it becomes "set" or fixed against the thoracic wall in preparation for movement. From 30° to full elevation, for every 15° of movement about 10° occurs at the glenohumeral joint and 5° at the scapulothoracic joint. The scapula must rotate upward as well as forward around the chest wall. The early part of this movement occurs as a result of elevation at the sternoclavicular joint, as well as movement at the acromioclavicular joint, such that its angle narrows (looking from above) and the scapula rotates slightly upward on the clavicle. This close-packs the acromioclavicular joint but also draws the coracoclavicular ligaments tight, because of the downward movement of the coracoid relative to the clavicle. Thus, between, say, 90° and 120°, motion stops at the acromioclavicular joint. Further elevation from scapular rotation is possible only because the coracoclavicular ligaments pull the clavicle into long-axis rotation.

The S-shape of the clavicle becomes oriented superoinferiorly such that the distal end of the clavicle points somewhat upward, allowing the acromioclavicular joint to maintain apposition as the scapula continues to rotate upward. This clavicular rotation occurs, of course, at the sternoclavicular joint.

Since the convex humeral head is moving in relation to the concave glenoid cavity to allow upward swing of the humerus, it must glide inferiorly in the glenoid. The humerus must move out of the plane of the scapula in order to be elevated in the frontal plane; it must undergo an impure swing. As with any impure swing, a conjunct rotation occurs, in this case a medial rotation. However, the posterior and inferior capsular fibers cannot allow this amount of rotation, so in order for the humerus to come back into the plane of the scapula on full elevation, it must rotate laterally on its long axis. This lateral rotation is necessary for clearance of the greater tuberosity under the acromial arch.

The clinically important considerations are that elevation is impossible without appropriate sternoclavicular and acromioclavicular movements, especially rotation of the clavicle on its long axis, without inferior glide of the humeral head and without lateral rotation of the humerus on its long axis.

Furthermore, one must consider the motions occurring in the thoracic and lower cervical spines on shoulder movement. For example, bilateral elevation of the arms requires considerable thoracic extension; the person with a significant thoracic kyphosis will not be able to perform this movement throughout the full range. On unilateral elevation the upper thoracic spine must sidebend toward, and the lower thoracic spine must sidebend away from, the side of motion.

THE ELBOW

Component Motions

Extension

1. Superior glide of ulna on trochlea
2. Pronation of ulna relative to humerus
3. Abduction of ulna relative to humerus
4. Distal movement of radius on ulna
5. Pronation (inward rotation) of radius relative to humerus

Flexion

1. Inferior glide of ulna on trochlea
2. Supination of ulna relative to humerus
3. Adduction of ulna relative to humerus
4. Proximal movement of radius on ulna
5. Supination (outward rotation) of radius on humerus

HUMEROULNAR JOINT

Resting Position

Semiflexion: 70° flexion, 10° supination

Close-Packed Position

Extension

Capsular Pattern

More limitation of flexion than extension

HUMERORADIAL JOINT

Resting Position

Full extension and supination

Close-Packed Position

90° flexion and semipronation

Capsular Pattern

Flexion and extension are most restricted; supination and pronation are restricted.

FOREARM

Pronation–Supination

Proximal Radioulnar Joint and Radiohumeral Joint. This movement is essentially one of pure spin of the head of the radius on the capitellum and, therefore, one of roll and slide of the radius in the radial notch of the ulna and annular ligament.
Distal Radioulnar Joint. Here the radius is said to rotate around the head of the ulna, being largely a sliding movement. However, functionally the ulna also tends to move backward and laterally during pronation and forward and medially during supination. Therefore, component movements during pronation are as follows:

1. Palmar glide of the radius on ulna
2. Inward rotation of radius on ulna (looking palmarly)
3. Dorsal glide of ulna on radius
4. Outward rotation of ulna on radius (looking palmarly)
5. Abduction of ulna on humerus

The reverse would naturally occur on supination.

PROXIMAL RADIOULNAR JOINT

Resting Position

70° flexion, 35° supination

Close-Packed Position

5° supination

Capsular Pattern

More limitation of supination than pronation

DISTAL RADIOULNAR JOINT

Resting Position

10° supination

Close-Packed Position

5° supination

Capsular Pattern

Involvement of the distal radioulnar joint produces little limitation of movement, but there is pain at the extremes of pronation and supination.

THE WRIST

Radiocarpal Joint

Palmar Flexion

1. Dorsal movement of proximal carpals (scaphoid and lunate) on radius and disk
2. Distraction of radiocarpal joint

Dorsiflexion

1. Palmar movement of proximal carpals on radius (the scaphoid also spins—supinates—on the radius at full wrist dorsiflexion)
2. Approximation of scaphoid and lunate to radius and disk

Radial Deviation

1. Approximation of scaphoid to radius
2. Ulnar slide of the proximal carpals on the radius (this movement is quite limited and is somewhat increased by the tendency for the scaphoid to extend [slide palmarly and supinate] on the radius)

Ulnar Deviation

1. Distraction of scaphoid from radius
2. Radial slide of proximal carpals on radius

Ulnomeniscotriquetral Joint

The ulnomeniscotriquetral joint is primarily involved with pronation and supination of the forearm. During pronation and supination, the disk moves with the radius and carpals and must therefore sweep around the distal end of the ulna. During flexion and extension, the disk stays with the radius and ulna and movement occurs between the disk and the carpals. In this situation the disk acts as an ulnar extension of the distal radial joint surface to become, functionally, part of the radiocarpal joint.

During wrist radial deviation there is considerable distraction of the triquetrum and pisiform from the ulna, with approximation on ulnar deviation.

Midcarpal Joint

Palmar Flexion

1. Dorsal slide of hamate and capitate on triquetrum and lunate
2. Palmar slide of trapezoid on scaphoid

Dorsiflexion. From full flexion to neutral, the reverse of the above takes place. At neutral the hamate, capitate, and trapezoid become close-packed on the scaphoid, and these four bones tend to move together in a palmar slide and supinatory spin on the radius, lunate, and triquetrum. **Note:** The scaphoid acts as a proximal carpal from neutral into palmar flexion and as a "distal carpal" from neutral into full dorsiflexion. Also note the supination and radial deviation that tends to occur on extreme dorsiflexion of the wrist.

Radial Deviation. There is some ulnar slide of the hamate and capitate on the triquetrum and lunate, with considerable distraction of the base of the hamate from the lunate.

The trapezoid slides radially on the scaphoid.

Ulnar Deviation. This is the reverse of radial deviation. **Note:** The entire carpus might be divided into four functional units: (1) Hamate, capitate, trapezoid always acting as distal carpals; (2) scaphoid, acting as proximal carpal into flexion and distal carpal into extension; (3) triquetrum and lunate, always acting as proximal carpals; and (4) trapezium, acting primarily in its articulation with the first metacarpal of the thumb, playing little part in movements at the wrist.

Resting Position

Semiflexion: near neutral with slight ulnar deviation

Close-Packed Position

Of the wrist as a whole, extension (dorsiflexion) with radial deviation

Capsular Pattern

Equal limitation of palmar flexion and dorsiflexion

THE HAND

"Intermetacarpal Joints"

Although these are not true synovial joints, movement does take place between the heads of the metacarpals on grasp and release.

Grasp. The metacarpals form an "arch" through the following movements:

1. Palmar movement of second relative to third, fourth relative to third, and fifth relative to fourth metacarpal head
2. Supination of fourth and fifth metacarpals, perhaps slight pronation of the second

Release. The arch is flattened through the reverse of the above movements.

Component Motions of the Metacarpophalangeal Joints

Flexion

1. Palmar glide of the base of the phalanx on the head of the metacarpal
2. Supination of the phalanx on the metacarpal, especially with grasp or pinch
3. Ulnar deviation of the phalanx on metacarpal, especially with grasp or pinch
4. Approximation of the phalanx and the metacarpal

Extension. Reverse of flexion

Radial Deviation

1. Radial slide of the base of the phalanx on the head of the metacarpal

Ulnar Deviation

1. Ulnar slide of the base of the phalanx on the head of the metacarpal.

Component Motions of the Interphalangeal Joints

Flexion

1. Palmar glide of the base of the more distal phalanx on the head of the more proximal phalanx
2. Distraction of the distal phalanx on proximal phalanx
3. Supination of the distal phalanx on the more proximal phalanx (more at distal interphalangeal than proximal interphalangeal joint)
4. Radial deviation of the distal phalanx on the more proximal phalanx

Extension. Reverse of flexion

Component Motions of the Trapeziometacarpal Joint

This is a sellar joint with the trapezium concave in the plane of the palm and convex perpendicularly.

Extension. (radial deviation). There is ulnar slide of the base of the first metacarpal on the trapezium. A slight amount of lateral rotation (supination) occurs.

Flexion. Opposite of extension

Abduction. (away from the plane of the palm). Palmar slide of the base of the first metacarpal
Adduction. Dorsal slide of the base of the metacarpal
Opposition. This is a combined movement with considerable conjunct rotation as a consequence of the impure swing and is easily visible by the rather marked medial rotation that occurs, allowing the thumb pad to oppose the pads of the fingers. It is typical for relatively more conjunct rotation to take place at a sellar joint such as this or at the interphalangeal joints or humeroulnar joint than at ovoid joints.

Resting Position

1. First carpometacarpal: Neutral position
2. Metacarpophalangeal (2–5): Semiflexion and ulnar deviation
3. Metacarpophalangeal (1): Semiflexion
4. Interphalanageal joints: Semiflexion

Close-Packed Position

1. Most intercarpal joints: Full extension
2. First carpometacarpal: Full opposition
3. Metacarpophalangeal (2–5): Full flexion
4. Metacarpophalangeal (1): Full extension
5. Interphalangeal joints: Full extension

Capsular Patterns

1. Trapeziometacarpal joint: abduction and extension limited, flexion free
2. Metacarpophalangeal joint: more restricted in flexion than extension
3. Interphalangeal joints: more restricted in extension, some restriction of flexion

THE LOWER EXTREMITY

HIP

Component Motions

Flexion. Posterior and inferior glide of femoral head in acetabulum
Abduction. Inferior glide of femoral head in acetabulum
External Rotation. Anterior glide of femoral head
Internal Rotation. Posterior glide of femoral head

Resting Position

The hip is flexed to approximately 30°, abducted to approximately 30°, and slightly externally rotated.[12]

Close-Packed Position

Internal rotation with extension with abduction

Potential Close-Packed Position

The hip is flexed to about 90°, abducted and externally rotated slightly (see Biomechanics, Chap. 13, The Hip).

Capsular Pattern

Internal rotation and abduction are most restricted; flexion and extension are restricted; external rotation is relatively free.

KNEE

Component Motions

Flexion

1. Medial rotation of tibia on femur during first 15° to 20° flexion from full extension
2. Posterior glide of tibia on femur
3. Inferior movement of patella
4. Inferior movement of fibula

Extension. Reverse of flexion
Analysis of Knee Motion. The knee primarily moves about a single axis that lies horizontally in the frontal plane. If the tibia moves on a stationary femur, roll and slide occur in the same direction; but in the case of the femur moving on a fixed tibia, roll and slide occur in opposite directions. Toward the last 10° to 20° extension, almost a pure roll takes place, the rolling phase being somewhat longer on the lateral side. Moving into flexion, the rolling motion between the joint surfaces gradually becomes more and more a sliding motion. Thus, the articular contact point on the femur gradually moves backward (while moving into flexion); the articular contact point on the tibia moves backward during the first phase of flexion, then gradually narrows to a point (in the case of the femur moving in the tibia).

A length rotation also occurs between the femur and tibia during flexion and extension at this joint. This rotation is a necessary part of the normal joint kinematics and may be lost in certain pathologic conditions, such as a torn meniscus or adhered capsule. Considering the case of the femur moving on the tibia during the last, say, 30° extension, the femur must rotate inward in order for close-packing and full extension to occur. There are many explanations for this phenomenon. Most include the fact that because the lateral femoral condyle is smaller, it reaches its close-packed congruent position in extension before the medial condyle does. In order for the medial condyle to continue movement, it must slide backward around an axis passing somewhere through the lateral femoral condyle. The resultant rotation of the *lateral* condyle forces the anterior segment of the lateral meniscus forward over the convex lateral tibia condyle such that the lateral femoral condyle is no longer congruent and may continue into somewhat more extension. Of course, this all happens simultaneously and continues until the knee becomes locked in its close-packed position of full extension (about 5° hyperextension). In this position, the cruciates are pulled tight and twisted so as to prevent internal rotation of the tibia on the femur. The collaterals also become twisted relative to each other (the medial ligament passing downward and forward, the lateral ligament passing downward and backward) so as to prevent outward rotation of the tibia on the femur. Both sets of ligaments prevent further extension with help from the soft tissues posteriorly.

Resting Position

Approximately 25° knee flexion[12]

Close-Packed Position

Extension with lateral rotation

Capsular Pattern

Flexion is most restricted; extension is somewhat restricted.

ANKLE (MORTISE)

Component Motions

Dorsiflexion. Backward glide of talus on tibia; spreading of distal tibiofibular joint
Plantar Flexion. Reverse of dorsiflexion

Resting Position

The foot is in approximately 10° plantar flexion and midway between maximal inversion and eversion.[12]

Close-Packed Position

Dorsiflexion

Capsular Pattern

Dorsiflexion and plantar flexion are both limited, plantar flexion slightly more so unless the heel cord is tight.

SUBTALAR JOINT

Component Motions

The subtalar joint is essentially bicondylar. Of interest is the fact that the posterior facet of the talus on the calcaneous is a concave on convex surface, while the combined anterior and medial facet forms a convex on concave joint.

On eversion of the calcaneous on the talus, the posterior joint surface of the calcaneus must glide medially while the anterior and medial facets must glide laterally.

Resting Position

The foot is midway between maximal inversion and eversion with the subtalar joint in neutral.

Close-Packed Position

Inversion

Capsular Pattern

Inversion (varus) is very restricted; eversion (valgus) is free.

TRANSVERSE TARSAL JOINTS

Resting Position

The midfoot is midway between pronation and supination.

Close-Packed Position

Supination of the forefoot relative to the calcaneus, such as decreasing the normal longitudinal arch, as happens when standing with feet wide apart.

Capsular Pattern

Pronation is most limited.

FOREFOOT

Resting Position

Metatarsophalangeal joint in 10° extension; distal and proximal interphalangeal joints in slight flexion

Close-Packed Position

Metatarsophalangeal and proximal and distal interphalangeal joints in maximum extension

ORIENTATION OF JOINT AXES

Remember that in the developing embryo the lower limb started out abducted and externally rotated so

Fig. A–1. Scheme to illustrate the six degrees of freedom of vertebral segments. (White AA, Panjabi MM: Clinical Biomechanics of the Spine, p 38. Philadelphia, JB Lippincott, 1978)

that the sole of the foot faced forward. During development, the leg must rotate medially and adduct. As a result, the femoral condyles are rotated inward (about 10° in the adult) in relation to the neck of the femur, and the shaft of the femur is adducted (forming an angle of about 125° in the adult) with respect to the femoral neck.

The shaft of the tibia is rotated about 25° outwardly so the axis of the ankle mortise is 25° outwardly rotated, relative to the knee.

The axis of the subtalar joint runs about 20° from back and out to front and in.

THE SPINE

In three-dimensional space, the spine has six components (degrees of freedom) of the vertebral segments.[20] A vertebral body can move in six different ways (Fig. A–1):

1. Forward and backward in the sagittal plane (anterior and posterior translation)
2. Forward and backward tilting on a frontal axis (*i.e.*, flexion and extension)
3. Laterally, in the frontal plane by a slight translation or gliding motion (*i.e.*, lateral translation)
4. Lateral tilting or rotation around a sagittal axis (movement in the frontal plane) or sidebending
5. Rotation in the horizontal plane, around a vertical axis
6. Compression or distraction in the longitudinal axis of the spine

A vertebra may rotate or translate along any of these axes or move in various combinations of these motions (longitudinal, vertical, and sagittal). Pure movement in any of these three principal planes very seldom occurs. The facet joints act to guide and limit these motions; the plane of the facet determines the direction and amount of motion at each segment.

The torsional stiffness of the spine is largely determined by the design of the facet joints.

CERVICAL SPINE

Lower Cervical Spine (C2–C7)

The only pure motions that exist in the cervical spine from C2 through C7 are that of flexion and extension in the sagittal plane because lateral flexion and rotation are combined motions. The site of maximum motion in flexion and extension occurs between C4 and C6. In the combined movements of lateral flexion and rotation, the spinous processes of the vertebral bodies move toward the convexity of the curve or opposite to rotation of the vertebral body. The direction of physiological rotation combined with lateral flexion appears to be the same regardless of whether the cervical spine is in flexion or extension. When we laterally bend from one side, we automatically get some physiological rotation to that side; and when we rotate to one side, we automatically get some lateral flexion to the same side. According to Brown,[4] there are two degrees of coupled axial rotation for every three degrees of lateral bending. Between C2 and C7 there is a gradual cephalocaudal decrease in the amount of axial rotation that is associated.

Occipital-Atlanto-Axial Complex (Occiput–C1–C2)

It is generally agreed that the atlanto-occipital joint permits primarily a nodding motion of the head (i.e., flexion and extension in the sagittal plane around a coronal axis).[1,13] Although there is some dispute as to whether any rotation occurs between occiput and atlas, a small amount of rotation may be felt between the mastoid process and the transverse process on passive testing. During lateral flexion, the occiput moves in a direction opposite to that in which the head is laterally flexed.[3]

Motion at the atlantoaxial joint includes flexion, extension, lateral flexion, and rotation. Approximately 50% of the total rotation of the cervical region occurs at the median atlantoaxial joint before rotation in the rest of cervical spine. When the atlas pivots around the dens at the median atlantoaxial joint, the skull and atlas move as one unit. The lateral atlantoaxial joint serves to guide the rotation, which is about 45°.

LUMBAR SPINE

The lumbar region is the pivot point for most general movements of the trunk, with movements of the lower lumbar spine being the most free. The large lumbar intervertebral disks potentially allow free flexion, extension, and lateral flexion. However, these motions are limited in the lumbar spine and the direction of the movement is controlled by the orientation of the facet joints. Because of the shape of the facets, rotation in the lumbar spine is minimal and is accomplished only by a shearing force.

The lumbar region shows certain cross-coupling of spinal motions. Two types of motion may occur at the same time, and frequently three motions will simultaneously take place during normal physiological movements.[7,8,10,14,17]

Forward bending (flexion) and backward bending (extension) may be considered relatively pure movements to a degree. Both flexion and extension reduce the range of sidebending and rotation. Flexion sometimes slightly reverses the lumbar curve from the L3 segment upward. However, rotation and sidebending are not considered pure spinal movements—the performance of one results in the excitation of the other. Rotation restricts both flexion and extension and is invariably accompanied by a degree of sidebending.

Stoddard[18] stated that the direction of axial rotation varies depending on whether the lateral flexion was performed with the lumbar spine in flexion or extension. He suggests that the axial rotation is to the same side when lateral flexion is performed in flexion and to the opposite side when lateral flexion is performed in extension. Fryette[9] stated that axial rotation occurs to the same side if the segments are in full flexion or extension with the facets engaged; in neutral, without locking of the facets (erect standing), rotation is to the opposite side as sidebending. According to Edwards,[7] the direction of axial rotation is in the opposite direction to which the lumbar spine is laterally flexed regardless of whether the spine is in flexion or extension. Although these combined movement tendencies require further investigation, they offer a useful objective examination tool.

Resting Position

According to MacConaill,[15] flexed spinal joints are loose-packed and movement is limited by soft tissue contact. The anti-close-packed position is exteme flexion with minimal convexity of the lumbar portion of the column and minimal kinking of the lumbosacral junction.

Close-Packed Position

The close-packed position is that of full extension. In this position there is maximum forward convexity of the lumbar and cervical portions of the column and maximum kinking of the lumbosacral junction. At the thoracolumbar junction region, a mortise effect is produced on full extension by engagement of the articular facets. This is one of the few articular mechanisms in the body where a practically solid lock occurs at the extreme of movement.[6]

Capsular Pattern

Bilateral Pattern of Restriction. As in many synovial joints, movements toward the close-packed position are the most restricted and the earliest restricted in cases of capsular tightness. Thus the capsular patterns of restriction in bilateral facet joint involvement are as follows:

1. The occipital-atlanto joint presents with equally limited extension and lateral flexion.
2. From C2 through C7 there is considerable limitation of extension and moderate limitation of sidebending, with rotation and flexion being relatively free.
3. With respect to the lumbar spine there is marked and equal limitation of lateral flexion and rotation and limitation of flexion and extension.

Unilateral Pattern of Restriction. In general, motion loss will be most noticeable in sidebending opposite of and in rotation to the involved side. Thus if the right facet should become restricted, there will be:

1. Considerable limitation of sidebending left and rotation to the right
2. Moderate restriction of forward bending (swings to the right)
3. Mild to slight restriction of sidebending right, and rotation left

REFERENCES

1. Basmajian BE: Primary Anatomy, 7th ed. Baltimore, Williams & Wilkins, 1976
2. Barnett C, Davies D, MacConaill MA: Synovial Joints, Their Structure and Mechanics. Springfield, IL, Charles C Thomas, 1961
3. Braakman R, Penning L: Injuries of the Cervical Spine. Amsterdam, Excerpta Medica, 1971
4. Brown L: An introduction to the treatment and examination of the spine by combined movements. Physiotherapy 77:347–353, 1988
5. Cyriax J: Textbook of Orthopaedic Medicine, Vol 1, Diagnosis of Soft Tissue Lesions, 8th ed. London, Bailliere Tindall, 1982
6. Davis PR: The thoracolumbar mortise joint. J Anat 89:370, 1955
7. Edwards BC: Clinical assessment: The use of combined movements in assessment and treatment. In Twomey LT, Taylor JR (eds): Physical Therapy of the Low Back, pp 175–198. New York, Churchill Livingstone, 1987
8. Farfan HF: Muscular mechanisms of the lumbar spine and the positions of power and efficiency. Orthop Clin North Am 6:135, 1975
9. Fryette HH: The Principles of Osteopathic Technique. Carmel, CA, Academy of Applied Osteopathy, 1954
10. Gregerson GC, Lucas DB: An in vivo study of the axial rotation of the human thoracolumbar spine. J Bone Joint Surg 49(A):247–262, 1967
11. Hesse JR, Hansson JR: Factors influencing joint mobility in general and in particular respect of craniomandibular articulation: A literature review. J Craniomandibular Disord 2:19–28, 1988
12. Kaltenborn F: Manual Therapy for the Extremity Joints. Oslo, Olaf Norlis Bokhandel, 1986
13. Kent BA: Anatomy of the trunk: A review: I. Phys Ther 54:722–744, 1976
14. Loebl WY: Regional rotation of the lumbar spine. Rheumatol Rehab 12:223, 1973
15. MacConaill MA: Joint movement. Physiotherapy 50:359, 1964
16. Osborn JW: The disc of the human temporomandibular joint: Design, function, and dysfunction. J Oral Rehabil 12:279, 1985
17. Rolander SD: Motion of the lumbar spine with special reference to the stabilising effect of posterior fusion: An experimental study on autopsy specimens. Acta Orthop Scand Suppl 90:1–144, 1966
18. Stoddard A: Manual of Osteopathic Technique. London, Hutchinson, 1962
19. Warwick R, Williams P (eds): Gray's Anatomy, 35th ed. Philadelphia, WB Saunders, 1973
20. White AA, Panjabi MM: Clinical Biomechanics of the Spine. Philadelphia, JB Lippincott 1978

Appendix B: Modified Low-Dye Strapping

Low-dye strapping or taping is used primarily to reduce strain on the plantar fascia and medial arch structures to help control excessive pronation.[1,2,5] It has been found to be a useful adjunct in common "overuse syndromes" that present with excessive or prolonged pronation, such as medial arch strain, plantar fascitis (particularly in the early stages), and posterior tibial tendinitis (shin splints). At this time, much of the information regarding adhesive strapping is empirical. The ability of the low-dye taping method to modify forces on the medial arch during weight-bearing has been clearly demonstrated by Scranton et al.[7] This method is felt to medialize heel strike forces and diminish duration of forces under the midfoot, as well as medializing the anterior forefoot forces resulting in diminished strain on the medial plantar fascia and plantar-tarsal ligaments.[7] In effect, external and mechanical support to the arch is provided. This taping procedure should be meticulously applied and may be used with or without heelcups and orthoses during activity. It is especially useful in controlling pronation in dancers and gymnasts where orthoses cannot be utilized. Light elastic tape is preferable in activities such as gymnastics, whereas heavier tape can be utilized in most other activities and sports. Tape should be placed directly on the skin for maximum support. However, even with underwrap, proper taping will provide additional stabilization even after strenuous activity.[3,4] Low-dye strapping should be avoided in metatarsal stress fractures and metatarsalgia since this type of taping is seen to shift the forces anteriorly to the forefoot more rapidly and these conditions may be aggravated with the production of increased forefoot stress.[6]

I. Rationale for Use
  A. To stabilize the head of the first metatarsal by plantar flexion

  B. To decrease pain

  C. To determine need for an orthotic

II. Materials
  A. Moleskin strapping

  B. Tape adherent (*e.g.,* Tuf-skin)

  C. Tape—1 or 1½ inch

III. Procedure
  A. Preparation

    1. Shave, clean, and thoroughly dry the forefoot.

    2. Apply tape adherent to dorsal, plantar, and medial aspect of forefoot.

    3. Place small piece of adhesive moleskin below the first and fifth metatarsal heads to reduce abrasion on these areas.

    4. Cut a 2-inch wide adhesive moleskin strip to size of foot, measuring from the first to fifth metatarsal head. Cut a 3-×½-inch angled piece from both sides of midportion of the moleskin (Fig. B–1).[8]

  B. Tape application

    1. An anchor strip of 1-inch adhesive tape is applied loosely on the dorsal and plantar aspects of the foot just proximal to the metatarsal heads (Fig. B–2).

    2. Peel away the backing of the moleskin strip. Place one end on the head of the fifth metatarsal and secure it along the lateral aspect of the foot. Continue around the posterior aspect of calcaneus (Fig. B–3).

    3. Ensure that the foot is in subtalar neutral (see Fig. 15–18). Stabilize the lateral four rays by placing your hand on the lateral aspect of the foot with your thumb on plantar aspect of the foot. Plantar flex the first ray with a lesser finger before securing the rest of the moleskin to the head of the first metatarsal (Fig. B–4).

Fig. B-1. Preparation of adhesive moleskin tape.

Fig. B-4. Positioning of foot in subtalar neutral and securing rest of moleskin to metatarsal head.

Fig. B-2. Application of anchor strip to metatarsal heads.

Fig. B-5. Scissor applications of figures-of-eight from base of little toe.

Fig. B-3. Application of moleskin strip around calcaneus and lateral sides of foot.

Fig. B-6. Anchoring horizontal strips, dorsoplantar surface of foot.

Note: If tape is used in place of the adhesive moleskin, second and third strips are placed around the foot partially overlapping each other.

4. With 1-inch adhesive tape, strap the longitudinal arch with the "scissor" method or figure-of-eight. Half a figure-of-eight is performed by starting at the base of the great toe, angling across the longitudinal arch around the heel, and returning to the base of the great toe. The other half is reversed, using the base of the little toe as the starting position (Fig. B–5). The steps are repeated once or twice.

5. A closing anchor is placed on the dorsum of the foot over the original anchor. Additional anchor strips may be placed on the plantar aspect of the foot with horizontal strips applied from one side of the moleskin to the other, along the entire length of the foot. These horizontal strips are placed, pulling gently medially, from the heel to the ball of the foot (Fig. B–6).

Care must be taken to account for the expansion of the foot on weight-bearing. When the strapping is correctly applied, the great toe will be plantar flexed at the metatarsophalangeal joint and the medial longitudinal arch will be heightened and well maintained. A felt pad or a post under the medial aspect of the forefoot can be incorporated in the taping if a large deformity is present. The patient should be advised to keep the strapping dry. When weight-bearing, shoes should be worn to help prolong the life of the strapping. The foot and extremity posture should be reevaluated in stance and gait.

REFERENCES

1. Appenzeller O, Atkinson R: Sports Medicine. Fitness, Training Injuries Ed 3, pp 467–480. Baltimore, Urban S. Schwarzenberg, 1988
2. Duggar GE: Plantar fascitis and heel spurs. In McGlawry ED (ed): Reconstructive surgery of the foot and leg, pp 67–73. New York, Intercontinental Medical Book, 1974
3. Glick J, Gordon R, Nishimoto D: The prevention and treatment of ankle injuries. Am J Sports Med 4 : 136–141, 1976
4. Laughman RK, Carr TA, Chao EY, et al: Three-dimensional kinematics of the taped ankle before and after exercise. Am J Sports Med 8 : 425–531, 1980
5. Newell SG, Miller SJ: Conservative treatment of plantar fascial strain. Phys Sports Med 5 : 68–73, 1977
6. Scranton P: Metatarsalgia. Diagnosis and treatment. J Bone Joint Surg 62(A) : 723–732, 1980
7. Scranton PE, Pedegana LR, Whitesel JP: Gait analysis: alterations in support phase forces using supportive devices. Am J Sports Med 10 : 6–11, 1982
8. Whitesel J, Newell SG: Modified low-dye strapping. Phys Sports Med 10 : 280–281, 1980

RECOMMENDED READINGS

Bruggeman A, Bruggeman JH: Modifications in the treatment—program of the inversion sprain of the ankle. Int J Sports Med 5:42–44, 1984

Kosmahl EM, Kosmahl HE: Painful plantar heel, plantar fascitis, and calcaneal spur: Etiology and treatment. J Sports Med 9:17–24, 1987

Marshall P: The rehabilitation of over-use foot injuries in athletes and dancers. Clin Sports Med 7:175–191, 1988

Roy S, Irvin R: Sports Medicine: Prevention, Evaluation, Management and Rehabilitation, pp 55–77. Englewood Cliffs, NJ, Prentice-Hall, 1983

Index

Page numbers followed by an f indicate figures, numbers followed by t indicate tabular material.

ISBN 0-397-54805-2

90000

9 780397 548057